Advanced Aseptic Processing Technology

DRUGS AND THE PHARMACEUTICAL SCIENCES

A Series of Textbooks and Monographs

Recent Titles in Series

Generic Drug Product Development: International Regulatory Requirements for Bioequivalence, *edited by Isadore Kanfer and Leon Shargel*

Proteins and Peptides: Pharmacokinetic, Pharmacodynamic, and Metabolic Outcomes, *edited by Randall J. Mrsny and Ann Daugherty*

Pharmaceutical Statistics: Practical and Clinical Applications, Fifth Edition, *Sanford Bolton and Charles Bon*

Generic Drug Product Development: Specialty Dosage Forms, *edited by Leon Shargel and Isadore Kanfer*

Active Pharmaceutical Ingredients: Development, Manufacturing, and Regulation, Second Edition, *edited by Stanley H. Nusim*

Freeze Drying/Lyophilization of Pharmaceutical and Biological Products, Third Edition, *edited by Louis Rey and Joan C. May*

Advanced Aseptic Processing Technology

Edited by

James Agalloco
Agalloco and Associates, Belle Mead, NJ

James Akers
Akers Kennedy and Associates, Kansas City, MO

informa
healthcare

New York London

First published in 2010 by Informa Healthcare, Telephone House, 69-77 Paul Street, London EC2A 4LQ, UK.

Simultaneously published in the USA by Informa Healthcare, 52 Vanderbilt Avenue, 7th Floor, New York, NY 10017, USA.

Informa Healthcare is a trading division of Informa UK Ltd. Registered Office: 37–41 Mortimer Street, London W1T 3JH, UK. Registered in England and Wales number 1072954.

A CIP record for this book is available from the British Library.

Library of Congress Cataloging-in-Publication Data available on application

ISBN-13: 9781439825433

Orders may be sent to: Informa Healthcare, Sheepen Place, Colchester, Essex CO3 3LP, UK
Telephone: +44 (0)20 7017 5540
Email: CSDhealthcarebooks@informa.com
Website: http://informahealthcarebooks.com/

For corporate sales please contact: CorporateBooksIHC@informa.com
For foreign rights please contact: RightsIHC@informa.com
For reprint permissions please contact: PermissionsIHC@informa.com
Printed in the United Kingdom.

Preface

Advanced Aseptic Processing Technology: A Guide to Its Application in the Healthcare Industry is intended to provide a complete coverage of emerging aseptic processing technology, in particular those technologies that are reshaping the production of sterile health care products including: isolators, restricted access barrier systems (RABS), robotics, disposables, closed vials, and others. We are active in this area on a daily basis, and frequently find it necessary to explain the considerations associated with these newer technological advances to audiences that are largely unfamiliar or at times even uncomfortable with them. The new ideas and adaptations of older technologies that have emerged will likely have a profound impact on the global health care industry. In important ways, our industry has fallen behind other clean and aseptic industries in process design and control, and it is our profound desire that this book helps point the way forward. To bridge the gap between practices associated with more conventional aseptic processing and what is currently emerging in this area, we outlined this text as a means for transformation of concepts and practices for the next generation of aseptic processing.

At the onset, we recognized that this would be an ambitious undertaking particularly in an area experiencing continual innovation, which did not stand still while we were developing the text. This challenge is made even greater when we consider that a very well defined and rather rigid collection of process control strategies are in place for clean room–based aseptic processing. There has been a great temptation to bring these well-understood principles, which form the cornerstone of regulatory guidance in the area of aseptic processing, into the separative technology era. The current industry approaches and regulatory philosophies show that this temptation has not been resisted. We believe it is time to rethink our approach to aseptic process control away from the current heavy emphasis on microbiological monitoring that prevails in clean rooms to other approaches. To accomplish that will require a profound paradigm shift on the part of industry and the regulatory community. The shift we anticipate will take us from confirmation of acceptable environmental conditions through extensive monitoring of manned environments to installations where environmental control is accomplished by the elimination of contamination sources. Far more can be accomplished by designing the contamination out of the system, than by endeavoring to demonstrate its absence through extensive sampling and analysis.

At times, we wished we could somehow interrupt the passage of time, go off somewhere, get the book written, and then restart the clock an instant later with all of the information correct and complete. Well, that almost happened: under the stress of numerous competitive projects we suspended this effort for more than three years. When we returned to this text after that lengthy hiatus, we realized that two important things had changed.

First, and certainly foremost, we had to alter our scope rather dramatically to embrace technologies that either were not available at the onset of our original effort, or had not gained any measure of popularity as an aseptic processing option. Disposables, RABS, robotics, and automation were not considered really meaningful in the context of aseptic processing 10 years ago. The early efforts to incorporate them were minimally successful and their potential future impact was uncertain at that time. That vision has changed substantially, and as a consequence this book had to as well. The text has been transformed from one that was to focus solely on isolator technology, to one that would embrace more fully the more diverse improvements in aseptic processing made since.

Second, the passage of time has brought a clarity of purpose in many areas that was not previously available. A large part of the mystery associated with isolators had been eliminated, and they are better understood than ever before. Other technologies such as RABS have become established enough that they could be discussed based on substantial real-world experience.

Coming back to this project after our extended interruption, we recognized that for this effort to result in the resource we envisioned, we would have to work very aggressively in completing it in a timely manner. We wanted the book to be as current as possible, so that the reader would have a contemporary reference, rather than a historical tome. To that end, we revisited the list of chapters, eliminated a few that did not meet our new objective, and added a number that addressed subjects that were either out of scope or nonexistent at the beginning of this effort.

We charged each of the chapter authors (both original and those newly added) with a real sense of urgency to revise or prepare their chapters in an extremely short period of time. That they met our challenge is evidenced in the following pages. We are grateful to each of them for agreeing to participate in a project of extraordinary dimension over such a brief period. We both subscribe to the adage "If you want something done ask a busy person," and in this instance it seems to have served us and our contributors rather well.

Despite our desire to issue this text in a rapid and timely manner, we fully recognized that it is the quality of the information which is the true value of any document. To that end, we solicited contributions from individuals whom we believe are among the most knowledgeable in the subject matter. In the interest of time, and to provide greater continuity to the text, we also undertook the preparation of many chapters. We did this only where we believed we had technical background and requisite experience comparable to any potential outside contributor.

To provide for greater consistency in the chapters on decontamination technology, we asked the authors to use an identical outline where their subject matter was one of several parallel presentations. A similar approach was employed for the case studies, where a common outline for the various cases was also requested. We recognized that this was burdensome to the contributors, but we believed that the readers would derive improved utility with the final result.

This book is no small effort and would not have been possible without the efforts and support of a great many people.

First, we must thank the many individuals who attended our courses and presentations on aseptic processing and isolation technology over the years. We tested many of our ideas and concepts on them, and their interest in the subject is what prompted us to consider the development of this text in the first place.

Second, we must acknowledge those companies and individuals who have engaged our services over the years to consult on aseptic processing or provide hands-on project execution. The practical experience gathered from hands-on work with many of the aseptic processing systems described was invaluable in the preparation of this text (moreover it kept us fed as well).

Third, we must recognize the chapter authors, nearly all of whom we consider friends, and whose support to this text made it possible. Their contributions also appear in our efforts within this text, as each of them has contributed substantially to our knowledge of the subject.

Fourth, we acknowledge Bianca Trumbull and her associates at Informa. Bianca inherited this effort as the text neared its final stages and took on the important role of completing someone else's vision of what this effort would become.

Fifth, we must acknowledge our original editor, Sandra Beberman, whose patience in the early going was seemingly endless. Sandy's confidence that two very busy individuals would somehow find the time to complete a book of such scope must have seemed at times to be badly misplaced. With her support and persistence we were able to bring this substantial task near completion in a reasonable time frame. Sandy played a major role in making this vision a reality.

Last and certainly most of all, we must acknowledge our wives, Linda Agalloco and Colleen Kennedy. They allowed us to take time that could have been spent with them to prepare this text. Their continued emotional support was essential as well. Colleen also helped us administratively and provided input on subject material and author selection. Their love is a constant support to each of us.

James Agalloco
James Akers

Contents

Contributors

James Agalloco Agalloco and Associates, Belle Mead, New Jersey, U.S.A.

James Akers Akers Kennedy & Associates, Kansas City, Missouri, U.S.A.

David Barbault Sales Support Manager, Getinge–La Calhène, Vendôme, France

Harold Baseman ValSource LLC, Downingtown, Pennsylvania, U.S.A.

Bert Brabants Janssen Pharmaceutica, Brussels, Belgium

Jean-Marc Cappia Sartorius Stedim Biotech, France SAS, Aubagne, France

Mark Czarneski ClorDiSys Solutions, Inc., Lebanon, New Jersey, U.S.A.

Amnon Eylath Ariad Pharmaceuticals, Cambridge, Massachusetts, U.S.A.

Jorge Ferreira Jacobs Engineering, Conshohocken, Pennsylvania, U.S.A.

Richard L. Friedman Center for Drug Evaluation and Research, Food and Drug Administration, Silver Spring, Maryland, U.S.A.

Beth Holden Jacobs Engineering, Conshohocken, Pennsylvania, U.S.A.

David Hussong U.S. Food and Drug Administration, Silver Spring, Maryland, U.S.A.

Kunihiro Imai Shibuya Kogyo Co., Ltd., Kanazawa, Japan

Yoshi Izumi Shibuya Hoppmann Co., Elkwood, Virginia, U.S.A.

Maik W. Jornitz Sartorius Stedim Biotech, North America, Inc., Edgewood, New York, U.S.A.

Masahito Kawata Handai Biken, Osaka, Japan

Robert Keller DURECT Corporation, Cupertino, California, U.S.A.

Sterling Kline Integrated Project Services, Lafayette Hill, Pennsylvania, U.S.A.

Mamoru Kokubo Shibuya Kogyo Co., Ltd., Kanazawa, Japan

Jeff Kraft Jacobs Engineering, Conshohocken, Pennsylvania, U.S.A.

Brigitte Lechiffre Sales Manager, Europe, Getinge–La Calhène, Vendôme, France

Jack Lysfjord Lysfjord Consulting LLC, Minnetonka, Minnesota, U.S.A.

Paul Martin Pierre-Fabre Laboratories, Idron, France

Frank Mastromonica GE Healthcare, South Plainfield, New Jersey, U.S.A.

Didier Meyer Getinge–La Calhène Life Science, Tournefeuille, France

Yasusuke Oshima Shibuya Kogyo Co., Ltd., Kanazawa, Japan

David Pallister BioPharma Systems, LLC

Gary Partington Sales and Marketing Manager, Walker Barrier Systems, New Lisbon, Wisconsin, U.S.A.

Scott Pool Ellipse Technologies, Inc., Irvine, California, U.S.A.

Christopher Procyshyn Vanrx Pharmasystems, Inc., Burnaby, British Columbia, Canada

Daniel Py Chairman and CEO, Med-Instill Technologies, Inc., New Milford, Connecticut, U.S.A.

James Rickloff Partner/Scientific Director, Advanced Barrier Concepts, Inc., Cary, North Carolina, U.S.A.

Tsuguo Sasaki National Institute of Infectious Diseases, Tokyo, Japan

Kevin Schreier Jacobs Engineering, Conshohocken, Pennsylvania, U.S.A.

Brian Smith Skan US, Inc., Hanover, Pennsylvania, U.S.A.

Simon Steingart GE Healthcare, South Plainfield, New Jersey, U.S.A.

Morihiko Takeda Pharma Solutions Co., Ltd., Yokahama, Japan

Kazuhito Tanimoto Shibuya Kogyo Co., Ltd., Kanazawa, Japan

Angela Turner Med-Instill Technologies, Inc., New Milford, Connecticut, U.S.A.

Benoît Verjans Aseptic Technologies, Gembloux, Belgium

Souma Watanabe Shibuya Kogyo Co., Ltd., Kanazawa, Japan

David Watling Bioquell Ltd. (Retired), Westcott, U.K.

Valerie Welter Regulatory Compliance Associates, Inc., Kenosha, Wisconsin, U.S.A.

Julian Wilkins PharmaConsult Us, Inc.; Stevens Institute, Hoboken, New Jersey, U.S.A.

Jörg Zimmermann Vetter Pharma-Fertigung GmBH & Co., Ravensburg, Germany

1 An introduction to advanced aseptic processing technology

James Agalloco and James Akers

OVERVIEW

Aseptic processing is an umbrella term for a family of technologies that enable sterilized packaging components and products to be manufactured under conditions that mitigate contamination risk. In the healthcare product manufacturing fields aseptic processing is expected by regulation to be so effective at the reduction of contamination risk that the products can be labeled "sterile." It is widely used in the food, medical device, biotechnology, and pharmaceutical industries for the manufacture of products whose essential properties would be damaged by terminal sterilization processes using steam, radiation, or other means. There is universal preference for the use of terminal sterilization because of what is considered a superior assurance of sterility; however, the adverse effects of sterilization processes is such that an estimated 85% of sterile pharmaceuticals are made using aseptic processing (1–3).

Sterile products within the healthcare industry are considered relatively high risk, as they are customarily administered to patients in hospital and clinical settings where the patient may be immunocompromised. Should the product contain microbial contamination, there is a potential for patient injury, and in a worst-case situation even death. The criticality of concern is such that aseptic processing is subject to intense scrutiny in every application to assure that the aseptically produced healthcare product does not contribute to patient risk.

The origins of aseptic technique go back to Joseph Lister who introduced them to the medical profession in the 1860s to better manage infection risk in patients undergoing surgery (4). Lister's efforts revolutionized the way surgery was conducted and similar aseptic techniques spread to the then nascent science of medical microbiology and ultimately to the manufacture of sterile products and medical devices.

Early aseptically produced sterile products were crudely made, and a number of simple practices were adopted to improve their safety with the limited technological capabilities available. As late as the mid-1950s, sterile products were made without the benefit of HEPA-filtered air supply and many of the other practices that are today commonplace in most operations. Prior to this era, aseptically produced sterile products were manufactured using two similar methods:

- Manual/semiautomated assembly by gowned personnel in clean, but unclassified environments (the concept of room classification had not yet fully emerged).
- Manual assembly by personnel using a glovebox (a nonventilated sealed unit accessed via gloves).

The inherent limitations in these processes are historical facts; there were only limited available means for improvements in safety during the entire period from Lister's first efforts until the middle of the twentieth century, and these improvements largely focused on manual aseptic practices, a growing number of chemical disinfectants and perhaps most critically preservatives. The production of sterile products by aseptic technique, even without sophisticated means, employed the same principles of physical separation, and gowning in evidence today, although the gowns were quite limited in capability compared with those widely used today. It must be said that although the technology was comparatively limited and rather primitive, products of the pre-cleanroom era were effective and it is believed by and large safe. It is important to consider that hospitals, as is the case today, were confronted with even more daunting contamination control challenges. Therefore as is still the situation today, hospital practices in administering sterile products represented a greater risk to the seriously ill patients.

Industry's ability to control microbiological contamination improved significantly when the HEPA filter (developed for the Manhattan Project in World War II) was declassified and became available for use. The HEPA filter allowed entire rooms to reach levels of particle and microbial cleanliness not previously attainable and wholesale changes in facility designs and operating practices resulted. With large volumes of air effectively free of microbial contamination, it was now possible to dilute and/or remove from the environment human borne contamination that is always the greatest source of risk. The advent of HEPA filtration made it possible to use equipment inside a cleanroom to perform most, if not all, of the aseptic process, with gowned personnel in support. This encouraged the development of more automatic bottling and assembly equipment, resulting in the production of much larger volumes at lower cost with substantially less human activity, and therefore greatly reduced risk. Over the years, this operational concept evolved into the manned cleanroom that remains today the most commonly used environment for aseptic processing operations. The use of gloveboxes continued at a much reduced scale for nonsterile developmental activities of very potent compounds, but only very rarely for aseptic processing given the safety limitations inherent in the simple early designs, which were adapted from chemical and microbiology laboratory systems. The manned cleanroom became the industry preference for aseptic processing, because it was amenable to automated filling, inclusion of large-scale processing equipment, and could be easy adapted for supportive activities such as product formulation and component preparation. By the 1980s, cleanroom designs incorporated flexible plastic and/or rigid barriers to provide greater separation between operators and sterilized materials, products or components. This was the prevalent means for aseptic processing through the 1990s, and most of today's aseptically filled sterile products are manufactured in facilities that use these fundamental design principles. Throughout this period, as contamination control practices became more effective there was a growing understanding that personnel were the primary source of contamination in aseptic processing, and there were series of improvements introduced in manned cleanrooms that resulted in performance improvements (5).

Although the technological advances were significant, they were by no means sufficient. Regulatory pressures for continued improvement in aseptic processing performance were substantial, and a noted US Food and Drug Administration (FDA) inspector defined the problem with manned cleanrooms in a straightforward manner:

> It is useful to assume that the operator is always contaminated while operating in the aseptic area. If the procedures are viewed from this perspective, those practices which are exposing the product to contamination are more easily identified (6).

Clearly something beyond the manned cleanroom was needed, if aseptic processing was to improve further because even the most sophisticated manned cleanrooms were at the end of the day still manned cleanrooms, with all of the inherent limitations the operators presence creates. It had become obvious by 1990 that the future in aseptic processing lay not with continued incremental improvements in manned cleanroom operations, but rather the elimination of the need for human involvement altogether.

The early 1980s had witnessed the reemergence of the glovebox with substantial improvements that incorporated elements of cleanroom technology, novel transfer systems, and means for internal decontamination (7). Some of the manipulative and transfer technologies used in these newer gloveboxes or isolators came from the nuclear fuel industry, and this high-level contamination and containment technology was married with improved antimicrobial decontamination systems. The first pharmaceutical isolators were used for sterility testing where human-derived contamination from the analyst was a nagging concern. Their adoption for this purpose has spread across the industry, to where they are almost considered current good manufacturing practices in North America, Europe, and Japan for that purpose (8).

Success with isolation technology for sterility testing led to its adoption for aseptic filling and the first of these facilities became operational in the mid-1980s. Although skepticism abounded it was evident to the more progressive thinkers in the industry that the isolator was potentially an enormous improvement in contamination control relative to even the most sophisticated cleanroom designs then available. By the early 1990s, there were frequent reports regarding remarkable reductions in sterility test positives and the detection of airborne microbiological contamination in sterility-testing isolators. The ability to completely exclude personnel from the operating environment where sterilized materials are exposed was recognized as an enormous advantage over manned cleanroom systems. The widespread adoption of isolators for sterility testing emphasized to a remarkable extent the validity of the belief that human-borne contamination was not just a risk in aseptic processing, it was perhaps the only significant risk left to address. The first production isolators for aseptic processing began to appear with expectations comparable to that observed for sterility testing.

Some were so enthusiastic as to claim that sterility assurance equivalent to terminal sterilization would be possible with this new technology. This claim let to vigorous debate and had the unfortunate and unintended consequence of focusing attention away from the main advantage of human-free processing, which reduced product contamination risk. As with many technologies, implementation took time, especially in the very conservative pharmaceutical industry, and mistakes were made. Although some firms implementing isolator technology experienced considerable and well-publicized problems, there were more successes than failures (9). A number of firms frustrated by the lack of progress they encountered with isolator implementation (complaints ranged from difficulty with decontamination efficacy and cycle time; persistent leaks; changed ergonomics, limitations in access for operation and maintenance) sought other means to realize the operational performance improvements of isolators without the problems.

The result of these was the restricted access barrier system (RABS) concept, which although visually similar to isolators was conceived as a means to overcome the perceived operational hurdles (10). RABS is believed to provide the sterility assurance certainty of isolation technology with fewer technical complications of the types delineated above. The RABS is a highly evolved barrier system that builds upon the separative approaches used in manned cleanrooms through the use of material handling elements such as those used with isolators. RABS is derived from isolation technology, even though in some applications it may have more in common operationally with the manned cleanroom (Fig. 1).

In fact, RABSs are now further characterized as "closed" RABS and "open" RABS. The closed designation means that similar to the isolator, direct human intervention is not allowed in this particular style of RABS operation. In other words the "closed" RABS approach is from the separative perspective effectively identical to an isolator in operation. In contract "open" RABS as originally conceived contemplated operations in which the barriers were closed most of the time, but open-door interventions are allowed to correct certain manufacturing contingencies. The definitional difficulties for standard setting and compliance policy associated with this duality of operational control have proven to be difficult to resolve.

There are other newly introduced technologies available in use for aseptic processing, which bear mentioning. Closed-vial technology represents an entirely new concept for filling of containers that largely eliminates concerns relative to the background environment (11,12). Systems for covering vials post-fill during the lyophilization process are available and can improve aseptic processing by reducing contamination concerns during transfer to and loading

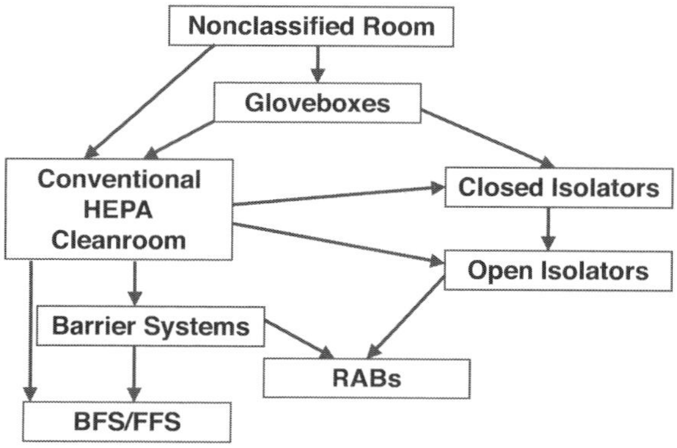

Figure 1
Aseptic processing family tree.

of lyophilizers. There are designs using either male–female connections systems or tube welders that allow for aseptic transfers in unclassified environments. These can be used with presterilized bags and tubing to allow for a variety of applications. Aseptic sampling systems are available from several suppliers, which allow for the removal of samples from closed equipment without the risk of contamination.

Blow-Fill-Seal and Form-Fill-Seal systems have been used for sterile production for many years, but these too have witnessed further improvement by the incorporation of RABS and/or isolator-type environments for the background. One of the newer designs in this area allows for the aseptic filling of small numbers of bags at slower speeds, which can be ideal for clinical/bulk subdivision/niche products of sterile fluids.

Another approach for improved contamination control in aseptic processing is the application of robots and automation. As the principal criterion necessary for improved contamination control is the elimination of personnel from the aseptic process, it stands to reason that automation can play an important role in this endeavor. Well over one million industrial robots are in use everyday in manufacturing operations throughout the world, and outside of secondary packaging operations their use remains relatively rare in healthcare product manufacturing. There are however, robots developed for use in isolators or cleanrooms, which are handling activities such as component supply on a routine basis. In addition, in other aseptic industrial bottling applications, for example beverage filling, isolator bottling/capping systems exist, which are so highly automated that they operate reliably without interventions and thus without gloves. It may be hard to believe for many industry professionals, but other aseptic industries are currently far more advanced that those used for the majority of healthcare products. The fact is our industries are only now beginning to consider levels of automation that have been commonplace in other industries for many years.

PERSPECTIVES ON ASEPTIC PROCESSING

Prior to the developments occurring over the last decade and a half, aseptic processing was almost always associated with manned cleanrooms in which personnel performed supportive activities related to set-up, environmental monitoring, and corrective interventions as needed. Recognition of the adverse impact the presence of personnel has led to the more evolved designs and processing equipment currently available. In looking at the newer aseptic processing systems, it is sometimes difficult to understand the technological distinction between them, as well as whether those variations result in meaningful performance differences.

In considering the technology options for aseptic filling, the means by which human contamination can be controlled must be the primary consideration. When a variety of technology options first became available to the healthcare industry, there was considerable confusion over what to call this new equipment. There were a variety of terms applied including isolator, barrier isolator, locally controlled environments, mini-environments, restricted access barrier systems, and separative enclosures. Not only was there confusing terminology, there were also meaningful differences in design and capability. As an industry, we were essentially speaking in "tongues," and confusion was rampant. We had to learn to speak in terms that everyone could understand what type of system was being described before we could consider the level of performance that could be expected from it.

One of the first necessary steps was to clarify what was an isolator system and what was a barrier system. Some basic definitions helped to clarify the system design and capability: (13).

Isolate—to set apart from others
Isolator—a piece of equipment that provides for complete separation between one environment and another
Bar—to obstruct or prevent passage, progress or action
Barrier—a material object which separates, demarcates or serves as a barricade.

Images that vividly portray this distinction are shown in Figure 2(A) and (B).

This proved adequate at a very basic level of understanding, but it was not really that simple to address the distinctions between the various designs present in the marketplace. The

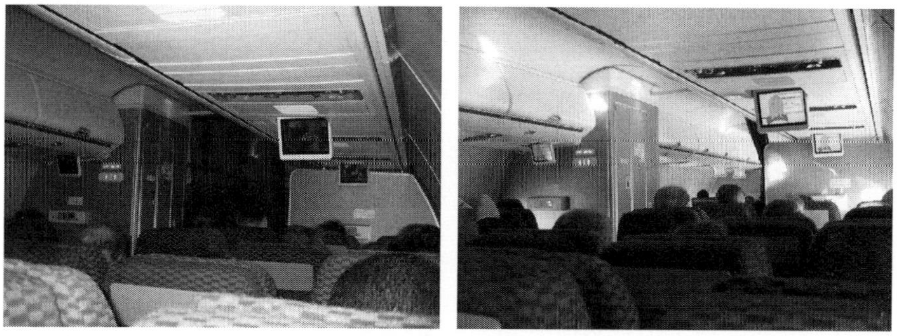

The separation between coach and business class is nowhere near as effective as the separation between the interior and exterior of the aircraft.

(A)

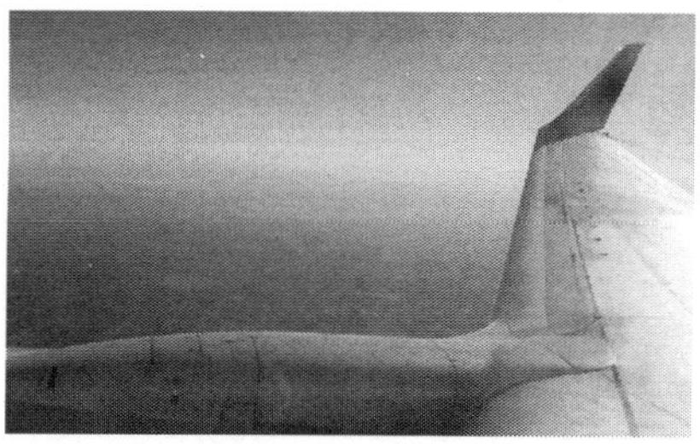

At 36,000 feet the interior of the airplane is maintained at conditions comfortable for the passengers despite –50°C exterior temperatures and atmospheric pressures of 0.25 in Hg.

(B)

Figure 2 (A) Airplanes as barriers. (B) Airplanes as isolators.

Parenteral Drug Association (PDA) developed a guidance document on "isolation technology," which included the following more comprehensive and explicit definition of isolator systems of two distinct types:

> An isolator is sealed or is supplied with air through a microbially retentive filtration system (HEPA minimum) and may be reproducibly decontaminated. When closed it uses only decontaminated (where necessary) interfaces or Rapid Transfer Ports (RTPs) for materials transfer. When open it allows for the ingress and/or egress of materials through defined openings that have been designed and validated to preclude the transfer of contamination. It can be used for aseptic processing activities, or containment of potent compounds or simultaneously for both asepsis and containment (14).

Some years later, as interest increased in the implementation of RABS, the International Society for Pharmaceutical Engineering (ISPE) developed a definition for those systems:

> A Restricted Access Barrier System (RABS) is an advanced aseptic processing system that can be utilized in many applications in a fill-finish area. RABS provides an enclosed environment to reduce the risk of contamination to product, containers, closures, and product contact surfaces compared to the risks associated with conventional cleanroom operations. RABS can operate as "doors closed" for processing with very low risk of contamination similar to isolators, or permit rare "open door interventions" provided appropriate measures are taken (15).

Both definitions rely substantially upon the operational characteristics of the system to define it appropriately, and each includes the option of operating in a "closed" and "open" manner. It might seem from the similarity of the definitions that these systems would have comparable capabilities. There are important differences between them that bear further discussion. The nuances of each design are briefly addressed in this chapter and at length later in other chapters.

Isolators

Isolators can be either "open" or "closed" depending upon their operational state and may operate at positive, neutral or negative pressures with respect to the surrounding environment. When "closed," isolators do not exchange unfiltered (HEPA or better) air with the surrounding environment. When "open," isolators should not exchange unfiltered air with the surrounding environment as air overpressure or overspill precludes the entrance of contamination. In fact, in many current isolator designs the opening or "mouse hole" is used only for the exit of fully sealed product. Thus, the performance differences between "open" and "closed" isolators with proper design and operation are negligible.

Isolators are customarily decontaminated using automated equipment that inject vaporous or gaseous sporicidal agents that can reproducibly render the interior of the isolator free of microorganisms. The result is what is an effective "germ-free" environment for aseptic processing. These sporicidal processes are typically used to treat parts or component supply hoppers and feed mechanisms in situ. At one time, this engendered a great deal of discussion regarding differences in concept between sterilization and decontamination. However, experience has confirmed that in practice the antimicrobial effects achieved on these parts supply systems are not a source of risk. In fact, treatment in situ is of less risk by far than sterilization, using a validated autoclave cycle followed by aseptic assembly in the critical zone by gowned human operators.

Isolators can be operated so as to maintain a pressure differential between the enclosure and the surrounding environment, which can be beneficial in ensuring operator/product safety. Isolators are intended to be operated without opening during use, the designation of "closed" or "open" with respect to an isolator relates solely to material in-feed/discharge in a batch (closed) or continuous (open) mode.

Restricted Access Barrier Systems

RABS provide many of the same operational advantages as isolators while eliminating what are to some the more challenging aspects of isolator design. RABS can operate in either a batch or a continuous mode just like an isolator. A "closed" RABS is one that is operated more like an isolator in that all activities are performed by operators located in the background environment. In an "open" RABS, the enclosure is allowed to be opened during the processing to allow direct access by aseptically garbed personnel. The performance of a "closed" RABS can be comparable with that of an isolator, whereas an "open" RABS is decidedly less capable, its performance may be only slightly better than a manned cleanroom.

RABS are prepared using high-level disinfection with sporicidal materials by aseptically gowned personnel. The treatment is preferably performed with the enclosure closed. A number of "high-level" disinfection methods have been employed and it is really in the area of decontamination where the greatest differences may be seen between isolator practice and "closed" RABS. Some users are opting to decontaminate both the RABS enclosure and the surrounding room with, for example, vapor phase hydrogen peroxide, which further blurs the distinction between isolators and "closed" RABS and to a lesser extent "open" RABS as well. There is even a special category of "closed" RABS called a C-RABS that is decontaminated in a manner identical to that used for an isolator design and then operated as a RABS with air-over spill to the background environment.

As with any new technology, the general descriptions of isolators and RABS mentioned above cannot fully accommodate the nuances of difference within and between each category of equipment. This was recognized early on by both PDA and International Organization for Standardization (ISO), each of which developed a visual continuum to explain the capabilities of the various systems. Neither continuum includes RABS as a specific point of clarification, and ISO does not mention isolators instead using a more general term "separative enclosures" (Fig. 3 and 4) (14,16).

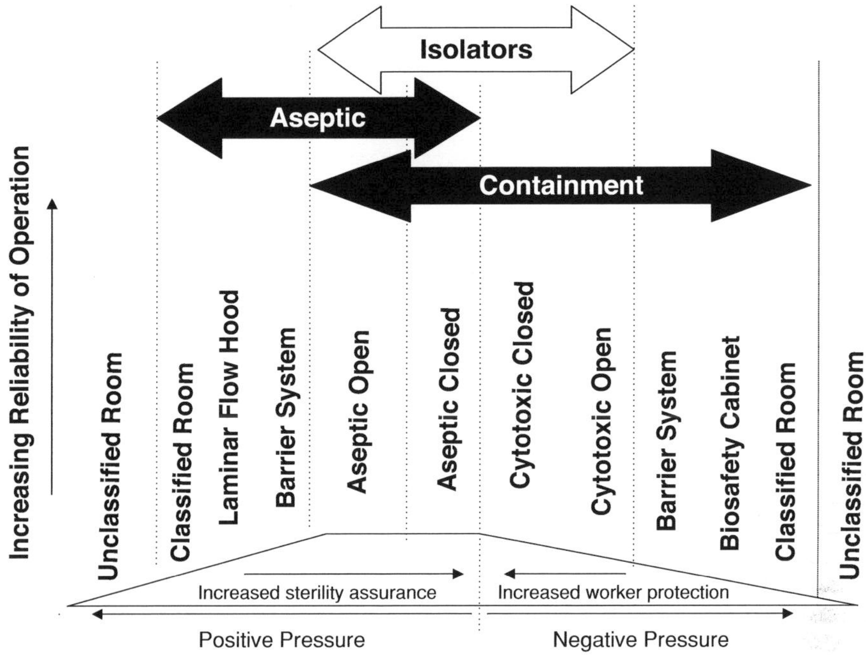

Figure 3 PDA's isolation continuum.

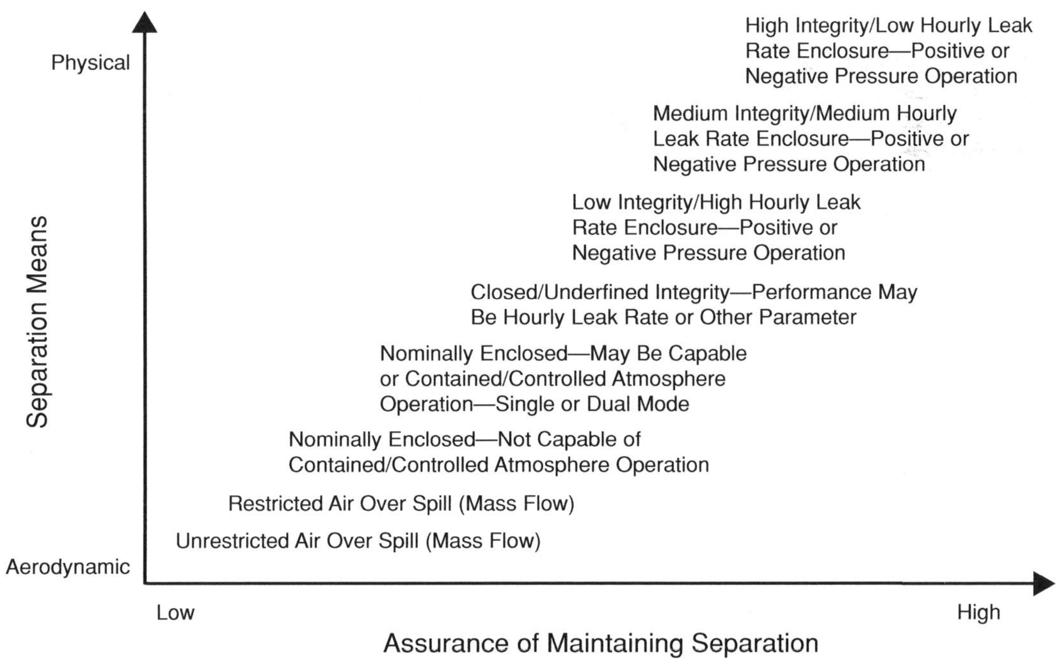

Figure 4 ISO 14644-7 continuum.

The emergence of these newer designs along with their improved capabilities led to the use of the term "advanced aseptic processing," which was widely rapidly adopted, but unfortunately ill defined for some period of time. Without a clear definition of what "advanced" truly meant in the context of aseptic processing, there were disparate claims made in a variety of areas. The authors of this chapter along with Russ Madsen offered the following definition in an attempt to establish a line of demarcation between "ordinary" and "advanced" aseptic processing systems:

> An advanced aseptic process is one in which direct intervention with open product containers or exposed product contact surfaces by operators wearing conventional cleanroom garments is not required and never permitted (17).

The focus on elimination of direct personnel intervention was consistent with the operational goal of many of the emergent technologies. An essential part of the definition was the establishment of a clear distinction, between what was and should not be considered advanced. Allowing gowned personnel to directly interact with sterile materials seemed to compromise the entire notion of 'advanced'. Since its publication in 2006, this definition has clarified the differences in technologies. The technologies described in this book are intended to meet the objectives of this definition to the fullest extent possible.

Why Advanced Aseptic Processing Technologies?

The driving forces behind the application of advanced aseptic processing technologies for sterile products relates foremost to improved separation between personnel and sterile materials, though that is certainly the most important reason (18). Other factors aiding in the transition to advanced technologies include:

- Improved separation between personnel and sterile materials, components, and equipment.
- Elimination of personnel from aseptic processing environments.
- Reduction in labor cost resulting from use of automated equipment.

When isolator technology is used, a number of added benefits are realized (18).

- The ability to create a germ-free operating environment.
- A substantial reduction in operational cost for the facility.
- A shortened time period from conceptual design to full implementation compared with standard facilities intended for the same process.
- Containment of toxic materials to an extent never before attainable.
- Substantial reduction in gowning requirements for personnel.
- Increased labor efficiency due to more flexible use of staff.
- Ability to produce in a campaign mode over extended periods.

When RABS technologies are used, a slightly different set of unique benefits are possible: (19).

- A means for evolutionary upgrade to existing facilities with reduced downtime.
- Lower capital cost when retrofitting an existing operation (this cost advantage for RABS, over isolators generally disappears when new production lines are specified).
- Easier implementation because practices and equipment are more like predecessor designs.

Many of these benefits were significant motivating factors in the case studies included in subsequent chapters.

The highly automated processing equipment now entering the market may further blur the environmental distinctions already described. Aseptic processing environments may virtually disappear in the midst of an automated machine. We are entering an era in which intervention free systems will become far more common. These systems can achieve a form of "electronic" separation. Therefore, in theory it would not matter whether these systems are installed in clean rooms, RABs enclosures ("open" or "closed" will be irrelevant) or isolators. Equipment designers and production experts will be free to choose the most cost-effective option because there would be no real production distinctions. If the aseptic beverage experience is any guide, it seems like that the solution could be a gloveless isolator with a far simpler air handling system than currently employed. Of course the advanced container closure systems described in this chapter could provide a similar level of performance and with automation the same flexibility in the choice of surrounding environmental system.

CONCLUSION

This chapter endeavors to introduce and in part promotes advanced aseptic technologies to the reader, many of whom perhaps already fully understand all that we have written to date. As all the technologies described in this text are relatively new, a great deal must still be learned about how to best apply them within our industry. Given the number of different designs, new terminologies, diversity of regulatory guidance, and the apparent similarity of many designs systems which may differ in performance, it is essential that we all attain a better level of understanding.

It is also vital that we be prepared to reconsider and potentially discard process control, environmental monitoring, and product analytical approaches that have been with us since the start of the manned cleanroom era and the introduction of process validation concepts. We may find that in the effectively germ-free environments that are becoming increasingly common, the use of traditional monitoring systems in association with the aseptic processing operation will be a non–value added activity. For the promise of an advanced aseptic processing future to be fully realized a true partnership among industry business management, regulatory professionals, analytical scientists, and process engineers is essential. We will all need to "think different" to borrow a popular marketing phrase.

REFERENCES

1. FDA. Guideline on Sterile Drug Products Produced by Aseptic Processing. 2004.
2. European Medicines Agency (EMEA). Annex 1. Sterile Medicinal Products, 2008.
3. PIC/S. Decision Tree for the Selection of Sterilization Methods. CPMP/QWP/054/098, 1999.
4. Lister, J. On the Antiseptic Principle of the Practice of Surgery. Vol. XXXVIII, Part 6. The Harvard Classics. New York: P.F. Collier & Son, 1909–1914; Bartleby.com, 2001.
5. Agalloco J, Madsen R, Akers J. Aseptic processing—a review of current industry practice. Pharm Technol 2004; 28(10):126–150.
6. Avallone H; FDA Field Investigator Training curriculum, circa 1985.
7. Bristol-Myers France, circa 1982.
8. Wagner C, Raynor J. Industry survey on sterility testing isolators: current status and trends. Pharm Eng 2001; 3:134–140.
9. Lysford J, Porter M. Barrier Isolation History and Trends. International Society for Pharmaceutical Engineering Washington Conference: Barrier Isolation Technology, June 2, 2004.
10. Lysford J. The ISPE RABS definition: an introduction. Pharm Eng 2005; 26(10):116–120.
11. www.medinstill.com. Accessed May 11, 2010.
12. www.aseptictech.com.
13. Agalloco J. Barriers, isolators and microbial control. PDA J Pharm Sci Technol 1999; 53(1):48–53.
14. PDA. Design and validation of isolator systems for the manufacturing and testing of health care products. PDA Technical Report #34. PDA J Pharm Sci Technol 2001; 55(5):supplement.
15. ISPE. Definition of a RABS. August 2005.
16. ISO 14644-7. Cleanrooms and Associated Controlled Environments—Part 7: Separative Enclosures (Clean Hoods, Glove Boxes, Isolators and Mini-Environments). 2001.
17. Akers J, Agalloco J, Madsen R. What is advanced aseptic processing? Pharm Manufact 2006; 4(2)25–27.
18. Agalloco J. Opportunities and obstacles in the implementation of barrier technology. PDA J Pharm Sci Technol 1995; 49(5):244–248.
19. Agalloco J, Akers J, Madsen R. Choosing technologies for aseptic filling—back to the future? Pharm Eng 2007; 27(1):8–16.

2 Getting started, establishing an aseptic processing systems technology group

Amnon Eylath

INTRODUCTION

Isolators, glove boxes, and restricted access barrier systems (RABS) technology are widely accepted as solutions to enhance product safety, protection of staff and facility from potent materials, and for cost-effective production of aseptic and powder drugs. Whichever specific technology used, we can loosely define these solutions as "aseptic processing systems" (APS). Currently, APS are in operation around the world in a variety of settings. The main users of APS are still large pharmaceutical and biotechnology companies that have had prior experience with this technology, and usually APS are used for minimizing the potential for false-positive result during product sterility testing. As the technologies involved in APS are becoming more commonplace, and as new process and product needs arise that require isolation, more companies are exploring and adopting the use of APS technology.

Implementation of APS technology can seem a daunting task for the group assigned this role. This can be done by following common-sense project-management techniques and using the existent knowledge and experience available from seminars, conferences, and training, as well as prior experience from the fabricators of APS systems and related components.

Identifying Needs

To promote, develop, and implement specific technologies, the company's needs must be evaluated. The implementation of APS technology must meet a current or prepare for a future need. Internal resources should be identified as sources of this information.

Following are some examples of internal resources for information. The process development group is involved in the development and introduction of new products and processes. Partnering with this group will identify the current products being developed and will also give the opportunity of process optimization by use of APS technology. Potent drugs may require containment to protect staff. For new substances with unknown properties, many environmental health and safety (EH&S) guidelines recommend treating all unknown as potentially hazardous until toxicology and bioavailability data are confirmed. In cases where a sterile final drug product cannot be terminally sterilized or sterilized by filtration, the only way to ensure sterile drug product is by processing the formulation and fill steps in a protected APS environment.

The clinical development group can identify new products in the pipeline, some of which may require either aseptic processing or containment, especially in the case of powder drugs that are potentially harmful to staff upon exposure. If there is a corporate planning group, they can contribute information on new facilities under consideration, where there is potential for APS use.

Quality assurance (QA) and quality control (QC) are also areas where there is a potential need for APS. If potent drugs are being developed or manufactured, then there is often a need for APS or containment for the analytical QA group developing the assays for the new product. QC-sterility testing is an area where the use of APS is well established in the pharmaceutical industry and being implemented now also in some of the larger biotechnology companies. Partnering with the sterility testing group will identify these needs.

Justifying to Management the Present and Future Corporate Needs

Obviously, the need to invest significant time and resources toward introduction of APS technology requires making a good case to company management. Some approaches that can be useful are listed as follows. Comparing APS technology to existing technologies, highlighting the safety benefits, cost savings (numbers help), enhances containment and the benefits in the design and operation of multiproduct facilities. A risk versus benefit analysis should be presented, based on actual company data, or on relevant models developed by other companies.

Assembling the Team

The team must be multifunctional, because implementation of APS technology spans a cross section of functions and skills, such as project management, engineering, manufacturing, documentation, QA/validation, process development, purchasing and environmental health and safety. Each representative to the team can bring in the knowledge and experience required assuring that all process, QA, regulatory and safety issues are addressed in real time and incorporated into the design and start-up of the systems.

Project Resources

A good evaluation of the resources required to implement APS technology is required to allow for accurate planning, budgeting, and allocation of these resources. There are obvious resources involved, such as the manufacturing and engineering group. I would like to list and highlight some of the resources that may not be as obvious to management.

The documentation department's involvement is in the issuing and circulation of draft standard operating procedures (SOPs) and then approval of the final SOP. The validation staff needs to apply resources in the validation of the completed system, and the QC-microbiology group will test any biological indicators as well as environmental samples from the APS, such as slit-to agar or settling plates. Good manufacturing practices (GMP)-compliance input is important to assure that the regulatory requirements for the planned use of the system are met. The purchasing group can assist in the procurement of equipment and components and also negotiate the contracts with the vendors. Process development must have a process that can be implemented in the APS, and also must define in advance the process parameters and environmental and storage conditions of in-process materials, so as to ensure that these considerations are incorporated into the system design and functionality. Environmental health and safety must define exposure limits for potent materials and solvents, as well as any plant safety considerations for flammable materials. A key to success of the design is direct and continuous involvement of the manufacturing staff that will actually operate the equipment. They are the most qualified ones to assist in the design from an ergonomic and from a material handling aspect.

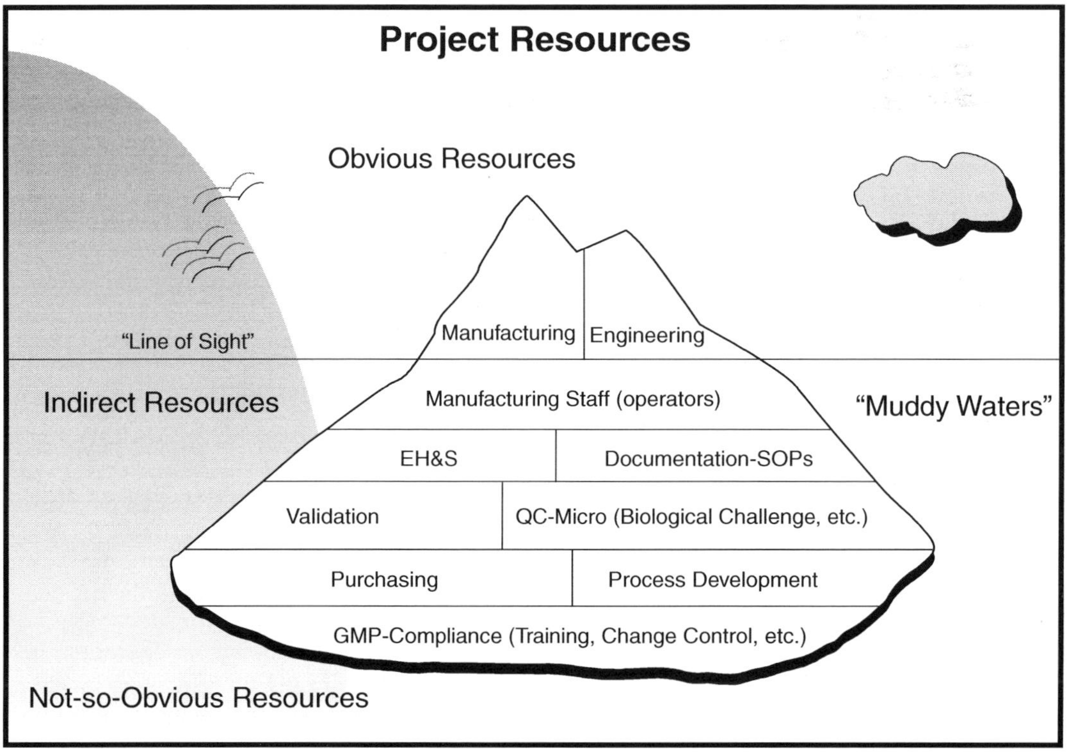

Identifying the Project Scope

A clear understanding of the project scope is necessary to plan for and identify the required resources, as well as the facility impact of the project. The following information is helpful in clearly defining and communicating the project scope to the project team and to the management. A description of the final process (or as close to the final process as is known) is crucial to assuring that the system and equipment design will actually meet the process requirements. A PFD (process flow diagram) is a useful tool for describing the process. The PFD can show materials flow and process steps, as well as necessary testing and holding steps in the process. If the process details are still being worked out, a process block diagram can be used to at least give a general description of the process. Process specifications will describe the parameters of the process, such as equipment requirements, room classification (Class 100,000, 10,000, etc.) for the surrounding room, presence of solvents, etc.).

Process safety requirements need to be evaluated by performing hazardous operations study. Based on the type of materials used in the process (potent drugs, solvents, etc.) and the local environmental, safety, and fire codes, the appropriate safety features can be installed and any required permits can be obtained.

Facility modifications may be minor, if the existing facility can meet the process requirements, or significant, as in the case of reclassification of rooms to meet environmental and safety regulations. If flammable or explosive materials are used, then the facility may need to be constructed to meet H1 or H2 requirement. Creating a class 100,000 area is not too difficult in most cases, but as the requirements become more stringent, the cost of air handlers and ductwork also increases.

Only after identification of these requirements can the overall capital costs and project schedule be developed. In some cases, an architecture and engineering firm can be enlisted to study these issues in detail and deliver a report of the projected costs.

Roles and Responsibilities

The following is a list of the major groups involved in the project and their individual roles and responsibilities.

Project Management

Coordinating the team's efforts is important for ensuring that all of the groups that contribute to the design and installation of the APS are working together in a team environment. By developing and effective project team duplication of effort and nonproductive activities can be prevented. By acting as a clearinghouse for information, the project manager can support communication among team members. Clear and accurate sharing of information is critical to the success of any complex project. The project manager needs to make decisions and bring about consensus among the team members. Consensus does not necessarily mean that all members are in agreement on every issue or detail. It means that decisions made by the team are supported actively by the team members. Tracking the timeline and budget are also important roles of the project manager. Project timelines are fluid and constantly being updated. By identifying potential delays, resources can be applied or redirected to specific project tasks. Keeping an eye on the budget is required to meet cost expectations for the completion of the project. If costs are projected to deviate from expectations, then early notice to management is required for approval.

Engineering

Developing specifications for the system should come first. The specifications should be based on the process and facility requirement: materials of construction, safety classification and alarms, and space considerations.

The engineering group will develop the conceptual design for the system, and the group on the basis of input from the project team and the vendor will oversee the delivery of the detailed design. The detailed design should contain all of the features and customization required supporting the process, utility requirements, and the appropriate ergonomics for operation. In-house safety requirements and design specifications should be incorporated into the vendor's proposal. An important part of this is the review of drawings and marking them up for final design.

Once the equipment is fabricated, engineering group will support the FAT (factory acceptance test) at the vendor, identify corrective actions and then supervise the installation in the user's facility. Once installed a site acceptance test should be performed, preferably while the vendor's technical staff is still present.

Manufacturing

Input from the manufacturing group is crucial in developing the conceptual and final designs. Because they are the end users of the equipment, all designs must meet the process's logistical and ergonomic requirements, as much as possible. The constraints should be based on the amount of time and money available, but by early involvement, most critical design parameters can be evaluated without causing delays for re-work later down the line.

The manufacturing staff must simulate the process in the mock-up, which will supply important information about the flow of materials, process details, on-line serviceability of the manufacturing equipment, and whether there are ergonomic issues to be addressed. Keep in mind that if it is difficult to operate and maintain the process, this will have significant negative impact on production efficiency and productivity.

With support of the FAT and installation, manufacturing staff have an opportunity to try out the equipment ahead of installation, and then learn about operation and maintenance as the equipment is being installed. As they learn to operate the equipment, EH&S can join in to develop training and safety procedures. Once the installation is completed, the manufacturing staff will operate the system in support of validation efforts.

Documentation/QA/Validation

If being implemented for GMP manufacturing, timely and comprehensive delivery of documentation is critical. Typically for validation to proceed, a SOP (at least a QA approved draft version) must be in place, as well as validation protocols for installation qualification, operation qualification, and process validation should be ready. Delays in these documents can delay operation of the equipment for production, regardless of whether the system is functionally ready.

The QA group needs to review these documents and approve them for use. Moreover, QA can offer useful input as to the content and suitability of the documentation. By having the QA group involved in the project from the outset, they will be better able to facilitate the approvals of the documents and design.

The validation group will develop a validation plan, issue validation protocols, and perform validation testing. A master plan for validation will help identify the resources, timelines, and milestones clearly so that they can be incorporated in to the mater schedule, without surprises. The participation of the engineering and manufacturing groups is critical if validation is to be appropriate and timely. Again, the earlier the validation is on board and involved, the better the plans and protocols will turn out to be.

Process Development

The process development group will define the process and work with engineering group to develop the technical solutions. They should participate in the design review, where they can identify critical parameters and control points for the process. Once a basic or pilot process is developed, it needs to be transferred to the manufacturing group for scale-up and implementation. If the process is unusual or exotic compared with the norm for the company, this relationship increases in importance, as all parties involved in the path from concept to qualified process need to communicate clearly and participate in all stages of the design and fabrication.

Purchasing/Environmental Health and Safety (EH&S)

Purchasing group will expedite contracts and agreements and track purchase orders. Often, the purchasing agent can negotiate for better prices and terms on the equipment.

EH&S reviews design and procedures for safety, develops and implements monitoring plan for exposure to potent and hazardous materials, if necessary.

The Design Team

Design of APS for aseptic processing can be subdivided into functionalities: aseptic for liquids, aseptic for powders, and combined aseptic/potent toxic hazardous containment. In order for the design to be functional and also meet specifications and regulations the design team should have representation and active involvement from various functional groups in the company.

Manufacturing staff's needs and preferences must be considered, as they are the ones to actually perform the process operations. The following are some of the key issues that manufacturing staff need to give input on: Interior space must be sufficient for the process. Location and positioning of glove ports and half suits are critical for ease of use. Ergonomics must be evaluated by having the operators model the process in a mock-up. Cleanability and ease of access are also important issues for the operators to evaluate.

Besides helping to develop the conceptual and detailed design, the engineering staff should review the functionality of the APS systems and the equipment to be installed in it. Other items for them to review are the materials of construction, the utilities and services required, and the turnover package (TOP) supplied by the vendors.

EH&S will give input into the containment level requirements for the APS as well as the arrangements for exposure-level air monitoring and liquid and solid waste disposal procedures. The exposure limits for any potent or hazardous materials should be discussed in detail with EH&S.

The Importance of Mock-Ups

Prior to final design of any APS system a mock-up of the APS must be evaluated. The purpose of the mock-up is to allow the project team to model the actual processes. Too often designs are approved based on drawings that can be misleading in regards to actual operations in the system. The more realistic you are the better you can determine the final design. It is recommended to use actual manufacturing staff for this process simulation as they are the true experts on the process. In addition, ergonomic problems can be detected and corrected. A system that is not ergonomically sound will be cumbersome to operate, leading to operation errors or process delays. Poor ergonomics will also contribute to repetitive motion, and other work-related injuries.

Choosing Vendors

Some useful criteria for choosing a vendor are the following: best design for your process, quality of construction, time of delivery, cost, installation support, validation support.

Prior experience with the vendor and references from clients using the equipment for similar applications is vital as part of the vendor bid review process. Check with other departments in the company as well as colleagues in the industry to get feedback on the responsiveness, timeliness, and quality of the deliverables from any given vendor. Lowest bids should be scrutinized carefully to ensure that the numbers can actually support delivery of the APS without the need for significant (10% or over) change in the budget. Choosing the second to lowest bid (if the other criteria are reasonably comparable) is one best practice in avoiding "bait and switch" low-ball bids.

Project Management

Regular team meetings are useful in bringing the groups together for brainstorming, following progress and coming to a consensus on design and implementation decisions. Detailed minutes are a must to identify assigned tasks and due dates and also so that information is not lost as the project progresses. Following up on action items (assign to people and give due dates) is important. If there are tasks that are not being performed, the causes can be identified as the following: lack of resources, assigned to the wrong person, due date is too far ahead, etc. Once the cause is identified, adjustments can be made. It is important to summarize milestones, to motivate the team, and to show progress to the project sponsors and management. A summary report can be issued to management periodically.

Being Cost-Effective

One can perform good work quickly if enough resources are applied (at a cost). One can perform good work with limited resources (at less cost) if enough time is allowed. One cannot be both quick and cheap if good results are expected. Therefore, a balance between cost and delivery time must be reached without compromising quality. By identifying the key drivers for the project, it easier to be cost-effective, which is not synonymous with inexpensive. If a short time to delivery is the objective, then quick identification of a reliable vendor is the key, as well as close and continuous supervision of the work. In a fast-track project, it is critical to identify any fabrication or design errors prior to the equipment leaving the vendor. When economy is the driver, much of the design work can be performed in-house, if the capabilities exist, and a close-to final design can be submitted for refinement by the fabricator. This will typically take longer, but will generate direct savings to the project.

The Importance of Networking

Networking with other people implementing APS solutions is your best source of up-to-date and honest information about vendors, technology, and practices. You can start an APS users group with your nearby companies or join one of the existing groups sponsored by the ISPE or PDA. A simple and inexpensive way of staying in touch with users is to create an e-mail discussion group, where nonproprietary information and solutions can be shared.

Applications in Biotechnology and Pharmaceutics

The potential applications of APS technology can be divided into four main areas: aseptic processing, potent and powder drug containment, containment of radiochemicals, and sterility testing.

Aseptic processing of parenteral drugs is a significant application of APS technology such as in the containment of the stages of the process that are vulnerable to contamination by viable and nonviable particulates. Examples are filling and aseptic processing of non-filterable materials in an APS classified for class 100 or better. This application reduces the risk of contaminating final product and increases the sterility assurance level. Where a sterile bulk drug must be used APS technology is crucial in ensuring protection of the bulk drug and sterile formulation.

The containment of potent and powder drugs is an area well established in the classical pharmaceutical field. With newer, more potent biotech and peptide drugs being developed, as well as biotech drugs that are filled in a powder form, the need for containment has increased. Containment is needed to protect the production staff and facility from exposure to the potent material, as well as reduce the risk of cross-contamination of multiproduct facilities.

Some therapeutics and tracing agents are radioactive; therefore the radioactive materials must be safely contained to protect the operators and the environment. High-level containment is critical for this application, as well as shielding with lead, lead glass, or other radioactivity barriers. Ease of decontamination is also a significant consideration for this application.

Sterility testing was one of the first applications of APS technology in the pharmaceutics field, typically using isolators, and its value in reduction of false positives is just as valid for the sterility and release testing of biotech products. This application is well established and usually implemented once lot throughput and size increase to a degree that makes this cost-effective.

3 Aseptic processing facility design

Sterling Kline

INTRODUCTION

This chapter focuses on advanced aseptic processing fill-finish facility design for sterile drug and biological product manufacture. The aseptic processing facility design is regulated to minimize particulate, pyrogen, and microbiological contamination to sterile products. Historically, the greatest potential for contamination comes from human intervention within the aseptic processing rooms. Recent advanced processing improvements including restricted area barrier systems (RABS) and isolation technology provide enhanced segregation of the operators from the product. These technologies reduce the risk of contamination versus the traditional aseptic facility design and are expected to effectively replace the traditional manned design over the coming years. The facility designs for RABS and isolation technology differ dramatically and therefore each is covered separately in this chapter.

One of the greatest difficulties in designing aseptic processing facilities is the current lack of harmonization of the regulatory requirements for operating area classifications. Later chapters in this book provide detailed discussions of the European Union (EU) and US Food and Drug Administration (FDA) requirements. This chapter identifies a practical solution to meet both the US FDA Guidance for Industry, Sterile Drug Products Produced by Aseptic Processing-Current Good Manufacturing Practices (1), and the European Commission EU Guidelines for Good Manufacturing Practice, Annex 1 Manufacture of Sterile Medicinal Products (2).

AREA CLASSIFICATIONS

To control microbiological particulate contamination, clean air classifications have been developed to define the conditions for all aseptic facility functions. The definitions vary between the EU and FDA, creating difficulty in designing facilities that are compliant with both sets of requirements. The primary design complications evolves from the EU identifying differing parameters for conditions at rest and in operation and the FDA in not differentiating between those states. Fortunately in the most restrictive condition, the Class 100-ISO 5-Grade A classification, for spaces that the product and/or components are exposed to in the environment, the regulations are in harmony because EU requires Grade A for both at-rest and in-operation conditions. Traditionally, Class 100-ISO 5-Grade A conditions exist over the filling operations and areas of local protection (at least from a particle count perspective) in the formulation and parts wrapping rooms. With isolator technology, the Class 100-ISO 5-Grade A filling operation is contained completely within the isolator. With RABS technology, current guidance includes an area of Class 100 airflow outside the RABS unit for a minimum width of the fully opened doors should those doors be opened during operation (a practice that is less than desirable). This requirement creates significant design complexities that are addressed later.

The second area classification is Class 10,000-ISO 7-Grade B that applies to spaces that are immediately adjacent to the aseptic filling line. This classification has traditionally caused the most confusion and is no longer an issue in isolation technology facility design. It still creates significant issues for RABS facility design.

The third area classification is Class 100,000-ISO 8-Grade C. This classification applies to aseptic manufacturing support areas and becomes the background environment for the filling room, and the predominant classification for all other spaces in isolation technology suites. The EU requirements for Class 10,000 conditions at rest can lead to more conservative air change designs then would be typical for meeting FDA requirements alone.

The spaces adjacent to the aseptic suite, including access corridors, quality testing laboratories, inspection rooms, and secondary packaging functions, have become defined controlled unclassified (CunC)-Grade D spaces. The EU requirement for Class 100,000 conditions at rest can lead to the addition of terminal HEPA filters depending on design solutions. These spaces are designed to provide controlled access to the actual production areas. All other areas in the aseptic processing facility are defined as unclassified and include areas such as offices, toilets, break rooms, warehouses, utility rooms, and mechanical support areas.

TRANSITION POINTS

To protect the integrity of each of the operating classifications, transition points are necessary between each distinct classification. The transition points perform two functions; first they provide the necessary pressure differential between classifications, and second, they provide a space for personnel to don additional protective coverings and for material to be prepared for transfer. All doors in and out of the transition points must be interlocked to maintain pressure differentials.

Personnel Transitions

Personnel typically transit from unclassified to CunC spaces through gender-specific locker rooms. Access is controlled by an identity device. The locker rooms have unidirectional personnel flow with operators changing out of street clothing into a dedicated plant uniform and proceeding to a shoe change room to don dedicated plant shoes. Hair nets and Beard covers are added at this point. Current designs customarily eliminate toilet functions from locker rooms and standard operating procedures require personnel to access toilets and break rooms only in street clothing.

The transition from CunC to ISO 8 typically involves donning additional shoe covers, hair nets, and beard covers if the CunC corridor supports a single aseptic suite; if the CunC corridor provides access to multiple aseptic suites and/or inspection and secondary packaging suites, an additional one or two piece overgown that is gathered at the wrist and ankles is added.

To access ISO 7 or ISO 5 spaces, a gowning area for donning complete nonparticulate shredding sterilized uniforms with sterilized shoe covers, full head gear including face shields and gloves shall be provided; this gowning process is time consuming, expensive, and a prime risk of contamination is there due to poor operator technique.

Material Transitions

Separate material air locks shall be provided at the transition to and from areas of different classification. On a smaller scale, the air lock may be in the form of a double door pass-through in the wall between the environments. To maintain material segregation, separate material in and material out air locks are desired. Sufficient space should be provided to wipe the material down or remove protective coverings. Personnel will leave material in and pick material up from air locks, and should never pass completely through a material air lock. Doors shall be interlocked to maintain pressure differentials between area classifications. Equipment is accommodated in a similar fashion through the same air locks.

THE ASEPTIC MANUFACTURING PROCESS

General Definition

Aseptic processing is reserved for products that are not capable of maintaining efficacy under the more stressful conditions of terminal sterilization. In the aseptic process, the drug product, fully closed product containers, and product contact parts are subject to separate presterilization methods and the drug product and container are brought together (the filling/sealing or assembly process) in a highly controlled environment. RABS and isolation technology control this environment by eliminating the greatest source of contamination, the human operator, from potential product contact.

The aseptic processing suite is composed of three primary functions and their associated rooms: (i) product preparation, (ii) component and product contact part preparation, and (iii) filling/sealing or assembly.

Product preparation is preformed in the formulation room that typically includes areas for weighing the ingredients, making ingredient additions into tanks, and formulating the product. Open additions of active product ingredients and excipients should occur under unidirectional HEPA-filtered air supply to minimize added bioburden. Tanks in excess of 300 L are generally fixed and hard piped to the filling line. Smaller tanks are portable and are connected directly at

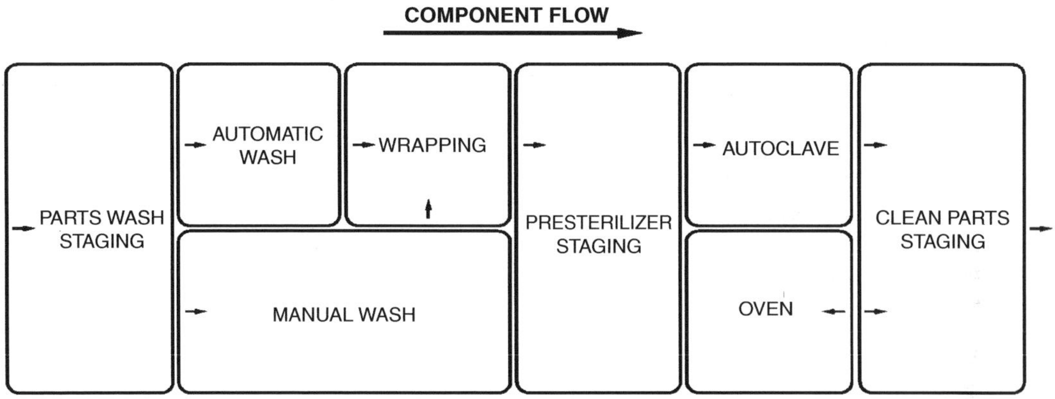

Figure 1 Component prep block flow diagram.

the filling machine with flexible stainless steel piping. On the smallest scale, the product can be supplied to filling in a disposable sterile container with integrated flexible tubing for product delivery. The product is customarily sterile filtered between the tanks and filling needles. The formulation room should be located as close as possible to filling machine to limit line losses of valuable product and reduce cleaning requirements. Fixed tanks are cleaned in place. Portable tanks can be cleaned in the formulation room or taken to a dedicated tank wash room usually adjacent the component/parts preparation area. The later is the preferred option for scheduling and product separation considerations.

Component and contact parts preparations are carried out in a series of rooms that typically progress in a unidirectional flow from the least clean to progressively cleaner spaces. (Fig. 1) The cleaning process begins by staging used parts in a prewash room.

They are washed in a two-door pass-through parts washer or manually in a sonocating sink in a continuous flow. The washed parts are transferred into a clean parts wrap area. This area is under local protection, which is defined as Class 100-Grade A air supply (100% HEPA-filtered unidirectional airflow). The intent is to minimize added bioburden to the parts prior to terminal sterilization. The wrapped parts are then transferred into a pass-through autoclave, sterilized, and withdrawn into a sterilized parts room ready for reuse. Another advanced trend currently gaining popularity is to use disposable parts that will limit the use of the parts cleaning suite.

Stoppers are typically the only components that are processed in this area. The amount of processing depends on how the stoppers are purchased. They are available as either unprocessed or ready-to-sterilize or ready-to-use stoppers. Unprocessed stoppers typically require washing, siliconizing, sterilizing, and drying. This process is often accomplished in a single machine. The most common current approach is to buy ready-to-sterilize stoppers that are introduced to the component preparation process immediately after the clean parts wrap area. They are then sterilized and dried if stopper moisture content is an issue. The ready-to-use stoppers are currently cost prohibitive due to first-time supplier validation costs.

The final space in the aseptic suite is the filling/sealing room where the product and components are integrated. For vials and ampoules, the glassware is typically washed, passed through a depyrogenation tunnel, filled, and stoppered in a continuous process. Small-volume clinical-scale facilities sometimes use separate washers and batch ovens. In the traditional clean room and RABS designs, this process occurs in a series of rooms of differing classifications. With isolator technology the continuous filling operation occurs in a single Class 100,000-ISO 8-Grade C room. In the case of ampoules and liquid-fill vials, the containers are sealed as soon as possible, in the case of lyophilized product the containers are transferred to the freeze-drier under ISO 5 conditions, prior to sealing. The capping process can occur outside the aseptic core with the additional requirements that the vials must be under Class 100-ISO 5-Grade A air supply until fully crimped. It is also recommended that a raised stopper detector and a vial reject station be installed just prior to the capper. For bulk syringes, the filling process is identical to vials through stoppering. For bagged nested syringes, presterilized stoppers are delivered in tubs to the filling line. Recently, some manufactures feel that the risk in aseptic technique in debagging the presterilized tubs is too great. They have added e-beam sterilization on line after debagging. It should be noted that the addition of the e-beam doubles the life cost of the nested syringe line.

Aseptic Suite Layout

The aseptic suite layout varies dramatically based on whether isolation or RABS technology is used. Aseptic suites using isolation technology are typically 30% smaller than RABS designs. These layouts are discussed in "RABS Technology–Based Aseptic Suite Design" and "Isolation Technology–Based Aseptic Suite Design" sections.

Aseptic Facility Layout

Although the aseptic suite is the core of the manufacturing process, it comprises only a small portion of the overall aseptic facility footprint. The aseptic facility also includes the remainder of the manufacturing functions including inspection, secondary packaging, material handling, product support including laboratories and documentation, administrative support, and both process and facility mechanical support.

The manufacturing function should have a unidirectional material flow proceeding from the receiving dock sequentially through material sampling, material warehouse, aseptic staging, aseptic processing suite, inspection staging, inspection, packaging staging, secondary packaging, finished product staging, and shipping (Fig. 2). As the materials proceed through this process, they must pass through a material air lock each time they transit into a new area classification. For biologic products, the staging and warehouse functions are typically in environmentally controlled 2°C to 8°C cold rooms.

A three-story design for an aseptic processing facility provides many advantages especially when using lyophilization. The aseptic processing suite is located on the second floor with all process utilities and the lyophilization mechanical support directly below on the first floor and the HVAC support located on the third floor. This configuration reduces the lengths for all ductwork and process piping. It also allows the process piping feeds from below thereby reducing the risk of leaks above the aseptic area ceiling. It also simplifies personnel controls by limiting the need for mechanics on the aseptic processing level.

RABS TECHNOLOGY–BASED ASEPTIC SUITE DESIGN

Aseptic processing suite design requirements are the same for traditional clean room and RABS technologies and both are addressed in this section. Figure 3 shows a typical RABS layout. The formulation room is typically Class 10,000-ISO 7-Grade B. The component preparation suite is typically Class 100,000-ISO 8-Grade C. The filling room is class 100-ISO 5-Grade A over critical operations with a Class 10,000-ISO 7-Grade B background. This classification configuration necessitates a minimum of three sets of gowning rooms, de-gowning rooms, and a minimum of three pairs of material air locks for each aseptic suite. Personnel must re-gown when going from one functional room to another.

Material access into the filling room is very complex for RABS-based designs. Change parts must access the filling room through a pass-through autoclave into a Class 100 staging area and then be transferred directly into the filling line. Stoppers will follow the same path with the potential additional drying step in an oven open to a Class 100 staging room. Glassware proceeds through the glassware washer and depyrogenation tunnel into the filling machine. In this traditional design, the washer and tunnel are in an adjacent Class 100,000 room with additional gowned operations personnel. Product will be transferred from the formulation tank through sterile filters into an additional tank in the filling room. For lyophilized vials, the stoppered vials exit the filling machine into a Class 100-ISO 5-Grade A lyo loading/unloading area. This area becomes large due to the lyo loading devices and must be curtained from the adjacent Grade B background. Automated laminar flow transfer tables can be a significant improvement over manual transfer by reducing the area and the risk of contamination due to manual interventions. Capping occurs in an adjacent Class 100,000-ISO 8-Grade C room; the stoppered vials must be under Class 100 air supply from the exiting point of the aseptic core to

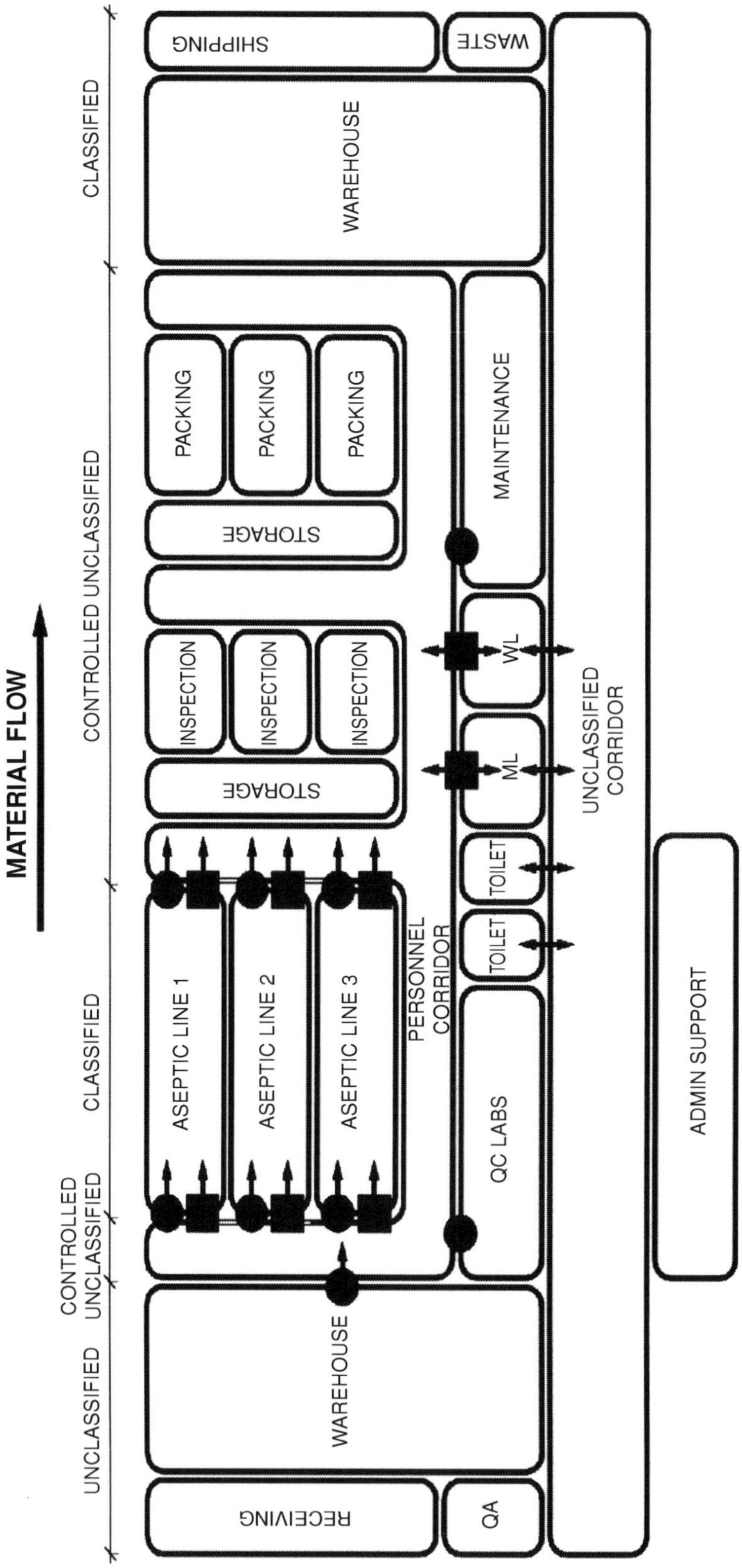

Figure 2 Aseptic facility block flow diagram.

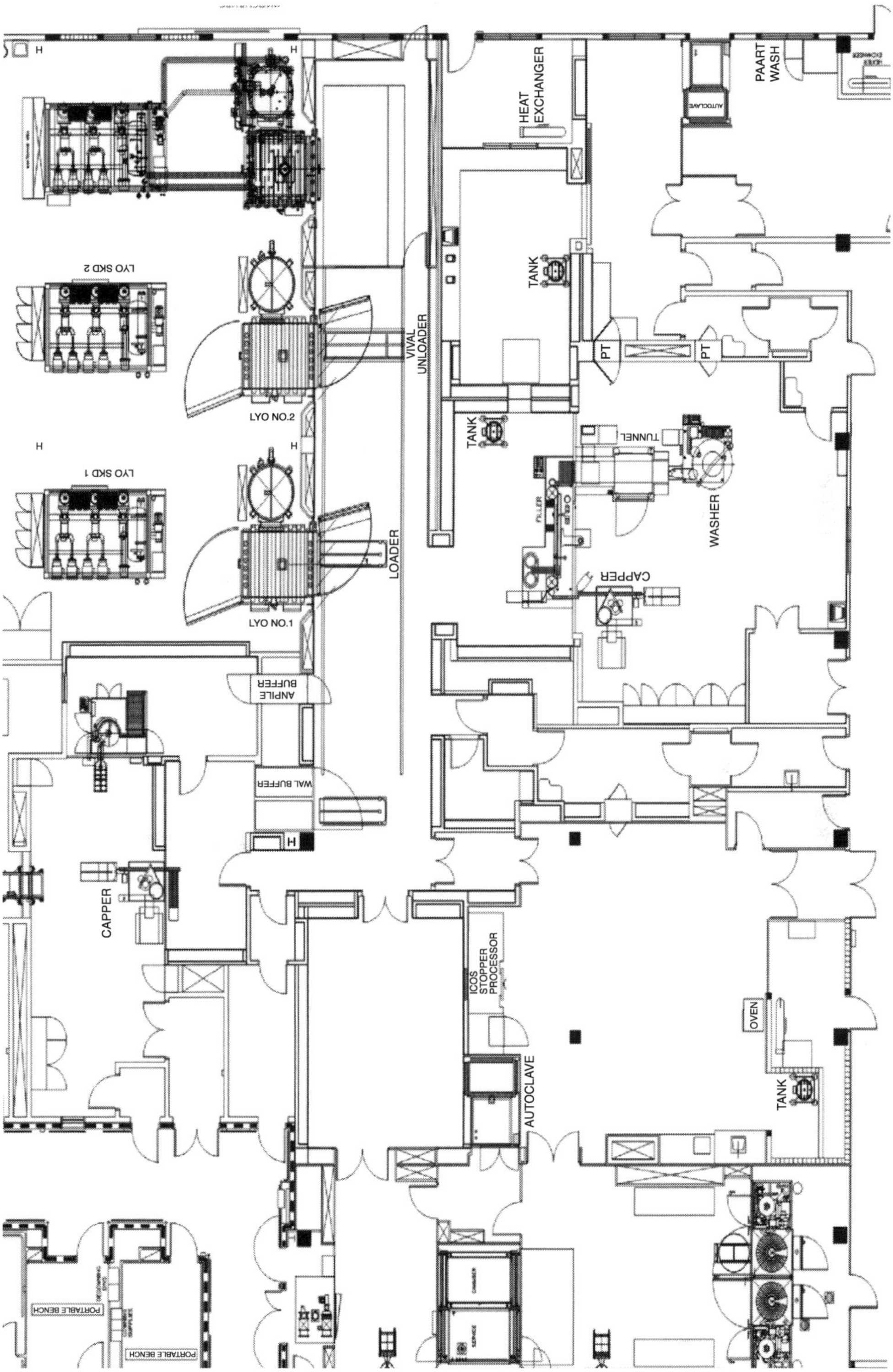

Figure 3 Typical RABS layout.

being fully crimped. The capping room typically requires additional dedicated gowning rooms and material air lock.

ISOLATION TECHNOLOGY–BASED ASEPTIC SUITE DESIGN

The use of isolation technology greatly simplifies the design of aseptic facilities.

The entire suite can be classified as Class 100,000-ISO 8-Grade C. There are now only single gowning, de-gowning, and material air locks per suite. In fact, depending on the products, single sets of transition points can serve several suites. All three aseptic functions, (i) product preparation, (ii) parts washing, and (iii) filling operations, can now be accessed by personnel without re-gowning. These facts allow isolator-based facilities to reduce the overall fill suites area by over 30% compared with a RABS and reduce the cost of gowning in time and materials significantly. Isolator-based aseptic suite design can be configured several ways. In early isolator facilities design, personnel and material proceeded through the transition points into a central corridor that connected to the product preparation area, the component/change parts area, and the filling room. This layout is still preferred for potent product design for containing potential contamination to the smallest area possible. Another design possibility connects the transition points directly to the central filling room that is adjacent to and connects directly to all of the other necessary rooms in the aseptic suite (Fig. 4). This design, which has been referred to as "the ballroom layout," can reduce the area of the suite by around 10% compare with the central corridor option. A third possible configuration for facilities that have multiple filling lines, shares the component/parts preparation area with multiple formulation/filling suites (Fig. 5). The optimum proportion is usually one parts-preparation suite for three formulation/filling suites, depending on throughput and number of products. This configuration is referred to as the parallel suite design and is a variation of the central clean corridor design. The aseptic isolator-based Class 100,000-ISO 8-Grade C facility parallel suite option can also provide an efficient design opportunity for leveraging support facilities for filling multiple product delivery systems. Examples exist where isolated liquid vial lines, isolated lyo vial lines, isolated nested syringe lines, terminally sterilized nonisolated vial lines, and/or blow-fill-seal (BFS) lines are in the same Grade C processing facility.

Another application for isolated filling technology is in the renovation of existing traditional aseptic suites. Typically older suites have Grade C–compliant product preparation and component/parts preparation areas but are at risk with Grade A/B filling room compliance. Design options for these facilities include converting space adjacent to the suite, if available, to a Grade C isolator filling room and abandoning the existing filling room once the isolated filling line is operational, or de-classify the existing filling room to Grade C and install a new isolated filling line. This renovation approach has significant cost benefit over a Greenfield approach.

It is desirable to locate the process equipment including parts washers, sterilizers, formulation tanks, and lyophilzers along the periphery of the Grade C suite, which can provide mechanical and process piping access from the adjacent CunC spaces. Integrating large fixed formulation tanks into the perimeter aseptic suite wall and locating all fixed pipe connections to the tank on the CunC side of the wall provide a formulation room that has compliant surfaces and is easily cleaned.

Ceilings are generally located at a height of 10 feet, which is fixed by the division between the HEPA/fan module and the air handler module of the filling line isolator. In isolator facilities, it is ideal to have a walkable ceiling to access the isolator mechanical systems and which allows for an option to replace worn-out HEPA filters and lamps outside the aseptic suite. This is an ideal application for the modular wall systems discussed later.

ARCHITECTURAL FINISHES AND DETAIL DESIGN CONSIDERATIONS

All surfaces in aseptic processing rooms shall be designed to facilitate cleaning. The following design standards are accepted current good manufacturing practices (cGMP):

- All surfaces in aseptic processing rooms shall have smooth, durable monolithic finishes. They should resist aggressive cleaning/sanitizing agents.
- All inside corners shall have approximately three inch radius corners.
- All door frames and windows shall be flush with surrounding walls.

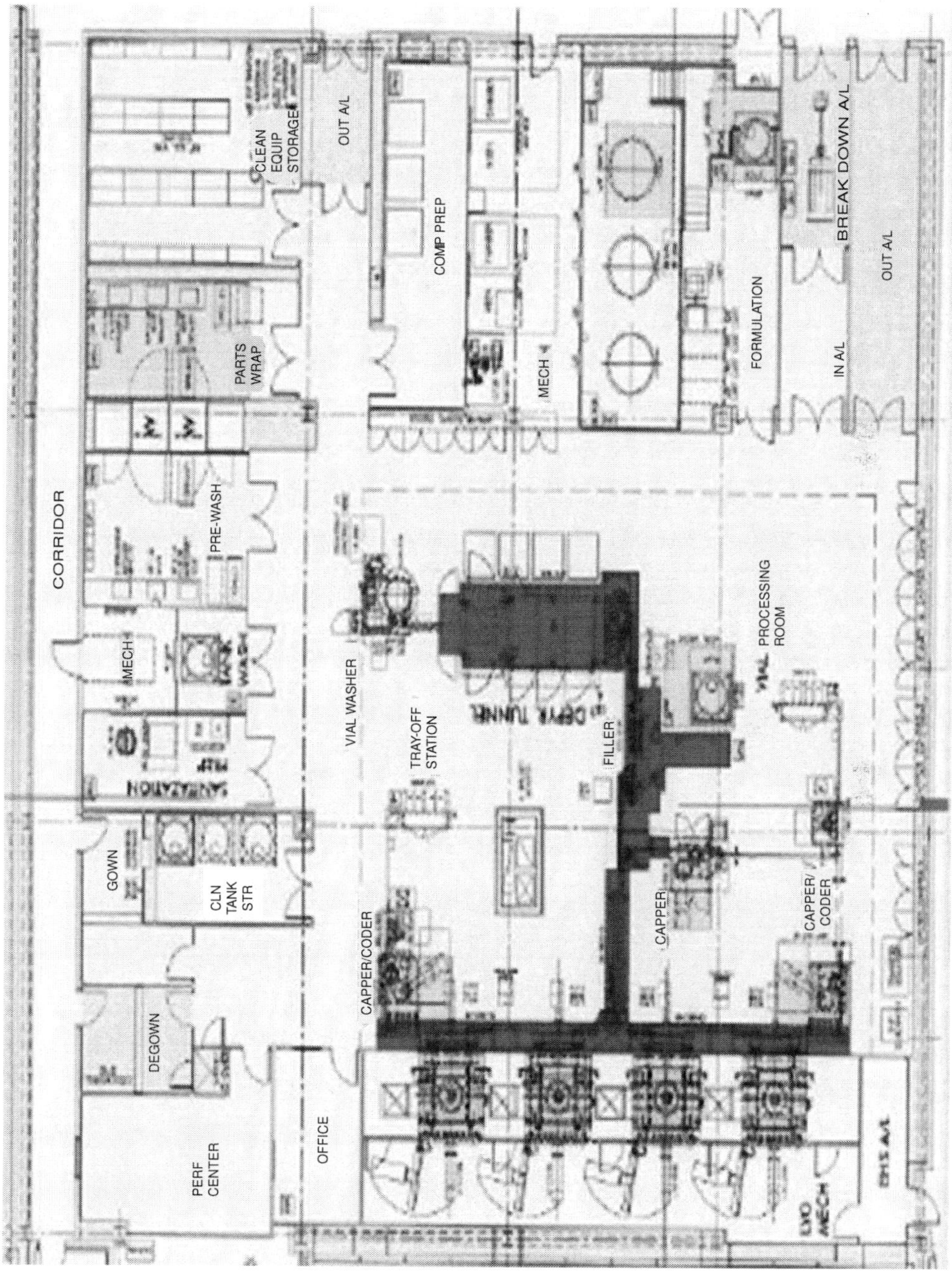

Figure 4 Isolator "ballroom" layout.

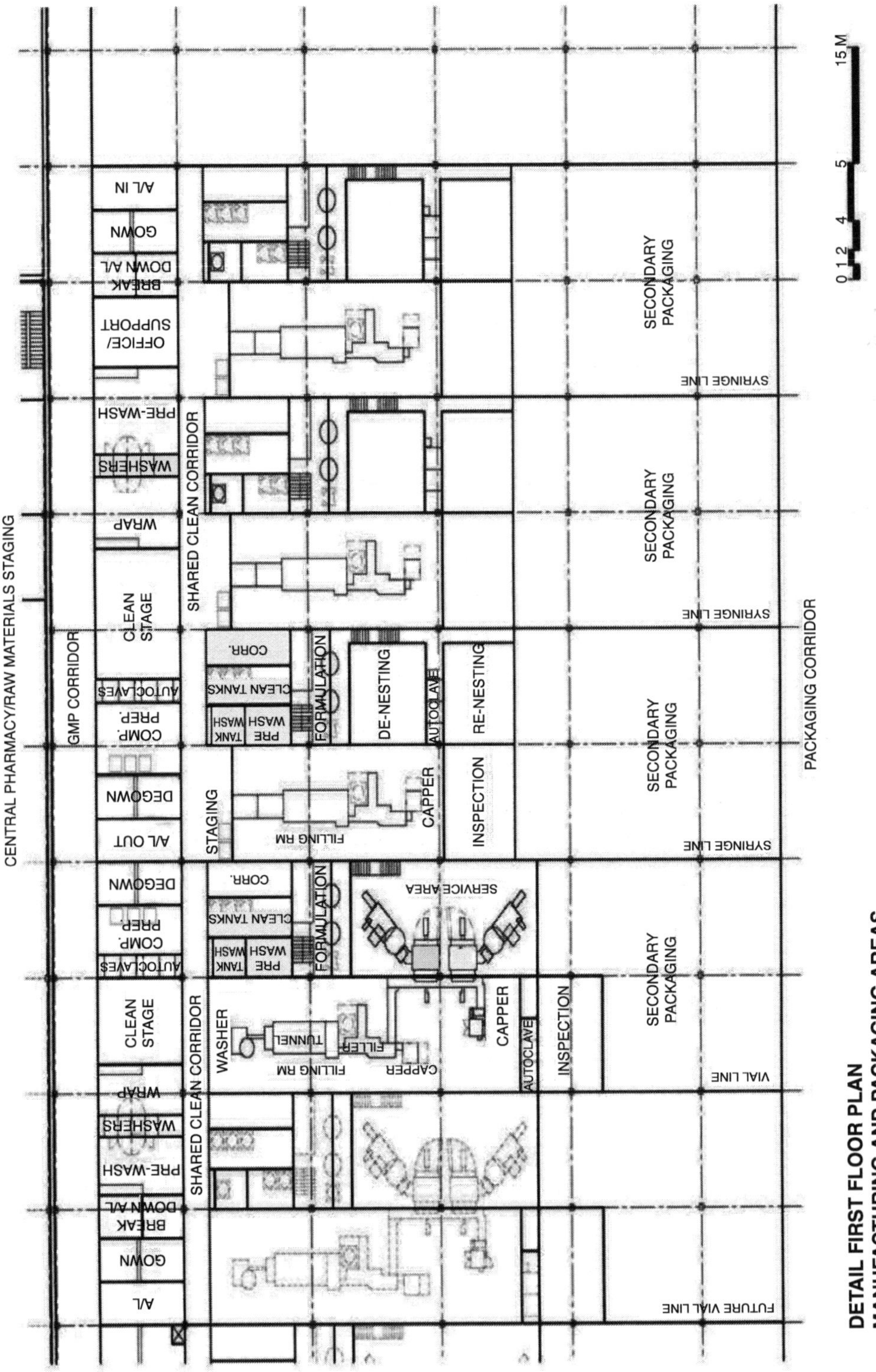

Figure 5 Isolator "multi-line" layout.

- Minimize the use of caulking. Caulking materials deteriorate over time or can be damaged easily by contact creating potential cavities that could promote growth. Use caulking only when no other material is viable to provide a seamless connection between two dissimilar materials.
- Avoid the use of drywall, especially when using isolators. The drywall installation generates particulates during construction, which creates issues when integrating simultaneous installation with the filling lines. Drywall construction also maximizes the need for caulking at connections.
- Recess all fixtures, panels, and equipment to be flush with the wall surface. Avoid all potential horizontal surfaces. Provide flush closure panels around all equipment and cabinets that do not meet walls, floors, or ceilings.
- Provide radius floor sweeps at all low-wall returns. Avoid louvers as they are difficult to clean and they conceal the dust that accumulates at the bottom of the duct returns.

The ideal material for aseptic room walls and ceilings is proven to be chemically welded modular panels. Beware of panel systems that use "batten" mechanical connections with square corners that are imposable to clean. There are currently three-door options that provide completely flush surfaces and can be easily cleaned: frameless glass, molded frameless PVC, and stainless steel.

Unfortunately, there are currently no ideal floor/base materials. The monolithic options are seamless vinyl sheet goods or epoxy flooring. The vinyl flooring cannot withstand wheel torque from heavy carts or pallets and the epoxy floors wear out and become porous over time. The epoxy floor is also more susceptible to poor workmanship.

Color is also a critical factor in aseptic facility design. Cool whites and blue tones give the perception that surfaces are clean. Warm whites and yellow and brown tones give the perception that surfaces are old or dirty. The use of the blue tones is a no-cost option to superior design results. The modular panel companies have discovered this technique and provide these as their standard colors.

ENGINEERING CONSIDERATIONS

Structural Systems

A steel frame structural design is preferred over a poured concrete design based on flexibility for mechanical and piping penetrations through the slabs. Spray fire proofing can be a disadvantage for steel frame installations due to material particulating issues; the fireproofing can be eliminated in many cases by reducing the area between fire separations. A 24 ft by 36 ft bay generally works well, avoiding conflict with equipment layouts. Because steel columns for this arrangement are typically 22-inch square, they can easily be integrated into mechanical chase walls limiting the number of inside corners in the classified rooms.

Mechanical Systems

Mechanical system design requirements for filling rooms vary dramatically between RABS- and isolator-based facilities. The major differences are the requirements for large volumes of Class 100 air supply in RABS facilities and the integration of the isolator air system with the room air system in isolator facilities. The first time cost as well as the life cost is significantly less for an isolator facility. With the current focus on green design, the RABS option is undesirable.

In RABS design, current guidance requests Class 100 conditions over the entire filling operation and Class 100 unidirectional airflow over open RABS doors. The unidirectional airflow requirement passing the doors is practically impossible to meet within a RABS filling room with a Class 10,000 background. Two major design issues limit the vertical airflow: (i) the low-wall returns are typically at a distance that causes horizontal airflow vectors above the bottom of the doors and (ii) the airflow exiting from the base of the RABS unit creates turbulence at the doors. Historically, flexible plastic curtains have been used in an effort to direct the air vertically; however, they tend to generate particles as the operators pass through, and that tends to be when the doors are open for an intervention. The low-risk solution is to provide Class 100 background in the entire filling room. This is obviously cost prohibitive.

Isolated filling lines are typically located in Class 100,000-ISO 8-Grade C rooms. The most common design is to use room air to supply the isolator. This room air should be returned to the isolator supply through low-wall returns for good room air profiles and to reduce the extreme air noise that has occurred when ceiling returns have been used. Typically isolator-based aseptic suites are designed for 25 to 30 air changes per hour, which translates to about 20% HEPA ceiling coverage.

Another consideration in aseptic facility design is the requirement for pressure differentials and air cascade from higher to lower classified rooms. The cumulative affect of the pressure differentials in RABS facilities between the various adjacent classified areas can be excessive pressure on doors and the need for complex control and monitoring systems. In isolator suites with all of the processing rooms at the same classification, the only required pressure differentials are across the transition points. Common practice in many recent isolator-based facility designs provides airflow from the filling room and clean component staging to the formulation room and the component preparation areas.

Plumbing Systems

The major current plumbing issue is providing an air break between equipment and drains and providing back flow prevention at floor drains. This is easier when the aseptic suite is on an upper building floor versus on grade.

Electrical Systems

The major electrical concern in aseptic facility design is maintaining continuous power supply (CPS) to critical systems during the production process. With the high value of the new aseptic products, use of redundant systems including uninterrupted power supply, emergency generators, or CPS systems become prudent business options.

Process Systems

Process system design primarily addresses the formulation process, process water systems and clean in place/sterilize in place (CIP/SIP) systems design. The process technologies tend to be the most difficult to manage during start up and continuous operation. This is one case where the simpler the better. The major complications arise around the CIP/SIP process for the product contact lines from fixed formulation tanks to the filling needles. Using portable tanks with direct aseptic connections to the filling machine with a completely disposable product path (including needles) is becoming the preferred option for many manufacturers to minimize the need for the CIP/SIP systems.

CONSTRUCTABILITY CONSIDERATIONS

The primary constructability issue particular to advanced aseptic processing facilities is the delivery and installation of the large process equipment. The three-story option previously referenced greatly simplifies access and rigging issues for the process water systems and other utilities located on the ground floor level. If possible, lyophilizers should be located along an exterior wall with the condenser and compressor skids on the ground floor and the chamber above. In this configuration, the lyophilizer will determine the ground to second floor ceiling height.

The most difficult installation access is generally for the filling line, the parts washer and the parts autoclave which by definition are located in the aseptic core of the facility. Modular wall/ceiling panels provide a tremendous advantage over stick built construction during the equipment installation process because the ceiling and wall panel installation can be easily removed and reinstalled along the rigging path in a single day.

THE DESIGN PROCESS

The design process in aseptic facility design is as critical to the success of a project as understanding the design program. The duration of an aseptic facility project from inception through design, construction, and validation is typically 4 to 5 years. Cutting this project time can be worth millions of dollars for the owner. The following process includes techniques that optimize the project design effort.

The initial design focus is to lock the business plan and objectives. Because the facility will be used for 15 to 20 years, most of the products that will be made there have not yet been identified, so facility flexibility should be evaluated based on potential product profiles. The project variables of cost, schedule, and program scope should be prioritized to determine the best project delivery system. Once the business parameters are fully understood, the design programming effort can commence. Too often engineers begin the design before they have locked the program scope, which is the greatest single cause for redesign and project delays.

The first programming step is to define the product manufacturing process; remember the goal is to manufacture an aseptic product in a robust compliant manner not to build a signature building. For aseptic facility design, once the manufacturing process is defined, detailed gowning and material transfer procedures can be established. Next the process technology and equipment should be selected. In aseptic facilities, especially when using isolation technology, it is imperative that the equipment manufacturers and models be selected prior to commencing detailed engineering design. It is also important to order the process equipment at this point to ensure timely deliveries. With both RABS and isolator technologies, it is important to perform factory acceptance tests at the individual vendor sites as well as an integrated test usually at the filling machine vendor site. At this point the design process can proceed as in any other complex project with the architectural and engineering disciplines addressing the design requirements discussed in this chapter.

THE TREND

The advancements in aseptic facility design involve RABS and isolation processing technologies. Advanced aseptic facility design using isolation technology are proving to be simpler for personnel, material and equipment flows, area classifications, and operating procedures. Isolator facilities have become cost competitive to construct and are substantially less expensive to operate. Isolator-based facilities are much more energy efficient and a greener design option. The issues with early isolator designs including cleaning and change over times, and in-process interventions have been resolved with the new generation isolator designs. The advantages of isolators over RABS are so overwhelming that by comparison in the future, RABS may become known as a "ridiculous attempt being sterile."

REFERENCES

1. FDA. Guidance for Industry. Sterile Drug Products Produced by Aseptic Processing-Current good Manufacturing Practice. U S Department of Health Services. Food and Drug Administration, September 2004.
2. EU Guidelines to Good Manufacturing Practice Medicinal Products for Human and Veterinary Use. Annex 1. Manufacture of Sterile Medicinal Products, European Commission, EudraLex. The Rules Governing Medicinal Products in the European Union, November 2008.

4 Innovations in aseptic processing technology

James Agalloco and James Akers

INTRODUCTION

The preparation of many parenteral products must be accomplished by aseptic processing due to limitations of the formulation and/or container to withstand the conditions necessary for sterilization of the final dosage form. Considered in the simplest manner, the preparation of an aseptically processed product requires that the placement of a sterile material inside a sterile container, and securing that container with a sterile closure (Fig. 1).[1] In practice, the task is substantially more complex, and successful aseptic processing entails a substantially larger number of considerations all of which can influence the outcome of the process (Fig. 2). Aseptic processing can be defined as

> Handling sterile materials in a controlled environment, in which the air supply, facility, materials, equipment and personnel are regulated to control microbial and particulate contamination to acceptable levels (1).

Rearranging the elements of the Parenteral Drug Association definition into similar activities is perhaps more useful as they provide a means for understanding the major concerns that must be addressed to assure sterility of the materials being produced. Successful aseptic processing requires at a minimum the following:

- Suitably developed and validated sterilization processes for the components, formulation, and equipment product contact parts.
- Establishment/maintenance of a suitable environment in which microbial contamination is controlled appropriately to mitigate contamination risk.
- Defined methods for the set-up and operation of the sterilized equipment.
- Appropriately gowned and trained individuals to conduct the process in the prescribed manner.
- A monitoring program for the assessment of contamination control on an ongoing basis.

Those elements that are less subject to human variation should be validated to assure their continual acceptability for use. Where operators are central to success for one of the central requirements already listed the outcome is substantially less certain. There is consensus agreement that operators are the prime source of microbial contamination in aseptic processing, and as a consequence aseptic processing technology evolved to minimize the adverse impact of the operator contemporaneously with improvements in equipment, material, and automation (2,3). If interventions are to be avoided, as is now better understood, then designs that eliminate them can provide meaningful improvements in aseptic processing performance. The systems that resulted from this new understanding are the harbingers of a new era of "advanced aseptic processing," in which personnel as a source of contamination are eliminated to an extent not possible in conventional clean rooms. It can be defined as follows:

> An advanced aseptic process is one in which direct intervention with open product containers or exposed product contact surfaces by operators wearing conventional cleanroom garments is not required and never permitted (4).

Many of these new technologies were conceived with the express purpose of eliminating operator-borne contamination. Other changes in aseptic processing were developed by as component vendors and equipment suppliers that sought to expand their market penetration through vertical integration, technological advancement, or cost reductions.

[1] Some other containers do not require a separate closure component, that is, ampoules, plastic/metal tubes, and form-fill-seal (FFS)/blow-fill-seal (BFS), as the container can be secured by heat and/or pressure on the container materials to affect a seal. In all other ways, these containers are processed identical to those with separate closures.

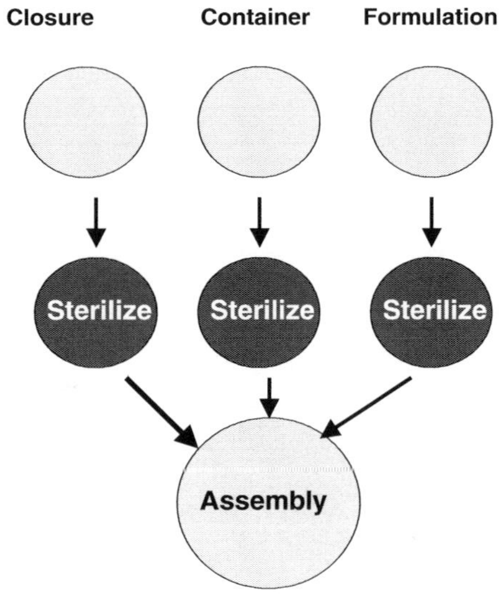

Figure 1 A simplistic view of aseptic processing.

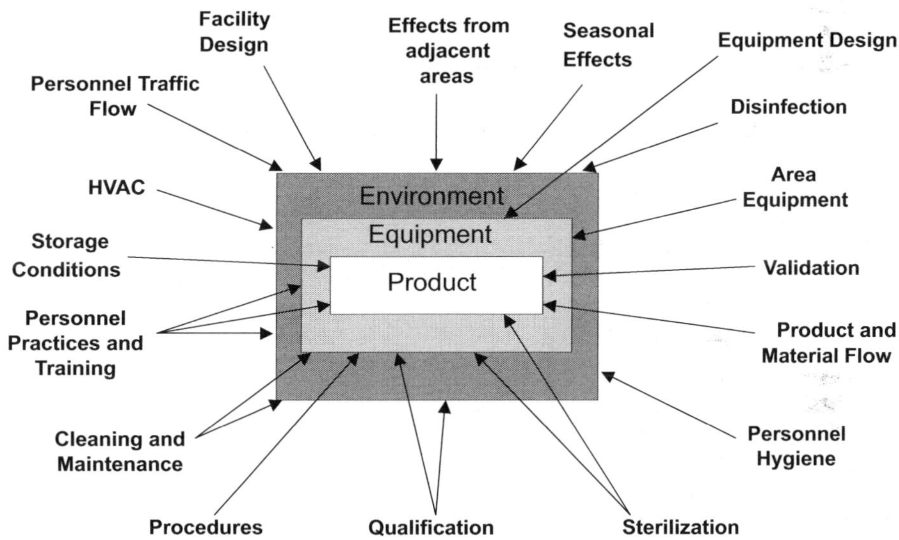

Figure 2 A more realistic view of aseptic processing. *Source*: Adapted from Leonard Mestrandrea.

The introductory chapter to this volume outlined how the methods for aseptic processing changed from the 1950s through the end of the twentieth century as significant technological breakthroughs enabled improved performance. The first of these advances was the HEPA filter, which allowed for filling and sealing equipment to be located in an aseptic environment. The early 1980s witnessed the first pharmaceutical isolators, which were made possible by the availability of a rapid transfer port (RTP). Both the HEPA and the RTP can be considered "disruptive" technologies, as each resulted in substantial changes to practices that transformed the manner in which aseptic processing was being performed.[2]

Aseptic processing has witnessed rapid evolutionary change since the RTP was introduced for aseptic applications. This chapter identifies some of the more prominent of the technology advances. Generic names are used wherever possible to avoid both confusion and commercial nomenclature. Structuring this chapter proved problematic, a series of tables has been used in

[2] Other "disruptive" technologies of recent vintage include personal computers, cell phones, and digital cameras.

which technologies are grouped by application to a core aseptic processing activity. It should be noted, that many of the items included could have been placed in multiple categories. There is also a strong synergistic element to the technologies; for example, the impact of plastics has been facilitated by the increased usage of radiation sterilization and the availability of reliable decontamination allowed for the emergence of isolation technology.

Plastic Materials

The classic 1967 movie, The Graduate, included a classic line, in which the hero of the film is given a single word as a harbinger of the future—"plastics." In the context of aseptic processing, it would seem that this notion was especially prophetic. The pharmaceutical and medical device industries have embraced plastics in many ways and as a result aseptically processed product delivery systems are both more varied and more versatile than they were in the recent past. The major benefits of plastics are their lighter weight, lower overall cost, and single-use capability. Plastics have also allowed more complex combination drug delivery systems that simply could not have existed using glass, rubber, and metal container closure systems. The biggest concerns with their expanded use are issues with respect to extractable and leachable materials that might be present, as well as the stability considerations for formulated materials.

Item	Application/change	Impact
Containers	For sterile filling of injectable drugs	Reduced requirements for washing of containers because they can be produced in cleaner environments; reduction in particles; replacement of dry heat depyrogenation with radiation sterilization; formulation compatibility; changes in potential extractables/leachables
Stoppers	Vendor provides valued-added steps for end user by supply of ready-to-sterilize and ready-to-use components; new formulations are radiation compatible.	Eliminates internal processing at end user site; shifts validation responsibilities to supplier; reduces cost; better suited to low-volume production facilities; raises concerns for package integrity during shipment; allows for terminal irradiation of filled units; reduce requirements for drying of stoppers; formulation compatibility; changes in potential extractables/leachables
Syringes	Increased usage for ease in administration (glass syringe usage has also increased)	Requires means for introduction of sealed containers into aseptic core; vendor responsible for cleaning/sterilization of syringes; formulation compatibility; extractables/leachables
Tyvek®	For wrapping of materials prior to sterilization by both component vendors and end users	Allows sterilization by varied means with improved container integrity; more reliable than paper wrapping or boxes for material introduction into aseptic core; usable with steam, gas and vapor sterilization; validation of agent penetration
RTP	For use with isolators and RABS systems; multiple- or single-use	Supports the introduction of items into RABS and isolators; used with some ready-to-use and ready-to-sterilize stopper systems; elimination of airlocks for material entry
Flexible bags	Replacement for tanks on largest scale; replacement of glass/plastic sample containers; single use	Elimination of cleaning / cleaning validation; reductions in water usage safer, lower overall cost; elimination of cross contamination potential
Disposable items	Assemblies of multiple components presterilized for use	Elimination of cleaning/cleaning validation; formulation compatibility; extractables/leachables; elimination of aseptic connections, consistency of design; worker protected from product residues
Filters	Filters capable of withstanding steam sterilization for extended periods enabling sterilization-in-place of large systems with ease	Simpler validation of large sterilization-in-place systems; greater reliability of sterilization-in-place compared with aseptic assembly; fewer interventions necessary

Room and Enclosure Environmental Decontamination

The need to control microbial contamination in aseptic processing has always existed. Until the 1980s, agents such as formaldehyde were widely used on a periodic basis to "fog" aseptic areas to reduce contamination risk in rooms and ductwork. The classification of formaldehyde as a carcinogenic agent ended the practice of fogging with this agent in clean rooms. In addition, many users became aware that formaldehyde fogging was difficult to control and worked most efficiently when humidity could be elevated to 60% or more. Unfortunately, there was no readily identifiable agent that could be used as a "fogging" agent for decontaminating environments. Replacement approaches have been dominated by manual application of sanitizing agents by using mops, buckets, sponges, and a substantial amount of manual effort. The frequency of treatment was varied with the criticality of the room being treated. These manual decontamination methods are time consuming, costly, and only as effective as the diligence of the personnel performing this rather arduous task.

The first pharmaceutical isolators implemented in the mid-1980s for sterility testing and aseptic processing were internally decontaminated with aerosolized Peracetic acid. This agent was effective, but the method of delivery, corrosive properties, and strong odor limited its utility (and may have slowed the introduction of isolation technology).

A significant change in decontamination approach came with the introduction of vapor phase H_2O_2 (VPHP) generators for isolator decontamination (unfortunately initially termed isolator sterilization), which changed first the means for treating enclosures and soon afterwards for entire clean rooms. VPHP provide a level of treatment superior to formaldehyde fogging processes, without the potential for adverse impact on personnel. With this new means at its disposal, industry's decontamination methods were being transformed once again.

Item	Application/change	Impact
VPHP	Decontamination of rooms, isolators, and closed Restricted Access Barrier Systems (cRABS) using automated means	Simplified and more effective decontamination of classified environments than is possible with manual methods; lower cost
Change in process objective	Decontamination, not sterilization, as the goal for isolators and other environments	Sterilization is an inappropriate objective when personnel are present or when the purpose of the treatment is environmental control; less aggressive treatments, shorter process cycles; less adverse impact on materials exposed to the treatment

Personnel

The production of sterile products required the direct participation of gowned personnel for much of the last 50 years. Although it had been recognized that personnel were the primary source of contamination, their presence was considered unavoidable because aseptic processing approaches relied heavily on the operator for many activities. Efforts to mitigate the adverse impact of personnel have been continuous and have culminated in designs that essentially eliminate their presence. For those older facilities there are measures available short of new equipment that can improve the impact of personnel on the aseptic process.

An important consideration in aseptic processing has been the difference between capability and expectation. Aseptically produced products are labeled rightly or perhaps wrongly "sterile." As a result, some regulators and a number of industry specialists came to think that the objective was to operate a "sterile" clean room and that personnel could, with proper control efforts, contribute no contamination to an aseptic environment. Recently, this tension point has become well understood to many practitioners and it is now generally accepted that there is no such thing as a manned "sterile" environment.

Beyond the accoutrements associated with personnel garb is the growing realization that interventions by gowned personnel however well designed are to be avoided (3). The elimination of personnel interventions can be accomplished in various ways: improved and redesigned equipment; tighter acceptance quality levels (AQLs) for components, automation/robotics. Alternatively, firms can adopt the more expensive, but certainly mire effective approach of advanced aseptic processing technologies.

Item	Application/change	Impact
New gown materials	Elimination of heavier fabrics better filtration properties	Outsourced sterilization at vendor; greater operator comfort
Helmets replace hood, mask and goggles	Lightweight combination helmet/hood with integrated HEPA-filtered air supply	Greater operator comfort; better vision; less difficulty with fogging goggles; more complex sterilization prior to use
New glove materials offer greater integrity	Polymers with greater resistance to decontamination agents used on isolators	Fewer glove failures; fewer deviations resulting from glove failure; higher cost offset by longer life
Isolators eliminate personnel within the aseptic environment	Isolators replace clean rooms primarily for new installations	Dramatically improved aseptic processing performance; decontamination and leak issues (initially, but no longer); operator protection from potent compounds; campaign operation simplified
RABS restrict personnel access to aseptic environment	RABS are used to provide a more complete barrier between personnel and the critical zone in an aseptic environment	Improved aseptic processing performance
Altered intervention perspective	Interventions are not inherently safe and should be minimized at all times,	New perspective on aseptic processing resulting in emergence of many new designs, practices and approaches for performing interventions; greater motivation for advanced aseptic technologies

Disposables

Until the 1990s, pharmaceutical equipment were considered clean on the basis of the completion of a cleaning procedure and satisfactory visual inspection prior to use. That all changed when US Food and Drug Administration began to expect validation of cleaning procedures. That requirement changed things dramatically, and as industry ramped up its efforts, the full impact of that expectation became evident. Cleaning validation proved to be no simple task, and firms continue to find it technically difficult, time consuming, and expensive to conduct. A production option that was dismissed as foolish before cleaning validation became a concern, the use of single-use disposable technology, has grown in appeal over the years, especially in biological processing. The "life cycle" costs associated with disposable equipment can be favorable compared to re-useable equipment that must be cleaned with each use, although this is by no means universally true. Disposable equipment can be found in a variety of configurations and sizes providing the end user with several important benefits.

Item	Application/change	Impact
Filter sets Fill sets Compounding sampling Connectors	Preassembled and sterilized single-use assemblies for use in variety of application	Eliminates errors and aseptic manipulations in assembly, less exposure of personnel to materials, elimination of cleaning, less chance of leakage, lower cost than reusable items when cleaning is considered; increased reliance on vendors; extractable/leachable issues to be addressed

Sterilization

The sterilization processes play an essential role in every aseptic process. Because aseptic processing entails the assembly of components that have been individually presterilized, there may be several different processes required. As the variety of materials being used in aseptic processing has expanded so have the means for effecting the sterilization of them. Radiation was once almost exclusively used for medical devices; however, the emergence of e-beam systems that can be located within a pharmaceutical facility and the VD_{MAX} dose setting method that allowed for smaller sample sizes has resulted in increased usage.

New gases for sterilization of materials may mean a return to in-house gas sterilization of items unable to withstand moist- or dry-heat conditions. The safety and environmental concerns associated with ethylene oxide (EtO) sterilization had resulted in pharmaceutical firms outsourcing EtO sterilization processes to contractors willing to provide the necessary controls to assure safe use.

Steam sterilization-in-place (SIP) has received greater attention as well. SIP allows for the in situ sterilization of complex piping systems. Where vessels, fluid handling, filtration, and filling systems were once sterilized as individual items and aseptically assembled, it is far preferable to preassemble these items, and steam them in place eliminating numerous aseptic interventions.

Item	Application/change	Impact
H_2O_2	Environmentally friendly, ease of use, nonheat process, more effective, lower cost	
New sterilizing agents	Availability of ClO_2, O_3 for sterilization of items	Replacement of EtO; in-house gas sterilization of items; potential application for isolator and room decontamination; gas processes are simpler than vapor processes
Increased use of radiation	Availability of in-house e-beam systems; integration of e-beam with isolators and RABS; VD_{MAX} dose setting method is better suited to pharmaceuticals than prior methods; Increased use of plastics required new methods	Allows for increased use of plastic and disposable items (see above); simple process to validate; lower dose increased flexibility of usage
Postaseptic treatments	Patient safety can be improved if a lethal treatment (however modest) follows an aseptic fill	Safer products, less concern about environmental excursions; simple addition of steam or radiation treatments to aseptically filled products
SIP for assemblies	Sterilization of assemblies rather than aseptic assembly	More reliable aseptic processes; elimination of aseptic interventions

Equipment

Processing and filling equipment have been essential to aseptic processing since the first HEPA-filtered clean rooms of the 1950s. The equipment provided the means for increased lots sizes and more reliable production than had been possible with the prior practices that were largely hand-fill oriented. The manned clean room is still the dominant means for aseptic processing, and although processing equipment has improved over the years, the gowned operator still plays an important role in its operation. With few exceptions, even the most modern equipment requires personnel for initial set-up, component resupply, and corrective interventions in the even of a malfunction or missfeed. Nevertheless, equipment improvements and innovations have reduced the need for operator intervention.

Item	Application/change	Impact
Changes in lyophilizer-loading methods	Automated and single height loading systems requiring less operator involvement	Substantially reduce personnel related contamination; increased reliability; higher throughput; worker protected from potent compounds
Single-use tanks	Disposable mixing/holding vessels for solution preparation and holding	Reduction in water consumption; lower "life cycle" costs; less exposure of operators to potent/toxic materials; elimination of cleaning validation
Tunnel cool zone	Dry-heat sterilization of the cooling zone of tunnels	Enhanced protection of the aseptic processing zone
Process analytical technologies	Integrated feedback systems that bring real-time analytical tools to the production floor for superior process reliability	Brings process control to the shop floor; the relocation of analytical instrumentation to control/evaluate processes as the are executed offers the potential for improvements in cycle time, and product quality
Mass flow	Adding mass flow sensors to individual fill needles affords a superior dosing and ease of SIP application	Improved dose uniformity by using a noninvasive approach
Neck hold	Replacement of bottom-drive conveyors with grippers that position vials by their neck.	Easier changeover; more accurate positioning; fewer jams; allows for 100% weight check at production speeds
Machine vision	Use of automated vision systems for in-process inspection of filled units	More reliable inspection without operators; higher speed inspection possible

Automation

The microchip was perhaps the most significant invention of the later half of the twentieth century. Its presence is almost ubiquitous in our society, yet only in the last 5 to 10 years has it become a major part of our industry. Its expanding presence in our industry has already fostered dramatic changes in operations. The following examples are just a few of the applications already in place.

Item	Application/change	Impact
Robotics	The use of robots to perform tasks customarily performed by operators	Elimination of gowned personnel; protection of workers from toxic or dangerous materials; elimination of personnel derived contamination, improved reliability of execution
Remote environmental monitoring of classified environments	Designs that bring the sample to a remote location outside the critical zone	No interventions with the critical zone; greatly reduced potential for sampling induced product contamination

Next-Generation Technologies

The methods used for aseptic processing have undergone dramatic change in the last 20 to 30 years beginning with the introduction of the isolator. A veritable avalanche of change has been witnessed as evidenced by the items briefly described earlier. Yet, the future appears to hold even more promising innovations that may further improve aseptic processing. The most prominent of these are closed vials technology (described in detail in chaps. 15 and 40) and the replacement of aseptic processing environments with machines (as described in chaps. 34 and 41).

CONCLUSION

Nearly 2500 years ago, the Greek historian Herodotus wrote the "The only constant is change" (5). Had he witnessed the last few years in our industry, especially in the area of aseptic processing he might have been even more emphatic. The changes our industry has already embraced have been substantial; those that are on the horizon are truly game changing.

REFERENCES

1. Parenteral Drug Association (PDA).TR # 22 Revision, Process Simulation for Aseptically Filled Products. Draft # 6 in preparation, 2009.
2. Agalloco J, Akers J, Madsen R. Current practices in the validation of aseptic processing—2001. PDA Technical Report 36. PDA J Pharm Sci Technol 2002; 56(3 suppl).
3. Agalloco J, Akers J. The truth about interventions in aseptic processing. Pharm Technol 2007; 31(5): S8–S11.
4. Akers J, Agalloco J, Madsen R. What is advanced aseptic processing? Pharm Manufacturing 2006; 4(2):25–27.
5. Heraclitus. The Histories, circa 450 BC. www:wikiquote. Accessed May 13, 2010.

5 Ergonomics in enclosure design

Brian Smith and David Pallister

This chapter explains some important points to consider for ergonomics in the design of aseptic processing enclosures. It discusses specific considerations for the product such as the scale of the operation, process flow, dedicated or multipurpose use, quantities being transferred, sizes of the containers, the method of transfer, characteristics of the materials, cleaning requirements, the method of sampling, and the manipulations required for the product.

Considerations for equipment are also reviewed for specific applications, interfaces to integrated equipment, the location and impact of external equipment, the visibility of critical items for the operator, and the need to study the ergonomics through the use of mock-ups. It is also pointed out that consideration of the facility is important in regard to the utilities available, waste disposal, and any support ancillaries.

On the basis of these topics, it will be evident that ergonomics is a critical component in the design of custom installations.

APPLICATIONS

In all design scenarios, each application should be reviewed in detail to assess how access to each component during operation and maintenance is achieved to ensure due consideration that system ergonomics is understood. This is a most important factor where the use of mock-ups becomes the only tried and tested method of understanding the needs of the system layout. Each application differs not just in relation to the operations that need to be addressed from an ergonomic perspective, but in addition, the space for installation also must be addressed. Many times the plant layout constraints or space available for the equipment installation affects the operational ability of the system. For example, filter discharge systems with reduced elevation or charging stations where head room is at a premium, the ergonomics of operation versus fit needs to be considered early in the design process.

Where equipment is interfaced as a part of the application, again the ergonomics of access to this equipment is also crucial, primarily to ensure that it can also be operated safely and easily as an integral part of the device.

EQUIPMENT/INTERFACE (RETRO-FIT VERSUS NEW)

For additional design considerations on this subject refer to chapter 6.

Along with the design considerations, an ergonomic study should be conducted. In some cases, when isolating an existing piece of equipment, it may be necessary to redesign/modify aspects of that equipment to make it easier to operate with or contain. When designing around new equipment, the best practice would be to involve the equipment supplier in the design evaluation. This includes both drawings and mock-ups. If involved early, the equipment supplier can work with the enclosure supplier and customer to contribute to a total solution to the containment application.

SCALE OF OPERATION

The scale of the operation is significant in regard to ergonomics of the ultimate system design. Small-scale applications such as laboratory-scale operations would typically be easier to achieve an ergonomic solution. This is a result of the comparatively small quantities of product processed and physically smaller process equipment in comparison with production applications. The need in the laboratory environment from an ergonomic perspective can be most challenging from the viewpoint of flexibility to ensure the laboratory staff have the range of movement and operation to accommodate all eventualities that may be created.

As the scale of operation and as the throughput increases from pilot processes through bulk and solid dosage form production, the ergonomics are further challenged by the space available, size of the process equipment to be interfaced with, as well as the physical quantity of material being handled. As in laboratory or development operations, flexibility is also a key with pilot operations. However, this is largely due to the potentially changing nature of the process. Although, production environments may appear more challenging due to the physical size of the items to be contained, the operations should be better defined in the form of a longer term solution where a defined product flow and standard operating procedures (SOPs) are established.

SOP/PRODUCT FLOW

During the early phases of the design process, and certainly at the time of initial mock-up assessment, the SOPs of the proposed system should be reviewed and accepted. This will help define a suitable and ergonomically sound product flow through the containment system.

Working with the mock-up and simulating the product flow from raw material/process entry through manipulations within the chamber and ultimate exit allows a thorough review of the operational procedures. This will allow the manipulations and access to take place in the most acceptable, ergonomic manner. The SOPs should define the product manipulations, cleaning, and reach for maintenance/component access, etc.

DEDICATED/MULTIPURPOSE USE

When considering ergonomic solutions, it is important for both the supplier and customer to fully understand the intended uses of the system. A detailed process description of the anticipated customer applications should be provided. After preparing the process description, a mock-up can be designed and built with the various process requirements. A mock-up review should be conducted for all different configurations. In general, it is easier to consider ergonomics, when the isolator is dedicated to a specific application. When the unit serves different purposes, more extensive ergonomic solutions may need to be applied.

CONTAINER SIZES

Enclosures traditionally had been designed to accommodate relatively small quantities of material and as such, small containers have been handled within the enclosure. As quantities of material increased the containers in which they are supplied have also increased. Therefore, the ergonomics of handling these containers need to be addressed more closely. The understanding of container sizes needs to provide a review of both input (raw material) containers in the form of drums, bags, intermediate bulk containers (IBCs), etc. and also the output (receiving containers) drums, liners, IBCs, etc.

The size of these containers dramatically affects the sizing of the system, especially if drum tipping is required for the larger drums and hence the ergonomics involved are critical. Early mock-ups during the design phase can provide significant input into the design process to ensure that the input and output containers interface with the logical sequence of operation required for the process.

QUANTITIES OF TRANSFER

Similar to the container sizes already referred to, the greater the quantity of material transferred, particularly manually, the more thoroughly the ergonomics of the design need to be assessed. The more "hands-on" transfers that take place, the greater the containment risk but also the more important is the ergonomic interface. Design considerations, such as the depth plus the height and width of the enclosure, can all be affected by container sizes, as well as the quantities and volumes of material being transferred.

Obviously any automated material transfers via conveyors, lifts, pumps, etc. will only help with ergonomics, but they all need to be considered during the cleaning phase. Access to and around these systems is important to understand and consider during the mock-up and design.

TRANSFER SYSTEMS

Chapter 6– (Transfer Systems section) provides specific details on transfer systems such as rapid transfer ports (RTP), split butterfly valves (SBV), other high containment transfer systems, bag-in/bag-out ports and air locks.

Automated transfer systems typically provide a better ergonomic solution. By using these, less physical intervention is required by the operator. An IBC with a SBV or RTP being moved by a post hoist is considered the most ergonomic way to connect to an isolator or RABS. Bag-out technology requires an operator to perform the bagging, clamping, and cutting steps exactly as the SOP describes. During design evaluation and mock-up review, the operation and access of these transfer systems should be a review point. Operators should fully understand the operations of transfer systems required of them before evaluating them on a mock-up. Access to transfer systems is only one part of the review. Simulated product or component transfers should be conducted.

MATERIALS

The volume and density of the material being processed require a thorough understanding and operational commitment. The design, sizing, and access requirements of the enclosure may be dependent on the product characteristics, such as dustiness or flowability. Hence, during design and mock-up phase, always consider the material type being processed to ensure that the unit can control and perform to the levels expected.

MANIPULATION CONSIDERATIONS

Movement or manipulations that take place both internally and externally warrants consideration at an early stage in the design. This in turn impacts the physical space, size, and access requirements in and around the system. Equipment, product, and process items contained within the system must be accessed for operation and cleaning. This should ideally be prior to mock-up evaluation, primarily due to cost impacts, for container sizes and handling requirements (integral drum tippers for larger bulk drums), as well as equipment/process movement (lid openings for baskets/filters, etc.). This may also impact and determine the need for exterior access platforms and the subsequent overall footprint of the unit. Ideally, this solution needs to be configured at the proposal stage as the inclusion of drum tippers and elongated chambers may be required to improve access. In addition, ergonomics can impact cost, lead time, and special requirements.

EXTERNAL ACCESS REQUIREMENTS

External access of the enclosure may be required for a number of operations. These access points and the operations involved need to be evaluated in the design phase and ergonomic study of the isolator. The access may include operator support structures, stand, steps, or even chairs or stools. Other equipment that may be required for product manipulation are posthoists and drum lifts.

In most applications, the height of gloveports from the floor while standing ranges between 48 and 50 inches. Due to design restrictions, this height may force the operator off the actual floor and a support structure under them may be required. These structures can be integrated into the design, but local safety codes will need to be reviewed with the end users' health and safety department. Railings, rigid, chain, or cable types, are a required feature of most platforms. Local building codes will dictate the design of both the platform and elevation systems.

Some installations are designed for the operator to work long periods of time. If it is feasible, consideration should be taken to design the system so that the operator can be seated in a chair or stool. The system might be designed with a height adjustable stand. This feature allows for the height differences of multiple operators.

When manipulating products in drums, intermediate bulk containers or in sizes or weights that are not manageable, mechanical assistance might be required. Again, check with the companies' Health and Safety department for lifting restrictions. When using a bag-out system for drums, the drum lift may not only be required to lift the drum, but it might also be required to tilt and advance it forward.

Other operations that require access to the external surfaces of the enclosure are routine maintenance and service. Maintenance operations could include cleaning, changing filters, and changing lights. Platform designs need to consider the maintenance as well as the operation of the unit.

VISIBILITY

Visibility within the enclosure is critical for quality operation and cleaning. Locations of windows should be carefully thought out in the design phase and confirmed in the mock-up phase.

At the mock-up review, altering windows sizes, shapes, and positions are more common occurrences. The system design evaluation team should always consider modifying the windows during the mock-up review. The time required is well spent to confirm that the operator can observe the process properly.

Lighting is another key to the visibility within an enclosure. Foot candle or lumen specifications within a stainless steel system need to be thoroughly considered. There is extensive reflection of light off the stainless steel. This reflection of light can reduce the foot candle values required and may need to be redirected to avoid interfering with the operator's sight.

If external lighting is insufficient, consider spot lights mounted through sanitary fitting at specific locations or "goose neck" fixtures that can be swung out of the way when not in use.

One visibility issue that is often overlooked is where the controls are located. The control display, switches, buttons, etc. should be a mock-up review agenda item. Local codes need to be reviewed for the locations. Many designs have the controls mounted above or below the chamber. Depending on the design and application, the best position will need to be determined. Another option to improve the visibility of the controls or display is to place them in a "swing arm". The swing arm permits, the controls and display to be moved into a good viewing position when necessary and out of the way when not in use.

CLEANING REQUIREMENTS

Chapter 6– (Cleaning Requirements section) provides for specific design considerations. When evaluating the application, understanding the cleaning requirements can be equally important to the process requirements. During the design and mock-up phases, it is important to review this part of the application.

In some cases, product contact components cannot be cleaned thoroughly inside the enclosure and therefore must be removed. How these items are prepared and removed must be determined. Can they be cleaned and bagged well enough to be removed?

In some cases where reaching is an issue, an automated cleaning system (spray nozzles, etc.) can be designed into the system.

The cleaning process should be written and simulated by the operators during the mock-up review. The actual cleaning tools such as vacuum and spray wands, wipes and brushes, should be provided for evaluation during the mock-up review. This will help confirm that the process can be accomplished within the enclosure.

Just as important as confirming the ability to conduct the intended process is the ability to clean the internal surfaces and equipment.

UTILITIES

During the ergonomic design and mock-up evaluation, a thorough review of external utility connections and internal operator access to those utilities is needed. For example, if the operator is required to make or break a quick disconnect to a liquid or gas line internally, the location and accessibility must be evaluated on the mock-up. For facility planning and maintenance, a review of the external utility connections should be conducted on the design and possibly the mock-up.

WASTE DISPOSAL

For waste disposal the position and access of bag-out ports and waste dump chutes should be considered during the design.

From a perspective of reaching out, the ease of access by the operators disposing of waste, as well as the position of the waste-out port and access must be ensured so as not to interfere or restrict the internally arranged equipment. Having a thorough understanding of the positions of equipment and containers within the unit at the design and mock-up stage will help position and more adequately size the waste disposal chute. The waste chute can often provide allowance for bagging out equipment for either remote cleaning or incineration, hence the size and position of the chute needs to be reviewed carefully.

SUPPORT ANCILLARIES

Support ancillaries typically include scoops for weighing and dispensing, sample thieves, croupier sticks, tongs, shelves, beakers, flasks, trays, etc. They also include stainless steel hoppers or funnels, o-rings, cable ties, cable tie hand tools, cable cutters, and shelves. The specification of those items and their availability is beneficial when conducting the ergonomic study during the design and mock-up phase. During this evaluation, it is important to explain to the operators why and how these types of support ancillary equipment are used.

SAMPLING

Just as with any of the equipment interfaces, to safely obtain samples in a contained manner the ergonomics of the design require due consideration. Not just access to and viewing of the sample, but also the storage and marking of sample jars and containers within the containment environment. This may require alteration of the shape and size to build in sampling capability. However as sampling and sample removal is typically an intrinsic part of the containment process, consideration in terms of ergonomic access and safe sample removal needs to be addressed during design.

MOCK-UP

For custom-designed installations it is highly recommended to conduct a mock-up evaluation before finalizing the specification and design. Depending on the complexity of the design, a mock-up can range in price from US $3000 to $25,000. They are typically constructed of wood, plastic, steel tubing, acrylic, or foam board. In rare instances, they may need to be fabricated of metal or painted because of restrictions of bringing exposed wood into a facility. The process of building a mock-up starts with the user requirement specification and concept drawing. After a thorough review and approval between the end user and supplier, fabrication of the mock-ups can proceed. As part of the mock-up process, it should be determined if actual components or equipment are available to be integrated into the mock-up. Examples would be process equipment such as a mill, granulator, sieve, blender, stir plate, oven, freezer, refrigerator, tank or vessel, pumps, filling machine, lyophilizer door, conveying systems, lyophilizer loading systems, accumulator tables, etc. Other smaller equipment/utensil components could include a balance, shelf, sample thief, beaker, flask, scoop, tongs, plastic bags, and anything else that may be a required part of the process. If any of these items are not available for integration into the mock-up, they should be fabricated, as best possible, to simulate their size and weight. Before fabricating these items, the supplier should understand how they operate and what items may need to be accessed while in containment. This applies to both the operation and cleaning of these items.

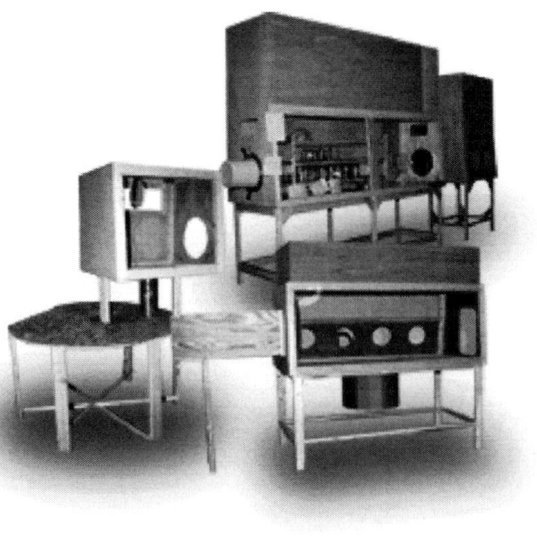

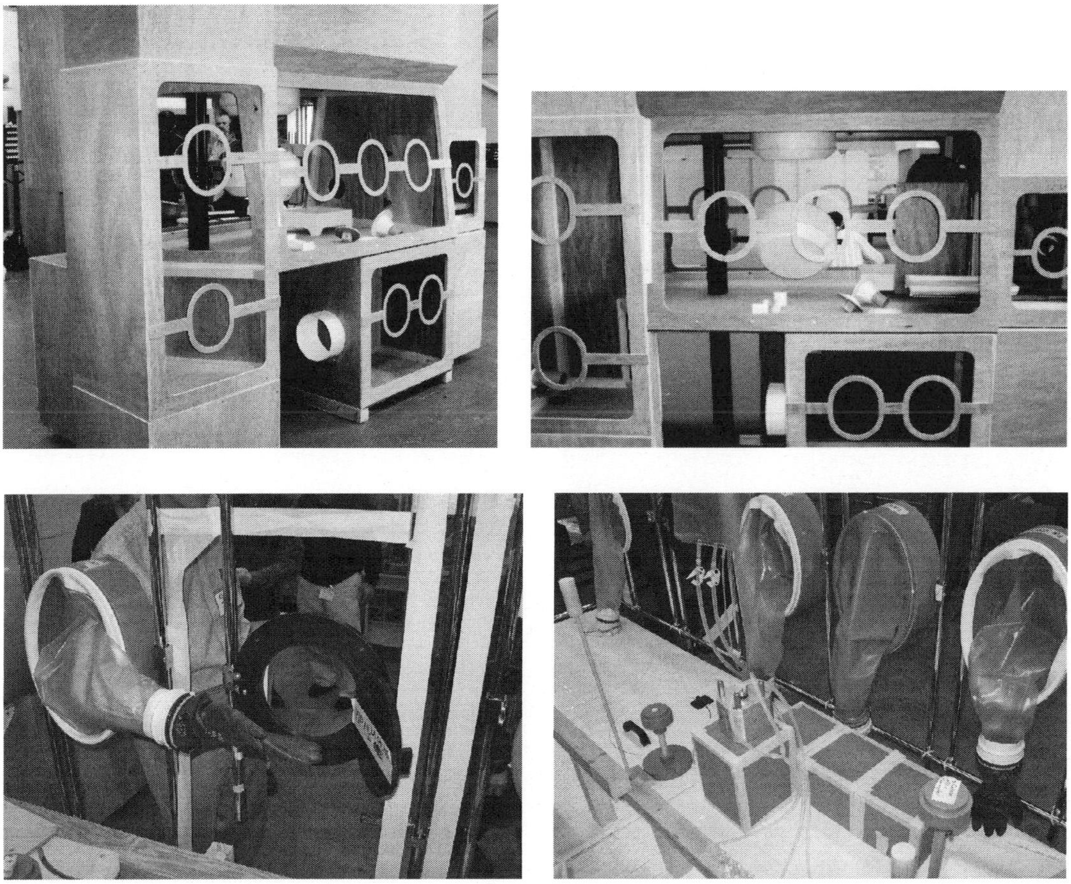

The mock-up of the physical system is built to the dimensions specified on the concept drawing. It should include all windows, gloveports, doors, transfer ports (RTP, containment valve, bag-out port), and air locks. Those components should all be located as specified on the concept drawing. Lights, controls, maintenance items, and platforms that require access on the exterior should also be incorporated into the mock-up and review.

As part of the mock-up process, it is necessary to determine where the evaluation will take place and who should participate. The location can be at the enclosure supplier, an associate equipment vendor, or at the customer's site. The attendees should include the supplier's project manager, the customer's project manager, at least one person from operations, and possibly a representative from validation, quality assurance, and health and safety departments. Having the actual operators evaluate the mock-up is a key to getting them comfortable with the use of the system. It gives them the opportunity to participate in the design and take ownership of it when it is installed. Participation by quality assurance and health and safety staff can help to underline the benefits of protecting the operators and the product.

When planning for a mock-up evaluation, the enclosure supplier should prepare a detailed agenda. The agenda should include a description of the purpose and operation of the isolator itself. It should also review the process being conducted. This process may be brand new or an enclosed adaptation of a process that the operators are already familiar with.

If handling powders or liquids within the enclosure, simulate those items with a placebo. Review the operators reach to all required components inside the system, such as fittings, ports, doors and shelves. Evaluate the visibility within the enclosure. It may be necessary to look into a vessel or tank and doing this may require extra lighting or a mirror. Review the disassembly and cleaning of all integrated equipment. Remember, the purpose of the system is to contain the process and cleaning of the integrated equipment ad components.

During the mock-up study, adjustments to the mock-up can be made such as moving or adding a gloveport or fitting to improve operator comfort. Once those changes are found acceptable, they can be noted on the concept drawing.

During the evaluation, it is important to record the results, both positive and negative. If negative comments are reported, a corrective action should be suggested. The copy of the system concept drawing marked with any changes is a major a part of the mock-up evaluation report. From that report, specification and drawing changes can be made and appropriate adjustments made to the scope of the project.

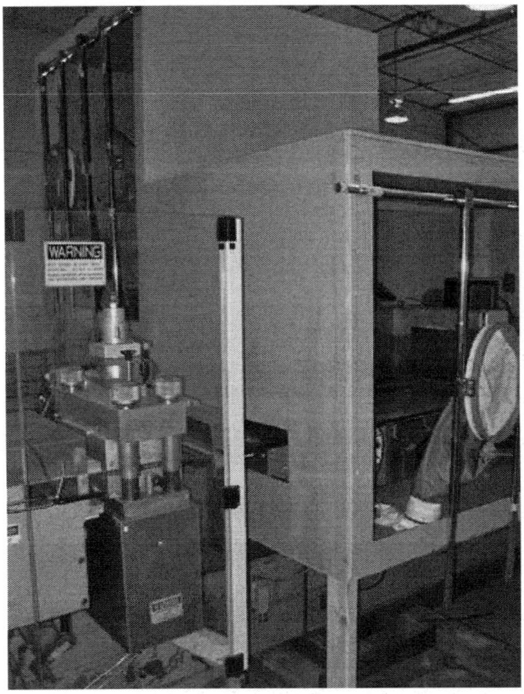

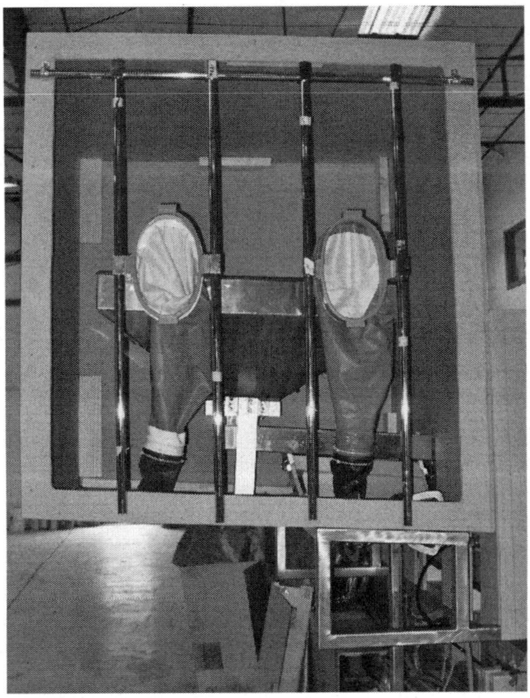

It cannot be understated that ergonomics is a critical consideration in the design of a custom design. Understanding the application of the system from the beginning to end of the process will help considerably with that ergonomic analysis. This analysis should be done by conceptual designs and mock-ups prior to finalizing the design of the system. The system needs to be designed for both operational requirements and for maintenance and cleaning. Whatever process is being enclosed, the supplier of the equipment must be part of the team to explain the maintenance and cleaning requirements if not already thoroughly understood.

6 Design and engineering—containment applications

Brian Smith and David Pallister

DESIGN AND ENGINEERING—CONTAINMENT APPLICATIONS

This chapter describes key points to consider in the design and engineering of a containment isolator. It specifically discusses considerations for the product such as operator exposure limits (OEL), the scale of the operation, process flow, dedicated or multiproduct use, dedicated or multipurpose use, sizes of the containers, quantities being transferred, the method of transfer, weighing requirements, the effect on materials of construction, the hazard classification (need for inert purging), cleaning requirements, and the method of sampling.

Considerations for equipment are also reviewed for specific applications and interfaces. Additional details of the containment systems are outlined for ventilation requirements, materials of construction, ergonomics, lighting, controls, monitoring and date acquisition, factory and site acceptance testing, and validation. It is also pointed out that consideration of the facility is important in regards to the installed location, the electrical hazard classification of the location, utilities available, waste disposal, and any support ancillaries.

On the basis of these topics, you will see there is much to consider for the design and engineering of custom containment isolators.

APPLICATIONS

With the development of more potent drugs that require aseptic processing, it is necessary to look at the entire drug manufacturing process. Numerous drugs contain potent ingredients that need to be formulated into the end product. Because of these processes, there are many applications for isolation technology in the containment arena. Each individual application needs to be considered in detail to assess the specific issues that impact the design of the isolator. Every application will have its own unique challenges in regard to the design of the isolator including such aspects as: ergonomic orientation, physical space constraints, and area electrical class. Listed below are some typical containment isolator examples and references to some of the key considerations to be made for each type.

- *Weigh/dispense*: Weighing ranges required and specifically methods for moving containers "in and out" of the isolator.
- *Charging* (vessel/process): Isolator interface with equipment and area electrical classification.
- *Formulation*: Quantities, accuracy and batch liquids
- *Process off-loading* (from dryer, etc.): Height constraints and volume/weight of off-loaded materials
- Tray dryer interface: Access requirements for tray 'reach' and dryer door design.
- *Milling*: Mill equipment size and output/loading method.
- *Compounding*: Vessel size and volume.
- *Filling*: Dispensing of sterile potent materials into containers (vials, ampoules, syringes, etc.)

The above-mentioned examples are by no means exhaustive and every application differs in complexity especially across the scale of operation. Production scale often has the benefit of fixed sizes and dimensions; however, the containers being handled can be quite large affecting ergonomics, where on a laboratory or development scale, flexibility is the key with smaller volumes usually being accommodated.

A thorough review of each application is required before embarking on a specific isolator design. In particular, undertaking mock-ups (see Ergonomics in Design section) will be essential to prove reach, integration, and accessibility as described is achieved.

OCCUPATIONAL EXPOSURE LIMITS

Another component that must be addressed at the design stage is the OELs of the compounds being handled or processed. Referring back to the application section, achievable OEL performance (containment performance) from any particular isolator operation is dependant on a number of factors that need to be considered during the isolator design.

1. Scale or quantities of material being processed could mean there is a greater risk of exposure during any given process operation when more potent materials are being handled in and around the isolator.
2. Material density and its tendency to become airborne as well as the degree of dust in a dry powder handling application calls for greater consideration to ensure ventilation is effective enough to handle potential exposure.
3. Duration of operation much like the scale of operation as well as a greater period of time exposed to potent materials accounts for greater exposure risk to the operator.

The above factors in along with the more physical design attributes of the isolator need to be considered during the engineering and design phase of the project.

These considerations will provide a basic assessment of the capabilities of any isolator design even before the potent material OEL is considered.

To summarize this section a low OEL potent material being handled in small quantities in a sampling application will have much less exposure risk to the operator than a less potent material being handled in kilogram quantities during dispensing and/or reactor charging. The application and material quantities significantly affect the achievable OELs for any given isolator system design.

EQUIPMENT/INTERFACE (RETROFIT VERSUS NEW)

Equipment/interface must also be considered when evaluating an application for containment. A key factor is whether the equipment being contained is new or existing. Once determined, each scenario has its own unique areas to address.

For new equipment it is important to identify the exact make and model of equipment being contained. It is best if the isolator manufacturer can contact that equipment vendor to determine if this equipment has been designed for containment or whether minor modifications can be made prior to that equipment's factory acceptance test (FAT).

For new equipment, common changes to standard practice are to relocate the controls, change fasteners to thumb screws or wing nuts, and generally remove any sharp edges that can cut the isolator gloves. The isolator needs to provide ventilation for safety and also to provide a physical barrier. Because of this physical barrier, some equipment shrouds can be considered for removal. Part of this consideration would be to install gloveports that can be locked out. Locking out gloveports can be done by various methods such as light curtains, interlocked covers or keyed lanyards. These methods of locking out the gloveports are electrically interlocked to the equipment so that if the lockout feature is tripped the machine will turn off.

Another key item to evaluate is if the equipment being isolated is leak tight if partially mounted inside the isolator. In some cases, the motor of a mill, mixer, or other rotating pieces of equipment is mounted outside the isolator. In those instances, a shaft seal will be required, by either the equipment vendor or the isolator vendor to prevent the escape of materials around the shaft. In other instances, equipment may be built with its own table top and the isolator is designed to sit on top of that table. The equipment vendor would be required to ensure that all table top penetrations are leak tight to isolator standards.

Often times with new equipment these evaluations and solutions can be worked out at both the equipment and isolator vendor's factory prior to factory acceptance testing. Usually with new equipment, it is standard practice to have it delivered to the isolator vendor for integration and testing, although, the isolator can be delivered and integrated at the process equipment supplier or even at the customer site.

For the retrofit of existing equipment, there are similar challenges along with others that are unique to a retrofit. Obviously, before receiving an order to contain an existing piece of equipment, there will be some field evaluation and concept presented to the customer by the isolator vendor. First and foremost to consider is can the equipment to be contained be delivered to the isolator vendor? If it can, determine if and when the customer can take this equipment out of service and for how long.

For the equipment that can be delivered to the isolator vendor, it is usually the isolator vendor who will make modifications (with the equipment vendor's approval) for containment. Again these could be, but are not limited to, relocating controls, lengthening cables, adding shaft seals, adding gaskets, changing hardware to glove-friendly type, etc. In some instances safety interlocks may be added or removed, depending on their purpose in a contained environment.

Certainly, some pieces of equipment cannot be taken out of service, due to either manufacturing requirements or sheer size constraints. For equipment that cannot be sent to the isolator vendor, allowances in both time and money should be made. Field integration is much more difficult and costly than doing this at the isolator vendor's factory. It should also be noted that for equipment returned to an isolator vendor, the customer will be required to certify that the equipment is validated clean and safe to work on.

Ultimately it is best for the customer, equipment, and isolator vendors to work together early and often in a containment project. That way expectations and responsibilities are clearly quickly conveyed to each other.

SCALE OF OPERATION

Careful consideration must be given with regard to the scale of operation. The greater the quantity of material being handled and processed within the isolator needs to be assessed in accordance with the items presented below.

Larger quantities of material will result in the following:

- Greater ergonomic considerations and the possible use of drum or container manipulators.
- Increased exposure potential to the operators and environment.
- Cleaning requirements will increase.
- Increased heating, ventilation, air conditioning (HVAC) requirements (HEPA filter changing, increased air volumes).
- Increased physical size of the isolator.
- Increased frequency of operator working at the isolator.
- Greater potential for operator fatigue.

Minimizing the quantities handled within the isolator may not always be practical in consideration of the above mentioned, depending on the process; however, being aware of the physical scale of the operation is a necessary step during the engineering design and ergonomic development phase of the project.

The typical small- to large-scale operations can be classified very basically into the following categories;

- *Lab scale*: Where material may be processed in smaller "gram" quantities.
- *Pilot/development/kilo scale*: Classified as medium "kilogram" quantities.
- *Bulk production*: Typically larger scale of operation, where the above bullet points on size and scale of operation need consideration during the design phase of the project.

Ergonomics, especially on the larger scale processes are important to address at the mock-up phase of the design to ensure maximum operating benefits and consideration of potential operator fatigue.

STANDARD OPERATING PROCEDURES/PRODUCT FLOW

Standard operating procedures (SOP) as well as product flow must be understood to aid in the design. All isolator design projects should commence with a thorough understanding of the product and process flow to achieve and develop the correct and most appropriate SOP for the application. SOPs will usually be defined in conjunction with the end user and isolator vendor, as both parties need involvement with this critical step.

The flow of the process will take step-by-step consideration of materials, containers, loading requirements, sampling requirements, equipment integration, process and original equipment manufacturer (OEM) items, ancillary support features, etc., to enable a thorough overview of the application steps to be understood. Upon completion of the process flow overview, the isolator design can commence, which will lead to the engineering mock-up. At the stage of the mock-up prior to any level of fabrication, an SOP should be developed. This SOP should cover aspects of operation, cleaning, and maintenance to ensure that containment is maintained during each part of the process flow. SOPs will also form and integral part of any factory acceptance tests as well as acceptance criteria when the equipment is finally to be accepted on site.

Process flow can very often be defined within a user requirement specification (URS); however, to establish a SOP during any design phase of an isolator project the steps within the process, from equipment set up to final cleaning need to be clearly defined.

INSTALLED LOCATION

The installed location of an isolator must be considered at an early stage in the design.

An isolator may have all of the best components, the most sophisticated features and be built of the highest quality, but if it does not fit in the room it is intended for, then it is useless to the owner.

An equally important design consideration is the room restrictions for the planned location. Although an isolator is often a small, classified area with ventilation and filtration requirements, the overall height is often overlooked. When designing an isolator the space required needs to be evaluated in three dimensions, length, width, and height.

The next most important dimensional consideration is the delivery path. The plan for delivering the isolator from a loading dock or point of delivery to the final installed locations needs to be reviewed for door openings, elevator restrictions, and sharp turns. This can be done electronically by inserting a plan view CAD file into an existing facility layout, but usually that confirms the fit for length and width. For more sophisticated projects a 3D model of the isolator can be moved through the 3D model of the building. In some instances the isolator can be disassembled prior to shipment to a point that may better suit the delivery restrictions. Other ways to get the isolator into its final location may be through hatches in the ceiling or roof or through windows.

If it is determined at the beginning of the design that the isolator will not be able to travel from the point of delivery to the final location, it may be possible to build the isolator in sections. If that is a possible solution, the re-assembly of those sections needs to be planned and designed. In some instances, flanged sections bolted together may be acceptable. In other cases, field welding the sections together may be required. Understanding the challenges of delivering an isolator is important for financial planning and scheduling.

Dedicated/Multiproduct

Determining whether the isolator will be used for a specific product or multiple products will have an affect on the design. Isolators can be designed for a dedicated product or for multiuse with different products. When designing an isolator for a dedicated product, you may not need to supply or have different components that are in contact with the product. Some of these components could include scoops, beakers, containers, bags, etc. An isolator may have a mill, sieve, or granulator integrated into it and may need different screen sizes. Consideration should be given for cleaning between products if extra change parts or components are required for different products, as cross contamination is always a concern. If components need to be introduced into a contaminated isolator, the method and space required for those items needs to be provided.

In some instances, the basic use of an isolator changes slightly for different products. For example, a weighing and dispensing isolator will most likely be used for numerous products. But those products might come in different bulk containers and may need to be dispensed in different amounts in different containers or bags. In this instance, the balance and the entry and exits ports need to be specified properly. Again, cleaning of the different products must be determined prior to the final configuration of the isolator. If different cleaning solutions are required, specific materials of construction for some components may be required. Obviously, if the isolator were dedicated to a specific product, the design would be less complicated but may not be practical. One of the benefits of isolation technology is the flexibility, as long as its intended uses are thought of well in advance of fabrication.

Dedicated/Multipurpose

Another consideration is an isolator that is dedicated to one purpose or process or one that may have multiple processes in it. Some isolators are designed for a small laboratory or production line. In these instances, laboratory or pilot-scale pieces of process equipment may be installed in a single isolator. For example, an analytical balance, small mill, and blender may be best put into one isolator. The advantage of a design like this would be to minimize the product transfers and to minimize the cleaning.

In some instances, a basic isolator may be required and different pieces of equipment used at different times. If that is required, consideration needs to be given on how the different pieces of equipment are brought into and taken from the isolator and where those items are stored when not in use.

Again, if each isolator were dedicated to a specific process, the design would be less complicated but that may not use the flexibility of isolation technology.

CONTAINER SIZES

An understanding of all of the "containers" to be used in conjunction with the containment process needs to be thoroughly considered during the isolator design activities. "Container" sizing and type affects ergonomics, materials handling requirements, space considerations for access, and overall isolator dimensions.

By "containers" we mean the following

- *Raw material drums/bags entering the isolator.* [Load in original container or via rapid transfer port (RTP).]. For RTP, see "Transfer Systems" section.
- *Sampling containers.* Specific sampling bottle sizes.
- *Receiving or exiting containers.* In a dispensary application, what are the containers and sizes of the containers being dispensed into?
- Sizes of any internal weighing 'boats' need to be considered.
- Filled vials, ampoules, syringes, cartages, etc. and the quantity be processed at one time.

A thorough understanding of the above will highlight the need for drum tippers in the case of material loading and also the ergonomics for each isolator dependant on the sizes of the compound containers being handled.

As isolators by their very nature reduce the amount of reach and movement around the product containers, to effectively enter raw material drums into the isolator to a position accessible by the operator, while still maintaining high levels of containment, manipulators may be required provide drum-handling capabilities for the materials being loaded. These drum manipulators can be mounted within the loading chamber or external to the isolator.

In applications where product is being subdivided from larger volumes and packed off into smaller volumes in a continuous liner, the size of the receiving container in the first instance dictates the elevations and space available for the incorporation of a suitable isolator.

Containers, the product liner sizes, volumes, and dimensions should also be considered in conjunction as even in the most ideal design circumstances, the raw material container or exit container should not be physically within the isolator to minimize surface contamination and cleaning requirements before removal. Therefore, in some cases the liners or bags containing product only will enter the isolator work area.

QUANTITIES OF TRANSFER

In conjunction with the container type, size, and product liner dimensions and also relating back to the achievable containment performance from the application versus isolator design, we need to ascertain an understanding of the quantities of the materials being handled or processed inside the isolator. This should highlight the weight and volume of the potent compound as well as the frequency of transfer, that is, production scale, laboratory scale, development batches, etc.

For example in a product off-loading application from a filter dryer, the batch quantity of the filter dryer should be ascertained to establish the amount of drums or containers to be filled from the dryer discharge nozzle. The reason that this is important is from a make–break standpoint. If multiple drums are to be filled and as such the make and break frequency is high, then the potential for exposure is increased if compared to the filling of one container only.

Similarly on the loading side of an isolator, if multiple containers are to be loaded as a part of a batch operation, the efficiency of the loading method needs to be carefully reviewed as again, multiple make and break connections if not mechanically controlled can lead to exposure.

Smaller laboratory-scale quantities or even simply reducing the container sizes to ease the method of loading the isolator will lead to improved exposure control and ergonomic considerations.

From an ergonomic perspective, minimizing the weight and volume of the product being handled is also an important consideration, which should be reviewed at mock-up stage of the design process. Some product volumes simply cannot be handled within a standard isolator arrangement in a single container due to size and ergonomic constraints; however, with modifications to the orientation of docking and using gravity where possible, these design obstacles can often be overcome.

TRANSFER SYSTEMS

In regard to transfer systems, most containment applications require that a potent product be transferred through or in/out of the isolator. There are various methods and devices available to accomplish these tasks. Some factors to consider when evaluating a containment application are target OEL for the product, type of product be transferred (liquid, powder, slurry, etc.), available space, quantity of product, previous or subsequent process step, and cost.

In today's market, it is believed that the RTP provides the highest level of containment. The basic concept of this device is that there are two ports (alpha/active and beta/passive) that dock together. Each port consists of a flange, a door or cell, and a gasket. Typically the alpha/active port mounts to the isolator and the beta/passive mounts to a container, bag, tube, vessel, or adjoining isolator. When the two ports are connected together, the two doors/cells and gaskets form a sandwich that can be swung open into the isolator. The gaskets prevent potent products from contacting the area in the middle of the sandwich of door/cell of the RTP and therefore provide the containment when disconnecting the ports at the end of the process.

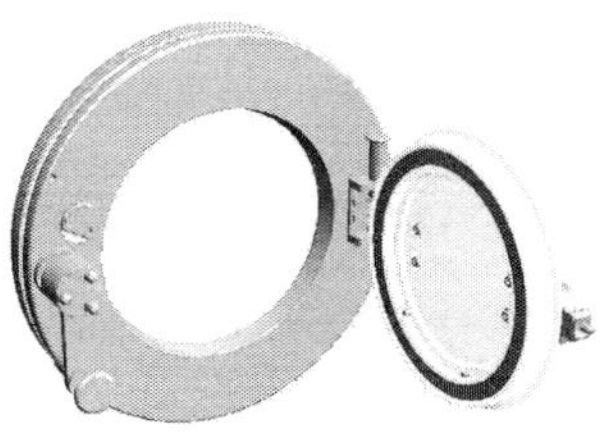

Alpha RTP with Door Open

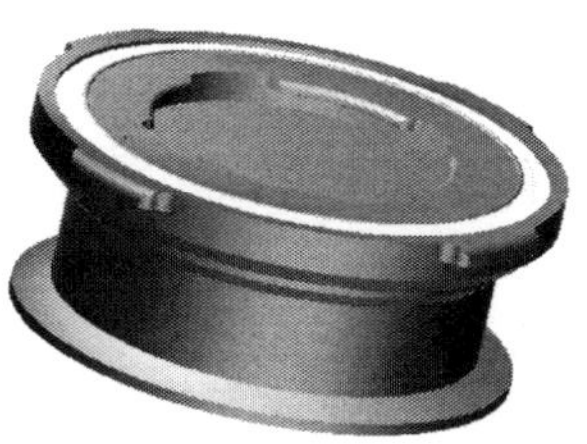

Beta Flange to Tri-clover Fitting

The RTP comes in various sizes ranging between nominally 4 to 13 inches in diameter. Their components are typically made of 316L stainless steel, polyethylene, polypropylene, silicone, and PVC. One important feature to consider is the lockout option. This feature prevents opening the alpha/active RTP when the mating beta port is not connected and it also prevents disconnecting the beta/passive port if the alpha/active is not properly closed. It is also recommended that when moving open products between the connected RTP, an adapter be locked in place. This adapter will protect the RTP gaskets from being directly contacted with the products.

There are other options available for the operation of the RTP, some of which include automatic docking, beta/passive port rotating, and alpha/active port rotating. The price of the RTP transfer systems is commensurate with their high level of containment.

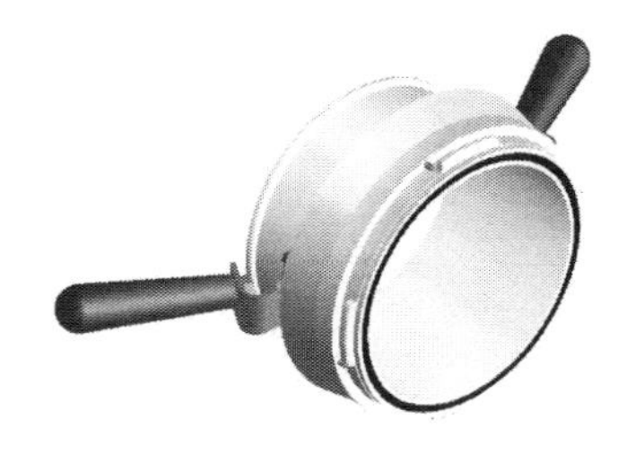

Inside Bagging Ring—for use when transferring powders through an open RTP

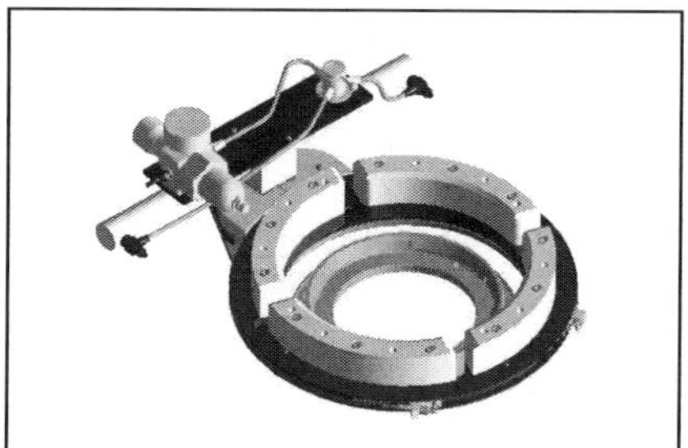

Beta Power Rotate Assembly—used for automatically docking a Beta Container to an Alpha Flange

Another type of transfer system is commonly known as the split butterfly valve (SBV) or high containment valve. Again, the basic theory behind this technology is that the valve consists of two halves, an active and passive. Each half has a flange that can be mounted to a mating flange (bolted or sanitary type are typical). In this type valve, the butterfly is actually made in two parts with a gasket on each half. When the valve is in the closed position, the valve can be disconnected. One half of the butterfly travels with the passive section and one half stays with the active half. With split butterfly valves, the active half usually is mounted on the most stationary piece of equipment (isolator, reactor, tablet press, mill, etc.). The passive half is mounted on the more mobile piece of equipment (intermediate bulk container [IBC], tote, mobile vessel, etc.). Some features of the SBV include a compensator for docking allowances, pneumatic or electric actuation, vacuum or air purge of the sealing surfaces during disconnect, integrated wash in place (WIP) system, and programmable logic controller (PLC) controls.

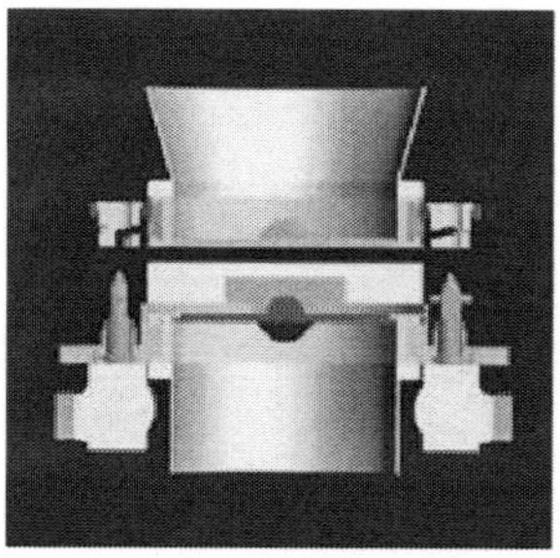

Undocked

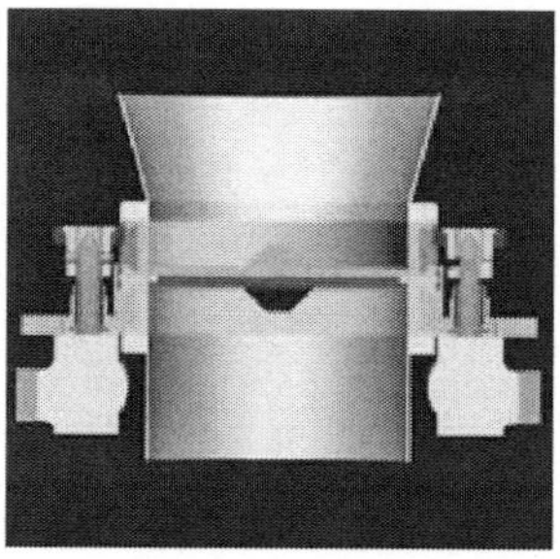

Docked and locked

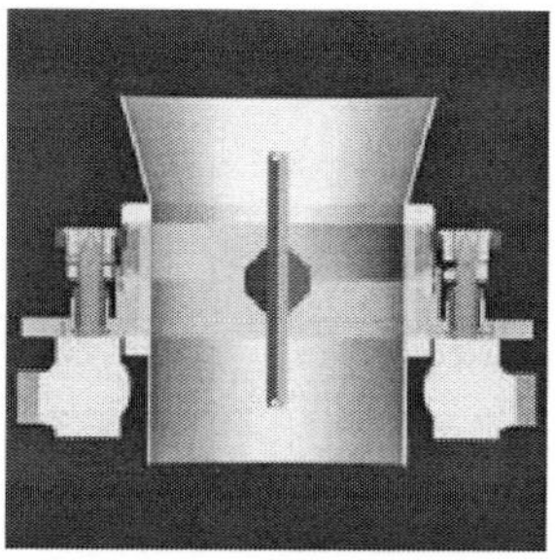

Docked, locked, and opened

One of the most cost-effective ways of transferring products into or out of an isolator is the bagging method or bag-in/bag-out transfer. This method is a more manual way of transferring than the devices already described, but the hardware costs are minimal. The basic concept is to have a flange with two ribs or grooves on the outside of an isolator. Typically, but not always, this port will have a sealed door on the inside of the isolator. In some designs the port may also have two ribs or grooves on an internal flange. This is used when double or triple bagging of the product is required. The size of the port will need to be determined by the maximum size of product or items that need to pass through. The bag that attaches to the port can be of any length, but of weight of material and stress on the bag should be considered.

The following diagram shows the steps of the bagging transfer method:

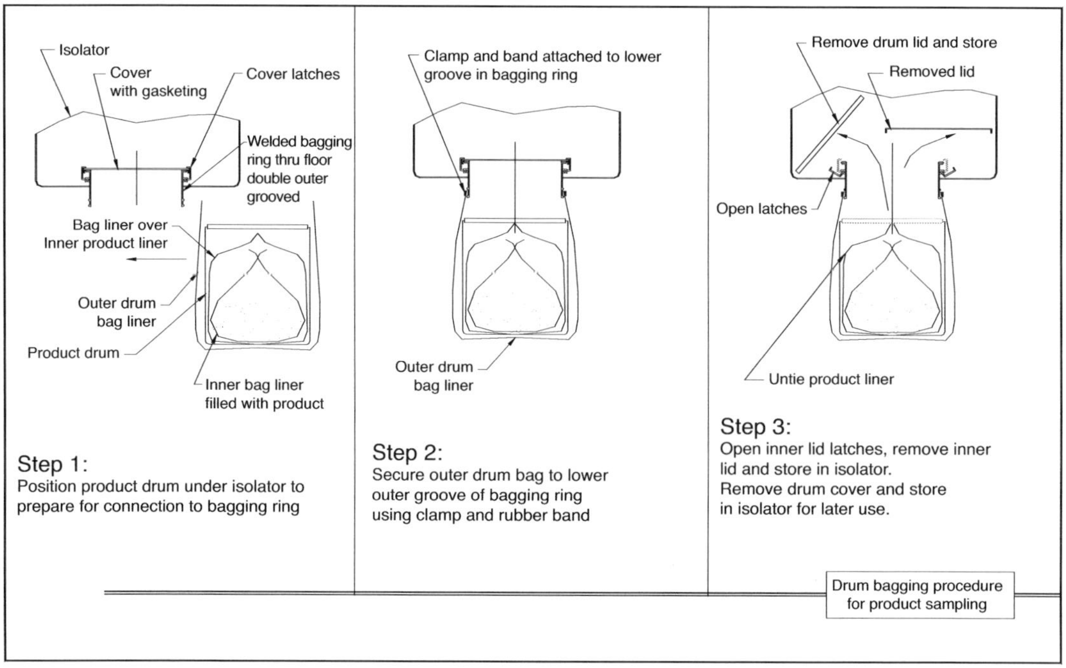

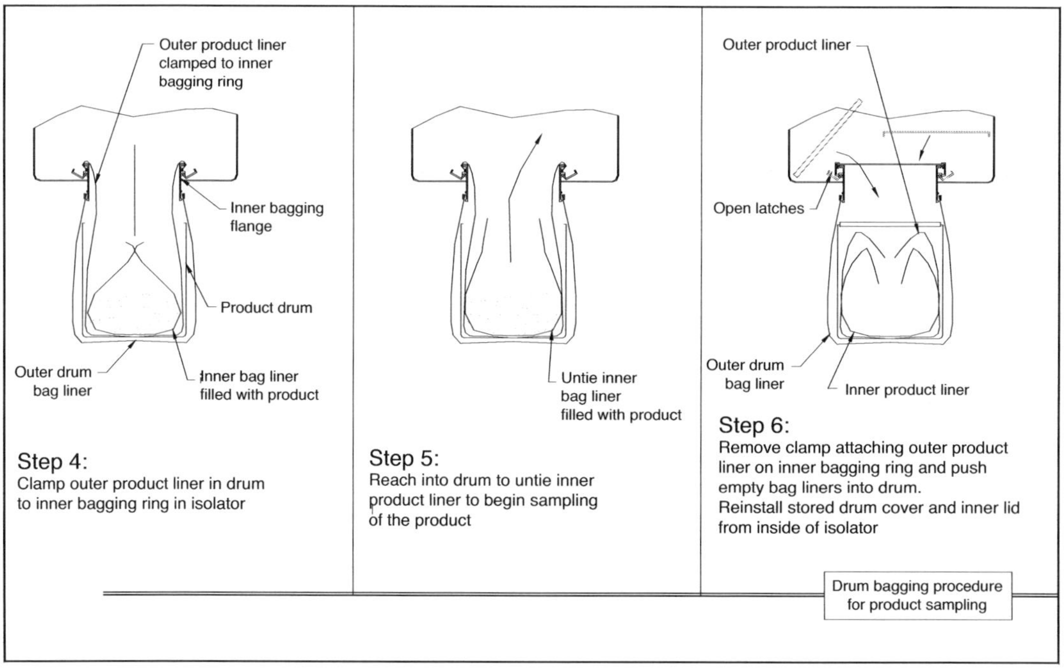

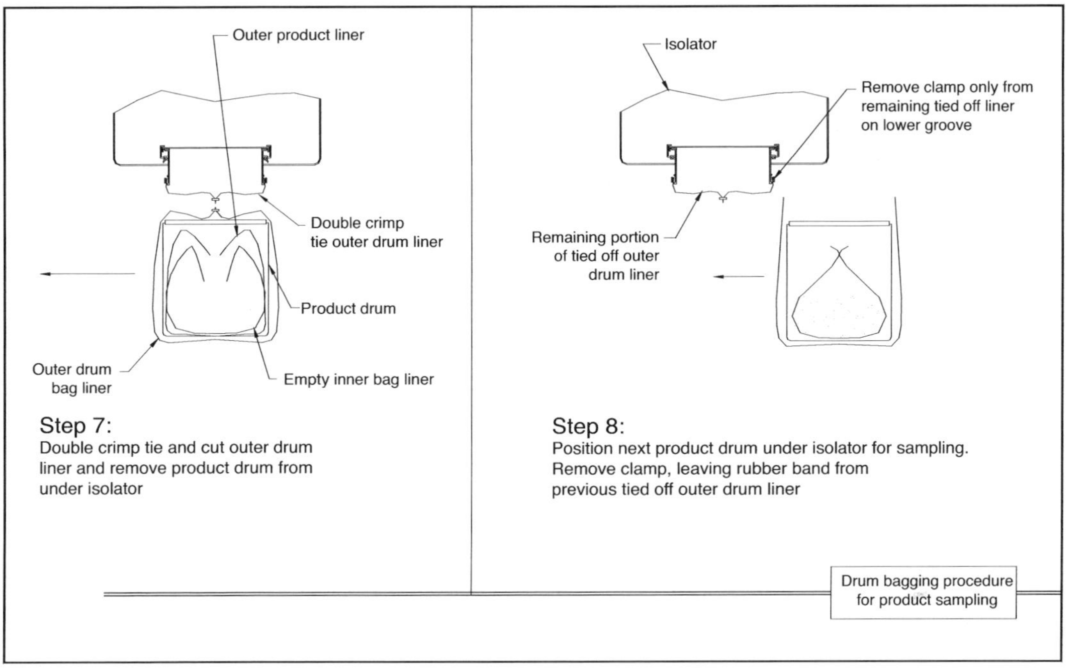

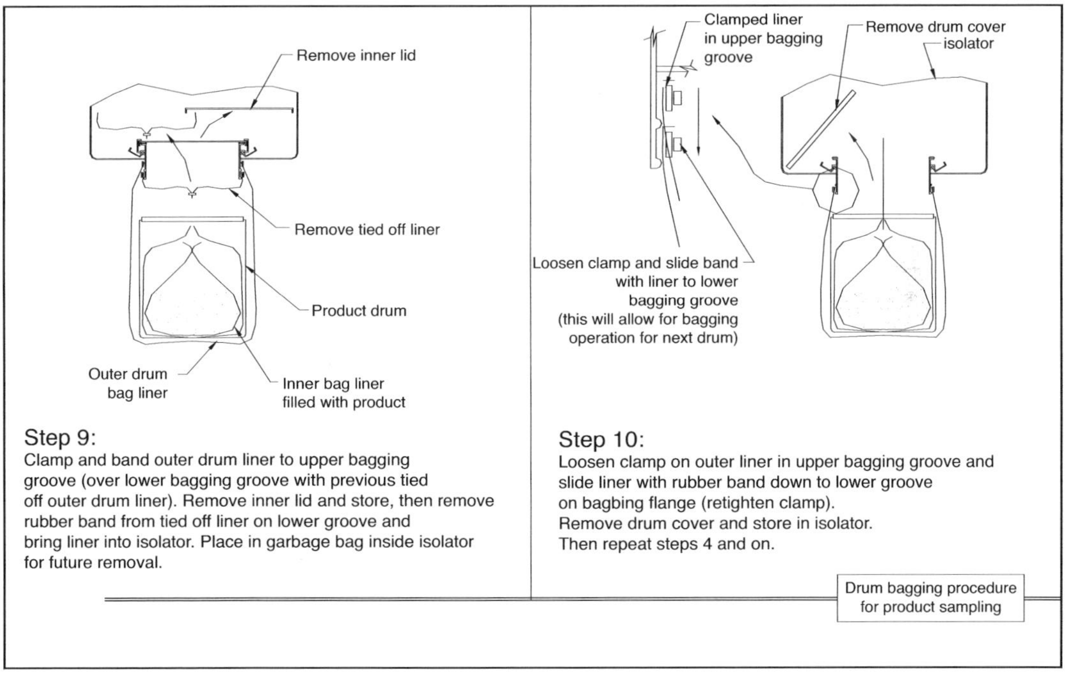

Note that when cutting the bagged product from the bagging port by the "umbilical style," the tighter the umbilical the better. The use of a banding clamp and associated tool can improve the security of the operation.

A similar method, but more automatic type, is the use of a drum-charging head or pack-off systems. These systems can be used for charging of powders into unlined or lined containers or with continuous liner system. They would be designed for the attachment to the underside of a piece of process equipment. They can be placed inside or outside the isolator depending on the containment level required. Various styles of seals are available, outward inflatable, downward inflatable, compression style, and molded versions. Again, depending on the containment level required the bag or liner can be simply clamp onto the discharge head or detached by means of the umbilical style.

The most basic type of transfer is the air lock system. This system is a chamber that is mounted to the isolator with doors on each end. The air lock can be made of any size and shape and can include numerous features. Some of those features include windows, gloveports, negative pressure control, humidity control, WIP systems, vaporized hydrogen peroxide systems (for aseptic decontamination of materials being transferred), drains, and door interlocks. These are typically used for entering product into an isolator that is in use. With the air lock door in the isolator closed, an operator would open the outside airlock door. The operator would then place the item to be transferred into the airlock and shut the outside door. The operator could then open the door in the isolator and transfer the item into the isolator. Once this procedure has been done it is important to know that the airlock must be considered that it is contaminated. Before the outside door on the air lock can be opened again, the interior of the airlock and any items transferred from the isolator must be cleaned.

WEIGHING REQUIREMENTS

Weighing requirements are a significant part of the detailed design of the system.

When weighing is to take place as part of a contained process, various aspects of the weighing steps are to be identified as follows: It would also be beneficial to involve an appropriate weighing system supplier for compatibility of the various specifications listed by the customer in the URS.

- Assessment of scale capacity, tare weight, and accuracy should be checked with the relevant scale vendors as some scale platforms and indicators are only compatible within certain conditions.
- Is weighing control of product feed required (i.e., outputs from scale) in the form of a set-point? If so, need to ensure communication method and safe area positioning.
- Can the weigh scale platform be positioned outside of the isolator and the receiving container positioned on this external scale? If so, how is the connection to the isolator made to ensure containment and weighing accuracy? With the scale outside of the isolator, it minimizes the contamination potential and need for cleaning but the container connection is critical.
- Should the scale platform be positioned within the isolator, need to ensure that is has wash down capabilities for decontamination, especially in larger weighing applications.
- If not able to wash down in place, need to ensure that the scale can be removed from the isolator under containment (bagged out or similar) for remote cleaning and/or maintenance.
- Need to identify weighing range and tolerance including the tare weight of the container.
- Should the scale base, and/or scale indicator be positioned in an explosion proof environment, due to products handled either within the isolator or external room classification, need to ensure compatibility of the same. Also if this scenario applies, need to consider weighing tolerances and accuracy, as some scales cannot be supplied with wash down/explosion proof capability as well as precision weighing, due to the electronics of the scale base.
- Positioning of the weighing indicator is critical from an ergonomic perspective plus reach for tare control. A tare control that can be operated from a foot switch if of benefit.
- These weigh scale items (base and indicator) should be assessed for positioning at mock-up stage early in the design process.

VENTILATION REQUIREMENTS

The ventilation requirements for the isolator are fundamental in the design stage.

Typically, containment isolators will be designed for operation with a single-pass or once through dedicated ventilation system; however, recirculation with exhaust back to the room space via double HEPA filters is also a frequent consideration.

The ventilation systems are usually provided as a part of the isolator vendor's scope of supply and will feature a local skid or onboard (the isolator) mounted blower and control package suitably rated for the room electrical hazard classification.

The control package as a minimum will be provided with an automatic fan speed control system in the form of a variable frequency drive to ensure that the isolator design conditions (negative/positive pressure and air change rate) are maintained during the operation.

For powder applications, the exhaust fan system is typically sized to maintain a minimum of two to five air changes per hour within the working chamber of the isolator to minimize the "contaminated" air volume to be handled and also minimizes Nitrogen consumption should a low oxygen or dry environment be required for the specific nature of the materials being processed. The sizing of the fan is also designed around the gloveport sizing to ensure that in breach conditions, via the variable frequency drive and with the loss of pressure, the fan will draw at its maximum to generate an inflow through an open gloveport at a rate between 100 and 200 ft/min (0.5–1.0 m/sec). Again, this airflow specification needs to be clearly defined during the engineering phase of the isolator.

It is important to know if there is any airflow required for the equipment being isolated. For instance, is there an external vacuum source as part of stopper placement, the washing and drying of vials in an external vial washer and most importantly the airflow from the depyrogenation tunnel and mouseholes. If there is, the isolator's ventilation system will need to compensate for that "loss" or "gain" of air. This again is an example of thoroughly knowing what the process is and how the equipment functions.

Similarly, some designs of larger isolator systems where drums are introduced into a separate loading chamber, the inflow velocity at the open door is sized around 68 ft/min (0.3 m/sec) to generate an air in-draught when the loading compartment door is opened for additional safety. The sizing and capacity of the filters need to be considered when designing flow and overall airflow requirements, as filters will require safe change capabilities, especially on the exhaust side of the isolator system.

For true aseptic isolators that handle potent product the ventilation system typically operates in positive pressure. Potent particles are control by different pressure cascades. A tunnel can provide a buffer to the room or if there is a vial accumulator section this can be a lower pressure than the filling zone. The following diagram shows an example of the pressure cascade from filling to lyophilizer loading.

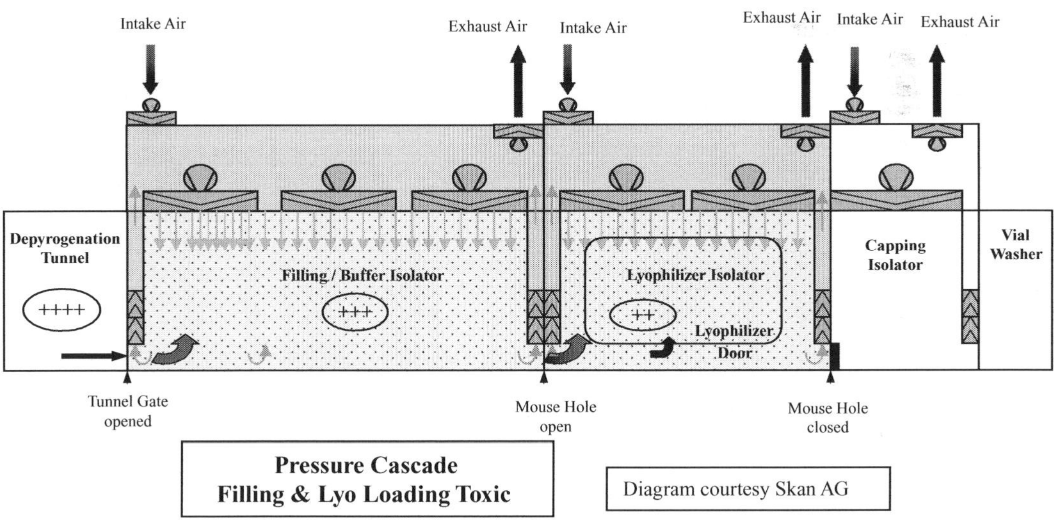

By designing a pressure cascade system, the system can safely contain the open filled vials. The major risk of exposure is postlyophilization and this can handled by switching the pressure in the lyophilizer-loading isolator from positive (during loading) to negative (during unloading). For potent filling the capper is placed in an isolator for containment purposes. The capping isolator operates in negative pressure airlock that operates at a greater negative pressure than the lyophilizer-unloading isolator. Typically after capping, the vials enter an external vial washer and this can also have a negative pressure ventilation system.

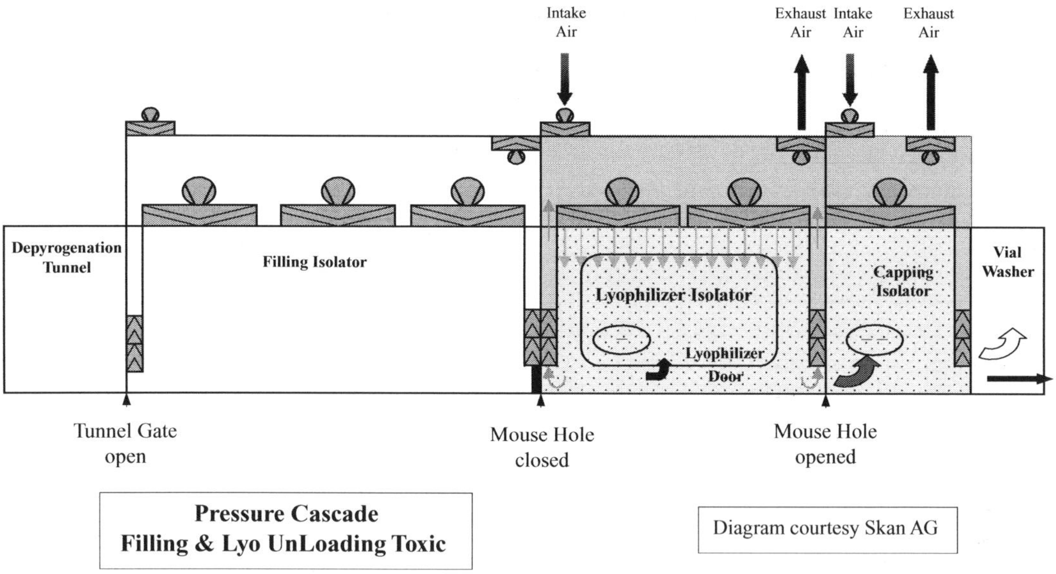

Safe change filtration can be either internally accessed HEPA filters located within the isolator and accessible for change via the gloveports (push–push HEPA filters or inline HEPAs for example) or bag-in/bag-out filter cells. The most recent filter is the FIBO® system (filter box). These are HEPA-filter quality and are designed for large air volumes. They are in a rigid plastic housing that can be changed without tools.

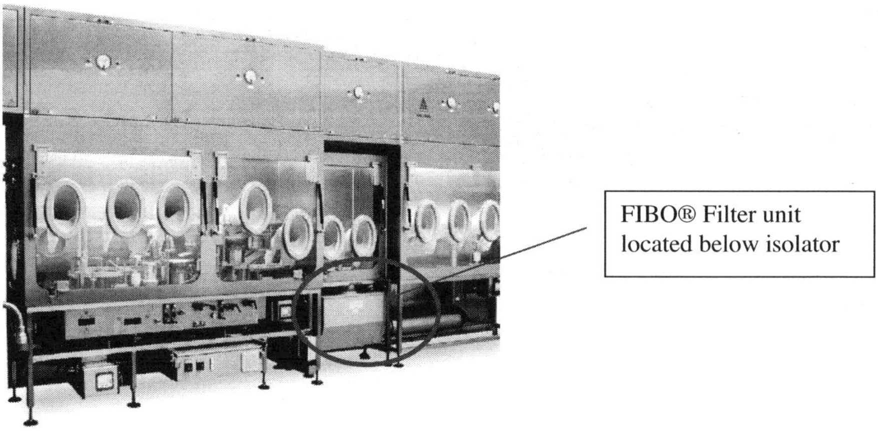

Larger scale isolators using larger material quantities may necessitate larger capacity filter cells in the form of bag-in/bag-out filtration. As the exhaust air may be more laden with particulate in these situations due to the volume of material being processed, a 93% prefilter is often installed prior to the HEPA to prolong its life.

In the case of nitrogen purge designs or isolators handling flammable materials either during operation or cleaning will have a dedicated once through ventilation system that will exhaust the contaminants via the exhaust filtration system to atmosphere.

MATERIALS

The type of potent materials being processed in the isolator, irrelevant of container sizes and physical quantities need to be evaluated for the design.

Some materials are skin sensitizers requiring consideration for maintenance of the filters (safe change—push–push or bag-in/bag-out styles) as well as specific methods of loading and unloading the isolator to ensure the operator does not become physically exposed to the material.

The compatibility of the gloves, window seals, and gaskets need to be considered when handling compounds containing solvents. Note that these components also need to be considered relevant to the cleaning materials used on the isolator, which may also relate back to the potent material type being processed. There may be no solvent in the potent material however solvents may be necessary to clean the material from the contact surfaces within the isolator.

Explosive materials may require low oxygen concentrations within the isolator (see "Nitrogen (Inert Gas) Purge" section) and similarly, purging with dry N_2 will also control internal conditions within the isolator allowing hydroscopic materials to be processed.

In all cases, knowledge of the specific features of the materials being handled within the Isolator is necessary to ensure effective isolator design accommodation.

CONSTRUCTION AND MATERIALS

With regard to construction and materials, isolators are typically fabricated of a stainless steel shell with a stainless steel stand and glass windows. Most often the shell is 316 L stainless steel polished to an internal finish of $\leq$22 Ra. In some cases, it is acceptable to construct the shell and stand of 304 or 304 L stainless steel.

When a highly corrosive product is being handled, parts of the isolator can be constructed of Hastelloy. Typically, only direct product contact components would be constructed of Hastelloy, due to the cost considerations.

Viewing panels or windows are constructed of glass (laminated safety or tempered) and of polycarbonate. Glass is specified most often, but when weight or breakage is a concern, polycarbonate is the usually the first option. The polycarbonate materials can be purchased with coatings to improve the scratch resistance or to dissipate the static electricity. They can also have ultraviolet (UV)-inhibiting characteristics. If UV light is a concern with glass, a film can be applied to reduce the UV light entering the isolator.

A wide range of elastomers can be used inside the isolator for seals, O-rings, bellows, or other flexible connections. Silicone, neoprene, EPDM, butyl, nitrile, and viton are just a few of the possible materials that can be used. Again, numerous plastics can be used, such as PVC, ABS, nylon, polyethylene, polypropylene, polyurethane, and teflon. Note that the use of nylon is not permitted in an isolator that has a vaporized hydrogen peroxide system and the use of all plastic should be minimized.

When selecting the materials of construction, it is important to evaluate the chemical compatibility of those materials with the products being processed and the agents being used to clean the isolator.

Ergonomics (Glove Location)

When designing an isolator it is important to make sure that the operator can perform all of the tasks that are required within the isolator. The operator can only do this if the ergonomics have been properly evaluated.

At a minimum, the gloveports should be located such that all internal equipment and doors can be reached. At best, the gloveports should be located so the operator can reach all surfaces of the interior. In some cases, this may not be possible due to restrictions incurred from the placement of the isolator in the room or from integrated equipment. If all surfaces cannot be reached with the gloves, hand held tools may be required for cleaning.

When evaluating the gloveport locations and isolator design, consider the process being performed. In some instances, it may be laboratory-type operations such as pouring liquids, measuring powders, and operating a test instrument. In other cases, operations may include moderate lifting, opening doors, operating valves, or changing parts on a piece of equipment. A thorough understanding of the process flow is required at the beginning of the design phase.

LIGHTING

In considering proper lighting to an isolator while challenging is crucial. In some applications, there is not much space available or the space available may not be in the best location. When designing an isolator, the area where the operator needs to work most frequently is where the lighting should be located or directed towards. In most cases, the best location is from the ceiling directly down on the work surface. Other options may be from the rear wall or from the end walls. Rarely, is it from the front window, as this could interfere with the operator unless a "gooseneck" fixture is used and can be swung out of the way when not in use.

Typically, the lights are mounted on the exterior of the isolator and shine through windows. This is done to keep the fixture out of the isolated environment, which reduces cleaning requirements within the isolator. Where hidden areas need to be illuminated, a handheld light stick can be hung inside the isolator. Typically, the power cord would pass through a compression fitting in the wall.

In most applications, fluorescent light fixtures are acceptable, but halogen or other types may be used because of space restrictions. When specifying light levels in foot-candles, consider that the light will be shining in a polished stainless steel chamber and there may be reflection/glare that will result. Special features that can be provided for lights are ratings for hazardous conditions, UV protection, and yellow filters for light-sensitive products.

Again, it is important to fully understand the processes within the isolator and the operator's vision requirements.

CONTROLS

Containment isolators can have a wide range of controls systems and features. Depending on the performance requirements of the isolator, the product being processed, the equipment being contained and the budget constraints, controls can vary from the truly manual to completely automated.

The most basic control system could have isolator pressure controlled by connecting the filtration system (usually HEPA) to either the room or dedicated exhaust. The pressure would be monitored by a magnehelic gauge and controlled by the positioning of manual valves on the inlet or outlet of the isolator. This system neither allows for variation in the exhaust airflow or pressure changes due to glove movement, nor does it allow for an increase in airflow through an open glove port in case of a "glove off" situation.

The next level of control would be one that is a single-loop control system. A standard system would contain a single-loop control to control pressure, manual valves, switches for phase/mode selection, a digital controller (this is not a PLC), pilot lights, and audible alarms. An option for this system would be a purge system for classified environments. This purge system pressurizes the enclosure so that combustible gas vapors are prevented from entering the enclosure. This system is typically used for basic isolators. It can also be easily integrated into a Class I, Division I environment. This control design type has limited capabilities and options. It would have the capability of sensing a loss in pressure and increasing the blower speed to compensate for a "glove off" situation.

Advancing another step in controls would normally entail a PLC system. PLC controls have many features and greater flexibility for future capabilities. A standard system would contain a small, analog touchscreen (with some printing capabilities), a PLC, pneumatic or electrically actuated valves, an emergency stop button, automatic control of all features, and PID loop tuning. Some options could be a purge system for classified environments, humidity control, oxygen control, temperature control, and ammonia leak test pressure control. It would also have the capability of sensing a loss in pressure and increasing the blower speed to compensate for a "glove off" situation.

The most sophisticated controls would be a higher level PLC system. This provides the highest level of control and capabilities. This control system would contain a large, analog, active matrix, touchscreen/computer, and PLC with PC-based human-machine interface (HMI), which gives the ability to store data, pneumatic or electrically actuate valves, emergency stop button, and automatic control of all features. It would also have process and instrument diagram (PID) loop tuning, phase/mode recipe creation, datalog capabilities, alarm record capabilities, user logon, web accessible, a purge system for classified environments, humidity control, oxygen control, temperature control, and ammonia leak test pressure control.

Some additional options could be facility SCADA interface and complex auxiliary equipment integration. It might also have the capability of sensing a loss in pressure and increasing the blower speed to compensate for a "glove off" situation.

PRODUCT HAZARD CLASSIFICATION

A primary consideration in the design and engineering of containment solators is the OEL of the product being handled or processed. There are various classifications and rating systems that are generally individual company based. Some companies have classifications 1 through 4, 1 through 5, A through D, or A through E. Generally the classification 1 or A is the least potent products and the classification 4, 5, D and E are the most potent products.

As there are various scales and categories for the different classifications, the following is *an example* of typical OEL (potency TWA-exposure limits);

Class 1 = 1–5 mg/m^3
Class 2 = 0.1–1 mg/m^3
Class 3 = 1–100 $\mu g/m^3$
Class 4 $<$ 1 $\mu g/m^3$
Class 5 $\ll$ 1 $\mu g/m^3$

The need for containment devices would apply to Classes 3, 4, and 5. Containment devices for these applications would range between directional dust control devices such as downflow booths coupled with specific ventilation of exhaust systems. They could be closed systems with containment valves, isolators with gloveports and RTP and isolators without human interface, such as conveyors with robotics.

When designing an isolator or containment system, it is essential to determine what the OEL of the product is, what is the customers required containment technology, and how is it being processed.

Electrical Hazard Classification

As with all equipment, consideration for safe electrical operation needs be reviewed during the specification development phase of an isolator system design.

If required by room or internal isolator conditions, intrinsically safe electrical components may need to be specified. Note that electrical components are classified "intrinsically safe" because their power usage is lower than the level required to cause an explosion within a specified hazardous area. In addition, "intrinsically safe'" components are not capable of storing sufficient amounts of energy which might trigger an explosion when discharged.

Both, Underwriters Laboratories and Factory Mutual Research, as well as the American National Standards Institute (1) apply the same definitions for a hazardous area. These areas are defined as Class I (combustible gas and liquids), Class II (combustible dust), and Class III (combustible fibers). Class I is subdivided into groups A (acetylene), B (hydrogen and butadiene), C (diethyl ether, ethylene, isoprene, and UDMH), and D (acetone, gasoline, lacquer solvent, styrene, propane, and natural gas). Class II is divided into Groups E (metal dust), F (carbon black, coal, and coke), and G (flour, starch, and grain dusts).

All classes include two divisions. Division I covers electrical equipment directly exposed in an explosion atmosphere of the material of a specific group. Division II covers electrical equipment in an explosive atmosphere only when accident or fallout occurs, or in a properly vented direct exposure.

Remember the "explosion-proof" rating is given only to a single piece of equipment (isolator) for a specific class, division, and group. Equipment installation is the sole responsibility of the end user.

Again, when developing isolator specifications, it is critical to know the product being handled and the cleaning procedure. Some products contain solvents and some cleaning procedures required solvents. The electrical hazard classification of an isolator should be evaluated for those details.

NITROGEN (INERT GAS) PURGE

In some isolator applications, there may be a need for the internal environment to be nitrogen or inert gas purged or controlled to a low oxygen level. The need for this feature may be product sensitivity to oxygen or for safety reasons to reduce the oxygen level to a safe level (below that able to support combustion).

There are various ways to design and operate in a nitrogen or inert gas purged environment. The most basic is to manually purge the chamber during start-up and to provide make-up with only nitrogen. In a negative pressure isolator, the validation of this type system would involve operating the isolator during the purge phase at a greater negative pressure than standard (but less than the validated leak test pressure). During this phase, the air being drawn out by the negative pressure ventilation is replaced by nitrogen that is connected and regulated on the inlet of the isolator. As there are no controls for this method, it will need to be validated at a certain flow rate for a certain time to obtain the proper levels required. In normal use, the operator would be required to closely follow a SOP and record the specific flow and duration. With this system, there would not be any alarms for high oxygen levels.

The next more sophisticated system would be to automatically control the flow of nitrogen and the duration of the purge digital controllers. Both of these two systems assume a leak tight isolator and that there is no other source of oxygen capable of entering the isolator. There could be independent oxygen alarms with the addition of an oxygen sensor. Specific oxygen levels cannot be controlled.

The most sophisticated system would actually monitor the oxygen level and the isolator pressure simultaneously. With this system, the purge rate (flow and time) is fully programmable so that the optimum time and nitrogen consumption can be determined in validation. This system has both oxygen and pressure sensor that continuously monitors the levels and adjusts them to the set point. If the oxygen level approached a high level the system would automatically add nitrogen and increase the blower speed to maintain the pressure set point. Conversely, if the isolator pressure dropped to low level, the system would automatically add pressure by adding nitrogen to the isolator. These type systems can be purchased as a complete package or configured by the isolator vendor. The fully automatic oxygen analyzing and control system will be equipped with both high and low oxygen and pressure alarms.

MONITORING/DATA ACQUISITION

With respect to monitoring and data acquisition isolators should have the capability to provide local or remote monitoring and control where required of the operating parameters and internal conditions generated within the unit. This is particularly important for compounds that may need to be processed under strict environmental control (temperature, oxygen level, humidity, etc.) from a product integrity standpoint.

The following parameters can be monitored using standard isolator control features however some dedicated probes and sensors will be necessary should temperature and humidity monitoring be necessary within the isolator work environment. When choosing a suitable detection probe, cleaning, and area electrical class compatibility need to be addressed.

- Chamber pressure monitoring and output facilities from pressure transmitters for data acquisition.
- Supply and exhaust filter differential pressure indication. (Monitored across individual filters). HEPA filters will also need filter integrity test ports and scanning ability where large filter cells are employed.
- Nitrogen supply flow rate.
- Exhaust oxygen concentration. Monitoring and recording as required from process.
- Internal work chamber temperature.
- Internal work chamber humidity.
- Weighing system outputs. Local and duplicate readouts for remote monitoring.
- Blower run conditions. (Critical if exhaust flow is integrated with room HVAC system.)

- Ancillary equipment monitoring. (Equipment mounted within isolator, or operated in conjunction with the isolator may need to be monitored along with the isolator parameters.)
- For aseptic isolator, air velocity for unidirectional airflow can be monitored.
- Also vaporized hydrogen peroxide (H_2O_2), both high and low concentration inside the isolator and low concentration in the room can be monitored.

All monitoring expectations should be advised at as early a stage as possible by the user team to establish the parameters critical to the process in question. Sophisticated monitoring packages are available by many vendors to readily address the above data collection and system monitoring requirements; however, as per most systems of this nature, the needs of every system differs in some way hence the aspect of critical monitoring and data collection should be addressed as a part of the engineering design phase of the isolator.

CLEANING REQUIREMENTS

Cleaning requirements of both the interior and exterior of the isolator along with the equipment or components inside the isolator are vital.

When designing an isolator determine the materials that are being handled and the best chemicals to achieve a validated "clean" isolator. If the product is water soluble, then simply provide a device or method to deliver the water into the isolator. If it is determined that another solution or solvent is required, determine the chemical compatibility of the chosen liquid and the materials of construction of the isolator. In some instances, it may be required to enlist the services of an third party to do a cleaning study on the specific compounds to be cleaned. Typically, isolators constructed of 316L stainless steel are compatible with most cleaning solutions, but occasionally a dilute bleach solution may be the best. In those cases, it is important to determine the duration of the cleaning process and the impact on the stainless steel.

The main areas of concern for chemical compatibility are the elastomers used in the isolator. Those components include gaskets, O-rings, gloves, sleeves, and other seals. In some instances, it may be best to replace gloves or the flexible components, rather than to try to clean them. Gloves come in a limited choice of materials; the most common are neoprene, hypalon, butyl, and viton.

The typical methods of delivering the cleaning solutions include spray bottle, spray wand/gun, and spray nozzles. When using spray nozzles to wash the inside of an isolator, you may also want to again use the services of a third party to help determined optimum locations for the nozzles. It should also be noted that spray nozzles alone inside an isolator would not be able to hit every surface. It is recommended that a spray wand also be included to address the areas that the nozzles do not. A riboflavin test can be performed during validation to help determine the coverage of the spray nozzles and pinpoint the areas that need to be addressed by the spray wand.

When using considerable amounts of liquids for cleaning, a drain of some type should be included in the isolator. The typical drains are flared holes with a sanitary fitting and a valve. This valve is typically a ball or diaphragm style. Another choice is a flush mount sanitary diaphragm valve welded into the isolator floor.

For aseptic toxic isolator, the cleaning methods need to be different since the isolators have the added features of unidirectional airflow with more HEPA filters. Some of the styles of cleaning aseptic toxic isolators included having the isolator design with round or square return ducts (instead of double-pane windows. In these designs the return ducts would be protected by a HEPA filters that were positioned at the bottom of the isolator. Return air was pulled through those HEPA filters and therefore preventing toxic materials from contaminating the return ducts and the ventilation above. The difficulty with these systems is to get adequate capacity of HEPA filters at the bottom of the isolator to meet the airflow required.

Another design was to have bag-in/bag-out HEPA filters at the top of the return ducts. These would be located in the technical area above the isolator and could be changed out from there. The return ducts would not be protected from below and therefore needed to be cleaned. To clean these ducts, a WIP system would be required. This WIP requires validation to ensure that all toxic materials could be washed away.

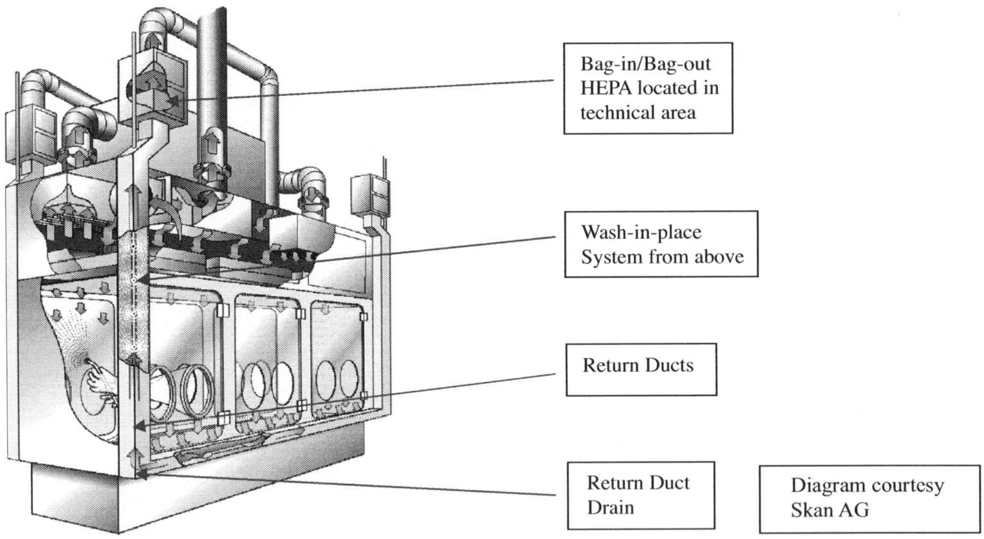

More recently another design has been used. This uses the FIBO® HEPA filter system. FIBO® filters are placed in parallel along the bottom of the isolator and based on capacity they feed multiple return ducts. The advantage of this design is that the filters are high capacity and can be changed from within the production room.

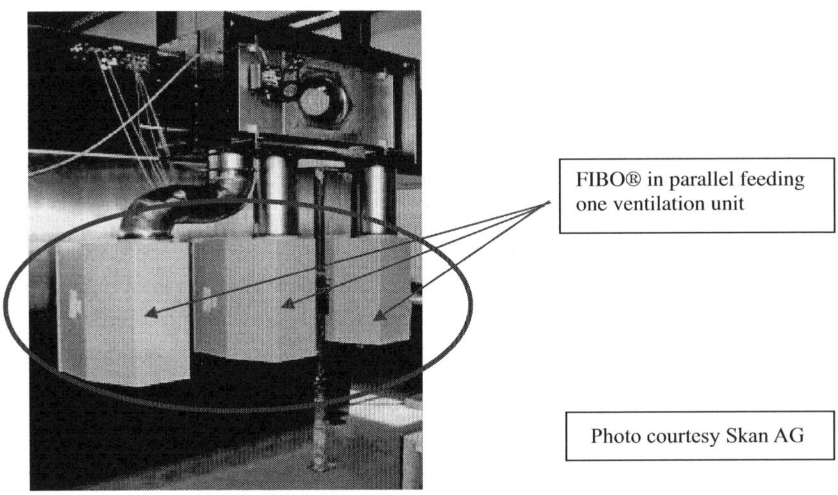

UTILITIES

For the proper operation of the isolator and equipment integrated into the isolator, it may require various types of utilities be supplied to the isolator.

- Power to operate the isolator control and lighting systems.
- Power to operate integrated equipment such as balances, instrumentation and laboratory equipment.
- Compressed air to actuate valves or to operate integrated equipment.
- Conditioned air to maintain specified temperature and humidity levels within the isolator during operation or for preconditioning for decontamination.
- Water for spray wands or wash in place systems, or for integrated equipment.

- Compressed dry air to use in spray wands and wash in place systems to dry the isolator after washing or to reduce the humidity within the isolator.
- Compressed dry nitrogen can be used to control oxygen levels or reduce humidity levels within the isolator.

It is important to verify with the owner what utilities are available in the room where the isolator will be located. It will be necessary to determine what utilities are required for the operation of the isolator and the processes being run. It may be necessary to have utilities added to the room if the existing specifications do not meet the equipment requirements.

WASTE DISPOSAL

In the engineering design consideration needs to be given to the removal of waste material components from the isolator in a safe and contained manner.

Solid waste, in the form of cable ties, drum liners, cleaning cloths, broken or rejected glassware, components, etc., would typically be removed from the isolator in the following ways:

- *Bag-out disposal port*. Typically attached to the side of the isolator would be a disposal chute, welded into the wall, which would retain a bag support cage. Over this cage would be located a continuous overbag for holding and removing waste from the isolator. Waste would then be removed via double tying and cutting the continuous overbag containing the waste materials.
- *Air lock*. In the same way that product and components may enter or exit the isolator, an air lock may be used to remove the waste. The waste would be placed in a bag or container within the isolator. The exterior surface of the container would then be cleaned before exiting via the air lock.
- *RTP/SBV container*. Waste, per the air lock version above may be removed from the isolator in the same way as components and materials enter the unit, that is, in this case via a split butterfly or RTP container system. Please refer to "Transfer Systems" section of this document. Waste then ultimately needs to be removed from the transfer container in a remote location.
- *Exit drum*. In large-scale applications where drums and liners are used to load the materials into the isolator, the same drum or liner, after being emptied, may be used to remove the waste generated within the unit after operations are complete.

Waste could also be considered as "liquid waste" following cleaning, which would be removed by drainage from the base of the isolator as advised in the "Cleaning Requirements" section.

SUPPORT ANCILLARIES

In most containment isolators, some support ancillary equipment is required within the isolator or located conveniently on the outside.

When reviewing the process or operation being performed within the isolator, it is important to list those types of support equipment. Once a list is determined, specifying the exact size and type will be necessary. What may have been acceptable in a normal process may not work in a contained process within an isolator.

Some examples of support ancillaries are scoops for weighing and dispensing, sample thieves, croupier sticks (to extend the operator reach), tongs, shelves, beakers, flasks, trays, etc. For security, some of these may need to be attached to the isolator structure with a chain or cable so that they cannot accidentally fall into a vessel, drum, or other open container.

In weighing isolators, stainless steel hoppers or funnels may need to be designed. In some instances, a specific size screen will be required in the hopper or funnel.

When using the bagging method of transfer, O-rings, cable ties, cable tie hand tools and cable cutters will be required. To ensure proper technique is used, those items must be stored near the isolator.

Some designs may require that a printer or chart recorder be mounted on the isolator. Shelves will be required and their location should be evaluated during the design and ergonomic study phases.

SAMPLING

Product sampling may be periodically required during operations with the isolator whereas at the same time, maintaining containment for remote testing and analysis. Samples may either be manually collected from product containers with suitably sized sample thieves and augers or automatically collected via a sample valve and retrieval system. In any event, containment needs to be maintained during sample collection and removal from the Isolator.

In open powder-handling operations within a containment isolator, manual product samples are typically collected in a sample pouch or jar and removed from the isolator via the most appropriate transfer system described in "Transfer System" section. These include RTP/SBV and container, continuous liner, removal drum, air lock, etc.)

More automated sampling systems are available, for example to collect in-flight material during a contained pack-out system that would extend, via a tube and shuttle system, into the product feed chute and withdraw a predetermined sample (designated by collection size and time) which would be discharged with the aid of vibration into a collection jar. This collection jar, dependant on the level of containment required may be located within a continuous liner for additional protection or positioned within the isolator itself for maximum protection to the operator and environment during sample retrieval.

As per all isolator considerations, discussions with the end user of the isolator is required to assess sampling requirements and frequency; however, appropriate systems are available to ensure containment is maintained during these activities.

TESTING (MECHANICAL, ENVIRONMENTAL, FUNCTIONAL, AND PERFORMANCE)

Performance testing is an important aspect of any isolator project from both the end users' and vendor's perspective. The mechanical, functional as well as performance testing of the containment isolator system, both on- and offsite as well as both parties' expectations should be met for that testing.

These "expectations" need to be addressed early in the project design phase and should be highlighted on the project schedule plan as these activities are significant milestones as well as potential timeframes in any successful project.

Mechanical functional and predelivery performance testing would commence at an FAT at the vendors site to address the following items:

- Note that the testing scope needs to be identified and written into any user requirement specification.
- General construction quality, mechanical checks and dimensions (backed up with drawing and documentation review).
- Surface finish checks.
- Airflow volume and control in the event of failure.
- Overall operation.
- Interface with OEM equipment. Either as part of scope of the isolator vendor or "free issued" (ordered by customer and delivered to the isolator vendor).
- Alarms and interlock tests.
- Loop checks.
- Ergonomics
- Lighting levels
- Noise levels
- Oxygen levels
- Temperature levels
- Humidity levels
- Smoke tests
- Pressure decay testing (negative pressure)
- Helium-leak testing.

- Personal dust in air sampling and surface swab testing (predelivery performance tests)
- CIP/WIP systems testing (predelivery performance tests)

Upon successful completion and acceptance of the above-mentioned points, the unit would be prepared for shipping and delivered to site and tests repeated/operational qualification undertaken to assess the necessary parameters as part of a site acceptance procedure with the following additional undertakings.

- Control system set point checks.
- Site loop checks.
- Interface with site installed OEM equipment. (Part of scope or "free issued")
- Calibration of gauges and transmitters.
- Filter pressure drops and gauge reference set point check.
- Motor run tests.
- Site performance tests for dust in air and surface contamination during operator training.

Mechanical and performance testing is a considered "norm" at site acceptance testing phase; however, increasing tests are now being undertaken at FAT to ensure the most satisfactory piece of equipment is delivered to site.

These tests need to be agreed between vendor and end user as soon as practically possible.

VALIDATION

In the end accountability warrants that validation is considered at the design phase.

Validation is the confirmation by examination and provision of objective evidence that a particular requirement for a specific use can be consistently fulfilled.

The validation of a containment system shall also include demonstrations that the hazardous materials are adequately contained.

Benefits of a properly validated and controlled process during design will:

- Yield fewer out of specification products, produce increased output
- Achieve enhanced performance
- Lower exposure of operators to materials being contained

Information generated during the validation and design processes can, if required, provide important information during investigations of inadequate performance of containment equipment.

Process is each stage of a project: generation of specification, design, build, installation, testing, and maintenance of a containment device/system should be clearly documented.

Key stages in the validation process are the following:

Preparation of a validation master plan;

Design qualification (DQ): verifying that the design documentation correctly specifies the required system (highly recommended for large projects, may be omitted in smaller efforts, and required by some firms in either case);

Installation qualification (IQ): verifying that the system is built and installed in accordance with the design documentation;

Operational qualification (OQ): verifying the system functions as required;

Performance Qualification (PQ): verifying that the outputs from the system (e.g.: products or intermediates) conform to requirements;

Computer systems validation: verifying that software components of the system function as required.

A team approach should be applied to ensure that all validation issues are identified during the design phase of the project and appropriate action undertaken. The following people should be involved in some form during the process:

Project manager;
Production representative;
Quality assurance (QA) representative;

Technical representative;
Maintenance representative;
Safety representative;
Occupational hygienist.

For a review of the validation process to be undertaken, the constituent elements DQ, IQ, OQ, and PQ must be completed and in place consisting of the following:

DQ report
IQ report
OQ report
Computer validation rationale
Computer test protocols, with results
Source code review
PQ report

All these documents are to be reviewed for compliance with validation requirements, the status of which shall be recorded in a validation review report.

The validation review report provides a final statement of acceptance or rejection of the specified process.

In conclusion, there are many areas to consider when evaluating the design of containment isolator projects. These items listed above cover most of the critical and obvious areas, but as the technology and regulatory requirements expand, other items may need to added to design and engineering considerations.

REFERENCE

1. National Fire Protection Association. NFPA 70: National Electrical Code®. 2008 ed. Quincy, MA: NFPA, 2008.

7 Design and engineering of isolators

Didier Meyer

DEFINITION OF AN ISOLATOR

The definition of an isolator is almost an existential question for anyone who has to decide to buy or to design an isolator. The official definition is actually given by a regulatory body ISO 14644–7 regarding the "separative enclosures" in which the isolator is described among other means of separative devices. To clear the view of the readers we can use the definition given by James Akers in June 1995 (1): "Isolators are devices that provide for total separation between one environment and another. An isolator does not directly exchange air with the surrounding environment and all air must enter through a HEPA or ULPA filtration system. All transfer of material into the isolator must be accomplished while maintaining complete environmental separation." The key words to be taken in account in this definition are "total separation." This definition does not emphasize that although the operators are physically inside the isolator, they are biologically outside through means of manipulative devices such as gloves, half or even full suits.

To have "total separation between one environment and another" the enclosure that constitutes the body or shell of the isolator must be "leaktight" that is to say to provide for minimal passage between the internal and external environments. Isolators can also be used for containment purposes to protect the operators and the environment from highly toxic or potent products because of the limited ability for exchange of air from inside to outside.

According to James Agalloco, the isolators can be either "closed" when the process inside is in a batch mode or "open" when the process has a continuous ingress and/or egress mode (2). In the case of an "open" isolator, it's design would include at least one opening each for the ingress and egress of materials. These "holes" include protective dynamic systems to avoid cross contamination with the surroundings during the production process. The design of an isolator is closely related to the process for which it is intended and that is one of the major differences between isolators and manned clean rooms.

The key acronym is URS (user's requirements specifications). The design of the isolator generally begins with a stepwise description of the process from which the isolator is intended and the critical points for which neither experience nor dedicated equipment are available. The optional solutions for the critical points should be explored for potential integration into the project development. The isolator(s) should integrate the necessary functions in a process flow diagram.

An isolator can be used either to protect the product (operating in a positive pressure relative its surroundings) or to protect the operator (working in a negative pressure mode). The intrinsic leak rate of the isolator and any potential accidental leakage provide the rationale for this technological choice. In theory, where a perfectly leaktight isolator to exist, the choice would not be of any consequence. Due to real (however slight) and potential leakage, there is a priority given either to the product (positive pressure for aseptic processes) or to the environment (negative pressure for toxic processes). The choice is more difficult in the case of an aseptic processing of a toxic product. The two possibilities are a positive pressure isolator in a class D surrounding environment or a negative pressure isolator in a class B surrounding. Both of these approaches have been successfully validated (3,4). A rational way to choose between them would be to use a hazard analysis of control of critical points (HACCP) approach. This method takes into account factors such as toxicity, quantity of material, open exposure in the enclosure, filling speed, number of operators, construction of the isolator, type and frequency of transfers, cleanliness class of the surrounding, etc. Ranking of the hazards and development of a decision tree can help make the proper choice and to explain it both internally (operator, safety engineer, quality assurance and externally, auditor, insurance consultant, inspector).

The routine usage of isolators in the pharmaceutical industry follows the usual steps to produce medications:

- Fine chemical production
- Weighing, mixing, and compounding
- Aseptic filling
- Final testing

ACTIVE PHARMACEUTICAL INGREDIENT PRODUCTION

The isolator for the fine chemical process is often connected permanently or semipermanently to a process vessel. The working zone must often be explosion-proof and thus the components of the isolator must be as well. That makes it, generally speaking, difficult to have an electronic follow-up as accurate as in the other parts of the process due to explosion-proof area. Any connection to a tank or to a dryer must take in account the differential working pressures of these elements and the isolator to properly install the required safety devices. The fine chemical step produces the active pharmaceutical ingredient that often has to be transferred and/or shipped and/or stored before the next step of the process. A sampling of the product must be completed under the same conditions either during the process itself or prior to its transfer. The next step is often weighing of the powder that may have to be performed in the same explosion proof atmosphere. The main concern with the weighing is to get accurate results. The scale can be either fully inside the isolator, or the electronics can be outside with the display and printer. Whatever the choice, the weighing operations must take in account the internal pressure of the isolator. When the collecting container or vessel is installed underneath the isolator, an outside scale or weighing device may be used.

The mixing of the powder with a solvent to obtain the final solution can be completed inside the isolator for small quantities or in an attached vessel for larger quantities. The introduction of the solvent should use appropriate in-line filters (one inside the enclosure, one outside); when the solvent cannot be filtered a RTP (rapid transfer port) connection is necessary (5). The ingredients and fluids for compounding must enter the isolator with appropriate treatments to preclude the entry of any unwanted materials able to cross contaminate the final preparation (particulates, bacterias, etc.). Preventing their introduction should be driven by compatible protocols.

ASEPTIC FILLING OF CONTAINERS

Two distinct processes of filling have to be considered inside an isolator: manual and semiautomatic process (to a maximum throughput of 30 containers per minute) where the machine is installed within the isolator on one side and the automatic process where the machine is integrated with the isolator on the other side (6). The filling machine has to be loaded with empty containers, the drug to be filled, and stoppered/capped in the case of vials.

For manual and semiautomatic machines the autoclave (for stoppers and product contact fill parts) and the oven (for glass containers) can be directly connected to the isolator. The alternative is the use of an RTP-equipped transfer isolator to transfer the materials from an autoclave-isolator or oven-isolator. The choice of the first solution avoids an extra sterilization of the outside of the packaging. The use of a directly connected autoclave or oven to the process isolator can also be used for the egress of materials from the isolator. In the case of automatic filling line of glass containers, a depyrogenation tunnel is permanently connected to the entrance of the filling isolator; the egress of the filled containers should be protected against any ingress from the external atmosphere into the isolator. When the product is toxic an external cleaning of the container is usually necessary after the sealing or capping. This part of the filing process has to be related to the removal of toxic materials and to the protection of the operators and surrounding environment.

In the case of plastic containers, they are ordinarily gamma irradiated and then introduced into the isolator after the decontamination of the outside surface of their bulk packaging. As an alternative in-line decontamination of the bulk package can be performed instead (7). One mean is using disposable or reusable RTP beta flanges mounted on autoclavable or irradiated sterile bags.

STERILITY TESTING

The final testing for sterile medications and devices includes sterility testing. This test is defined in the various pharmacopeias. A "false-positive" result is to be avoided to prevent the unnecessary loss of otherwise acceptable materials. The use of a closed system for the membrane sterility test has resulted in a significant decrease in the incidence of "false-positive" results. The use of isolator in addition of such a closed system results in an almost zero the level of "false positives." In addition, the isolator provides an easier investigation in the event of a failure to determine whether the positive result is due to an operator error. Another concern can be a "false-negative" result if decontamination of the sample container exterior results in penetration of the decontaminating agent into the sample container. In such a case, a fertility test under the conditions of the sterility test has to be provided (8,9). To avoid this risk, when possible, the samples can be transferred from the production area to the sterility testing isolator within an empty sterile RTP container or bag.

CONTAINMENT

The pharmaceutical industry uses more and more potent and toxic products as the active part of the drug delivered to the patient. These potent and toxic products are produced by the fine chemical industry. The industry must protect its operators and has tended to build closed designs including vessels for the various steps of the product developments (crystallization, mixing, filtering, drying, etc.). At certain stages, solutions or powders have to be added or extracted. Where low operator exposure limit (OEL) products ($<1\ \mu g/m^3$) are being processed, these operation must be performed in an isolator (10). The purpose of this isolator is to protect the operators and environment so it must operate under negative pressure relative to the surrounding room. The designer must exercise caution regarding explosion proof requirements, which are not always compatible with the electronic service and monitoring, and with the pressures of the vessels. The pressure should be stabilized before the opening in isolator (11). Negative pressure containment is used when the toxic or potent product is in its powder stage. After mixing with a solvent under negative pressure, the OEL often allows the operators to work in positive pressure isolator, if necessary, for aseptic production of injectable drug (12).

ASEPTIC PROCESSING

The aseptic process is acceptable only where the package or product cannot tolerate terminal sterilization. The use of an isolator is in these cases is a significant plus relative to the manned clean room technology as the operator stays outside the aseptic environment. An isolator is far preferable for the formulation of a sterile product that cannot be membrane filtered (i.e., emulsions, suspensions) and for the filling of liquids, powders, and other sterile dosage forms. When the liquid is to be freeze dried, an isolator can be placed in front of the freeze drier.

Liquids whether membrane filtered (13) or not (e.g., emulsion) (14) can be transferred through a dedicated RTP system. For batch processes (low speed or manual process) the work flows between "closed" isolators linked and/or connected to single-door (e.g., freeze drier) or double-door processors (i.e., autoclave, oven). The use of RTP connections helps solve the problem of multiple connections between the sterile enclosures (15). The risk in case of contamination of one of the isolators is the transfer of this contamination. In case of a continuous filling process (high speed), special care has to be given to the ingress and egress of the components without disturbing the quality of the atmosphere within the isolator. A pressure cascade between the surrounding environment and the various sections of the isolator(s) may help avoid contamination that could compromise the quality of the product. Some components (i.e., stoppers, caps, etc.) require introduction through a double-door autoclave, chemical lock chamber or ultraviolet lock chamber. One solution is the use of outside RTP bag delivered with its sterile components (16). For microbiological monitoring, disposable devices can be introduced into the isolator during the process without contamination through interlocked chambers, RTP isolators or RTP bags.

Special care has to taken for installations used for the aseptic filling of toxic products. In this case the RTP connection must be bidirectional and stay leaktight in both directions. The comparative risk assessments personnel/product can be estimated by a HACCP type of method

Table 1 Classification of Containment Enclosures According to Their Hourly Leak Rate from ISO 10648-2

Class	Hourly leak rate, T_f hr^{-1}	Example
1[a]	$\leq 5 \times 10^{-4}$	Containment enclosure with controlled atmosphere under inert gas conditions
2[a]	$<2.5 \times 10^{-3}$	Containment enclosure with controlled atmosphere under inert gas conditions or with permanently hazardous atmosphere
3	$<10^{-2}$	Containment enclosure with permanently hazardous atmosphere
4	$<10^{-1}$	Containment enclosure with atmosphere which could be hazardous

[a]The classification of leaktightness required for a particular application under classes 1 and 2 shall be decided by the designer and user and licensing authorities. Normally, class 1 will be applied for technical reasons when higher gas purity is required.

to decide whether to use containment (negative pressure isolator in a class B environment) or to aseptic process (positive pressure isolator in a class D environment).

The understanding of the monitoring is essential both for the physical measurements and the microbiological controls.

LEAK TIGHTNESS

A key aspect of isolators that is by no means absolute and induces questions of importance, level, location, and measurement is the "leak rate." Agalloco mentions, when comparing barrier system and isolator (2), that the isolator even the "open" ones have to be essentially leaktight during their decontamination process. The magnitude of the leak rate has to be realistic relative to the materials of construction and the leak test method used. The sleeves to which the gloves are attached are a part of the isolator wall. The risk of a leak has to be evaluated relative to its location and materials including gaskets. Several means of measuring the leaks are available and/or possible for either quantitative or qualitative measurement (Table 1). When considering the user's typical requirements and available equipment, the principle methods are the following:

- Pressure decay for the positive pressure isolator
- Pressure increase for the negative pressure isolator and RTP container
- Oxygen concentration for the glove on positive pressure isolator
- Detection of an indicator gas (helium, ammonia, freon) outside the isolator
- Ultrasonic detection of leak locations

Some potential acceptable values for the pressure increase/decay of the isolator (with its filtration system) are given in Table 2 according to the materials of construction of the isolator. It is evident that flexible wall isolators have generally superior performance relative to rigid construction due to the absence of gasket and locking devices. The leak rates are expressed in percentage of the isolator volume per hour. Another possibility is to use pascals per minute as in Microbial Safety Cabinet Class 3 that at a test pressure of 500 Pa has an allowable maximum pressure decay of 50 Pa in 30 minutes. Other than prior to each decontamination

Table 2 Table of Types of Isolator and Corresponding Pressures/Leak Rates from La Calhène Standards

Isolator type	Mechanical test pressure (Pa)	Leak test pressure (Pa)	Leak rate (% vol./hr)
Soft wall	150	100	0.1
Soft wall with Stainless Steel base	150	100	0.1
Rigid wall 1 piece plastic	150	100	0.1
Rigid wall on Stainless Steel base	150	100	0.5
Stainless Steel + hinged window	300	150	0.5
Containment box	500	500	0.1

(a very sensible time at which to perform the leak test), leak testing is desirable in conjunction with production processes and needs to be completed quickly and easily. The selection of a commercially available device for leak testing makes leak control easier (17). The isolator gloves that are widely recognized as the weakest part of the isolator can be leak checked with the isolator before the decontamination process. The most important risks associated with leaks occur during the production process carried out inside the isolator. The in-process leak check should be performed without compromising the inside quality of the enclosure as a part of the test. For any isolator intended for sterile operations, this requirement essentially eliminates any leak test method that might introduce nonsterile air from the outside of the sleeve or glove. The oxygen leak test method that reverses the glove within a tight chamber filled with nitrogen allows a precision measurement without risk of backward contamination (17).

The beta half of the RTP is the mobile head of the system to which a volume is attached. The shape, construction materials of the gasket and the volume itself depend upon the use of the RTP connection. The leaktightness of the beta assembly depend upon the volume and the beta head. The leaktightness of the volume is measured as already described, that of the beta head, which includes a flange, a lid, and a gasket can be measured as a whole with a pressure increase (17). Comparative values of the leaktightnesses of various parts of an isolator shows that the DPTE® Betapart (DPTE® is one of the available RTPs) is substantially more leaktight than the constitutive shell of the isolator (17).

ERGONOMICS

One's first look at an isolator often results in an impression of a "cumbersome environment" with a "jungle of arms." In fact the main feature provided by the designer is to provide access to the whole inside volume and surface through sleeves/gloves and/or half-suits fluid and easy. The operators, who are physically inside but biologically outside, must always work against the resistance provided by either positive or negative pressure. The operators have to be able to reach the critical parts of the isolator without being obliged to open it. The designers should insure that the atmosphere inside is not mixed with the outside if the isolator to provide the proper protection to the product and/or the operator. The manipulation means sleeve, half-suit or full-suits with their gloves are the most important and the most fragile part of the isolator. It is essential that the gloves are properly sized for the hands of the operator, strong enough to be resistant to leaks and resistant to the decontaminating agent. At the same time they must also be light enough to allow full sensation. The gloves should be exchangeable without breaking the integrity of the isolator to accommodate various sizes of hands as well replacement of any that might develop a leak.

The half-suit and the full-suit must be provided with enough filtered air for the operator to work comfortably for extended periods without interruption. Additional gowning of the operators may include undergloves and face masks for hygienic purposes.

STERILIZATION OR DECONTAMINATION?

Isolators in the pharmaceutical industry were originally considered as "mini clean rooms" and were only wiped with disinfectant solutions prior to use in aseptic processing or sterility testing. Beginning in the early 1980s, one of the goals of isolator users was the attainment of a more reproducible biologically lethal treatment for the internal environment. To demonstrate the effectiveness of these treatments, isolators are challenged with resistant spores prior to a liquid spray or evaporation of a chemical sporicidal agent (18). At first the only available sterilant was diluted peracetic acid. Since the beginning of the 1990s, evaporation of aqueous solution of H_2O_2 has become the method of choice. The byproducts of H_2O_2 degradation are water and oxygen. A recently introduced treatment uses gaseous ClO_2 (19). Ozone is seeing increased use as a sterilant in water systems and also has potential for use with isolators. All of these sterilants are accepted by the various pharmacopeias (20). The spores used for validation of the microbial treatment depend on the mode of sterilization and the sterilant itself. The carrier on which they are placed can be paper, plastic material, or stainless steel (21). The placement of inoculated carriers in the isolator, the concentration of spores (10^3 to 10^6), and its resistance (D value) depends upon the agent chosen and the process objective (22).

The use of the term "sterilization" appears in the recently issued USP <1208> (20). As the process is only a surface and atmospheric treatment (23), some regulatory bodies are reluctant to use the term "sterilization" as is often associated with more lethal destruction of microorganisms throughout an object. For this and other reasons, use of the terms "decontamination" or "biodecontamination" are becoming increasingly widespread. Whatever the treatment mode or terminology, one important and essential consideration is the risk for the operators. The process should always be performed inside a "closed" isolator having a minimal leak rate. The leak rate is for closed isolators less than 0.5% of the internal volume of the isolator per hour. The 8-hour time-weighted average OEL for H_2O_2 (for example) is 1 ppm and the concentration inside the isolator during the process is often in the range of 400 to 1300 ppm. For isolators with a high leak rate (sometimes as high as 10% of the volume/hour) the operators may have to leave the surroundings of the isolator during the biodecontamination and the air renewal of the room has to be taken in account to assess the risk for the environment. The time required for agent removal (generally by air replacement) is one factor of the selection of treatment mode, as well as in isolator design (24).

Materials of Construction

A choice must often be made according to the requirements of the application. The choice between flexible or rigid wall is often considered a competition merely of the two modes of construction notwithstanding that the manipulation devices (glove, sleeve, half-suit, full-suit) are always flexible. The choice of materials is based on the following:

- The use of the isolator
- The pressure mode
- The ventilation mode
- The decontamination agent

Sterility testing isolators are quite often with flexible walls to provide the operator with better comfort and a broader use of the natural light of the room. Automatic filling isolators are predominantly stainless steel walls allowing for continuity from the walls to the filling machine itself. Negative pressure isolators are usually made of rigid materials, avoiding the need for reinforcement of a flexible wall design. Where unidirectional flow is required with rather complex recirculation systems it is preferable to use rigid walls. Recirculation can be provided using either air return chimney's located on the outside of the enclosure or between double walls of the isolator. Continued recirculation of the air (at 90 cfm) makes cooling mandatory in order to maintain the operating temperature around 20°C. Turbulent flow air with between 5 and 40 air changes per hour can be readily installed on both flexible and rigid walls isolators.

Some plastic materials have a tendency to adsorb and then desorb the sterilant especially H_2O_2. One of the factors to use or not to use plastic walls and windows is the risk of permanent chemical residues that can cross contaminate the product or influence microbiological results (25).

A LOGIC APPROACH TO DESIGN

The primary functions of the isolator must be taken into account when designing it: Manipulation, transfer, ventilation-filtration, bio-decontamination and isolation/containment.

The result must be a piece of equipment that is compatible with the process and current regulatory recommendations. It is important to consider the space around the equipment. It should be large enough to allow the operators and transfer items to freely circulate. The classification of the surrounding environment is generally expected to be at least Grade D for aseptic production purposes. This means that the exterior of the isolator must like the interior be easily cleanable to meet the class requirements.

Sterility Testing

Sterility testing as a regulatory defined application is perhaps the only widespread use of isolators for which it is possible to use a standard equipment design. This application was one of the very first for isolators in the pharmaceutical industry beginning in the early 1980s. As the operating procedures are essentially the same for all users, the isolators and appended equipments use the same basic principles, that is; as it is a predominantly a manual activity proper lighting and ergonomics for the operators are essential. The choice of a half-suit equipped workstation with transparent flexible walls often provides a superior material-handling capability with fewer constraints. Even with a half-suit, the flexible walls of the isolator permit excellent sound transmission. Their transparency and extent allows the operator to feel "integrated" in the surrounding room rather than isolated from it.

- In many installations, there is a workstation isolator in which the test is performed and a transfer isolator where the outside surfaces of the samples, the media and the test units are bio-decontaminated.
- H_2O_2 decontamination has introduced concerns relative to adsorption/desorption on flexible walls, sleeves and half-suits. To avoid "false negatives" due to residual H_2O_2 remaining after the decontamination is complete there is a growing tendency to use rigid wall transfer isolator to decrease the post bio-decontamination aeration time.
- The ingress of the samples and the egress of the solid and liquid wastes can be done through appropriate RTP sterile containers or bags working bi-directionally while avoiding chemical and microbiological cross-contamination.

The number and the frequency of testing and the volumes of the required media, utensils and other equipment must be considered in sizing the isolators, as well as the choice of the manipulation devices (gloves and/or half-suits) and the routine processing procedures. The choice of the decontamination method (Hydrogen Peroxide, Peracetic Acid, Chlorine Dioxide, etc.), is an important factor impacting decontamination dwell periods and the extent/speed of aeration required.

Other Applications

Aside from sterility testing most other uses for isolator are process specific to their application and require customized isolators operating in classified rooms. The logic means to their design includes the following:

- Knowledge of the process steps
- Choosing between positive and negative pressure
- Choosing between open (continuous process) or closed (batch process) isolators
- Deciding upon unidirectional or turbulent flow
- Selecting the appropriate continuous or batch transfer systems for the ingress and/or egress of components
- Fabrication of a essentially identical mock-up of the finished isolator
- Simulating the process with full consideration of fatigue factors
- Identifying the materials of construction
- Preparation of a detailed functional description include detailed drawings

An important aspect is the selection of realistic leaktightness criteria for the isolator, consistent with process requirements and fabrication capability. Although it might seem that the isolator should have a "zero" leak rate, that is certainly not possible, and the smaller the acceptable the rate the more difficult time the firm will have in both initial qualification and ongoing maintenance to maintain that capability. The leaktightness should be evaluated both "at rest" and "in operation" especially when moving parts are concerned, as well as during the decontamination process.

Gaskets used to join walls and windows can be of various profiles with either inflatable or noninflatable designs. The chemical compatibility of these materials is as important as it is for the manipulation components (gloves, sleeves, and half-suits). The materials compatibility should be considered relative to the use concentration rather theoretical data from vendor literature.

A LOGICAL APPROACH TO QUALIFICATION (VALIDATION)

Qualification of isolators proceeds through a series of stages: design qualification (DQ), installation qualification (IQ), operational qualification (OQ), and performance qualification (PQ) and have been well defined in the literature (26). DQ, IQ, and OQ are customarily provided by the manufacturer of the isolator(s), validation services firm or architect and engineering (A&E) firm in charge of the project. The PQ is usually performed by the end user sometimes with the assistance of outsiders for the cycle development/performance qualification of the decontamination process. The PQ may include a media fill test (MFT). The number of containers to fill for the MFT depends upon the level of confidence desired (27). The expected result of the MFT should be zero contamination.

There is no standard format for the qualification documentation. Most of the DQ, IQ, and OQ protocol requirements can be satisfied during either the factory acceptance test (FAT) completed at the isolator manufacturer's site isolator or the site acceptance test (SAT) performed at the end users' site. The logic means to organize these activities is to follow the user requirements specification (URS) and clearly indicate the specific design elements/operating features associated with the key points of the process.

WHO MUST BE INVOLVED IN QUALIFICATION AND WHEN?

Isolator technology permits the operator to be positioned closer to the materials used in the process as never before. Thus, the production department must be involved at the very beginning of a project and provided with training on isolation technology if it is their first exposure to it. If they already have sufficient experience, it can prove extremely helpful in the implementation of the technology.

Depending on the scale of the project several other departments on the end users' side must also be involved, the sooner the better. As a general rule and without being exhaustive, we can identify the following:

- Production
- Engineering
- Quality assurance/quality control
- Maintenance
- Training

REGULATIONS/RECOMMENDATIONS TO FOLLOW

From a short chapter in *Pharmacopeia* (1985) introducing the technology, numerous publications are available from many other sources:

- USP <1208> Sterility testing—Validation of isolator systems (20)
- USP <1116> Microbiological evaluation of clean rooms and other controlled environments (28)
- European Pharmacopeia: Environment when using isolator for sterility testing (29)
- Isolators for pharmaceutical applications from the UK Isolator Group, available at HMSO London (30)
- ISO 10648-1 and ISO 10648-2 upon the containment enclosures
- ISO 14644-1 to 8: Clean room and associate-controlled environments
- PIC/PICS: "Recommendations for the inspection of isolator technology"(31)
- PDA TR#34 (32)
- 2004 FDA aseptic processing guide
- 2003/2008EU Annex 1 on Sterile Medicinal Products (33)

These references define many relevant elements of the technology:

- The URS process is explained in ISO/DIS 14644-4
- The isolator environments are depicted differently:
  - EP: Grade D for aseptic production and no requirement for sterility testing
  - USP <1116>: for aseptic production depending upon the design
  - USP <1208>: for sterility testing no requirement
  - PIC/PICS: Grade D as a minimum depending upon the design
  - UK recommendations: depending upon the accuracy of the transfer systems
  - PDA TR#34: Conventional and class 100,000
  - 2004 FDA (Class 10,000 to 100,000)

- Decontamination of the isolator
  - EP: use of PAA or H_2O_2 with a 10^6 spores log reduction
  - USP <1116>: use of PAA or H_2O_2 with a 10^6 spores log reduction
  - USP <1208>: use of PAA or H_2O_2 with a 10^6 spores log reduction
  - PIC/PICS: "sanitisation" with PAA or H_2O_2 to get a 10^3 spores log reduction
  - UK recommendations: use of PAA or H_2O_2 with a 10^6 spores log reduction
  - PDA TR#34 : 10^3 spores log reduction
  - FDA 2004 : 10^6 spores log reduction
- Qualification and validation
  - ISO 14644-4: detailed tests procedures for acceptance
  - USP <1208>: details of IQ, OQ, and PQ
  - PIC/PICS: details of IQ, OQ, and PQ
  - UK recommendations: tests to be done before operations
  - PDA TR#34: details of IQ, OQ, and PQ
- Monitoring
  - USP <1116> and <1208>: monitoring of the integrity: gloves and microbiological tests
  - PIC/PICS: Microbiological tests inside and outside
  - UK recommendations: frequencies of the monitoring
  - PDA TR#34: Limitations of microbiological monitoring
  - 2004 FDA: Inclusion of microbiological monitoring
- Operators
  - USP <1208>: documented training of the operators
  - PIC/PICS: formal training programme for manager, operator, engineer, and maintenance staff
  - UK recommendations: Validation of the operator on the glove change procedure
  - PDA TR#34: Aseptic techniques and caution with sterilant
- Frequency of the validations
  - USP <1208>: No precise figure given
  - UK recommendation: Once a year
  - PDA TR#34: Twice a year

Future guidelines combined with a broader use of isolation technology will undoubtedly bring to the end users more logical and unfortunately more stringent recommendations.

FINANCIAL MATTERS

Are isolators less expensive than clean rooms? This question that is often raised with each new technology has been matter of some discussion over the last 10 years (34,35).

Are these two technologies really comparable? Is an airship really that much like an airplane? As the isolator operator will never be in direct contact with the product makes for a major difference that will benefit the product, in many cases the operator and ultimately the patient as well. Initial investment and operating costs are the two primary criteria that form the basis for financial comparison. The figures to date (Tables 3 and 4) indicate that the capital investment for a production isolator system is equal or higher than the equivalent installation with clean room technology, while conversely that the operating costs are much lower with the isolator.

Table 3 Capital Cost Comparison (Thousands of Dollars)

Line type	Fill line cost	Facility cost	Total cost
LCE	2700	378	3078
Advanced conventional	1600	1044	2644
	1100	666	434

Abbreviation: LCE, locally controlled environment.
Does not include start up (expense) costs.
Source: From Ref. 35.

Table 4 1997 Annual Cost Savings

LCE-related savings	One line (£K/yr)	Four Lines (£K/yr)
Reduce filling personnel	85	340
Reduced utility costs	40	160
Increase filling shift from 360 to 405 minutes	24	96
Eliminate sterile gowns	11	44
Eliminate equipment preparation	27	108
Modify environmental testing	5	20
Increased maintenance costs	60	240
Total savings ($K/yr)	132	528

Source: From Ref. 35.

PERSONNEL MANAGEMENT MATTERS

Even if the operators are not biologically within the isolator, they will conduct the process using the glove/sleeve and/or half-suit and therefore they must be properly trained. This training includes basics on isolators, differences from clean rooms, safety practices, aseptic technique, and any other particulars of the isolator such as changing gloves without breaking containment. The completion of training can coincide with the start of MFT for aseptic isolators that can confirm to acceptability of the installation and certify the operators.

PROS ANS CONS VERSUS CLEAN ROOMS

This debate has been driven by several factors: patient needs, personnel capabilities, and finance. The major technical factor in favor of the isolator is of course the total segregation of the operator that serves to protect the product during aseptic production: the environment/operator in containment applications, and the patient, product, operator and environment when used for sterile cytotoxic products. Regulations/recommendations should normally help in requesting, for instance, a zero growth for the MFT, which is difficult to reach on a routine basis within a manned enclosure.

REFERENCES

1. Akers J, Kennedy C, Agalloco J. Experience in the design and use of barrier isolator systems for sterility testing. Proceedings of Parenteral Drug Association International Symposium. Basel, Switzerland. Parenteral Drug Association, 1994:221–231.
2. Agalloco J. Barriers, isolators and microbial control. PDA J Pharma Sci Technol, 1999; 53(1):48–53.
3. Martin P. The use of barrier isolator technology for a sterile anti-cancer drug. In: Advanced Barrier Technology: A Joint PDA/ISPE Conference, Atlanta; January 17 and 18, 1995.
4. Gold PM. Maintaining containment during the processing of a highly potent potentially toxic aseptically filled drug product. In: PDA Annual Meeting, Philadelphia; November 10–14, 1997.
5. Wilkins JJ. Potent powder charging and discharging. In: A joint PDA/ISPE Conference, Atlanta; January 17 and 18, 1995.
6. Woodworth A. Isolator for Sterile Filling of Intravenous (IV) Solutions into Flexible Containers. Zurich: ISPE, 1997.
7. Khoury J-M, Orsato J. Validation of a continuous feed syringe filling isolator using real time monitoring of vapour phase hydrogen peroxide (a case study).
8. Millipore Technical Brief. The effect of peracetic acid on Steritest® sterility testing devices. TB1012EN00.
9. Millipore Technical Brief. The effect of vaporous hydrogen peroxide on Steritest® sterility testing devices. PF1017EN00.
10. Ryder Martin. Design Requirements Criteria for Containment Device Selection. Amsterdam: ISPE, 1999.
11. Rowell V. Methodoly for Design Procurement and Testing of High Containment Devices. Amsterdam: ISPE, 1999.
12. Leblanc AJ. Compliance and Regulatory Issues Associated with Parenteral Manufacturing of Cytotoxic and Potent Compounds. In: PDA Annual Meeting, Philadalphia; November 10–14, 1997.
13. Heldner M. Automatische GT—Beschickung und Entladung in Isolatortechnik. In: Concept Heidelberg, Mannheim; May 12–13, 1998.

14. Brossard J-P. Components Transfer for Filling Isolators. In: ISPE Conference, Rockvile, MD; June 1–3, 1997.
15. Nottingham J. Evalution of the Potential Bacterial Contamination Release from the La Calhène DPTE® Rapid Transfer Port when Challenged with Airborne Suspension of Microorganisms. In: PDA, Basel; February 23–25, 1998.
16. Norton PH. Aseptic Transfer Device for Barrier Isolators. In: PDA Annual Meeting, Philadelphia; December 5, 2000.
17. Rivière J-M. Routine Integrity Testing of Isolators During Their Use. In: PDA, Basel; February 14–16, 2000.
18. Davenport SM. Design and use of a novel peracetic acis sterilizer for absolute barrier sterility testing. J Parenter Sci Technol 1989; 43(4):158–166.
19. Eylath A. Successful sterilization using chlorine dioxide gas. BioProcess Int 2003; 1(7):2–5.
20. USP <1208>. Sterility testing—validation of isolator systems.
21. Kokubo M. Resistance of common environmental spores of the genus bacillus to vapour hydrogen peroxide. J Parenter Sci Technol 1998; 52(5):228–231.
22. Davenport SM. Sterility Assurance and the Use of *Bacillus stearothermophilus* as the BI for VHP Decontamination of Isolators. In: PDA Annual Meeting, Washington DC; November 30 to December 3, 1999.
23. Klapes NA. Wesley D. Vapour phase hydrogen peroxide as a surface decontaminant and sterilant. Appl Environ Microbiol 1990; 56(2):503–506.
24. Agalloco J, Akers J, Madsen R. Isolation Technology Regulatory Highlights from PDA TR 34 USP <1208> ISO 14644-7 PICS PE-b 004-1. In: PDA Annual Meeting, Washington, DC; Dec 3–7, 2001.
25. Lang G. On-Line Anlysis of Vapour Hydrogen Peroxide for Isolation Barrier Technology. In: ISPE BIT Conference, Rockvile, MD; June 1–3, 1997.
26. Rombauts R. Technical Validation of Isolators. Antwerp: AUDITS, 1999.
27. FDA. Aseptic Processing Guide. 1987.
28. USP <1116>. Microbiological evaluation of clean rooms and other controlled environments.
29. European Pharmacopaiea, 2.6.1. Sterility precautions against microbial contamination. Pharmeuropa 2000; 12(2).
30. Midcalf B, Lee G. Isolators for Pharmaceutical Applications: Practical Guidelines on the Design and Use of Isolators for the Aseptic Processing of Pharmaceuticals. HMSO, 1994.
31. PIC/S. Isolators used for aseptic processing and sterility testing. PE-004-1, Draft 4.
32. PDA. Technical Report N 34. Design and validation of isolators systems for the manufacturing and testing of health care products. June 2001.
33. Delattin R. EU status of GMP for sterile products. PDA J Pharm Sci Technol 1998; 52(3):82–88.
34. Brader WR. Impact of implementing barrier technology on existing aseptic fill facilities. Pharm Eng 1995.
35. Porter ME. Merck barrier isolator cost analysis revisited. In: ISPE Conferences, Rockville, MD; June 2, 1997.

8 Definition of restricted access barrier systems

Jörg Zimmermann

INTRODUCTION

RABS—restricted access barrier systems—were developed to advance the aseptic processes that were previously carried out in conventional clean rooms.

Traditionally, the protection of product from contamination by the operator was achieved by putting the filling equipment under laminar airflow units. Manual interventions, operators operating directly over open product, uncontrolled airflow patterns and frequent sterility test failures, and media fill failures were common then.

It was widely acknowledged that the concept of isolators for aseptic filling was nearly immediately understandable, while the design concepts and ways of operation for RABS were somewhat more difficult to understand. Several attempts were made to exactly define RABS, some of them creating perhaps more confusion than actually helping to understand the technology.

In 2005, triggered by a request from the US Food and Drug Administration, a group of industrial professionals within ISPE (International Society of Pharmaceutical Engineering) worked out a concise definition of RABS (1). The main building blocks of this definition were the following:

- Rigid wall enclosure
- ISO 5 unidirectional airflow environment
- Gloves for set-up and interventions
- Automation of the process wherever possible
- Sterilization of all equipment
- High-level disinfection (i.e., sporicidal disinfection)
- Rare open-door interventions

The open-door interventions need to be under a defined protocol with line cleaning/line clearance and local sanitization. The appropriate documentation for this intervention is also mandatory. When this definition was published, the debate continued on the inclusion of "rare open-door interventions." This was seen as a way out of proper aseptic technology, allowing for inclusion of bad practices.

In this chapter, an attempt is made to define the different variants of RABS in a more appropriate manner.

Passive RABS–Active RABS

The terms "passive" and "active" RABS refer to the way in which the RABS air supply is designed within the core aseptic area. Generally, a passive RABS has air supply through HEPA filters that are part of the clean room (Fig. 1) (2).

For a passive RABS to work properly, the HEPA-filter surface has to be larger than that of the machine. This is due to the open space between the top of the machine cover and the filter surface. If this is fully aligned, air ingress from class B cannot be avoided due to the Venturi effect.

An active RABS has air supply through HEPA filters, which are integrated into the ceiling of the machine barrier (Fig. 2) (2).

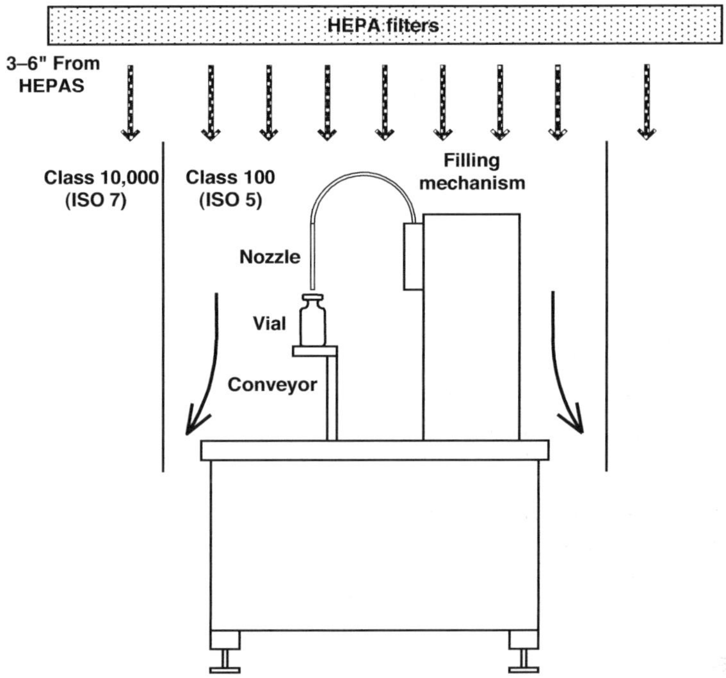

Figure 1 RABS (Passive) Restricted Access Barrier System. *Source*: From Ref. 2.

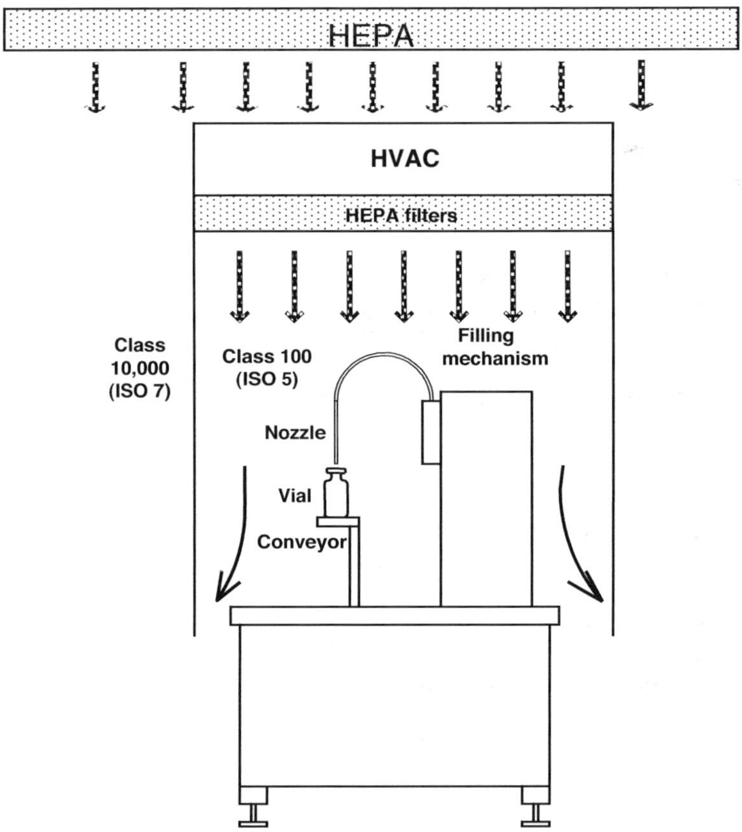

Figure 2 RABS (Active) Restricted Access Barrier System. *Source*: From Ref. 2.

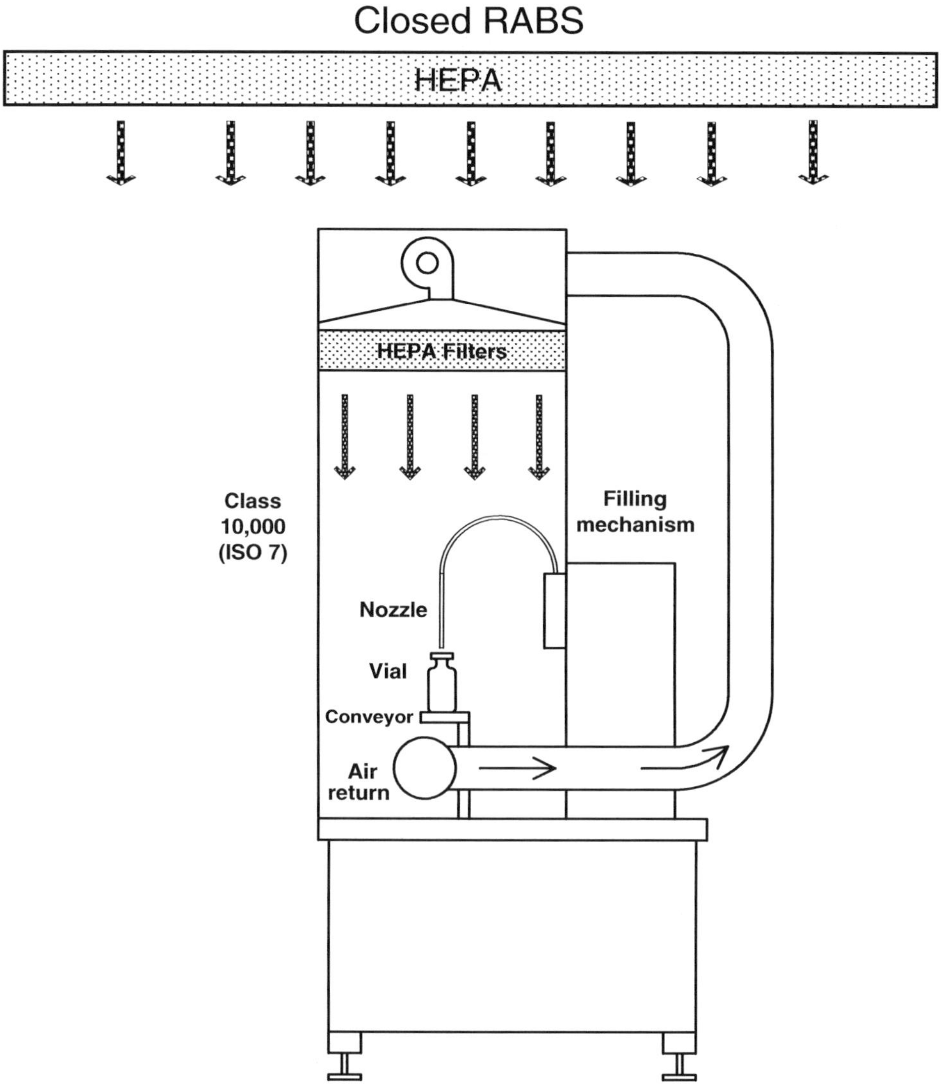

Figure 3 RABS (Closed) Restricted Access Barrier System. *Source*: From Ref. 2.

Open RABS–Closed RABS

The terms "open" and "closed" RABS refer to the manner in which the airflow at the bottom of the machine is designed. An "open" RABS therefore is a RABS where the air spills over into the room and is recirculated into the room heating, ventilation and air conditioning (HVAC) system through central return air channels.

A "closed" RABS has the air recirculated into the HVAC system that is part of the machine. Air overspill into the room is avoided through hermetic seals. This brings a closed RABS almost to the level of an isolator, but usually without automatic decontamination (Fig. 3) (2).

RABS for Containment

A RABS used for the filling of highly potent drugs where operator protection becomes equally important as product protection can be designed by adding clean-in-place equipment.

Operation of a RABS

All of the above-mentioned RABS variants can be operated as a best-practice RABS where open-door interventions are strictly prohibited. When this is combined with frequent high-level disinfection, proper aseptic technique and monitoring, a very safe and robust process is achieved.

CONCLUSIONS

As always, product requirements, dosage forms, and economic considerations have to be aligned when a new filling room is designed. Following the original ISPE–RABS definition and combining it with the simple distinctions between active/passive and open/closed RABS, one should easily come to the right conclusions as the design and operation of RABS.

REFERENCES

1. Lysfjord J, et al. Restricted access barrier system (RABS) for aseptic processing. Pharm Eng 2005; 25(6):116–117, 120.
2. Lysfjord J. Aseptic Processing: Advancements in Manufacturing—RABS & Isolators. PDA Conference on Risk Management, Bethesda, MD, May 15–16, 2008.

9 Rapid transfer port system: the key element for contained enclosures in advanced aseptic processing

Brigitte Lechiffre and David Barbault

INTRODUCTION

Contamination is an important consideration in risk analysis in classical aseptic processing areas. Open processes, which require direct human intervention, represent a greater risk for contamination than closed processes. As a matter of fact, implementation of isolator technology has dramatically reduced the impact of the contaminated surrounding environment upon the critical zone of aseptic processing. Although isolators when properly validated and operated can reduce risk from environmental contamination to a level approaching zero, the transfer of materials (Fig. 1) in and out of an isolator [or other types of separative technologies such as restricted access barrier system (RABS)] represents the most probable reason for the loss of separative enclosure environmental integrity. The more secure the transfer system, the less threatening the external environment becomes, and therefore, results in more effective risk management.

RAPID TRANSFER PORT

The most commonly used double-door transfer port system is the well-known rapid transfer port (RTP) extensively developed by La Calhène in the 1960s for the movement of highly toxic radioactive materials between process glove boxes and cells. This device marketing under the name DPTE®—*Double Porte de Transfert Etanche* in French—was adopted for use in biological and pharmaceutical manufacturing and testing in the 1980s and remains in wide use today.

RTP designs with interlock systems provide the safest systems for tight, sealable, and reliable transfers that are not operator dependent. The RTP is considered the key element in the development of isolators for aseptic processing and containment applications. The DPTE® transfer port system has become an industry standard worldwide and is a key element in the development of pharmaceutical isolators to address the need for containment and protection against contamination.

The patenting of the DPTE® system (Fig. 2) by La Calhène was followed by the development of several different transfer systems for isolator applications, all using the same original concept. Two types of RTP systems are available in the market: the most common one is the rotating docking systems that are supplied by La Calhène, CRL, ACE, Ingénia, and Ostermeier. These RTPs are based on the mechanical interaction of two separate units—an "alpha" flange that is static and typically mounted on an isolator wall—Fig. 3) and a "beta" that is mounted on a mobile transfer device of many possible designs and functions. Each RTP is composed of three major parts, which are the flange, the door, and the seal. The major differences among the different vendor designs are concentrated in the different seal mechanical features and available sizes, which are typically given as opening diameter.

Another RTP system developed in the 1990s by IDC is a nonrotating system known as the Biosafe® port system. It is based on a magnetic connection and is available in only one diameter.

It is vital that any user contemplating the specification and use of RTPs consider such variables as size requirements, maintenance, testing, and customer support. Among the key considerations in customer support are technical data supporting safe use of the RTP system, regulatory compliance information, and perhaps validation support.

SAFE, STERILE, AND CONTAINED ASEPTIC TRANSFERS

Aseptic processing areas such as isolators or RABS must comply with stringent regulations. US Food and Drug Administration (FDA) Guidance for Industry, Sterile Drug Products Produced

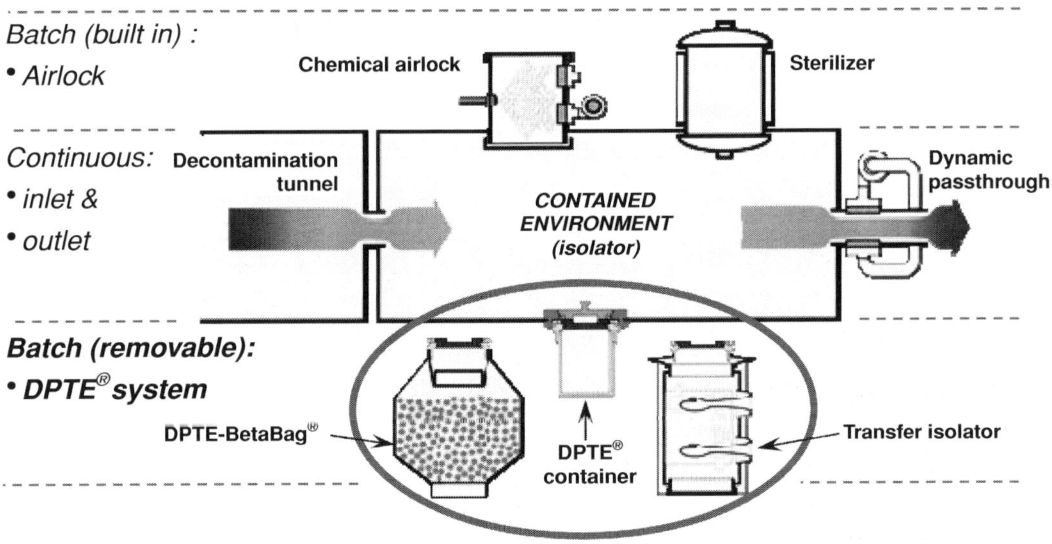

Figure 1 Various transfer systems on isolator. *Source*: From Getinge La Calhène.

by Aseptic Processing—Current Good Manufacturing Practice, September 2004, clearly states that the "integrity of a decontaminated isolator can be affected and impacted by the design of transfer ports" and that some RTPs may have "significant limitations, including marginal decontaminating capability." The choice of an RTP design must be considered at an early stage in an aseptic processing project. A RTP alpha flange must be mounted on the enclosure or barrier in a manner that ensures that its seal surface can decontaminated during the sporicidal treatment of the enclosure with vapor-phase hydrogen peroxide or another agent chosen by the

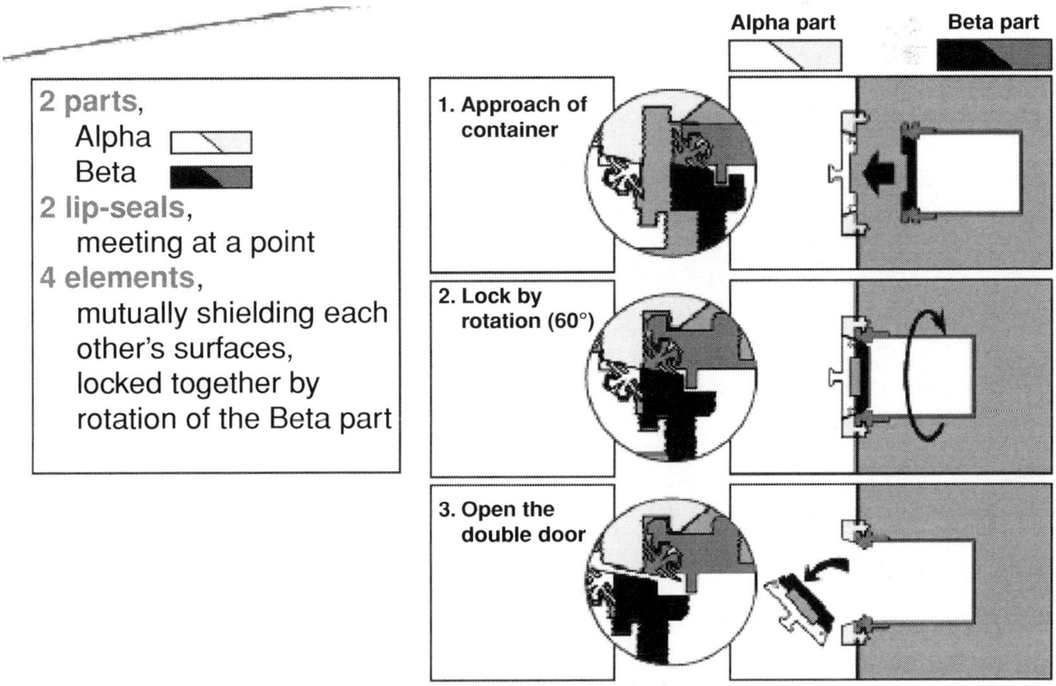

Figure 2 DPTE® principle. *Source*: From Getinge La Calhène.

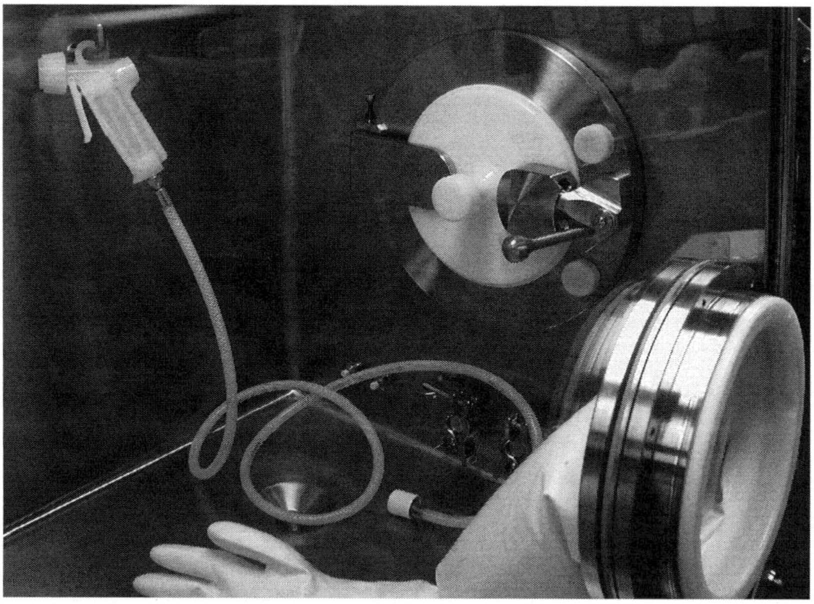

Figure 3 DPTE® alpha part. *Source*: From Getinge La Calhène.

user. The use of a so-called "false" or "dummy" beta container, which allows contact of gas or vapor decontaminating agents with the RTP seal whereas at the same time containing the agent for environmental safety is therefore compulsory.

Dry-heat sterilization and ultraviolet light decontamination have been used to address the seal decontamination issue, which is commonly called the "ring of uncertainty." However, these secondary decontamination systems require additional proof of concept and validation. Therefore it remains far more common to use a dummy container during decontamination, rather than adding an often complex secondary decontamination process. Further production of the seal area (ring of uncertainty) can be accomplished by using a protective chute or sleeve that covers the seal during transfer. Of course the user should have well-written procedures describing the use of protective chutes/sleeves; in addition, some users have chosen to add a tertiary level of risk management that involves periodic manual treatment of the seal ring using gloves mounted on the isolator/barrier.

In the late 1990s, La Calhène performed extensive validation of their DPTE® transfer system; the system was challenged with airborne suspension of microorganisms under defined "worst-case" conditions. Bacterial contamination release was measured during intensive use of DPTE® in an enclosure where the pressure gradient was opposite to the normal positive pressure gradient within the isolator. These validation studies revealed that the tight mechanical tolerances, the correct overlapping of the surface, and leaktightness performances of the system were factors that effectively prevented penetration of bacteria under "worst-case" evaluative conditions.

In addition, La Calhène evaluated the containment ratio or efficiency ratio of DPTE®, that is, the level of particulate contamination released when using a DPTE® in an environment with a known level of contamination. By using "worst-case" conditions favoring contamination, the test study challenge features included uranine injection, a differential pressure of 120 Pa between two enclosures, and transfer sequences comprised 15 and 30 transfers. In addition, both stainless steel and polyethylene DPTE® containers were used in the study. Swab tests on the DPTE® alpha part seal and continuous air sampling methods were used on DPTE® container seal to evaluate the efficiency of the seal system under these worst-case challenge conditions. The results established that the containment or efficiency ratio for the DPTE® system was 6.10^6 $\pm$ 30% and that compared to an HEPA filter of 99.999% efficiency for 0.3 μm particulates, this

RTP provided filtering coefficient of 10^5. Therefore, one can easily see that the risk generated by a DPTE® RTP is significantly lower than that of a "five nines" HEPA filter.

RTPS APPLICATIONS IN ADVANCED ASEPTIC PROCESSING

The applications of RTPs in advanced aseptic processing are quite extensive. Dimensions of the RTP must be appropriate to the required manipulations and transfers. For most of the projects, mock-up studies are a "must" to evaluate all steps and ergonomics of the production process. Selecting an RTP type is also a crucial step as the RTP is a critical part of the production process that may cause issues if the functionality is not perfectly reliable and if it does not fulfil the required specifications for transfer. The RTP should be viewed not just as a component but as a key function of an enclosure—RABS, isolator, or even clean room. In fact, RTP items can be complemented by various accessories to make working conditions easier for the operator. Among the various RTP systems, Getinge La Calhène's DPTE® port system provides the widest range, with accessories, and represents the most advanced technology available on the market today.

MATERIAL AND SMALL EQUIPMENT TRANSFER

Filling machine pumping and dosing systems can commonly be sterilized in place using cleaning in place–sterilization in place (CIP–SIP) methodology. However, for some types of production, such as biotechnology, vaccines, and cytotoxics, pharmaceutical manufacturers may perform cleaning and sterilization of critical parts outside the machine and enclosure in view of the cross-contamination risk. Sterilization is performed in a steam autoclave with autoclavable containers of large dimensions, commonly 270 or 350 mm nominal diameter. Autoclavable RTP-equipped containers (Fig. 4) can be fitted with dedicated accessories such as rails with supports with a smooth finish to be compliant with requisite cleanliness and sterilization levels. Stainless steel autoclavable containers are also commonly used to transfer all kinds of small items of equipment required, monitoring devices, etc., when the aseptic processing area is not in direct interface with an autoclave. In some specific cases, outlets of the enclosure are also managed via stainless

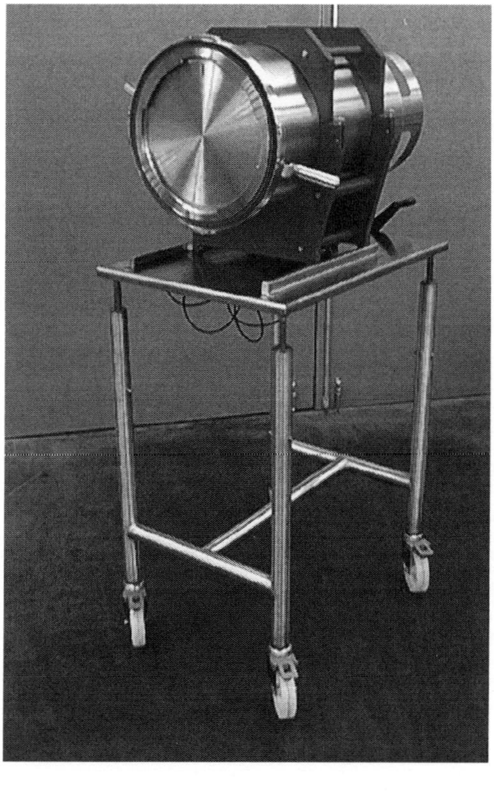

Figure 4 DPTE® autoclavable container on mobile transportation trolley. *Source*: From Getinge La Calhène.

steel containers, that is, waste, rejects, and production samples. Autoclavable containers provide flexibility for the producer and RTP manufacturers have made some major improvements in recent years including weight reduction for stainless steel units, adding rollers to reduce the docking torque, supplying internal perforated baskets, etc., to make usage much easier for operators. In the case of large and heavy RTP containers, mobile transportation trolleys are a useful dedicated accessory that is nearly compulsory in docking situations for larger items.

STERILE LIQUIDS

For the transfer of sterile liquids into the aseptic processing area, it is common when dealing with large production volumes to use fixed piping directly connected to the filling machine. This typically includes a filter skid, filling reservoir, and surge vessel, all of which can be CIP–SIP treated in a process that generally also includes filling pumps and nozzles. In the case of multiple products and/or small batches, pharmaceutical manufacturers may instead introduce the sterile liquid via a RTP container directly linked to a buffer tank that has been previously CIP–SIP or cleaned/sterilized out of place. The RTP guarantees the required flexibility and sterility assurance. In the case of autoclave sterilization, RTP container design and dedicated internal accessory enable the product sterilization filter, hose, and nozzle to be sterilized together with the filling piping (Fig. 5). Such RTP containers are mainly designed in small dimensions—105 or 190 nominal diameters—and can be equipped with various types of inner baskets and supports.

Currently, RTP containers meant for liquid product transfer (Fig. 6) are customized to meet the end user's requirements arising from a range of variables including length of pipes, number of pipes, and fitting diameters that will affect the container diameter and length as well as the corresponding accessories.

When SIP sterilization is preferred, RTP containers are designed to meet Pressure Equipment Directive 97/23/EC in EU and thus need to be equipped with pressure covers during the sterilization cycle. Two types of pressure covers are available: the simple pressure cover that is positioned onto the RTP door of the container and will avoid any movement of the door and the seal, and the lifting pressure cover (Fig. 7) that will also disengage the beta door and allow a flow of steam between the beta door and seal; the latter is considered by the industry as the "state-of-the art" system to eliminate potentially occluded zones at the gasket during the sterilization process. These pressure covers are commonly used on stopper processing systems fitted with RTPs.

It is increasingly common to consider the requirements for disposable systems for the transfer of highly toxic products or small volumes in biotechnology production and therefore avoid the costly validation and processes as well as the time-consuming cleaning and sterilization steps required for re-useable equipment. Several products are on the market to meet

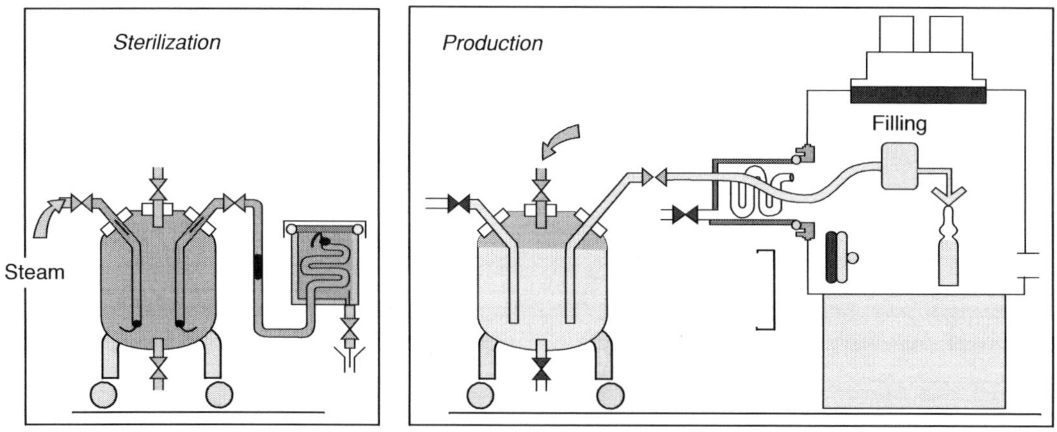

Figure 5 Example of SIP DPTE® container on mobile vessel *Source*: From Getinge La Calhène.

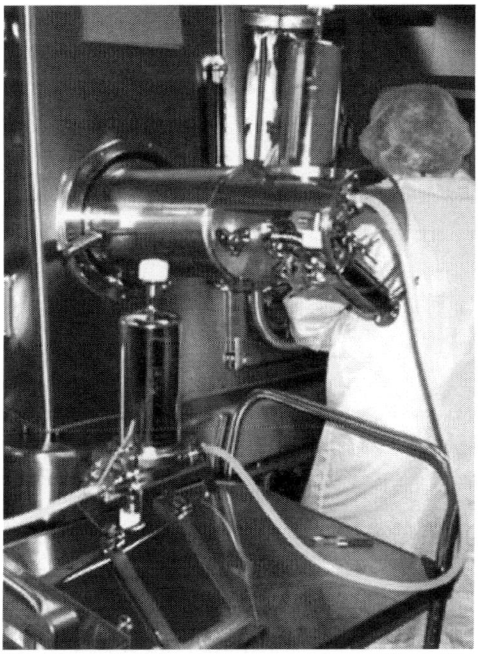

Figure 6 DPTE® container for liquid transfer. *Source*: From Getinge La Calhène.

an increasing demand, such as the Biosafe® and SART system from Sartorius Stedim, PALL Kleenpak sterile connectors and the DPTE-BetaBag® system from GETINGE La Calhène.

INTERFACE CONTAINERS

The same containment and sterility assurance requirements exist when the aseptic enclosure must be interfaced with either a formulation tank or process equipment such as stopper processing systems. In this case, the tank will need to be equipped with a beta part. The sterilization method—SIP or autoclave—will determine the choice of beta part; if SIP is used then a pressure cover is required.

These large tanks or containers require proper and safe connections to the sterile enclosure. Depending upon the product type, the operator, the product, or both must be protected. Again in this case the transfer between the environments must be secured using RTPs. However, simple RTPs will not be compatible in such situations. For such specific applications, the so-called "DPTE® alpha rotating system" (Fig. 8) was developed and introduced about 15 years ago. This type of RTP allows for rotation of the alpha flange instead of the typical rotation of the beta flange as a normal condition of use. In addition, flexibility for approach and insertion was

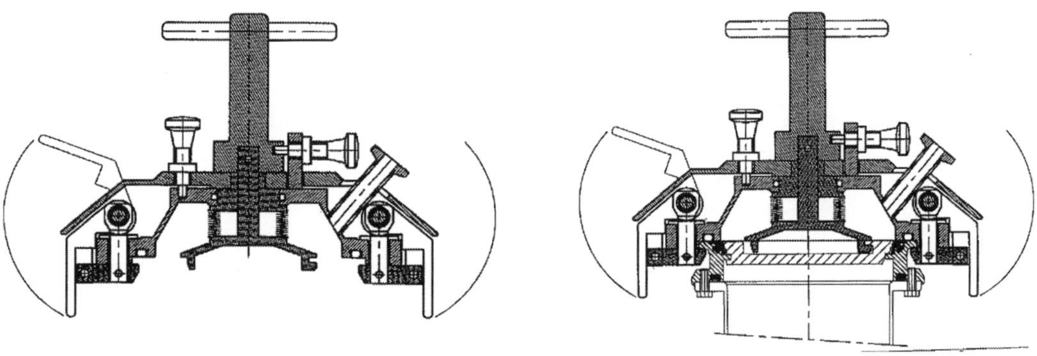

Figure 7 Lifting cover pressure for DPTE® container. *Source*: From Getinge La Calhène.

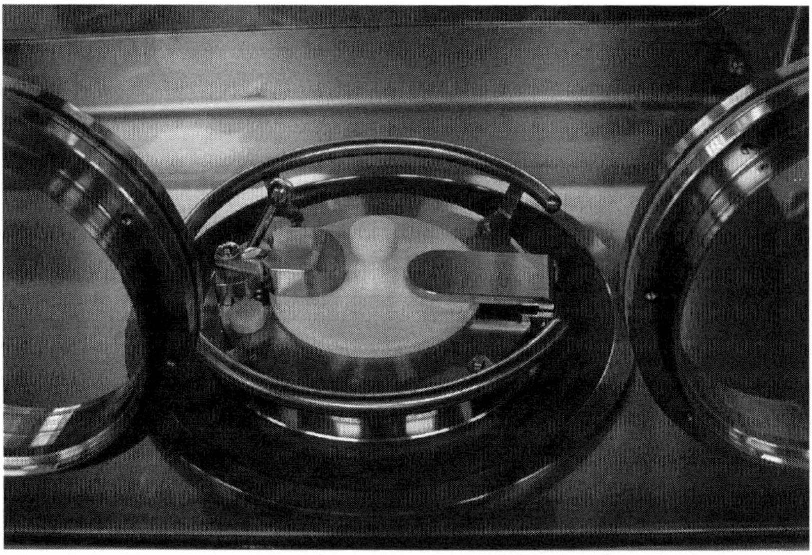

Figure 8 DPTE® alpha with rotating system. *Source*: From Getinge La Calhène.

a necessity; thus the use of flexible EPDM or silicone membranes was developed and became the preferred solution.

For some specific applications, RTP manufacturers have developed an "automatic RTP door" to avoid the need for an operator to use a glove merely to open the RTP door after the beta part has been docked. Although the idea appears to be potentially advantageous as a result of time savings, reduced enclosure space, and reduced risk of contamination from glove manipulation, this feature has not come into wide use. This is likely because another manual intervention is typically required anyway, such as the fitting of a chute, the opening of the inner sleeve, and the transfer of components, for example.

SOLIDS AND CLOSURES

The production of parenterals in vials or syringes requires the introduction into the filling line of presterilized closures such as tip caps for blow fill seal vials, stoppers and caps for vials and pistons, or plungers for syringes, cartridges, or pens.

For syringes and vials, H_2O_2 sterilization tunnels are commonly used. Electron beam technology can be applied for the introduction of prefilled syringes in tubs.

Closures are either steam sterilized at the vendor's production site in their own moist heat sterilization systems or gamma irradiated at a contract radiation sterilization firm. In the case of steam sterilized items, two different solutions have proven effective, depending upon the closure quantities required, handling necessities, the manufacturer's preference to outsource stopper preparation prior to sterilization or both preparation and sterilization.

The first option is processing in bulk quantities. Closures are received raw or prerinsed in bags and the manufacturer will manage their complete treatment locally, that is, have them cleaned, depyrogenated, siliconized, sterilized, and dried in a closed processing system. These closure processing systems can be directly linked to the filling machine and allow direct feeding of closures. In this case, the supply tank of the closure processing unit is connected to the filling line either by a fixed connection or via an RTP. This approach is often chosen for high-throughput production lines as well as those used for campaign style manufacturing.

Sometimes the producer has a single closure processing system for the treatment of all their closures to be distributed to several filling lines of different generations. In these circumstances, the treated sterile closures are discharged via an interface isolator and packed into simple bags that are then relocated to the appropriate filling lines and transferred in a traditional manner, that is, opening doors and pouring the closures into the feeding bowl. More commonly now, due to current good manufacturing practices requirements, simple bags are being replaced by

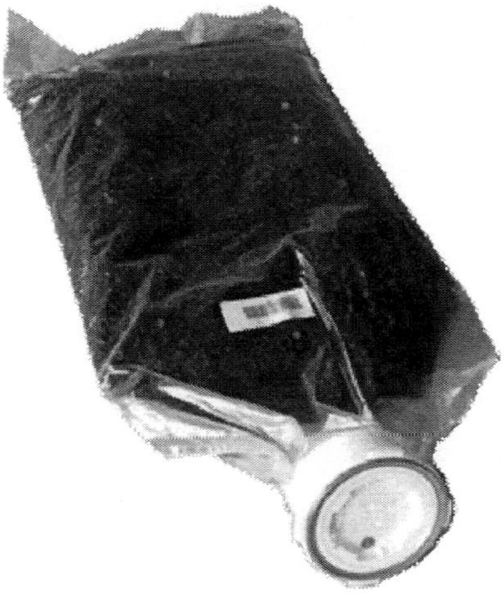

Figure 9 DPTE-BetaBag® filled with stoppers. *Source*: From Getinge La Calhène.

port-bags such as presterilized empty DPTE-BetaBag® units that can be docked onto the alpha part of various aseptic filling lines.

The second option is ready-to-sterilize (RTS) or ready-to-use (RTU) closures. Closures and more widely, stoppers of all kinds, are packed by the closure manufacturer into the appropriate port-bags either with Tyvek® or polyethylene bags fitted with an RTP. Tyvek® bags fitted with an RTP and filled with stoppers are delivered to the pharmaceutical producer. They are called RTS port-bags because the pharmaceutical producer needs only to perform and validate the steam sterilization at his production site. With polyethylene bags fitted with an RTP and filled with closures, the closure manufacturer is also responsible for the gamma irradiation of a whole batch of port-bags. The closure vendor also assumes responsibility for the stopper quality, the high quality packaging, the port-bags integrity and the validation of the sterilization of a full batch. In this case, stoppers are delivered RTU because the pharmaceutical producer has chosen a full package product service, that is, high cleanliness level for stoppers (several cleaning steps, appropriate siliconization, etc.), proven packaging and transfer technology, and validation package. They can use the stoppers directly in the various production areas with no need for any preparation step.

There are two port-bag systems currently used for the transfer of closures into isolator or RABS aseptic filling lines and more significantly for pistons for syringes and stoppers for vials: Biosafe® port-bag and DPTE-BetaBag® (Fig. 9).

These port-bag systems allow for safe material transfers and avoid the risk of cross contamination. The port-bag or BetaBag systems have a good track record for safe performance and are widely used in a number of validated aseptic production lines.

POWDER TRANSFER

The safe and aseptic transfer of powder, sterile and/or toxic, is increasingly a requirement in the fine chemical and pharmaceutical industries, due to the use of ever more potent drugs that have an extremely low operator exposure level (OEL) and a very high cost. The RTP is probably the only transfer system available on the market for leaktight connection of two sterile and/or toxic environments (isolators, flexible, or rigid individual bulk containers (IBC), bags, process vessels, etc.) inside a clean room. For toxic powder transfer, compared with split butterfly valves and other systems, a well-designed RTP system does not require any additional external features (vacuum protection, CIP, etc.) to reach nanogram levels of containment. Standardized measurement of equipment particulate airborne concentration (SMEPAC) tests have confirmed the ability of RTPs to obtain an OEL < 10 ng. However, to reach this very low value, the primary containment of the product line must be well designed. The RTP is not designed for direct transfer of power with the double door opened.

When powder is transferred directly, traces of powder (Fig. 10) have been found, after RTP disconnection, visually on the outside of the RTP, on the lip seals of the beta flange and

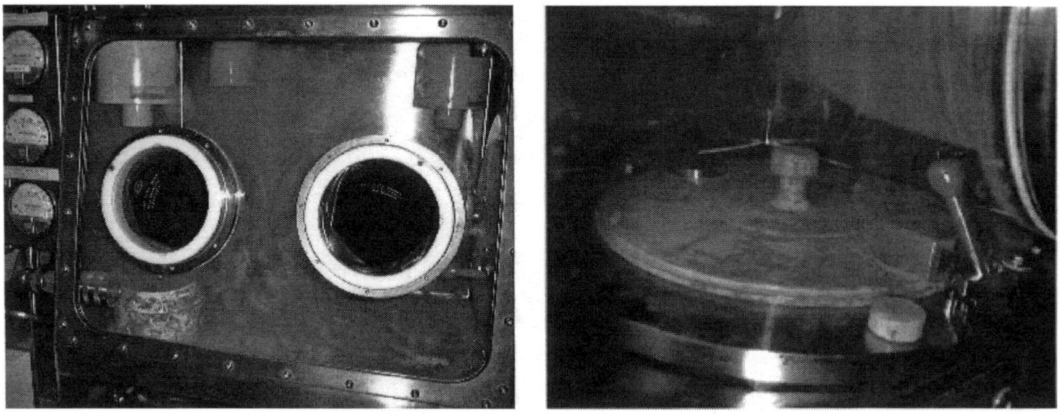

Figure 10 Example of large powder dispersion/lack of primary containment. *Source*: From Getinge La Calhène.

on other parts of the system as well. The explanation is clear: volatile powder very difficult to contain and easily dispersed, even into the "heart" of the transfer system! It is therefore essential to direct the powder flow using a primary containment feature, which can simply be a funnel or bag/inner sleeve (Fig. 11), or in the case of an IBCs connection it can be composed of a plastic or stainless steel chute with gasket and silicone to compensate for potential alignment issues (see photo).

Care must be taken with the design of the beta flange attached to the IBC or vessel, and of the corresponding chute which will fit the beta flange when the double door is opened, Also, considerable care must be taken with the corresponding "powder" gaskets, as it is of critical importance to prevent powder from reaching active parts of the RTP (from inside the isolator) and also it is critical to keep powder transferred into the IBC or vessel from backing up into the isolator and onto the active parts of the RTP. For these reasons in some cases the chute has to be fitted with an appropriate vent filter (or prefilter).

This kind of accessory has to be customized according to the process and the design of the isolator. One must carefully consider the isolator's inlet and outlet ports and connections as well. It is important to keep in mind that these details are vital to the successful completion of a project requirement a high level of containment.

The second key for a successful project is to optimize, the size of the transfer system, ideally this means keeping this system as small as possible. The smaller the gasket diameter

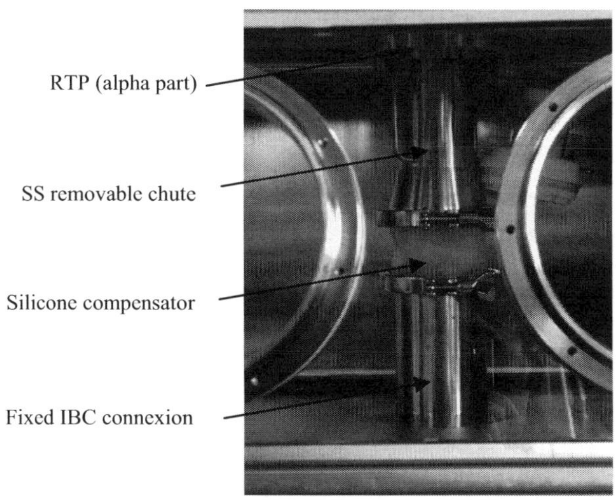

Figure 11 Primary containment example. *Source*: From Getinge La Calhène.

used, the lower the risk of leak or contamination. Experience has shown that the design of the beta flange is not just a is a critical feature for passing SMEPAC tests (see ISPE Good Practice Guide, Assessing the particulate containment performance of pharmaceutical equipment), but also a key factor in successful validation and ongoing operation.

FURTHER READING

1. FDA. Guidance for Industry, Sterile Drug Products Produced by Aseptic Processing—Current Good Manufacturing Practice. September 2004.
2. ISO 10648–2, Containment Enclosures—Part 2: classification according to leak tightness and associated checking methods.
3. Validation of sterility assurance of sterile stopper transfer using 270 and 105 mm diameter DPTE (Rapid Transfer Port) attached to a flexible film isolator. Eurostar Technology Ltd. Canterbury, UK: 1996.
4. Nottingham J, Dabard J. Evaluation of the potential bacterial contamination release from the La Calhène DPTE® rapid transfer port system when challenged with an airborne suspension of micro-organisms. PDA Congress, Basel, Switzerland, 1998.
5. DPTE® micro-biological qualification report NTA 3003/57. La Calhène, 2000.
6. DPTE® qualification report for particule contamination NTA 3003/58. La Calhène, 2000.
7. DeSantis F, Amsberry K, Folks JL, et al. Aseptic formulation and filling using isolator technology. Pharmaceutical Technology, Outsourcing Resources, 2003.
8. Friedman RL. Design of barrier isolators for aseptic processing: a GMP perspective. Pharmaceutical Engineering, March–April 1998.
9. Byrne T. The use of a RABS enclosure to provide a sterilized environment for the aseptic filling of vials. UK Parenteral Society, November 2005.
10. Assessing the particulate containment performance of pharmaceutical equipment, ISPE good practice guide, 2005.
11. FDA Guidance for Industry, Q7 A, Good Manufacturing Practice guide for Active Pharmaceutical Ingredients, August 2001.

10 Aseptic processing transfer systems

Gary Partington

An important consideration when designing an enclosure is how to enter/exit items from the enclosure. There are times when the integrity of the enclosure cannot be compromised and other times when this is not important. This chapter reviews several transfer systems from the most basic to the more complex, which can be used in aseptic and/or containment applications.

SIMPLE TRANSFER SYSTEMS

Hinged Doors

Hinged doors may be used in either aseptic or containment isolators as well as in restricted access barriers (RABs). As shown in Figure 1, this door is a simple hinged door made of stainless steel or plastic, which is opened to permit loading of the chamber prior to the task operation. It can also be used to unload the chamber after task operation, as long as the containment isolator has been thoroughly cleaned, and is safe to open or when the product is sealed in an aseptic isolator.

Often these doors are equipped with safety interlocks to prohibit the door from being opened during operations.

Similarly, the simple door in the right end (Fig. 2) is used in a RABs system to allow entry of components such as empty vials and stoppers and to exit filled and stoppered vials.

Hatchback Windows

As is the case with hinged doors, hatchback windows provide another method of loading or unloading an isolator or RABs, but provide a much larger opening to pass material or process equipment through. This type of transfer system is popular in R&D isolators in which flexibility may be required when using different types of process equipment. It is also useful in sterility testing when loading an isolator with test materials, product, media, etc., and filling machine isolators prior to operation. Hatchback windows are mainly used in aseptic isolators, but can be used on containment isolators if contact surfaces are verified as cleaned before opening the window. Hatchback windows can use inflatable and noninflatable gaskets to create the airtight seal on the isolator or RABs body. The transfer isolator shown in Figure 3 uses a hatchback window for easy loading.

Airlocks

Airlocks are typically small chambers attached to the end of the main enclosure. Airlocks use pairs of simple hinged doors that are located between the airlock and the main isolator and the airlock and the room. These doors can be interlocked such that one door cannot be opened unless the other is closed. This will help prevent exposure from/to the main chamber and the room. Airlocks are available in various sizes and often are equipped with a view window and a glove port (Fig. 4).

Airlocks can also be equipped with a pressure equilibration HEPA (high-efficiency particulate arresting) filter or its own ventilation/HEPA filtration system. Airlocks are used to enter/exit materials from the main chamber. These materials are generally larger than those that can fit within a rapid transfer ports (RTP) system, which is discussed later. Before the airlock door is opened to the outside room, the airlock must be completely cleaned of any residual potent materials so as not to expose the operators. If used in an aseptic application, the door between the chamber and the airlock cannot be opened until the airlock has been decontaminated with a sporicidal agent.

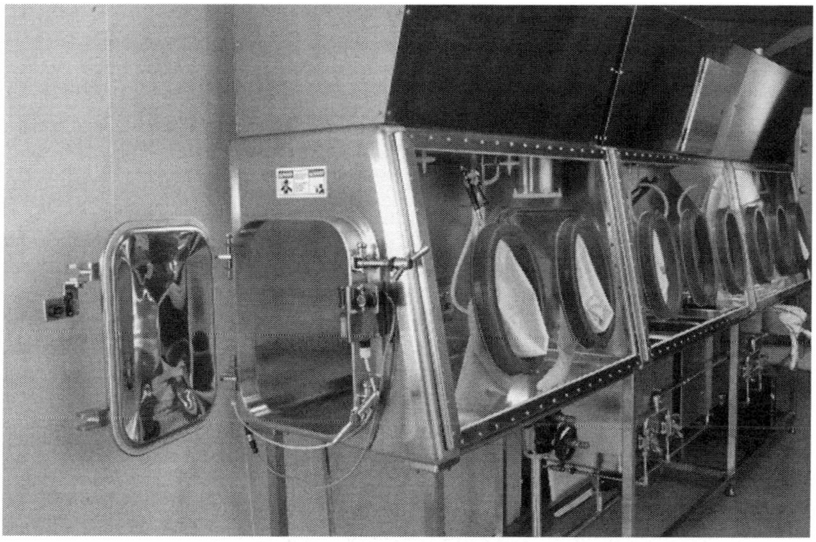

Figure 1 Hinged door. *Source*: Photo courtesy of Walker Barrier Systems.

Utility Panels

Often electrical cords for scales, mixers, stir plates, and other equipment can be passed out of the isolator through a utility panel. Similarly, vacuum, liquid, air, or other process utilities need to be brought inside the isolator. This can be done using a utility panel built into the body of the isolator. The panel is customized for the process being performed inside the isolator. The utility panel can consist of tri-clamp connections, bulkhead fittings, quick connects, hose bards, compression fittings, etc. The utility panel shown in Figure 5 shows a number of connections.

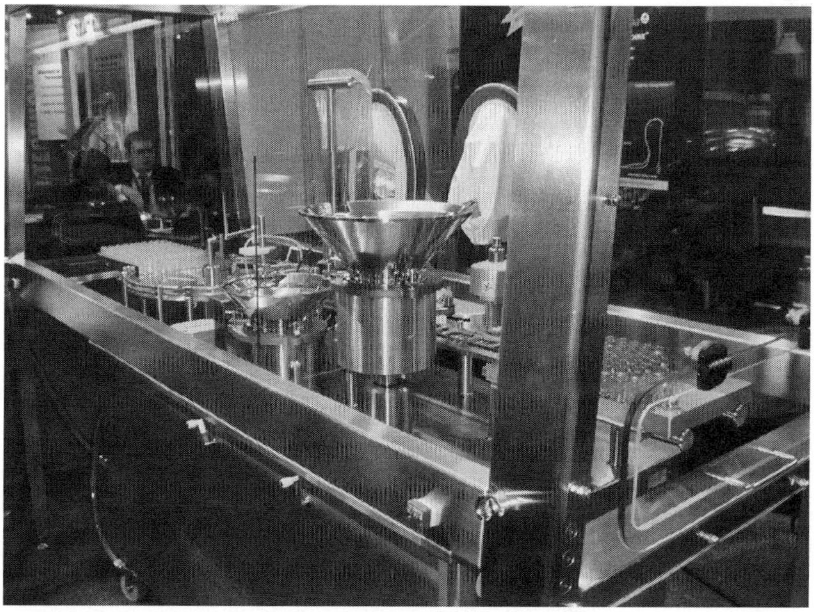

Figure 2 RABs door. *Source*: Photo courtesy of Walker Barrier Systems.

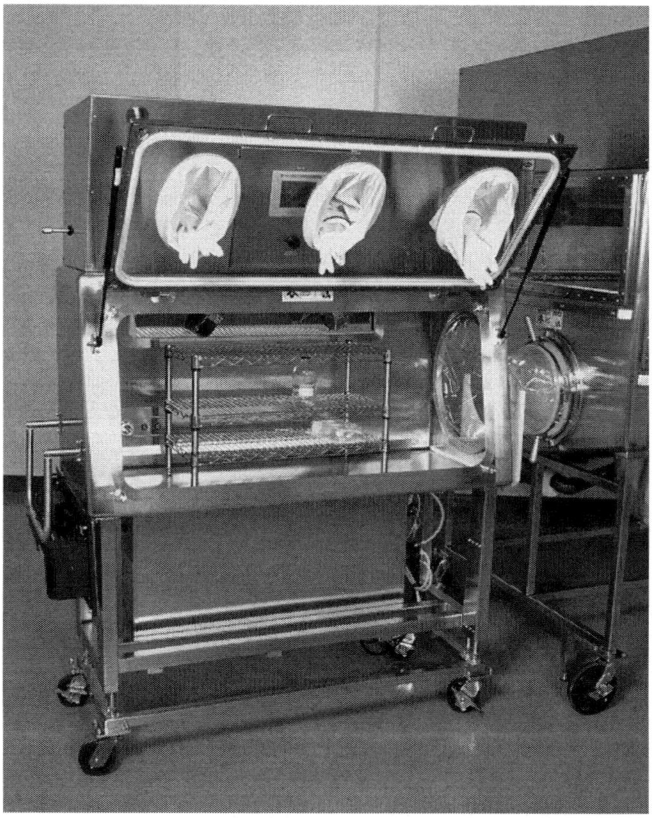

Figure 3 Hatchback window. *Source*: Photo courtesy of Walker Barrier Systems.

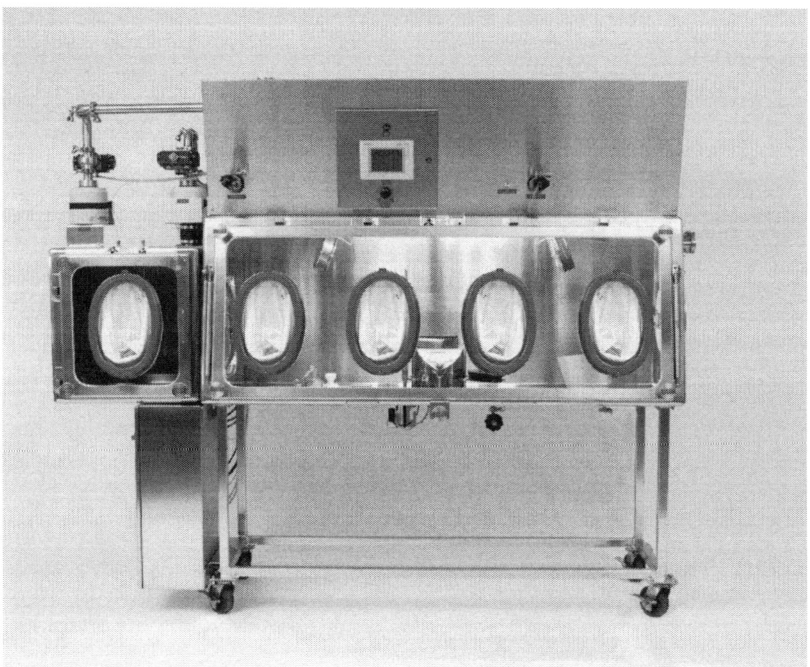

Figure 4 Airlock. *Source*: Photo courtesy of Walker Barrier Systems.

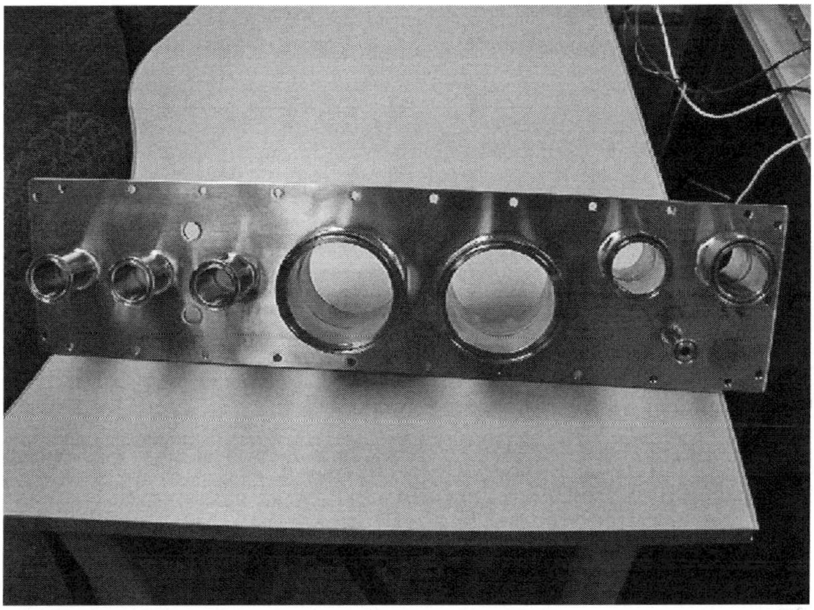

Figure 5 Utility panel. *Source*: Photo courtesy of Walker Barrier Systems.

Drum Doors and Bag Ports

A typical use for drum doors and bag ports is to connect large drums to an enclosure so that its contents can be subdivided and dispensed, under negative pressure, into smaller containers to protect the operator. As shown in Figure 6, the doors can be rather large, often 30 in. in diameter to accommodate large drums. The door needs to pivot on a hinge so that the enclosure depth can be minimized. This will allow the operator to reach the inner liner inside the drum, by using glove ports.

Drums are presented to the outside of the enclosure using a drum lift device.

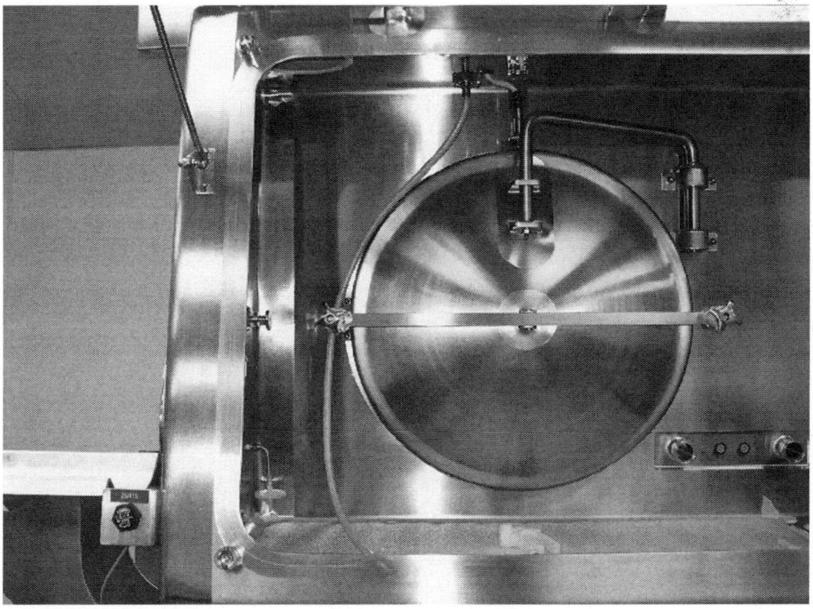

Figure 6 Drum door. *Source*: Courtesy of Walker Barrier Systems.

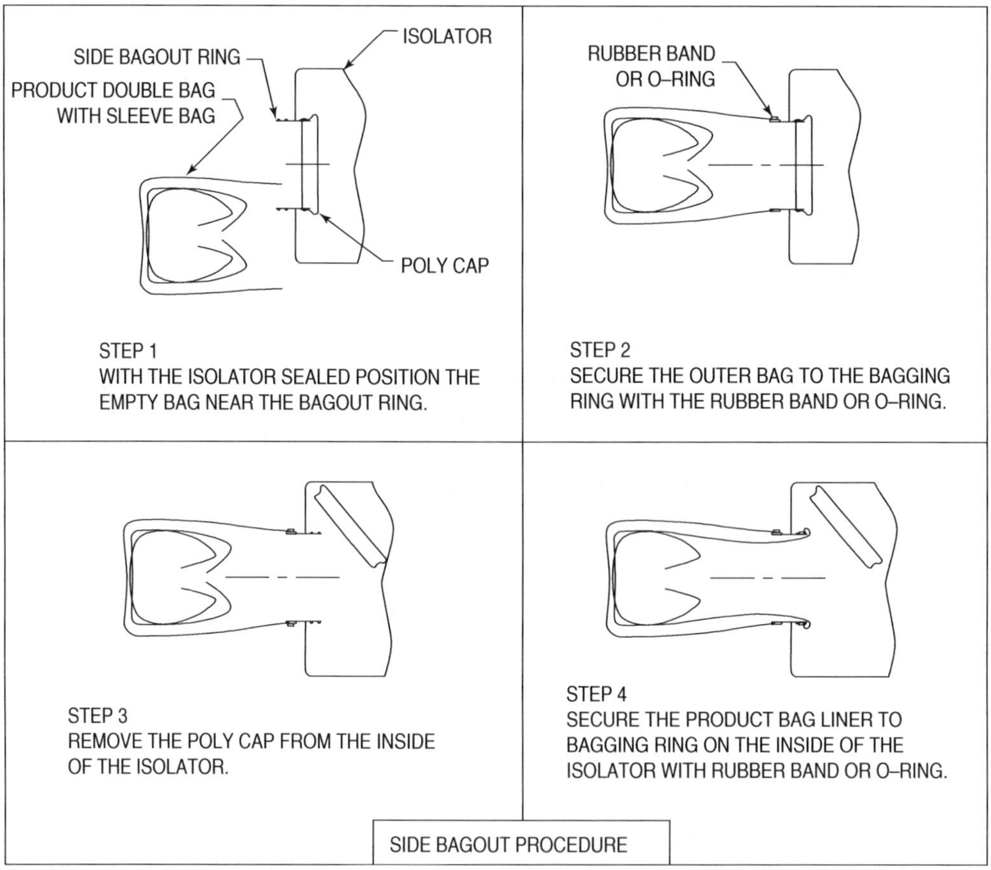

Figure 7 Bag out process drawing. *Source*: Courtesy of Walker Barrier Systems. (*Continued*)

The drum can be placed in a bag and sealed to the bag port, as shown in Figure 7, or can be sealed via an inflatable gasket inside the drum door, as shown in Figure 8.

When exiting smaller subdivided containers or product from an enclosure, smaller bag ports can be used. The procedure shown in Figure 7 can be used to remove items as well. If a drum is not used, the plastic bag can simply be sealed using a heat sealer or tie wrap method, which will seal both the bag and the resulting cap on the bag port connected to the chamber.

INTERFACE SYSTEMS

Process Equipment Interface

Parts, media, and glassware need to be entered into an aseptic enclosure without breaking the integrity of the environment. In this case, the vial tunnel, autoclave, or depyrogenation oven is directly connected and sealed to the enclosure. The process equipment are equipped with flange that is attached to the enclosure body with a gasket. Glassware is loaded into the "dirty" side opening of an oven or tunnel. After washing and/or depyrogenation, the vials enter the enclosure that has been decontaminated and is in the run mode. The door, shown in Figure 9, raises up via an air cylinder to allow vials from a tunnel to enter the enclosure where an accumulation table collects the vials. The door is sealed with an inflatable gasket during decontamination.

Pass through autoclaves are used to enter media into isolators for sterility testing. Both lab size (Fig. 10) and production size lyophilizers interface with aseptic enclosures so that loosely stoppered vials filled inside can be placed into a lyophilizer, without exposure to the outside room.

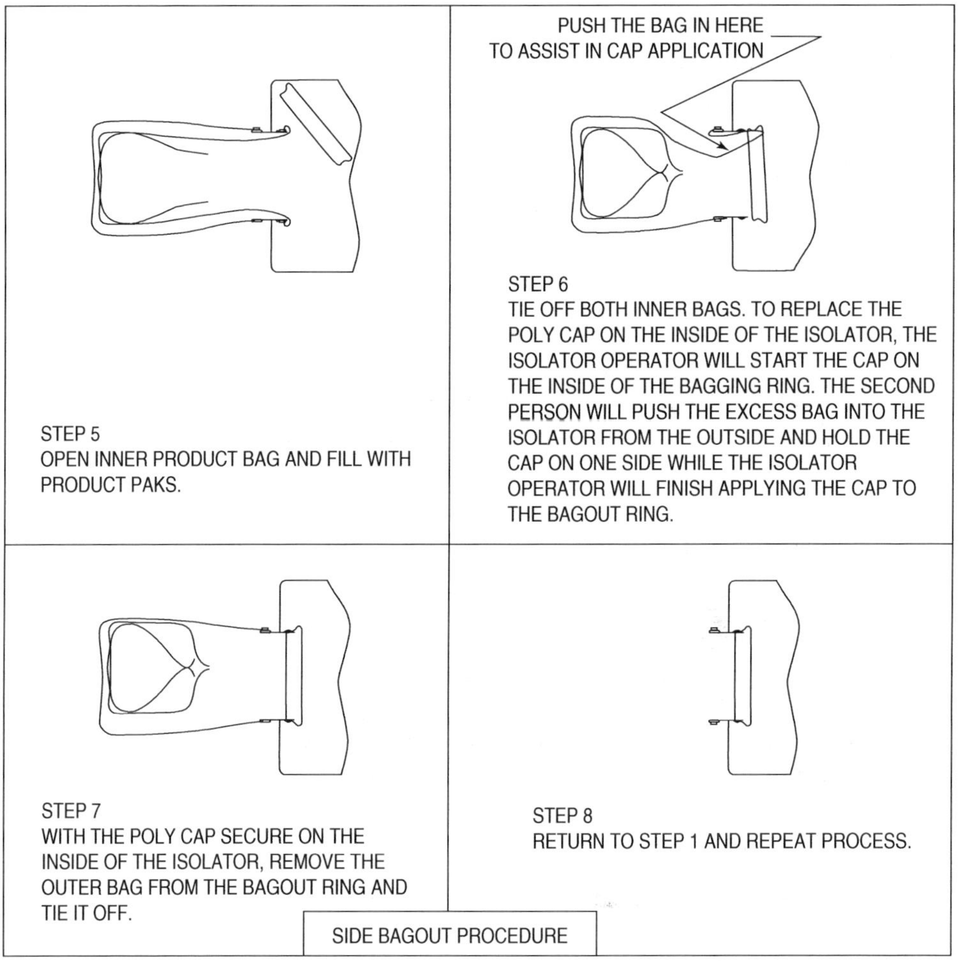

Figure 7 (*Continued*)

Other equipment such as Fitzmills (Fig. 11) and tray dryers (Fig. 12) can be interfaced to the isolator body. These are often used when processing potent powders. The mill motor and dryer heating systems are outside the isolator to prevent contamination.

SOPHISTICATED TRANSFER SYSTEMS

Split Butterfly Valves

Split butterfly valves are used primarily in containment applications. Transfer of potent powders from one area to another can be achieved using this technology. Split butterfly valves are available in various sizes and styles, with the ability to achieve operator exposure level (OEL) of <0.1 to 25 $\mu g/m^3$ (1). This is a two-part system, an active part and a passive part, each of which acts as an ordinary butterfly valve (Fig. 13). When these two parts are joined together, they form a single valve preventing any surfaces from being exposed to potent powder during the transfer. This technology can be integrated direct with process equipment. When used with an isolator, the active valve is integrated into the isolator. The passive valve is part of a container, individual bulk container (IBC), or other vessel. Product can be discharged either from the passive valve container into the isolator for weighing, milling, etc., or from the isolator into the container after it has been weighed, milled, etc.

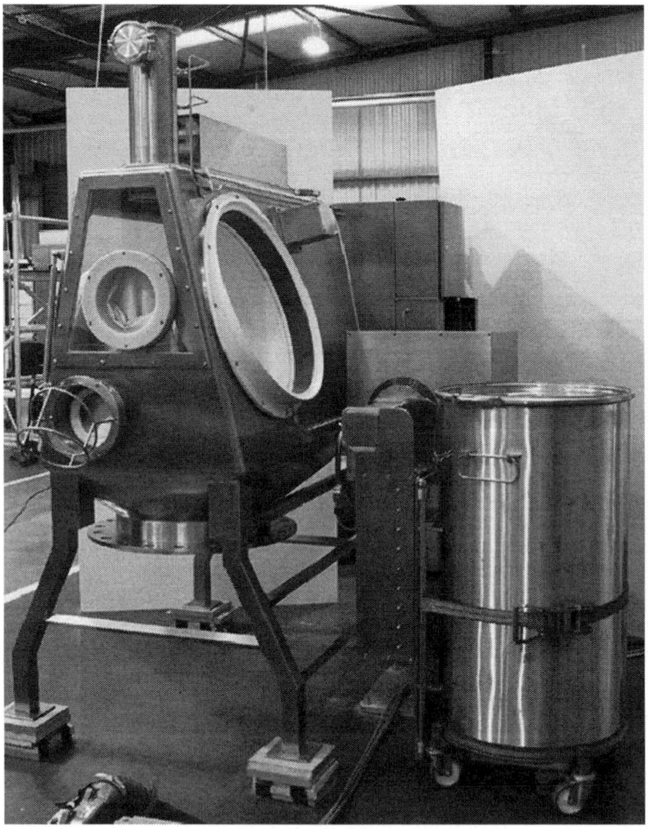

Figure 8 Inflatable drum seal. *Source*: Photo courtesy of Extract Technology.

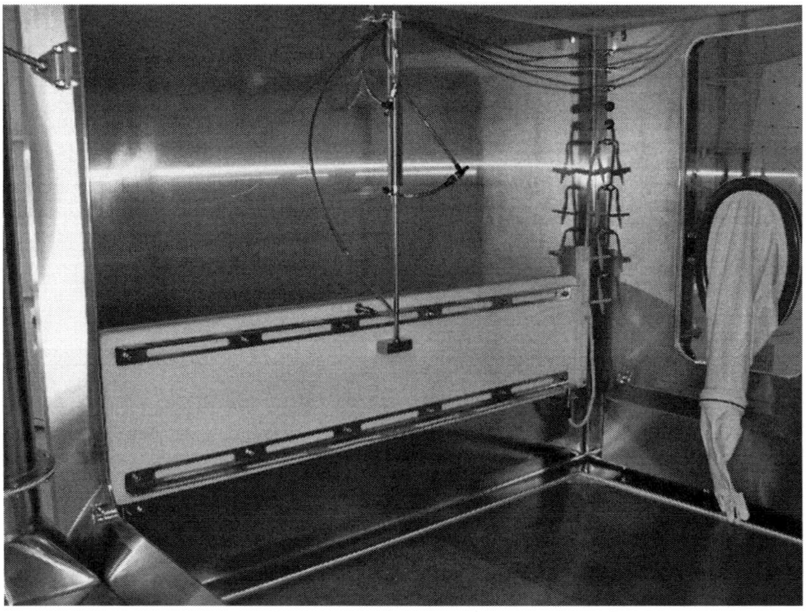

Figure 9 Vial tunnel door. *Source*: Photo courtesy of Walker Barrier Systems.

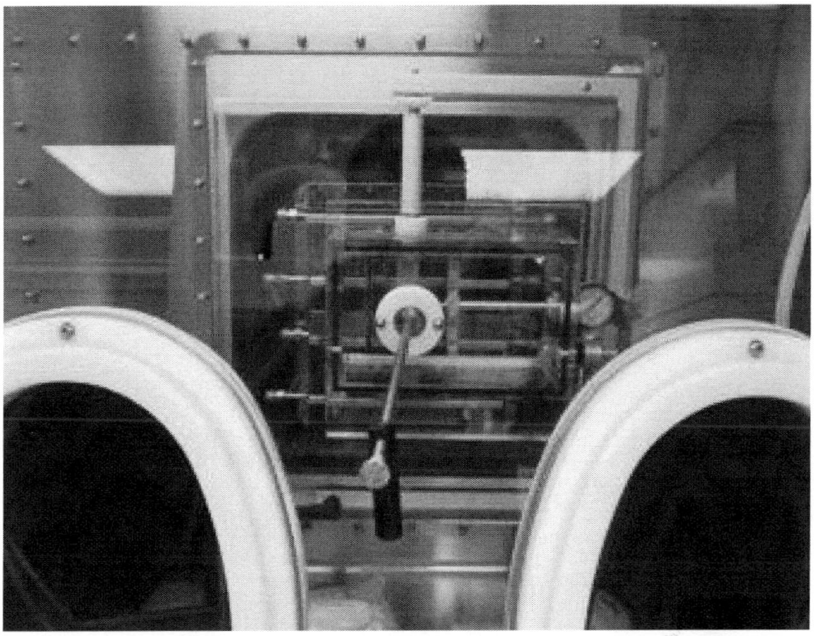

Figure 10 Lab lyophilizer isolator. *Source*: Photo courtesy of Walker Barrier Systems.

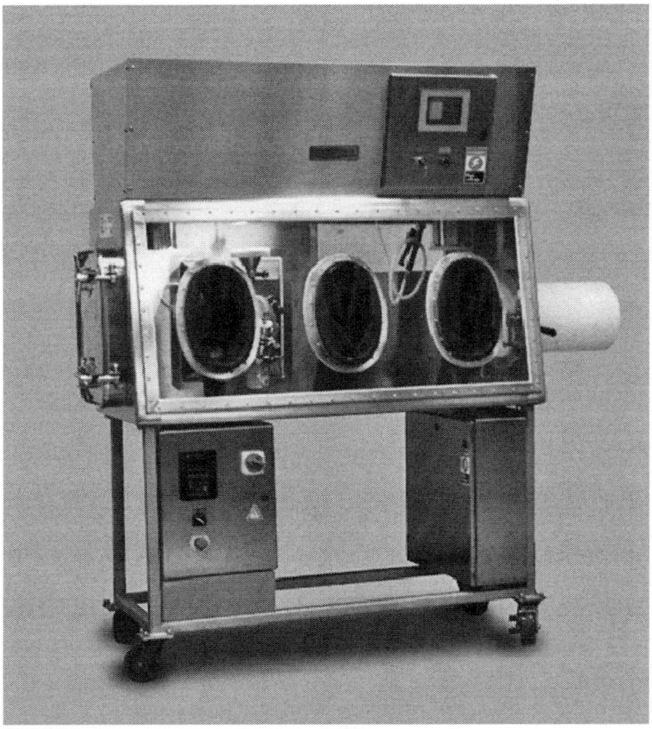

Figure 11 Mill isolator. *Source*: Photo courtesy of Walker Barrier Systems.

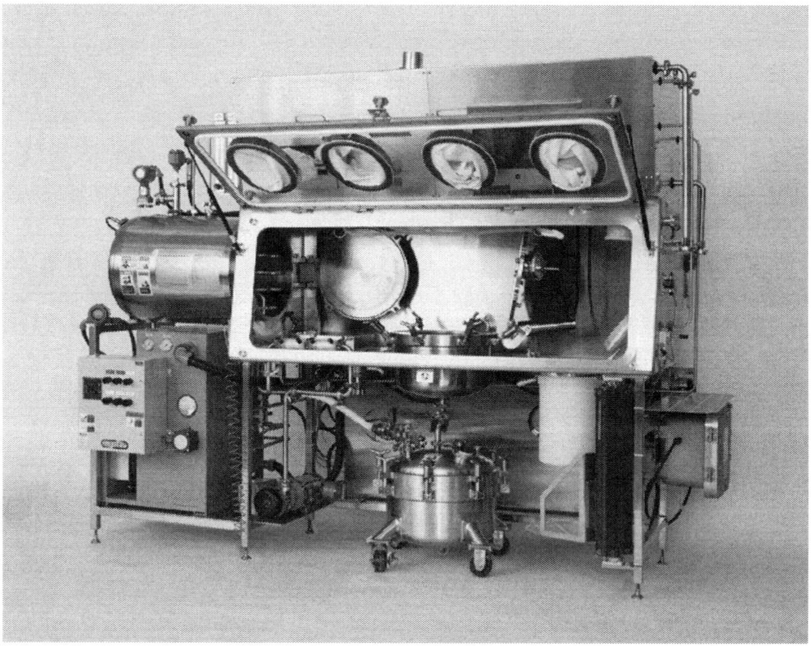

Figure 12 Tray dryer isolator. *Source*: Photo courtesy of Walker Barrier Systems.

Rapid Transfer Ports (RTP)

RTP (Fig. 14) can be used to protect both product and personnel in aseptic and containment applications. Air concentration of less than 1 $\mu g/m^3$ has been recorded using the RTP transfer system (2). The RTP system is made of the two parts typically called the alpha flange and beta flange. Diameters of the most popular RTP are 105 mm, 190 mm, 270 mm, 350 mm and some at 460 mm. Materials of construction are polyethylene or polypropylene and stainless steel.

The alpha flange (Fig. 15) is generally mounted on the body of the enclosure.

Depending on the process being performed within the enclosure, the alpha flange can be mounted in the floor, end wall, or ceiling. The beta flange (Fig. 16) can be connected to a transfer isolator or a container or to a piece of process equipment such as an IBC or tank. The beta flange is connected to the alpha flange by lining up the tabs in the beta flange to the slots in the alpha flange (Fig. 17).

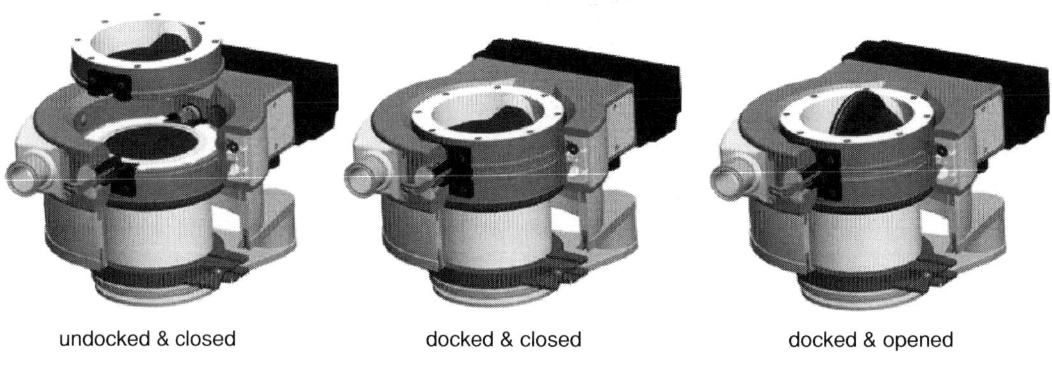

Figure 13 Split butterfly valve. *Source*: Photo courtesy of GEA Pharma Systems.

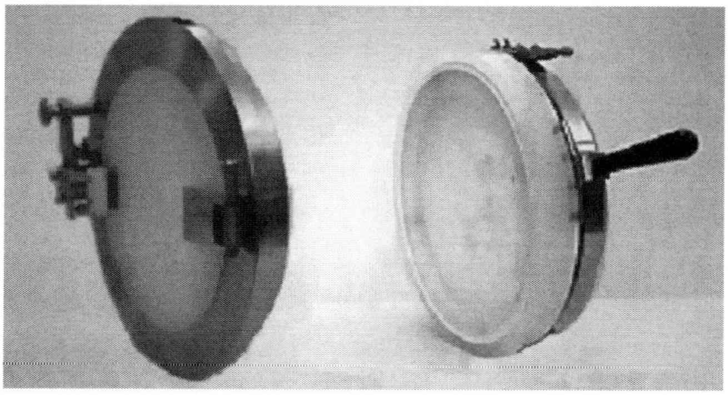

Figure 14 Rapid transfer ports. *Source*: Photo courtesy of Central Research Laboratories.

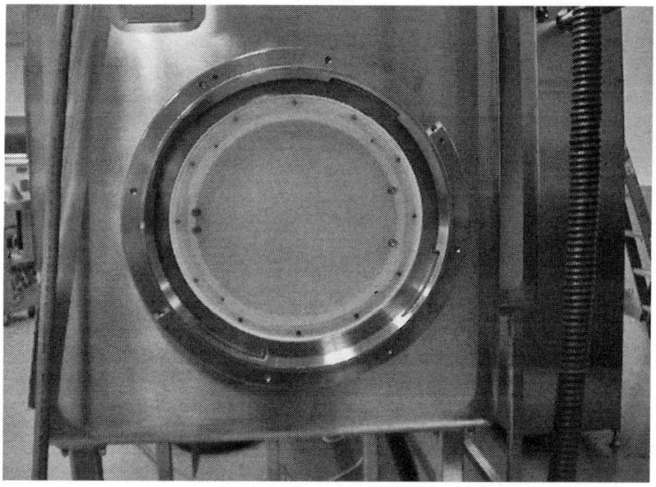

Figure 15 Alpha flange. *Source*: Photo courtesy of Walker Barrier Systems.

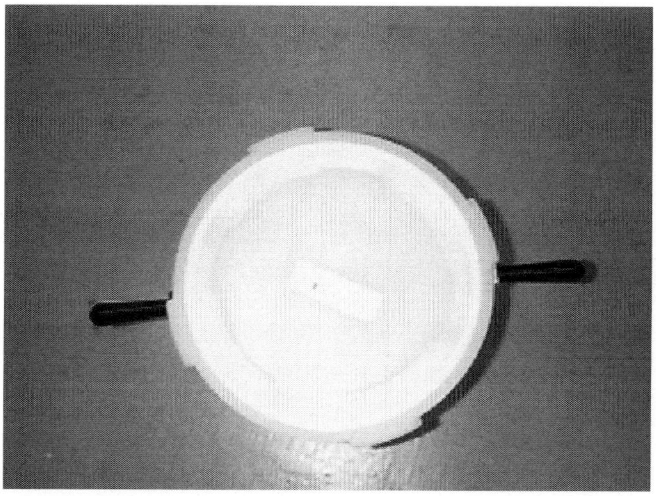

Figure 16 Beta flange. *Source*: Photo courtesy of Walker Barrier Systems.

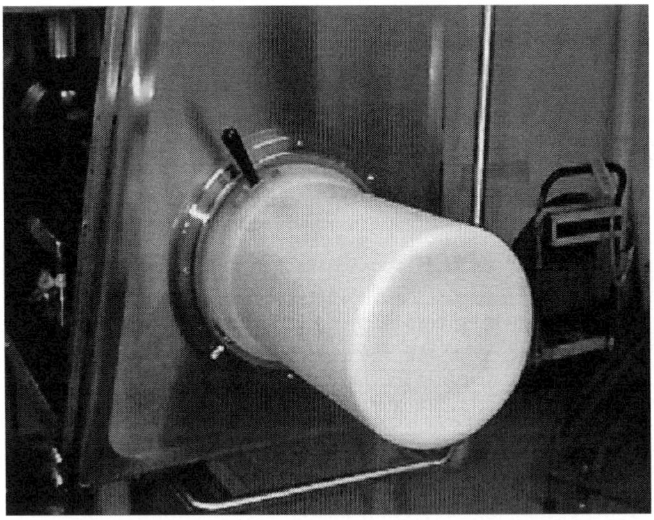

Figure 17 Container connected. *Source*: Photo courtesy of Walker Barrier Systems.

The beta flange is rotated at 60° clockwise, thus engaging both door halves together. The operator will open the combined flanges inside the enclosure via the glove ports or half-suit. The gaskets on the flanges seal the two door halves together and the beta flange to the alpha flange. Potent material or microbes can neither get in/out of the chamber nor in/out of the two door halves when they are "sandwiched" together (Fig. 18).

Items, product, parts, etc., can be transferred to and from the process enclosure without breaking containment or "sterility." While there is a line of contact when the RTP halves are mated together, there are funnels and inserts that can be used to protect the gaskets as well as eliminate possible product or component contact. There are also external gasket decontamination devices available. Beta containers made of stainless steel can be steam sterilized with components or supplies in an autoclave. It is then connected to a previously decontaminated isolator for transfer of sterile supplies into the enclosure. Beta flanges are also available with or

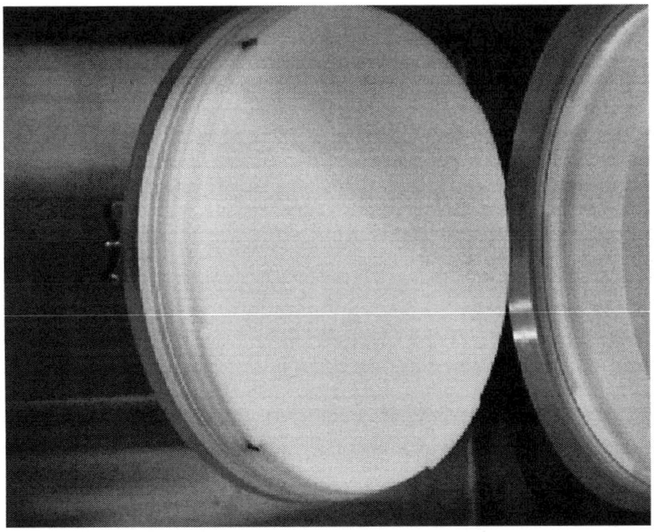

Figure 18 Opened RTP. *Source*: Photo courtesy of Walker Barrier Systems.

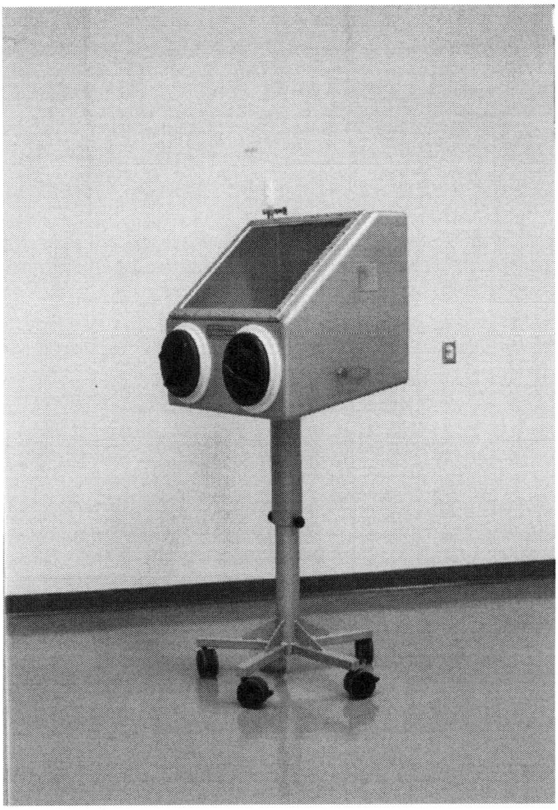

Figure 19 Document transfer isolator (front view). *Source*: Photo courtesy of Walker Barrier Systems.

for attachment of bags. Bags that can be sterilized can be used, for example, for stopper entry. Others are used to bag out waste of potent materials.

OTHER TRANSFER SYSTEMS

Document Transfer Systems

Document Transfer systems are being considered more in containment applications. Rather than risk passing contaminated paperwork into office areas or placing a fax machine in a highly potent process area, document transfer boxes are being employed. This is a small isolator with a RTP system, as shown in Figures 19 and 20. The alpha flange is mounted into the facility wall between the contained process room and the "uncontained" area. The beta flange of the document box is connected to the alpha flange. Paperwork can be passed through the connected RTP, allowing the operator to complete the paperwork via glove ports. The paperwork is not exposed to the potent materials in the process room and can be safely returned to the noncontained area.

Tray Transfer Systems

Tray transfer systems are often employed inside transfer isolators and airlocks. To facilitate passing materials through an airlock or through a RTP beta sleeve, a sliding tray can be provided. Material is placed on the tray, which is then slid through the airlock or beta sleeve on telescoping rails to the next position. Other tray handling devices include a lift system, which rises to various shelf heights where an operator can slide a tray of product to or from a shelf minimizing the risk of dropping the tray.

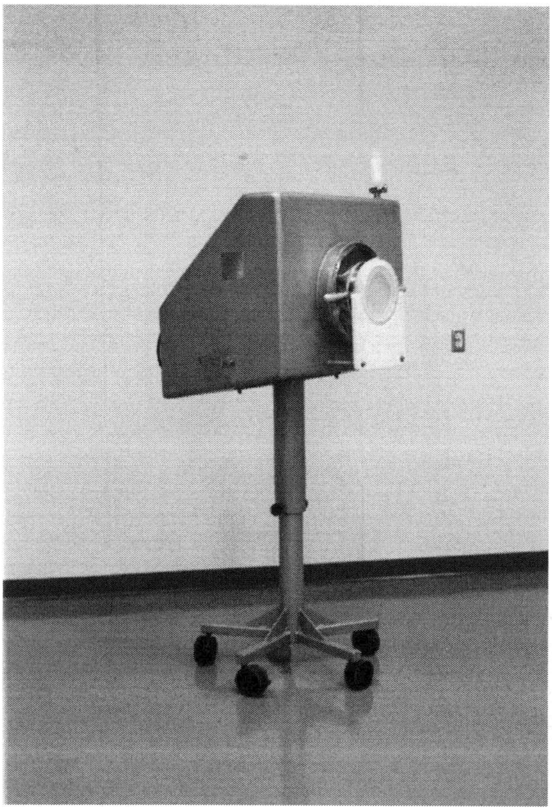

Figure 20 Document transfer isolator (rear view). *Source*: Photo courtesy of Walker Barrier Systems.

Sterile Liquid Transfer

During aseptic fill processes, a sterile liquid transfer container may be used to make an aseptic connection inside the enclosure. The container is made of 316 L stainless steel and is fixed with a RTP beta flange. Inside the container is a coil of tubing (Fig. 21).

This arrangement can be steamed in place. Once the RTP halves have been connected together and the filling isolator has been decontaminated, the RTP is opened. The coil of tubing is pulled from the container and connected to the filling nozzle.

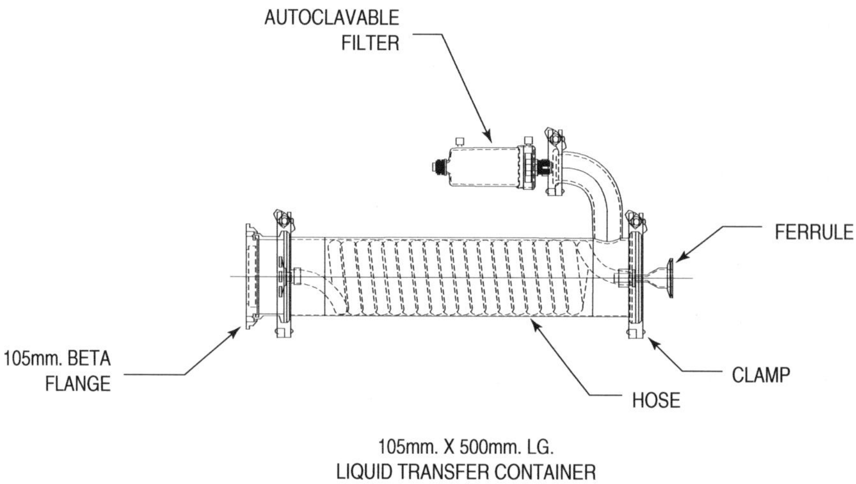

Figure 21 Sterile liquid transfer container drawing. *Source*: Courtesy of Walker Barrier Systems.

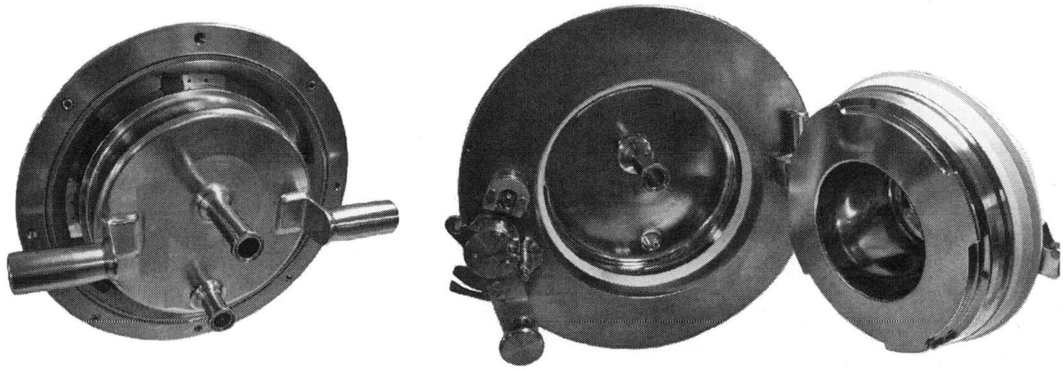

Figure 22 Sterile liquid transfer port. *Source*: Photo courtesy of Central Research Laboratories.

The sterile liquid transfer port (SLPT) (Fig. 22) uses a 190-mm RTP beta flange in 316 L stainless steel, which is equipped with tri-clamp fittings for product connection and condensate drain. The product tank in connected to the SLTP with flex tubing. The product tank and the SLTP are steamed in place together. Upon completion, the 190-mm beta flange is connected to the alpha flange in the wall of the enclosure. The door is opened and sterile tubing inside the enclosure is connected to the fill machine and to the SLTP. The product may now be delivered from the product tank to the fill machine through a sterile connection.

Another system uses plastic connectors that are made up of a male and female coupling that are compatible with gamma and autoclave. Once the single use, single actuation components are assembled together, a sterile fluid path is enabled. The components cannot be disassembled, reducing the risk of a sterility breach.

Pack-off Heads

Finally, pack-off heads are used to seal against drums, IBCs, and drum liners to provide containment when transferring potent powders from process equipment into containers. For highly potent powders, an outward inflating sealing head (Fig. 23) is incorporated inside an isolator.

A drum with a liner is brought inside the isolator. The liner is connected to the pack-off head. The seal is inflated and expands to seal against the liner in an airtight manner. Potent

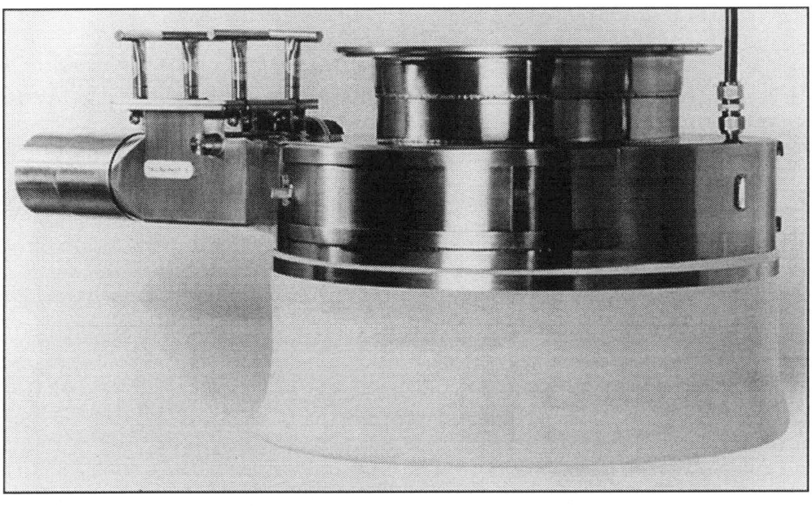

Figure 23 Pack-off head. *Source*: Photo courtesy of Extract Technology.

powder is discharged through the pack-off head and safely into the drum. The liner is tied off and the drum closed. Use of the pack-off head inside the isolator eliminates plumes of powder being scattered inside the isolator and keeps the drum clean.

CONCLUSION

Many solutions are available for transferring materials in/out of an enclosure. It is important to determine the criticality of maintaining the enclosure environment when selecting the transfer approach. It is also important to have a process plan in place along with sizes of materials to be transferred, frequency of transfer, weight, and duration. This will help chose the correct transfer system(s) as well as the design of the enclosure.

REFERENCES

1. GEA Pharma Systems. http://www.gea-ps.com. Accessed April 3, 2009.
2. Lahti C. 35097 Isolator surrogate test protocol and report. New Lisbon, WI: Walker Barrier Systems. 2009.

11 Disposable equipment in advanced aseptic technology

Maik W. Jornitz and Jean-Marc Cappia

DISPOSABLE UNIT OPERATIONS

Aseptic processing gains an increasing importance within the biotech industry due to the fact that sterilization by membrane filtration is the generally the only option to sterilize biological solutions. Any heat treatment would destructively affect the drug product and target protein. To more confidently assure that the sterile filtered product maintains its sterile state, sterile closed disposable process solutions are increasingly used to process or store the resulting filtrate.

Liquid Hold Bags

Fluid holding or storage bags are not new to the industry, but have been in use for decades in the form of blood bags or infusion solution bags, which were most often of relatively small volume. Yet, within a manufacturing process multiple fluid holding steps might be involved, storing either water, media, buffer, or the drug product. These holding steps were once are handled by stainless steel tanks or glass vessels. Nevertheless, the capital investment, footprint, and cleaning/set-up costs are a concern and the industry started looking for alternatives in the form of disposable bags of larger volumes. These bags range from 100 mL to 3000 L in volume and are available in either standard or custom configurations. Filled small volume bags are commonly stored in trays and can be interconnected to dispense larger liquid volumes. Small holding bags are convenient where large volumes of media or buffer must be divided into smaller volumes to be fed into either bioreactor systems (media) or wash/elution processes (buffer). Large-volume bags can be placed in plastic totes or more reliably in pallet tank systems. The pallet tank systems are design to avoid friction or pressure points or bag folding to avoid damage to the bag (Fig. 1). An additional benefit of the pallet tank system is the ability to stack these systems to reduce footprint requirements. Some pallet tanks have load cells included to be able to verify volume intake or outflow.

As hold bags are also used to store and transport bulk drug product, the design and construction of such bags is critical. Welds, dimensions, bag film thickness, and layering are specifically developed to provide superior mechanical robustness. The bag film is often a multilayer of different polymers to obtain low extractable levels by the product contact film, mechanical stability, and gas barrier by the different layers supporting the inner film. The inner film is most commonly a low-density polyethylene film, where polyamide provides mechanical strength and ethyl vinyl a gas barrier.

Mixing

Mixing within the biopharmaceutical industry is an essential step in multiple process operations. For example buffer and media mixing are very common unit operations. The cleaning of stainless steel mixing system is tedious and requires appropriate attention to avoid any contaminating residues. For this reason, disposable mixing systems were designed and widely accepted after their introduction. These systems can be interconnected with filtration systems and/or hold bags. Disposable mixing systems are available in sizes from 50 to 3000 L and are most commonly used for buffer and media preparation, pH adjustments, UF/DF loops, protein folding, product compounding, or final formulation purposes. Newer applications include viral inactivation by pH shift. Mixing bags use disposable potentiometric pH sensors to determine the necessary pH levels during the inactivation period. The pH shifting solution can be fed into the mixing system using disposable hold bags.

The typical mixing methods are recirculation, pulsation of the bag, magnetic impellers, stirrer bars or pads, and levitation mixer. The later is unique as the mixer does not come in contact with the bag material and floats on a magnetic field. This avoids any friction of the bag

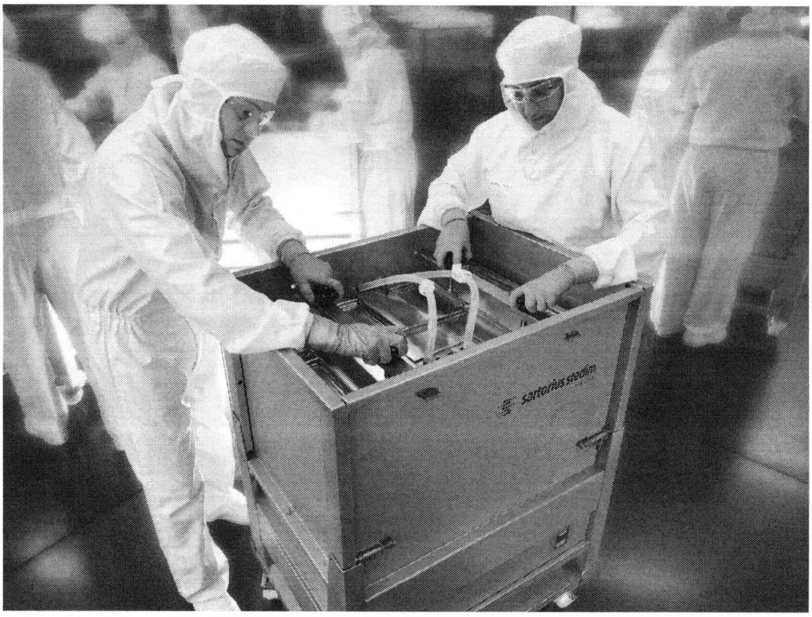

Figure 1 Example of a pallet tank.

material, while providing rapid and thorough mixing. The different mixing technology options are useful as the applications and complexity of mixing vary. Liquid/liquid mixing is among the easier mixing requirements, whereby liquid/powder mixing can be difficult and require careful design and mixing mode observations.

Liquid and Component Transfer

Within biopharmaceutical processes, bulk raw materials and process intermediates might be shipped over long distances or production processes require a product hold step due to downstream equipment bottlenecks. In both instances specific operations are required to avoid any protein degradation, which can happen due to enzymatic attack, temperature, pH, concentration, or gas conditions during the hold or transport step. To avoid such yield losses, the end users may use freeze steps to keep the product stable over an extended period of time. However, commonly used blast freeze steps are uncontrolled and can result in freeze concentration, pH shifts, aggregation, and ice crystals within the frozen material or hold bag damages. To avoid such damaging conditions, disposable controlled freeze/thaw devices have been designed. These devices use a hold bag within a frame and a freeze/thaw module that uses heat exchanger plates, which assure a unified controlled freeze and thaw process. The product hold bag with the frame is transferred into the freeze/thaw module and the heat exchanger plates move into position, pressing against the hold bag. The heat exchanger plates not only assure the temperature transfer, but also the uniform distribution of the liquid over the entire bag design. These devices are available in small-scale trial devices with a volume of 30 mL and process scale up to 16 L.

Component transfers, like rubber stoppers, can also be performed using disposable bags. The stoppers are placed into the transfer bag and the system is gamma irradiated. The transfer bag has an aseptic transfer port that allows the bag with the sterile content being connected to the transfer port installed on a production isolator. Once connected to the aseptic transfer port the bag is opened and the sterilized stoppers can be transferred into the hopper inside the isolator. The contaminated surface of the transfer port of the bag is covered by the counter connection on the port of the isolator, so neither the inside of the isolator nor the bag will come in contact with the surrounding environment.

Purification

Disposable process components within the purification process are available for tangential flow UF/DF steps, intermediate or column protection filtration and, limited though, capturing and polishing chromatography operations. The most commonly found disposable chromatographic separations are membrane adsorbers, which have proven to be an economical alternative to traditional resin and column-based operations (1). Microporous membranes with pore sizes ranging from 0.8 to 3 μm drastically reduce diffusion-related mass transfer effects and enable purification of large biomolecules (capturing) or the adsorptive removal of contaminants such as HCP, DNA, endotoxin, and viruses in flow-through mode (polishing). Membrane chromatography allows for accelerated flow rates and very low unspecific product binding. In a typical polishing application, a 1.5-L disposable membrane chromatography capsule can remove the contaminants downstream of a 10,000 L bioreactor, replacing a classical resin column that is more than 100 times larger. Although reusable resin columns require complex periphery including a packing station and a chromatography skid, this is not the case for disposable membrane chromatography, the impact of which can be verified by the utilization of process cost models (2). In addition to cost advantages, there are many additional benefits, including significantly shorter cycle times and superfluous carryover studies in process validation, making adsorptive virus clearance much more straightforward.

A broad range of functional chemistries, including various ion-exchange and affinity ligands, are currently available in disposable membrane formats with typical dynamic binding capacities of 30 g/L for proteins and up to 10 g/L for DNA. Protein A chromatography, although possible in membrane format, remains economically impractical at production scales, and the use of traditional resin-based columns is recommended. However, the trend toward disposable chromatography has just begun and will likely lead to a complete replacement of reusable systems in polishing with membrane capsules as part of the final filtration train. New formats of membrane chromatography, for example, include disposable direct capture devices allowing for processing of unclarified fermentor off-load. Other disposable chromatography systems are classical, prepacked, and presanitized columns. These units contain classical chromatography resins, but the end-user benefit is that the columns merely need to be connected into the fluid stream, without packing or testing. The sanitization agents used for such columns are either sodium hydroxide and/or isopropyl alcohol. As with membrane chromatography units, if disposability is not desired the systems can be cleaned and reused.

Another important step within the purification process is viral clearance. Integrated disposable mixing, filter, and bag assemblies are used for pH titration and low pH hold viral inactivation. The column eluate is titrated to a low pH by adding acid through a second filter to the eluate bag. The solution is then transferred via peristaltic pump to a second bag for low pH hold for viral inactivation. After the hold, buffer is added to raise the pH. A recently announced viral inactivation step is the use of UV-C. The fluid path around the UV-C burner is disposable so cleaning of the system is eliminated. The fluid is mixed within the disposable fluid path by Dean vortices to assure the entire fluid volume is subjected to the 254 nm irradiation. The benefit of the UV-C system is the precise control of the irradiation dose per fluid volume. However, UV-C has an effect on proteins; therefore appropriate process validation has to evaluate these effects on the target protein. Disposable virus filtration has been developed for the removal of relevant, as well as adventitious viruses. Virus filters are available in a variety of capsule sizes, making the processing of batch sizes of 1000 L or more possible. To protect the viral filter, a 0.1 μm viral prefilter is commonly used. The entire fluid path is disposable, including the viral prefilter, viral filter, collection bag, and all tubing.

Single-use concepts in cross-flow applications have become very popular in vaccine manufacturing and are currently being evaluated in monoclonal antibody production also. Ultrafiltration steps to diafilter and concentrate process intermediates are very common to exchange buffers and reduce fluid volumes. Cleaning of such membrane structures is tedious and requires thorough cleaning validation. It must be assured that all product and cleaning agent residues are removed form the ultrafilter membrane structure. Cross-flow systems with entirely disposable fluid paths are standard or customizable depending on batch size, concentration factor, and required processing time. Ultrafiltration membranes have molecular weight cut-off from 1 to 100 kDa.

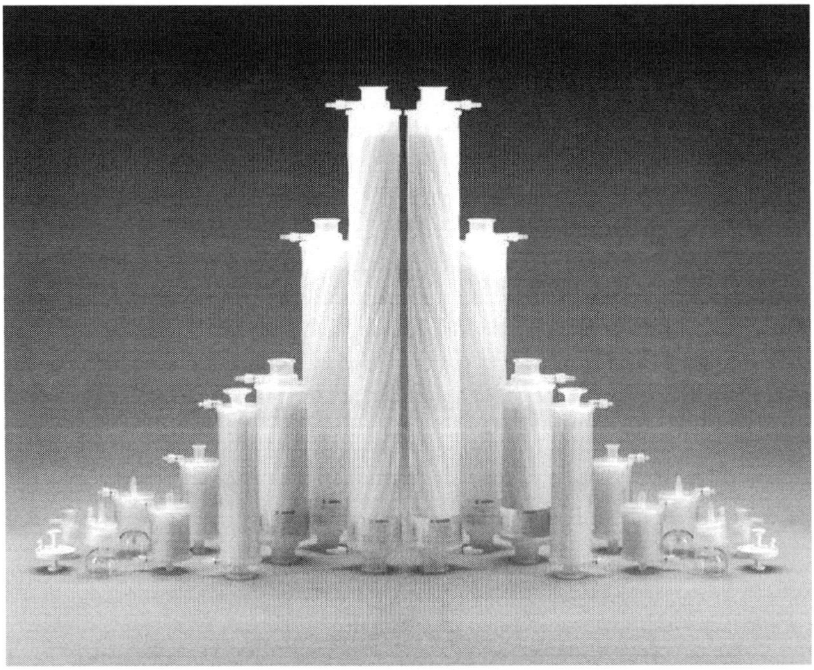

Figure 2 Different encapsulated filter devices: sizes and connectors.

Filtration

Disposable filter devices are commonly filter elements, membrane, and prefilter, which are encapsulated by a plastic housing (Fig. 2). These units are available in different sizes (filtration areas from 1.5 ft^2 to 30 ft^2), with different connectors (hose barb, sanitary flange, threaded) and design (in-line or T-style). These filter units are either supplied presterilized, (gamma irradiation or steam sterilization) or sterilizable by the end user. Because most manufacturers analyze the extractable release of such filters after sterilization and flush the filters within their production processes, these filters can be used without or limited rinsing. Limited rinse volume needs, the connectivity of filter capsules and the lack of filter assembly reduce the set-up time within the production process greatly. Furthermore, the filter units are often connected to tubing and aseptic connection devices, which reduce the possibility of filtrate contamination. Because the filter devices are disposable and encapsulated, the end user will not come in contact with the spent filter, that is, neither the filtered product, which could be cytotoxic or of elevated potency, nor the separated contaminants on the upstream side of the filter. End-user safety is therefore greatly improved.

Filter capsules are often regarded as cost-intensive devices, which require replacement after every filtration and therefore elevate the running costs. With disposable devices the capital expenses necessary for the purchase of stainless steel housings, depreciation and cleaning costs are avoided. Cleaning costs of filter housings, when analyzed appropriately, might exceed the cost of an encapsulated filter, depending on the flush volumes of water for injection (WFI), the manpower required, cleaning agent costs, and energy requirements to sterilize the filter system. These costs do not include any production capacity losses due to prolonged set-up time, which would be avoided with capsule filters. Cleaning validation, which needs to be performed with fixed equipment like filter housings, would be greatly reduced or eliminated.

Sterile connections

Commonly, assemblies of filter capsules and bags are connected via tubing and gamma irradiated. The assembly has to be connected to a feed stream, for example, a disposable mixing system or the hold bag could be connected to a bioreactor or fill line. In all cases, the goal is to connect the equipment or process units aseptically to achieve a high-sterility assurance. Fittings of all different designs, whether hose barb or sanitary flange may be used, but often do not address the criticality of the aseptic connection. The lack of appropriate aseptic connectivity has been recognized and addressed with newer more effective designs. These designs assure the connections are aseptic as these connectors are presterilized by gamma irradiation and the fluid path does not come in contact with the exterior environment. The integrity of those devices toward the external environment is ensured via either sterilizing-grade membranes or solid plugs. These aseptic connector devices are commonly 100% integrity tested after production by manufacturers. Aseptic connectors allow for the aseptic connection between two disposable systems without the use of a laminar airflow. They are available to fit on 1/4 , 3/8, and 1/2 inches tubing and can be sterilized by either gamma radiation or steam sterilization. To verify the appropriate functionality of these connectors, rigorous tests have been performed under worst-case operating conditions, for example bacterial ingress tests. Test data can be obtained from the vendor and might be useful within the user's own qualification process.

Other aseptic connections are performed by welding sterile thermoplastic tubing lengths together. The welding process cuts the tubing and welds the cut-ends together. Tubes of different diameters from 1/4 to 3/4 inches can be welded, each diameter requiring unique weld parameters programmed into the welder unit. The blade used to weld the tubing heats up to 752°F and thus is sterilized each time during the process. The welding process requires qualification within the end-user process to assure that the weld strength is according to specifications. Wet or filled tubing cannot be welded. The tubing must be dry to achieve an even heat distribution. Welders have been used for years in the biopharmaceutical industry with great success.

Filling

Single-use filling operations are mainly restricted to large-volume filling. Large-volume filling can be performed as a manual or automatic operation, whereas final drug filling is most often an automatic function. Large-volume disposable filling occurs in media or buffer preparations, which use disposable mixing tank. The mixed media or buffer volume is filtered through either a sterilizing or mycoplasma retentive filter and afterward distributed into a bag filling manifold, which apportions the bulk fluid into smaller volume fractions. Other large volume filling could be into bottles or drums. Large-volume filling ranges from 100 mL to multiple 100 L and is often found in upstream in a biopharmaceutical process or support service areas.

Small-volume end product filling remains an area of development needs. Attempts in the past were mainly in a small-scale, low-volume range, often with a lack of accuracy, which however is of utmost importance. More recent disposable filling introduced by established filling machine manufacturers hold promises that larger volume, high-speed fill lines could be established with fill precision experienced with the hard-piped machine versions. The pump action and design is the essential part for such fill lines and it has to be established whether all parts can be designed as disposable part. When this is accomplished, fill lines that are dedicated to a single product could be used for various purposes. Because fully disposable, high-speed fill machinery is still pending, some have resorted to hybrid designs, for example, only the fill needles are disposable, but the remainder of the line is hard-piped and stainless steel. This hybrid solution would require similar cleaning needs to the traditional fill line and the benefits of such fill machine options is questionable.

The hope for future fill lines will be designed with all drug product contact areas being disposable. Cleaning requirements would be greatly reduced, potential hazardous material filling would be eased, and fill line utilization would be optimized. End-user requirements are existent; the challenges of high-speed, large-volume, and strict accuracy filling result from the wear and tear of disposable polymeric parts being in constant motion. Hopefully engineering experts within the filling manufacturers will resolve these challenges and one will see such filling systems in the near future.

Plant Layout and Process Design

Disposable systems utilization creates the possibility to exploit either the entire or parts of the process for multiproduct processing purposes. Hard-piped processes, even when cleaned diligently, are often restricted to a specific product due to the potential risk of cross contamination. However, this also means that some processes, equipment or areas could be

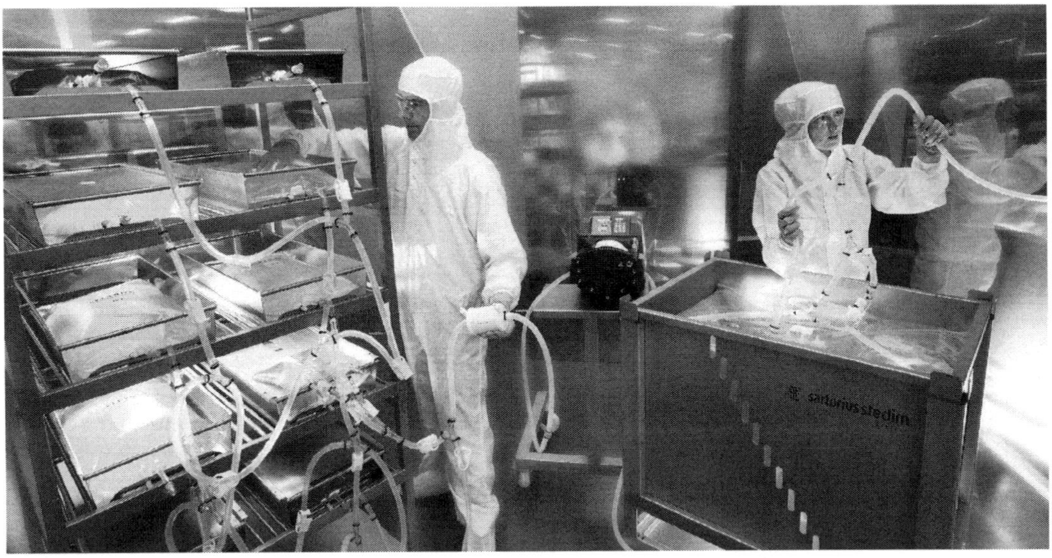

Figure 3 Example of a disposable process unit design.

underutilized, resulting in value losses. If a process step could be used by a multitude of product streams, a disposable version of this step would be advisable as cross contamination by the disposal of any product contact area would be eliminated. In addition, disposable systems can be self-containing and are qualified to assure that contaminant ingress from the environment is impossible. Depending on the disposable system set-up or unit operation, disposable systems could potentially be installed in areas of lower clean room classification. Process validation has to verify that the disposable unit operation works according to specifications within that clean room class, but the feasibility is there. With future advancements in disposability of process units, product site designs might change also as the disposable self-containment might allow the process units to run in a microenvironment while interconnected. Entire plant layouts would change with reduced clean room area requirements and therefore lower running costs. In addition, self-containment would reduce user interference and possibilities of contamination.

The most common and oldest disposable equipment assembly is a capsule filter connected to a bag to sterile filter a fluid into the holding bag for later use. Complex assemblies consist of disposable mixing systems, filters, manifolds of hold bags, sample bags, tubing, aseptic transfer systems, and connectors (Fig. 3). Such assemblies could represent a process unit within an entire process. If other process units are disposable and can be interconnected by aseptic connectors, a total disposable process is not improbable. All disposable assemblies or process units are usually presterilized by gamma irradiation and ready for use. Assemblies can be in standard configuration or designed as customized systems for individual user requirement specifications.

An important factor to be considered with assemblies, the qualification data exist only for the components of an assembly. Therefore the assembly itself requires qualification within the particular application or process step by the end user, because environmental, process, and fluid conditions vary from process to process.

REGULATORY AND VALIDATION REQUIREMENTS

The usability of particular components, like a capsule filter, depends on the requirements of the end user. Parameters of the application, such as flow, temperature, pressure conditions, and process will determine the rationale for specific design criteria and component choices. The user needs to have detailed knowledge of all process parameters to be able to predefine the needs of particular assembly designs and component robustness. Without precise user requirement specifications, a disposable assembly could be unsuitable for a process. Parameters that are critical for an assembly design are the following:

- Flow rate
- Pressure conditions
- Temperature conditions
- Filter pore size requirements
- Product volumes
- Filter size (established in previously performed throughput trials)
- Fluid properties (compatibility issues)
- Integrity test methods and needs

Bag Validation

Basically, the validation requirements for a disposable aseptic processing are no different than that of a traditional stainless steel process. Because single-use systems are preassembled and sterilized by vendors, there is a higher level of involvement of the supplier in the validation work. End users and suppliers work together at specifying the expected product performance for a given application and agree on the level of validation and certification required for the specific assembly. To be a qualified vendor of single-use aseptic processing therefore requires an in-depth understanding and the application of current regulatory and good manufacturing practices (GMP) requirements

Because most disposable devices are gamma irradiated, between 25 and 50 kGy short- and long-term stability studies with the irradiated devices should be performed. The irradiation commonly reduces the shelf life of such devices and it must be determined what the limits are. Furthermore, the irradiation step could accelerate the degradation of the polymeric substances used, which can impact leachable/extractable levels. To determine the effects of irradiation and the stability of the polymer used, manufacturer subject the devices to an extensive regimen of qualification tests before the device is launched. The qualification tests can be used as guidance by the end user and commonly encompass, but are not limited to, following tests:

- Biocompatibility testing
  - USP<87>: Biological reactivity tests, in vitro
  - USP<88>: Biological reactivity tests, in vivo
- Mechanical properties
  - Tensile strength
  - Elongation at break
  - Seal strength
  - Air leak test
- Gas transmission properties
  - ASTM D3985: oxygen
  - ASTM F1249: water vapor
- USP<661> Test for plastics
- E.P. 3.1.7.: EVA for containers and tubing
- E.P. 5.2.8. on TSE-BSE
- TOC analysis
- pH/conductivity
- Extractable/leachable tests with standard solutions
- Chemical compatibility testing
- Protein adsorption studies
- Endotoxin testing
- Gamma irradiation sterilization validation
- Bacterial ingress test

These tests are performed under standard settings with standard solutions. The data of these tests are available from the manufacturer. As qualification tests run under standard conditions, possible process-specific validation requirements need to be met. These validation studies can be supported by the services of the vendor. Process validation studies would,

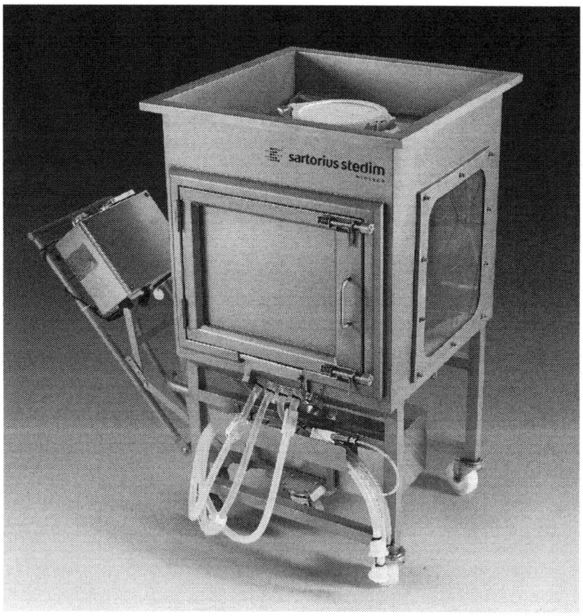

Figure 4 Example of a levitating disposable mixing unit design including a container, a mixing, and drive unit.

for example, use a model solvent and simulate the process parameters within the end-users specifications. Leachable testing with actual product cannot always be achieved as the product may cover potential peaks. For this reason, model solvents are often used, which are similar to the solvent used within the product stream. However, possible influences by the environmental conditions used within the end-users processes must be tested to assure that the disposable device performs to specifications (3,4).

The process validation steps vary as disposable devices have different purposes. Sterilizing-grade filters have to undergo a product bacteria challenge test under end-users process conditions. If the actual fluid is bactericidal or bacteriostatic, a placebo solution should be used. In any case, the influence of the process conditions and fluid toward the challenge organisms or separation mechanisms need to be determined. Product hold bags or mixing bags do not have to undergo bacteria challenge tests, but possibly bacteria ingress tests. Both filter and bags systems need to be tested for leachable or extractable components. As mentioned previously, the end users should take advantage of the vendor's services, which support by the qualification documentation and process validation.

Equipment Qualification

Disposable aseptic processing bag assemblies need to be installed in stainless steel or plastic totes to support the functional filling, draining, storage, transportation, and transfer operations. Jacketed bag holders may be required to provide thermoregulation and temperature control and other single-use sensors such as pH, conductivity, and dissolved oxygen probes can be necessary to control a single-use aseptic process. Also weighing load cells and automatic pinch valves can be integrated into these single-use units to offer filling and draining automation and controls. All process hardware, control devices, monitoring instruments, and probes used for the process will need to undergo the traditional installation qualification (IQ), operational qualification (OQ), and performance qualification (PQ). The approach is not different from that use to qualify traditional stainless steel systems, but the validation burden is significantly reduced as cleaning validation is not required and gamma sterilization is already validated by the supplier of the disposable assembly. Suppliers of single systems generally offer factory acceptance test, site acceptance test, and IQ and OQ services whereas PQ is the responsibility of the end user.

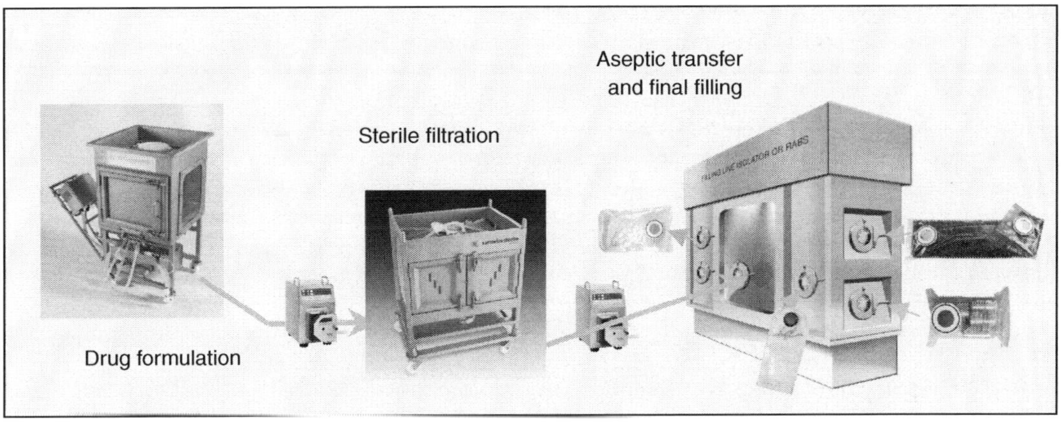

Figure 5 Disposable aseptic processing suite.

During IQ, and PQ, a validation expert team usually composed of personnel from the supplier and the end user ensure that the hardware, instruments, and disposable assemblies are designed and installed according to the user requirement specification. Critical dimensions, component design and part numbers, conformance to technical drawings and functionalities are checked and documented in a preestablished IQ/OQ protocol. Verification that the appropriate operating and maintenance documentation are available is also carried out. The calibration of instruments and probes is also checked during IQ/OQ. The equipment qualification is completed by in-depth training of the operators in charge of the system and the establishment of standard operating procedures (SOPs).

If a disposable filling system is used, filling accuracy and reproducibility tests using three different disposable set-ups will be required to qualify the filling equipment.

Mixing Qualification

Disposable mixing systems comprise a single-use bag and mixing device assembly and the associated tubing, sensors, filters, and connectors (Fig. 4). As is the case for disposable bags, single-use mixing systems involve a stainless steel or plastic container and a drive unit to actuate the impeller at the desired speed measured in rotation per minute (RPM). Thermoregulation, pH, and conductivity controls are commonly applied and monitoring instrumentation is often adjacent to single-use mixers. The mixing hardware, drive unit, instruments, and probes are subject to traditional IQ, OQ, and PQ procedures to verify that the system is installed and it operates according to manufacturer and user requirement specification and that it offers the expected end user mixing performances. Beyond classical equipment qualification steps, the major aspect of mixer qualification is the PQ carried out with the solution to be mixed or homogenized or with the powder to be dissolved. The PQ is performed under normal production conditions and will establish the mixing process parameters such as mixing time, temperature, and RPM that need to be observed during production. When in line monitoring is applied, the PQ will also define the pH or conductivity set limits to be obtained to guaranty the reproducibility of the mixing process.

Generally, three consecutive successful PQ test must be achieved to validate the disposable mixing process. Operator training and SOP development ultimately generate a fully validated process. No cleaning validation is required like with any other disposable unit operations.

Transfer Qualification

The final aseptic transfer of liquids and solid goods such as vial stoppers, syringe stoppers and plungers, monitors, and other items necessary for the aseptic process is certainly one of the most critical operations (Fig. 5). Disposable aseptic transfer systems made of a single-use connector and a bag that contains the components to be transferred (gamma sterilized by suppliers or by autoclaved at end users). The aseptic transfer door installed onto the isolator, the restricted access barrier system (RABS), or the wall of the clean room needs to undergo IQ, OQ, and PQ according to a predefined validation protocol. The IQ and OQ steps are generally supported by the supplier of the transfer door in collaboration with the supplier of the isolator, RABS, or clean room and the end user. Ideally, the qualification of the aseptic transfer system should be integrated with the qualification of the isolator or RABS to provide a completely qualified process solution. Dimensional checks, conformity to technical drawings, functional flow of components through the installed aseptic transfer door and integrity of the bag and the connection are the main qualification tests requirements. Following the qualification of the equipment and the disposable, three consecutive successful media fills must be obtained to demonstrate the transfer process together with the entire aseptic process. As multiple transfers can occur during a normal production campaign, it is critical that the maximum number of transfers is performed during the media fill validation so as to offer worst-case conditions.

All tests performed for the qualification of the aseptic transfer system, including the hardware and the disposable components are documented in a final validation report and signed off for approval by the quality and or validation management.

Filter Validation

Pharmaceutical and biopharmaceutical processes are validated processes to assure a reproducible product within set specifications. Equally important is the validation of the filters used within the process, especially the sterilizing-grade filters, which are used before the filling or final processing of the drug product (5). In its Guideline on Sterile Drug Products Produced by Aseptic Processing, 2004, the Food and Drug Administration (FDA) (6) describes that the validation of sterile processes is required by the manufacturers of sterile products. Sterilizing-grade filters are determined by the bacteria challenge tests (7). This test is performed under strict parameters and a defined solution (ASTM F 838–05, 2005) (8). New guidances, including FDA, nowadays require also evidence that the sterilizing grade filter will create a sterile filtration, no matter of the process parameters, fluid or bioburden found (9). This means that bacteria challenge tests have to be performed with the actual drug product, possibly native bioburden, if different or known to be smaller than *Brevundimonas diminuta* and the process parameters involved. The reason for the requirement of a product bacteria challenge test is threefold. First, the influence of the product and process parameters to the microorganism has to be tested. There may be cases of either shrinkage of organisms due to a higher osmolarity of the product or prolonged filtration times. Second, the filters compatibility with the product and the process parameters has to be tested. The filter should not show any sign of degradation due to the product filtered. In addition, assurance is required that the filter used will withstand the process parameters, for example, pressure pulses, should not influence the filter's performance. Third, there are two separation mechanisms involved in liquid filtration; sieve retention, and retention by adsorptive sequestration. In sieve retention, the smallest particle or organism size is retained by the biggest pore within the membrane structure. The contaminant will be retained, no matter of the process parameters. This is the ideal situation. However, retention by adsorptive sequestration depends on the filtration conditions. Contaminants smaller than the actual pore size penetrate such and may be captured by adsorptive attachment to the pore wall. This effect is enhanced using highly adsorptive filter materials, for example glass fiber as a prefilter or polyamide as a membrane (10,11). Nevertheless certain liquid properties can minimize the adsorptive effect, which could mean penetration of organisms. Whether the fluid has such properties and will lower the effect of adsorptive sequestration and may eventually cause penetration has to be evaluated in specific product bacteria challenge tests.

Before performing a product bacteria challenge test, it should be assured that the liquid product does not have any detrimental, bactericidal, or bacteriostatic effects on the challenge organisms. This is accomplished using viability tests (7). The organism is inoculated into the product to be filtered at a certain bioburden level. At specified times the log value of this bioburden is tested. If the bioburden is reduced due to the fluid properties different bacteria challenge test mode become applicable. If the mortality rate is low the challenge test will be performed with a higher bioburden, bearing in mind that the end challenge level should reach $10^7/cm^2$. If the mortality rate is high the toxic substance is either removed or product properties are changed. This type of challenge fluid is called a placebo. Another methodology would circulate the fluid product through the filter at the specific process parameters as long as the actual processing time would be. Afterward, the filter is flushed extensively with water and the challenge test, as described in ASTM F838–05 (8), is performed.

In addition to the product bacteria challenge test, tests determining the release of leachable substances or particulates have to be performed. Extractable measurements and the resulting data are available from filter manufacturers for the individual filters. Nevertheless depending on the process conditions and the solvents used, explicit leachable tests have to be performed. These tests are commonly done only with the solvent or diluent used, but not with the actual drug product, as the drug product usually covers any leachable/extractables during measurement. Often, such tests are conducted by the validation services of the filter manufacturers using sophisticated separation and detection methodologies, as GC–MS, FTIR, and RP-HPLC. These methodologies are required as the individual components possibly released from the filter have to be identified and quantified. Elaborated studies, performed by filter manufacturers have shown that there is neither a release of high quantities of extractables (the range is PPB to maximum PPM per 10 inches element) nor a release of toxic substances has been found (12).

Particulates are critical in sterile filtration, specifically of injectables. The USP (United States Pharmacopeia) and BP (British Pharmacopeia) define specific limits of particulate level contaminations for specific particle sizes. These limits have to be met by sterilizing-grade filters. Filters are routinely tested within the manufacturers release control, evaluating the filtrate with laser particle counters. Such tests are also performed with the actual product under process conditions to proof that the product, but especially process conditions do not result in an increased level of particulates within the filtrate.

Furthermore, within specific applications the loss of yield or product ingredients due to adsorption requires to be determined. For example preservatives, such as benzalkonium chloride or chlorhexadine, can be adsorbed by filter-membrane polymers like polyamide (13). Such membranes need to be saturated by the preservative to avoid preservative loss within the actual product. This preservative loss, for example, in contact lens solutions, can be detrimental due to long-term use of such solutions. Similarly problematic would be the adsorption of targeted proteins within a biological solution (14). To optimize the yield within an application, adsorption trials have to be performed to find the optimal-membrane material and filter construction.

Using the actual product as a wetting agent to perform integrity tests requires the evaluation of product integrity test limits. The product can have an influence on the measured integrity test values due to surface tension or solubility. A lower surface tension for example would shift the bubble point value to a lower pressure and could result in a false-negative test. The solubility of gas into the product could be reduced, which could result in false-positive tests. Therefore, a correlation of the product as wetting agent, by the filter manufacturer established, to the water-wet values has to be done. This correlation is carried out by using a minimum of three filters of three filter lots. Depending on the product and its variability, one or three product lots are used to perform the correlation. The accuracy of such correlation is enhanced by automatic integrity test machines. These test machines measure with highest accuracy and sensitivity and do not rely on a human judgment as with a manual test. Multipoint diffusion testing offers the ability to test the filters performance, but especially the plot the entire diffusive flow graph through the bubble point. The individual graphs for a water-wet integrity test can now be compared with the product-wet test and a possible shift evaluated. Furthermore the multipoint diffusion test enables an improved statistical base to determine the product wet versus water-wet limits.

SOP Development and Operator Training

Following the IQ, OQ, and PQ of hardware, disposable components and instruments involved in the different unit operations, the training of operators in charge of those operations, and the development of the associated SOPs will complete the validation work. Because disposable technologies such as bag assemblies, bioreactors, filling systems, or mixers are not yet broadly understood by operators who have historically been trained and certified to stainless steel process, operator training takes on a more critical importance. Validation scientists and application specialist from the key suppliers of disposable assemblies provide expert validation, SOP development, and training support to the industry.

The handling of disposable bags requires specific skills and hands-on experience to ensure that the bags are properly installed into their totes. The installation of the bag and the filling and draining processes are critical for the integrity of the disposable bag throughout the entire process. Well-documented IQ, OQ, and PQ, optimal SOP development and in depth operator training carried out in collaboration with expert suppliers will guaranty the safety and the robustness of the disposable aseptic process.

CONCLUSION

Most of process components, control devices, and monitoring tools necessary to operate an aseptic process in compliance with current GMP regulations are today available in a disposable form. This enables the design and implementation of flexible and ready to use aseptic processing suites that do not require any clean-in-place or steam-in-place operations. The latest single-use technology developments are focusing on disposable noninvasive process monitoring tools and process control devices to enable the monitoring and control of critical process parameters and the future automation of disposable processes.

Disposable powder bags that contain the active ingredient and formulation components can be connected to a disposable mixing unit to provide a complete disposable solution for the drug formulation unit operation. Single-use process monitoring tools such as pH and conductivity sensors coupled to noninvasive temperature probes are currently under final development to allow the monitoring and control of the formulation process step. Load cells are commonly used on bag containers to control the addition of powder and liquids during the drug-compounding step.

The sterile filtration of the formulated drug is processed with a disposable filtration unit that involves single-use filter capsules, tubing manifold, and sterile connectors. Peristaltic pumps coupled to disposable pressure sensors are used for transferring the sterile filter drug product into another disposable sterile receiving bag. Load cell installed on the sterile receiving bag are used to control that the complete volume of the formulated drug has been transferred. Disposable pressure sensors installed upstream of the filter act as a safety device to switch off the peristaltic pump in case of filter clogging.

The sterile holding bag is then connected to the final filling equipment via a set of single-use sterile connector and aseptic transfer to allow the final filling of the drug product under aseptic conditions in an isolator, RABS, or classical clean room. Further technology developments are in progress to offer a complete disposable filling system that will comprise single-use bag, tubing, precision pumps, and filling needles.

Future modern aseptic filling suites will rapidly become a reality as disposable technologies are now broadly used by the biopharmaceutical industry and well accepted by the regulatory authorities. The biopharmaceutical industry will then benefit of more flexible, faster to operate, safer, and more cost-effective aseptic processes by reducing turn around time, eliminating lengthy and costly cleaning and steaming in place processes and avoiding the risks of cross contamination.

The next challenge for the suppliers and users of disposable solutions will be the security of supply of the polymers, components, and assemblies. The security of supply combined with the reliability of products offered by single-use solution providers and their suppliers will be of utmost importance as drug producers will depend heavily on the ability of their vendors to supply their goods on time and with a consistent quality. Single-use solutions have been adopted in clinical phases and process developments and have given rise to a multitude of components and customized solutions. Because disposable solutions are now migrating into more critical process steps of commercial production they will need to be produced in a more rapid manner. Change controls for the polymer resins and the extrusion/molding processes involved in the fabrication of disposable components will become critical and could only be applied if a selected range of reliable components are used and assembled in increasingly standardized solutions. The rationalization of components and the standardization of disposable solutions are necessary steps for our industry to benefit of a long-term security of supply and a reliable quality.

REFERENCES

1. Gottschalk U. Bioseparation in Antibody Manufacturing: The Good, the Bad and the Ugly. ACS AICE 2008; BP070452G.
2. Sinclair A, Monge, M. Quantitative economic evaluation of single use disposables in bioprocessing. Pharm Eng 2002; 22(3):1–9.
3. Meyer BK, Vargas D. Impact of tubing material on the failure of product-specific bubble points of sterilizing-grade filters. PDA J Pharm Sci 2006; 60(4):248–253.
4. Uettwiller I. Testing and validation of disposable Systems. Genetic Eng News 2006; 26(3).
5. Akers JE. Microbiological considerations in the selection and validation of filter sterilization. In: Jornitz MW and Meltzer TH, eds. Filtration and Purification in the Biopharmaceutical Industry. New York: Informa, 2008.
6. FDA, Guidance for Industry, Sterile Drug Products Produced by Aseptic Processing, Center for Drugs and Biologics and Office of Regulatory Affairs. Rockville, MD: Food and Drug Administration, 2004.
7. PDA Technical Report 26. Liquid Sterilizing Filtration. Parenteral Drug Association. Bethesda, MD: 2008.
8. ASTM Committee F 838 05. Standard Test Method for Determining Bacterial Retention of Membrane Filters Utilized for Liquid Filtration. West Conshohocken, PA: ASTM, 2005.
9. PDA Special Scientific Forum Validation of Microbial Retention of Sterilizing Filters. Bethesda, MD: 1995:12–13.
10. Emory SF, Koga Y, Azuma N, et al. The effects surfactant types and latex-particle feed concentration on membrane retention. Ultrapure Water 1993; 10(2):41–44.
11. Tanny GB, Strong DK, Presswood WG, et al. Adsorptive retention of *Pseudomonas diminuta* by membrane filters. J Parent Drug Assoc 1979; 33:40–51.
12. Reif OW, Sölkner P, Rupp J. Analysis and evaluation of filter cartridge extractables for validation in pharmaceutical downstream processing. PDA J Pharm Sci Technol 1996; 50:399–410.
13. Brose DJ, Henricksen G. A quantitative analysis of preservative adsorption on microfiltration membranes. Pharm Technol Europe 1994; 42–49.
14. Hawker J, Hawker LM. Protein losses during sterilization by filtration. Lab Practises 1975; 24:805–814.

12 A comparison of capital and operating costs for aseptic manufacturing facilities

Jorge Ferreira, Beth Holden, Jeff Kraft, and Kevin Schreier

EXECUTIVE SUMMARY

Summary

Historically, the construction cost of buildings for core manufacturing areas in facilities using isolation technology is lower (reduced by 33%) than conventional aseptic processing areas, although it is offset by the higher costs of isolation equipment (greater than conventional equipment by 50%), resulting in a greater total capital cost. However, when validation and operation costs are considered, the cost–benefit analysis has been more difficult to quantify. When selecting the proper technology for a new project, it is important to weigh the advantages of increased sterility assurance levels (SAL) found with isolators against the overall increase in capital cost, while keeping in mind the overall lifecycle cost of the facility. It is the intent of this chapter to perform an analysis of capital, validation, and operating costs for a given facility scope, and to establish a more thorough comparison for the use of isolation and restricted access barrier systems (RABS) technology against conventional clean room design.

The floor area required for a conventional facility is typically larger than an isolator facility owing to several factors. To accomplish the subdivision required between cascading levels of cleanliness, conventional facilities require greater square footage for additional air locks, corridors, walls, doors, and mechanical space serving the larger Grade A/B environments. If more rigorous unidirectional flow is required, this size gap becomes even more divergent. In addition to the larger size, the higher dollar per square feet unit cost rate attributed to A/B areas in conventional aseptic clean room facilities consistently results in higher building costs for these conventional designs. However, the potential space reduction in an isolator facility does not compensate for isolator equipment costs.

RABS design solutions can offer some improvement in the SAL compared to conventional clean rooms and serve as an intermediate option between conventional clean rooms and isolators. The B3-type RABS used in the following examples is closer in cost to conventional clean room processing than to isolation technology.

The cost comparison can be illustrated as a set of multipliers to the base case, consisting of the conventional clean room facility. The basis of the analysis includes a formulation area serving two filling trains. One filling train consists of liquid and lyophilized vial filling, and includes automatic loading and unloading of the lyophilized vials as well as three lyophilizers. The second filling train consists of presterilized syringe filling.

Method

To provide a basis for comparison of conventional aseptic processing in a clean room and aseptic processing using RABS or isolation technology, a model process facility was designed to aseptically fill biopharmaceutical products, without any stated requirements for containment. The basis consists of a single formulation area serving two filling lines; one for liquid and lyophilized vials, using an automated loading and unloading system feeding three lyophilizers and a second for liquid syringes. As the bulk active cannot be filtered, it must be formulated as a sterile product. Also, once the filled units are sealed, they exit immediately from the facility. Downstream operations are not accounted for as part of this exercise.

In each case, including conventional clean room, RABS, and isolation technology selection, an equipment list and a conceptual layout were developed to serve as a basis for cost comparison. Each of the unit operations was estimated separately and can be viewed as a stand-alone operation. However, to understand the full impact of technology selection, support areas such as parts preparation and sterilization, and clean utilities were considered in the analysis. When comparing the total cost for each technology option, other costs, including support facilities, validation cost, and operation cost have been included.

It is helpful to define the terms "isolator" and "RABS." The following definitions are taken from ISPE (1):

> An isolator is a leaktight enclosure designed to protect operators from hazardous/potent processes or protect processes from people or detrimental external environments or both. A basic enclosure consists of a shell, viewing window, glove/sleeve assemblies, supply and exhaust filters, light (s), gauge (s), Input and Output openings (equipment door airlocks, Rapid Transfer Ports (RTPs), etc.), and various other penetrations. There are two types of isolators:
>
> 1. Closed Isolators—Isolators operated as closed systems do not exchange unfiltered air or contaminants with adjacent environments. Their ability to operate without personnel access to the critical zone makes isolators capable of levels of separation between the internal and external environment unattainable with other technologies. Because the effectiveness of this separation, closed isolators are ideally suited for application in the preparation of sterile and/or toxic material. Aseptic and Containment isolators are two types of closed isolators.
>
> 2. Open Isolators—Open isolators differ from closed isolators in that they are designed to allow for the continuous or semi-continuous egress of materials during operation, while maintaining a level of protection over the internal environment. Open isolators are decontaminated while closed, and then opened during manufacturing. Open isolators typically are used for the aseptic filling of finished pharmaceuticals.
>
> A Restricted Access Barrier System (RABS) is an advanced aseptic processing system that can be utilized in many applications in a fill-finish area. RABS provides an enclosed environment to reduce the risk of contamination to product, containers, closures, and product contact surfaces compared to the risks associated with conventional cleanroom operations. RABS can operate as "doors closed" for processing with very low risk of contamination similar to isolators, or permit rare "open door interventions" provided appropriate measures are taken.

In representative installations recently constructed, there are a wide variety of equipment configurations referred to as RABS. In construction detail, some approximate isolators in their level of segregation of the clean environment from the background environment, whereas other examples employ less rigorous segregation between the clean environment and the background room. For the purposes of this cost comparison, the quality of the RABS environment was defined at an intermediate level, a level 3. A level 3 RABS includes a dedicated fan and HEPA ceiling to create a Grade A zone. The air is supplied from the filling room heating, ventilation, and air conditioning (HVAC) system and exhausted into the filling room.

It is noted that capital costs are compared at the direct cost level and do not incorporate indirect costs such as engineering or construction management. Relevant validation and operating costs have been factored into the costs.

FORMULATION

Basis for Evaluation

Formulation of aseptic products requires, as a minimum, a Grade C area for the actual formulation operation, and then a sterile filtration into a holding vessel that is part of a closed presterilized system, to render the lot sterile. This methodology is acceptable for solution products that can be filtered, but if a product cannot be filtered in its final formulation, the formulation operation must provide for the addition of presterilized components in a high-level aseptic environment. A sterile suspension is an example of a product that cannot be filtered in its final form. This aseptic environment may be provided by a conventional Grade A/B clean room or by an isolator. In this case, the RABS case is essentially the same as the clean room case.

Formulation in Conventional Clean Room

In the case of a formulation process that requires aseptic additions, the liquid vehicle is usually formulated in a Grade C area. The excipients for the lot will be weighed in the raw material dispensing unit and delivered to the formulation area. The fluid will then be compounded for

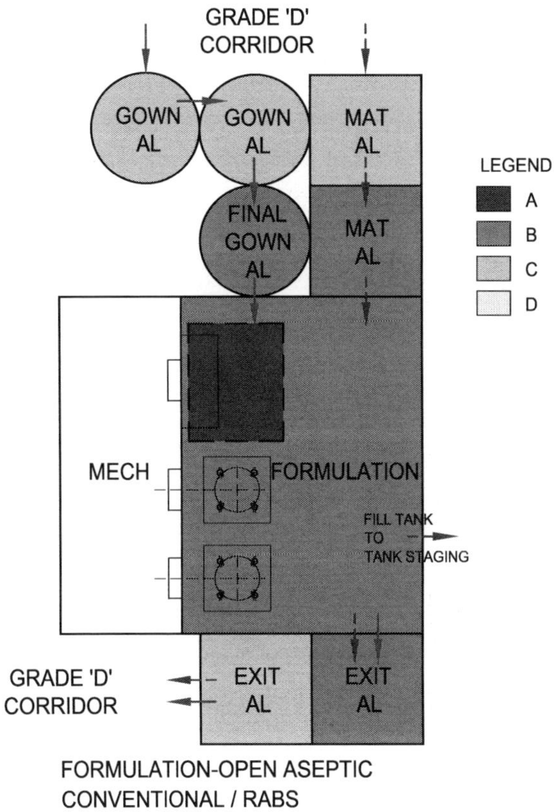

Figure 1 Formulation suite, conventional/RABS technology.

the lot. This fluid may be heat sterilized or sterilized by filtration and transferred to a Grade A/B area where the aseptic additions will take place.

In preparation for formulation, the presterilized ingredients will be brought to the formulation area for introduction to the system of airlocks leading to the aseptic formulation room. External coverings will be removed upon entrance to the Grade C area. Then the material will be transferred to the Grade B air lock where the externals of the container (or bag) will be wiped with a germicidal solution. If multiple layers of bags are used, the outer bag will be removed and the materials will be moved to the aseptic formulation room. The ingredients will be weighed in a Grade A flow hood then transferred to the sterilized vessel for addition to the lot, via a closed addition. The area used for open manipulations of product is a Grade A zone with air supplied by terminal, ceiling mounted HEPA filter modules. Figure 1 shows a schematic layout of the area.

Formulation within a conventional Grade A/B area requires full aseptic gowning of the operators as well as movement of materials through the required number of air locks for entry to the high-level clean room space. Operators will weigh the materials under Grade A conditions then add them to the formulation vessel. These operations require the operators to be in close contact with the aseptic components while maintaining good aseptic practice throughout the formulation process.

Formulation in RABS

In a RABS design, the formulation process occurs in the same way as the conventional clean room, with several enhancements. Prior to performing aseptic manipulations with sterile components, they are placed into a barrier system. This barrier, a level 3 RABS, is outfitted with glove ports, separating personnel from the open operation. However, formulation within a RABS environment still requires full aseptic gowning of the operators as well as movement of materials through the required number of air locks for entry to the high-level clean room space.

Operators are in close contact with the aseptic components and must maintain good aseptic practice throughout the formulation process.

Formulation in Isolator

The liquid vehicle is formulated in a Grade C area. The active ingredient for the lot will be weighed in the raw material dispensing unit and delivered to the formulation area. The fluid material will then be compounded for the lot. This fluid may be heat sterilized or sterilized by filtration. Once the liquid phase has been sterilized, aseptic additions may take place using an isolator docked to the holding vessel for the sterilized buffer.

In preparation for formulation, presterilized ingredients will be brought to the air locks leading to the formulation room. External coverings will be removed upon entrance to the Grade C area. Material will be placed into an antechamber, where it will be surface decontaminated, either by wipe down by gowned personnel using gloves, or by vapor phase hydrogen peroxide (VPHP). Once decontaminated, the material will be transferred into the isolator for weighing and aseptic addition. There are two common methods for transferring materials into the isolator. In one case, an air lock with a system of interlocked doors is used. The aseptic materials are moved into the air lock and the external surfaces of the container or wrapping are wiped with a germicidal solution. After allowing a measure of time for germicide exposure to outer surfaces of the container, the container is moved into the clean zone of the isolator. Another method for introducing materials into an isolator involves the use of rapid transfer ports (RTPs).

Once the aseptic materials have been introduced into the isolator, they are weighed and prepared for addition to the batch. The isolator provides the critical environment for the aseptic handling. The presterilized active and any other presterilized material will be added to the lot with agitation. The lot is then ready for the next operation. Figure 2 shows a schematic layout of the area.

The use of an isolator in a Grade C environment allows for more freedom of movement for people and materials than the use of a Grade A/B clean room. The isolator provides a mini-environment around the critical operation, excluding the operator except for interaction through gloveports. If an air lock is used to introduce materials into the isolator, the operations required

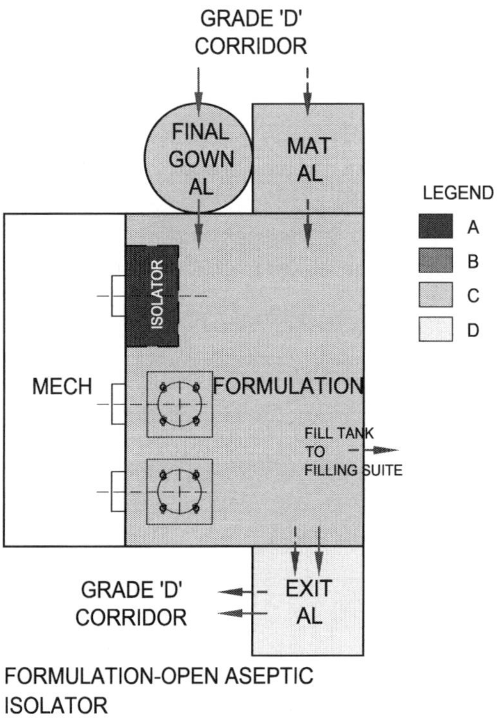

Figure 2 Formulation suite, isolation technology.

Table 1 Formulation Area

	Clean room	Isolator system	
Area classification	**Size (base case)**	**Size**	**% of Base**
A (Class 100)	90 ft^2	Via isolator	NA
B (Class 10,000)	850 ft^2	0 ft^2	0
C (Class 100,000)	430 ft^2	910 ft^2	212
D (Class 100,000 at rest)	0 ft^2	100 ft^2	NA
UAF (not included in subtotal)	0 ft^2	0 ft^2	NA
Total	1370 ft^2	1010 ft^2	74

to introduce materials are similar to those of a Grade A/B area. An RTP canister is a more robust way of introducing materials into an isolator. The use of an RTP canister requires that the materials have been introduced into canisters earlier in the process. This requires coordination with prior processing to provide compatible docking ports and canisters.

Comparison of Cost

The relative core facility sizes for each technology selection are included in Table 1.

The facility costs for these core classified areas are estimated in Table 2 along with the associated equipment costs [including factory acceptance test (FAT)].

In this case the isolated formulation area provides additional operational flexibility as well as a lower cost for facility and equipment.

Table 2 Formulation

	Clean room	Isolator system	
Direct costs	**Cost (base case)**	**Cost**	**% of Base**
Equipment	$ 751,000	$1157,000	154
Facility	$1299,000	$ 814,000	63
ST	$2050,000	$1971,000	96

VIAL FILLING

Basis for Evaluation

Aseptic filling must take place in a Grade A environment to protect the product from particulate and microbiological contamination. This critical, clean environment may be provided in several ways. In the first option, the environment is provided by means of a Grade A/B clean room with its associated system of air locks for entry and exit. In the second option, the clean environment is provided by means of a Grade A level 3 RABS unit with a Grade B background room. In the third option, this environment is miniaturized and provided as an integrated part of the filling system, in the form of an isolator.

An integrated filling line, running at approximately 300 units/min on 3 to 20 mL vials, will be used as the basis for this evaluation, as this is a common application. It is assumed that wetted path components are cleaned and sterilized out of place. Stoppers are supplied as ready to sterilize (RTS) and caps are gamma irradiated.

It is assumed that the vials will be supplied on in-house pallets with all particulate generating packaging (cardboard) removed prior to entering classified space. The vials to be washed will be brought into the air lock for the Grade D area where external wrapping will be removed. The pallets of vials will then be moved to a station located near the vial washer for loading onto the line. The packs of vials will be placed on a feed station, located in Grade D, where the final plastic wrapping will be removed. The vials are pushed onto an accumulating station to feed the washer and tunnel, which are both located in Grade C.

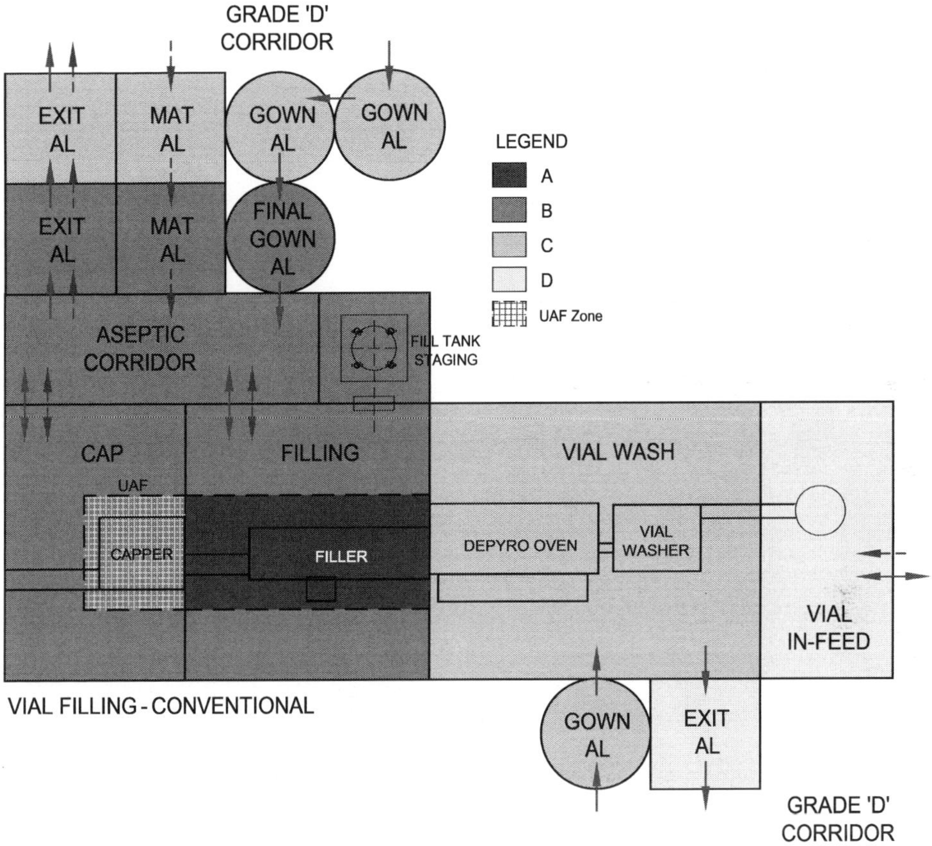

Figure 3 Vial filling suite, conventional technology.

The filling machine delivers the dose of product and places the stopper into the vial, and is located under Grade A. Capping occurs in an environment supplied with Grade A quality air. After capping, vials exit the facility. Operations occurring downstream, such as code placement, inspection or traying, are outside the scope of this exercise.

Vial Filling in Conventional Clean Room

In many cases, the washer and tunnel are located in a Grade C area with the tunnel being mounted into the wall of the Grade A/B area. When the vials exit the tunnel, they enter the Grade A zone of the filling room. The Grade A zone is created with terminal, ceiling-mounted HEPA filter modules.

The sterilized/depyrogenated and cooled vials exit the tunnel onto an accumulator and are fed into the transport section of the filler. Once filled and stoppered, the vials proceed to the capper for sealing and exit the fill line. Figure 3 shows a schematic layout of the area. The portion of the figure that shows the accumulation of vials for lyophilizer loading is not considered as part of the liquid filling case and is not added as part of the liquid filling area.

Filling within a Grade A/B area requires full aseptic gowning of the operators as well as sterilization of components and product contact parts. Operators will set up the filler, fill vials, and supply stoppers and caps to the fill line under Grade A conditions. These operations require the operators to be in close proximity to the aseptic filling process while maintaining good aseptic practice throughout the fill.

Vial Filling in RABS

The RABS unit case is very similar to the aseptic clean room case, except that the critical clean zone of the operation is provided by a HEPA-filtered unidirectional airflow unit integrated with

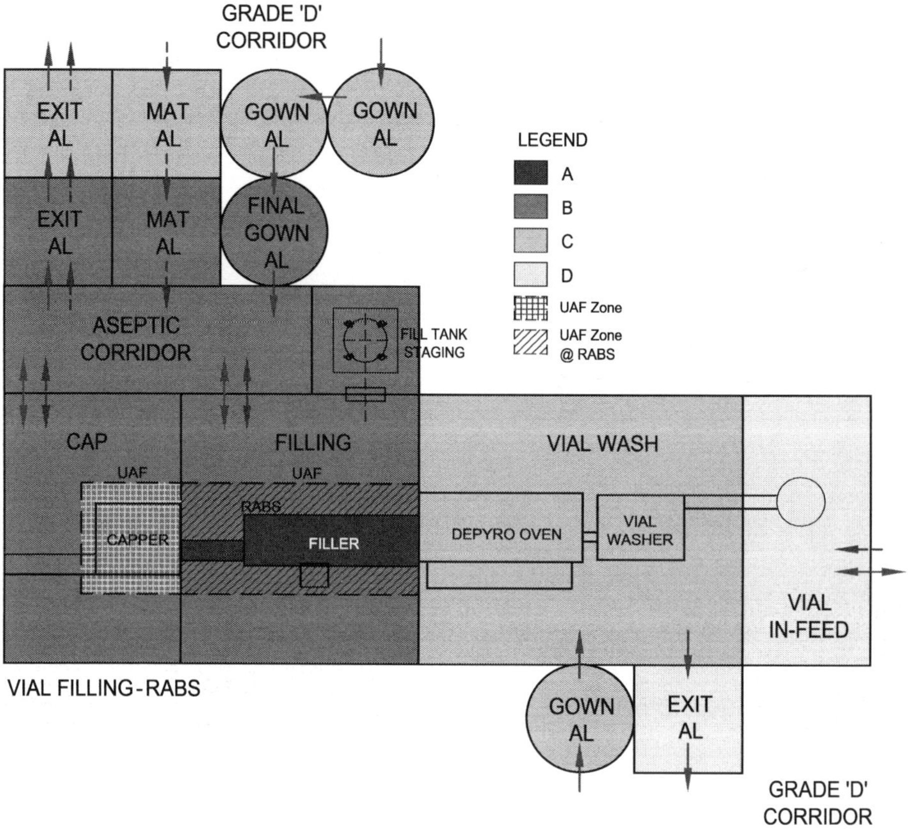

Figure 4 Vial filling suite, RABS technology.

the filling and capping machines. The RABS unit provides a more rigorous separation of the clean zone from the background environment. The clean zone is protected by solid panels or doors to minimize interaction with the background room (Fig. 4). Glove ports and RTP ports may be used to further limit the affect of the background area with the clean zone.

Stoppers may be introduced using an RTP port or other transfer device. Caps are supplied as presterilized or autoclaved in bags and supplied to the fill line. These too may be introduced using an RTP port or other transfer device. Operators will set up the filler, fill vials, and supply stoppers to the fill line under Grade A conditions. Caps will be added in an environment supplied with Grade A quality air. The RABS units provide a measure of separation for the operators from the aseptic zone. However, process upsets may lead to closer interactions of the operators with the clean zone.

Doors are intended to be closed during operation, as per ISPE guideline. The need for intervention during a fill batch should be minimized. If the barrier system of the RABS must be breached, it must be done under strict controls with the required safeguards built into the facility or the equipment. As the filling room is designed as a Grade B room, with Grade A level 3 RABS only over the machinery, any interventions requiring door openings must be planned for. Grade A areas will also be required over certain door swings to maintain the SAL during any intervention.

Vial Filling in Isolator

Filling within an isolator requires that robust equipment be present under isolation. The equipment must be capable of running with minimal intervention for successful isolator operations. Although the vial washer and tunnel operate much the same in an isolator line, as the filling

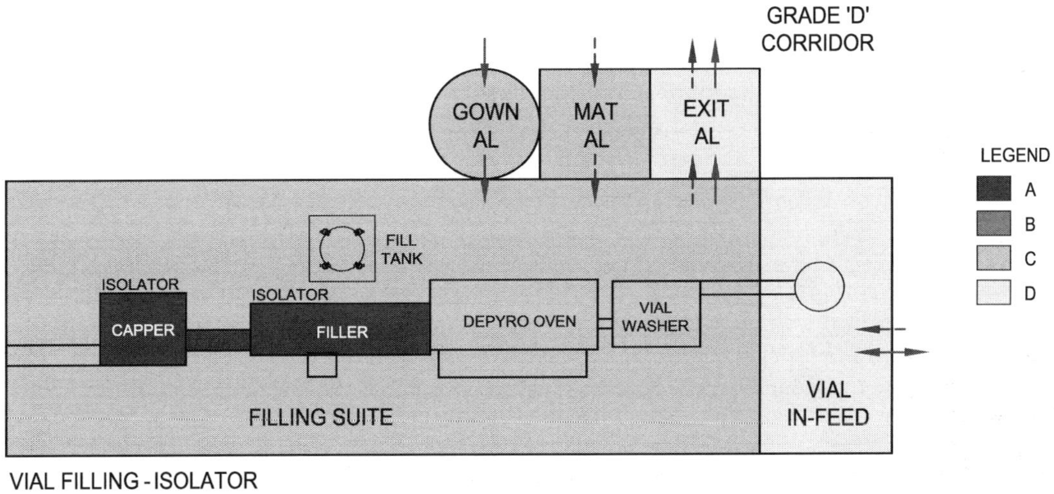

Figure 5 Vial filling suite, isolation technology.

isolator is decontaminated to a 6 log reduction, the cooling zone of the tunnel is considered to be an equivalent space, and is also decontaminated to this level. The discharge of the tunnel must also interact with the filling isolator to maintain pressure balance in the cooling zone of the tunnel and also to seal off the tunnel when the filling isolator undergoes decontamination with gaseous hydrogen peroxide. When the vials exit the tunnel, they enter the Grade A zone of the filling isolator, which contains an accumulator.

From the accumulator, vials are fed into the transport section of the filler. The filling machine delivers the dose of product and places the stopper into the vial. Stoppers may be introduced to the isolator using an RTP port, or other transfer device. Stoppers and caps are supplied as presterilized or autoclaved in bags and supplied to the fill line. Liquid fill vials then proceed to the capper for sealing and exit the fill line isolator system. Caps may also be introduced using an RTP port or other transfer device. Figure 5 shows a schematic layout of the area.

The isolator is located in a Grade C room. Operators are gowned appropriately for a Grade C area, which is less restrictive gowning than required for a Grade A/B area. The isolator and gloves provide the means to separate the operators from the aseptic filling process.

Comparison of Cost

The relative core facility sizes for each technology selection are included in Table 3.

The facility costs for these core classified areas are estimated in Table 4 along with the associated equipment costs (including FAT).

Table 3 Vial Filling Area

	Clean room	RABS		Isolator system	
Area classification	Size (base case)	Size	% of Base	Size	% of Base
A (Class 100)	230 ft^2	via RABS unit	NA	via isolator	NA
B (Class 10,000)	1400 ft^2	1630 ft^2	116	0 ft^2	0
C (Class 100,000)	1330 ft^2	1330 ft^2	100	1960 ft^2	147
D (Class 100,000 at rest)	400 ft^2	400 ft^2	100	400 ft^2	100
UAF (not included in subtotal)	100 ft^2	330 ft^2	330	0 ft^2	0
Total	3360 ft^2	3360 ft^2	100	2360 ft^2	70

Table 4 Vial Filling

	Clean room	RABS		Isolator system	
Direct costs	**Cost (base case)**	**Cost**	**% of Base**	**Cost**	**% of Base**
Equipment	$4051,000	$5255,000	130	$7747,000	191
Facility	$3021,000	$3159,000	105	$1856,000	61
Total	$7072,000	$8414,000	119	$9603,000	136

LYOPHILIZATION

Basis for Evaluation

Aseptic automated lyophilizer loading and unloading must take place in a Grade A environment to protect the product from particulate and microbiological contamination. This critical, clean environment may be provided in several ways, using different technologies. In the first option, the clean environment is provided by means of a clean room with its associated system of air locks for entry and exit. In the second option, the clean environment is provided by means of a system of RABS units with a Grade B background area. In the third option, this environment is miniaturized and provided as an integrated part of the filling system and automated lyophilizer loading and unloading system, in the form of a series of isolators. Both cart-based and conveyor-based technologies will be evaluated.

The example of an integrated filling line, running at approximately 300 units/min on 3 to 20 mL vials, feeding a loading and unloading system serving three at 25 to 30 m^2. lyophilizers will be used as the basis. The autoload system loads and unloads from one side, providing for mechanical access on the back side, and it is assumed that cycle times are sufficiently long to accommodate this design. Shelves are to be prechilled, requiring dehumidified air to be supplied at the lyophilizer slot door.

Cart-Based Approach

In the cart-based approach, the automated loading and unloading system consists of a transfer cart, with a load/unload table. Filled, partially stoppered vials will leave the filling machine on a conveyor and travel to the loading and unloading accumulation table (LUAT). As the vials enter this table, they will be lined up in long rows and accumulated in a large rectangular pack of vials suitable for loading onto a lyophilizer shelf. When this shelf pack of vials is formed, the transfer cart aligns and docks with the LUAT.

When loading, a rectangular transfer frame advances from the transfer cart to capture the shelf load of vials formed on the loading table. This transfer frame then moves the shelf pack of vials on to the transfer cart. The transfer cart then travels to the lyophilizer to be loaded and docks with a shelf. A Grade A zone with dehumidified air will be required over each lyophilizer slot door to provide coverage over the gap between the cart and the lyophilizer door. The transfer frame moves the vials from the transfer cart to the shelf of the lyophilizer. This process is repeated until all shelves in the lyophilizer are loaded. The vials remain in the lyophilizer for the duration of the lyophilization cycle.

When the lyophilization cycle is completed, the transfer cart travels to the lyophilizer for unloading, and docks with the shelf. The transfer frame moves to capture the shelf pack of vials, then moves them to the transfer cart. Then the transfer cart travels to the LUAT where the transfer frame delivers the shelf pack of vials. These vials exit using the unloading mechanism and are fed to the capper for sealing.

Cart-Based System in Conventional Clean Room

In the conventional clean room design option, the LUAT will have an integrated unidirectional HEPA-filtered airflow module, providing a Grade A area to protect the partially stoppered vials. The LUAT is located within the Grade A/B filling room.

The LUAT is positioned at the boundary of the filling room and the lyophilizer aisle, permitting the cart to dock up at the boundary of the lyophilizer aisle. This boundary serves

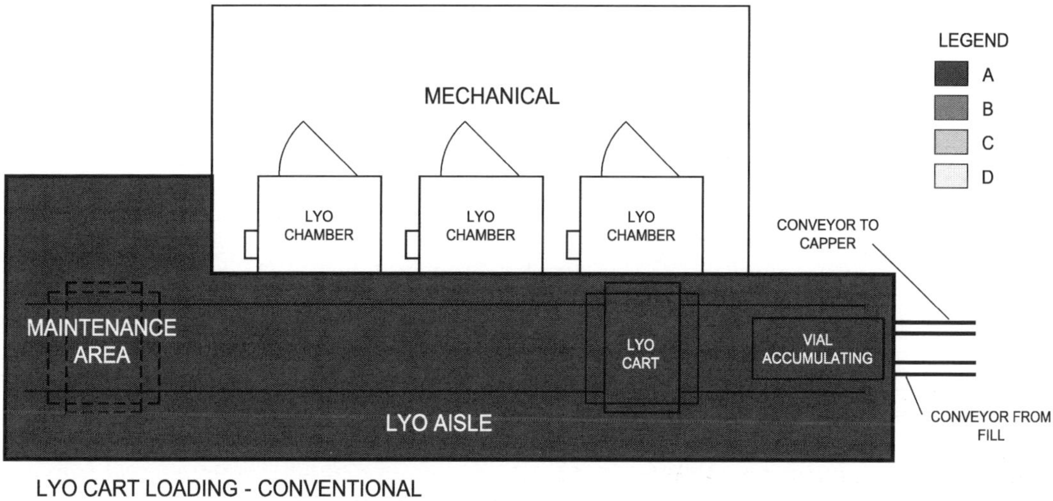

Figure 6 Lyo cart loading, conventional technology.

multiple purposes, including formation of a dedicated Grade A aisle for cart movement, as well as personnel safety. The Grade A zone is provided by terminal, ceiling mounted HEPA filter modules (Fig. 6).

Automated lyophilizer loading and unloading within a Grade A/B area requires full aseptic gowning of the operators as well as sterilization of components and product contact parts. Operators will need to enter the lyophilizer aisle for line clearance and cleaning.

Cart-Based System in RABS

The RABS unit case is very similar to the conventional clean room option, except that the critical clean zone of the operation is provided by HEPA-filtered unidirectional airflow units integrated with the LUAT and transfer cart. This series of level 3 RABS units provides a more rigorous separation of the clean zone from the background environment (Fig. 7). The clean zone is protected by solid panels or doors to minimize interaction with the background room. Glove ports and RTP ports may be used to further limit the affect of the background area with the clean zone.

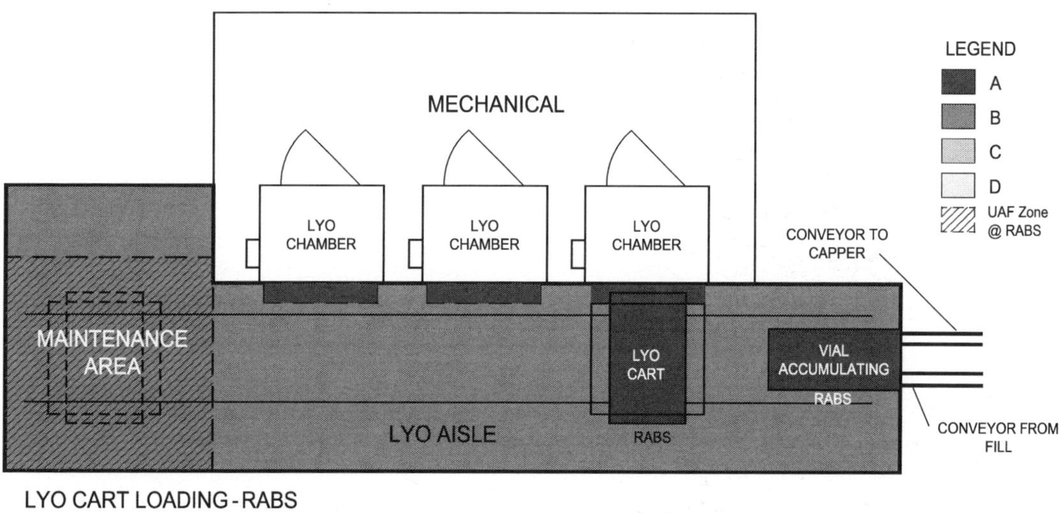

Figure 7 Lyo cart loading, RABS technology.

The lyophilizer aisle is designed as a Grade B zone, with Grade A zones over specific areas. Although the RABS units provide a measure of separation for the operators from the aseptic zone, process upsets may lead to closer interactions of the operators with the clean zone. Barrier doors are intended to be closed during operation, as per ISPE guideline. Proper equipment design should minimize the need for intervention during a fill batch. If the RABS barrier must be breached, it must be done under strict controls with the required safeguards built into the facility or the equipment. As the lyophilizer aisle is designed as a Grade B room, with Grade A level 3 RABS only over cart, any interventions requiring door openings must be planned for. A Grade A area will be required over the cart access doors, to maintain the SAL during for intervention. Additionally, a Grade A zone with dehumidified air will be required over each lyophilizer slot door to provide coverage over the gap between the cart and the lyophilizer door.

Cart-Based System in Isolator

In the isolator option, filled, partially stoppered vials will leave the isolated filling machine on an isolated conveyor and travel to the LUAT, which is equipped with an integrated isolator. When a shelf pack of vials is formed, the isolated transfer cart aligns and docks with the loading table by means of an RTP-type door. Once the vials are transferred to the transfer cart, it travels to the lyophilizer to be loaded, and docks up by means of an RTP-type door. The vials are then loaded into the lyophilizer. The cycle is repeated until the entire batch is loaded.

When the lyophilization cycle is completed, the lyophilized vials are unloaded back onto the transfer cart, which travels back to the isolated LUAT, and docks with the table by means of an RTP-type door. The transfer frame delivers the shelf pack of vials to the LUAT. These vials exit using the unloading mechanism and are fed to the isolated capper for sealing.

The loading and unloading system features an integrated isolator and is located in a Grade C area. The transfer cart is cleaned and decontaminated by docking with the transfer cart CIP station. Figure 8 shows a schematic layout of the area.

Although the LUAT is located in the fill room, the lyophilizer aisle is still maintained as a separate room, to maintain a physical barrier and satisfy safety concerns. Operators are gowned appropriately for a Grade C area, which is less restrictive gowning than required for a Grade A/B area. Most items introduced or removed from the isolators contained within RTP canisters or some other form of transfer device. The isolator and gloves provide the means to separate the operators from the aseptic filling process.

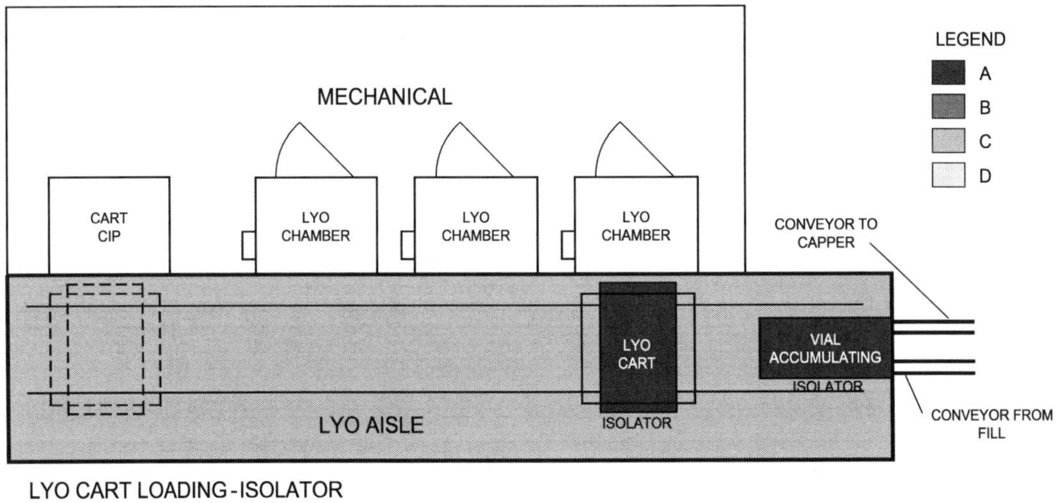

Figure 8 Lyo cart loading, isolation technology.

Table 5 Cart-Based Lyophilizer Loading and Unloading Area

	Clean room	RABS		Isolator system	
Area classification	**Size (base case)**	**Size**	**% of Base**	**Size**	**% of Base**
A (Class 100)	1560 ft^2	via RABS unit	NA	via isolator	NA
B (Class 10,000)	0 ft^2	1560 ft^2	NA	0 ft^2	NA
C (Class 100,000)	0 ft^2	0 ft^2	NA	1390 ft^2	NA
D (Class 100,000 at rest)	0 ft^2	0 ft^2	NA	0 ft^2	NA
UAF (not included in subtotal)	0 ft^2	370 ft^2	NA	0 ft^2	NA
Total	1560 ft^2	1560 ft^2	100	1390 ft^2	89

Comparison of Cost

The relative core facility sizes for each technology selection are included in Table 5; costs are given in Table 6.

Table 6 Cart-Based Lyophilizer Loading and Unloading

	Clean room	RABS		Isolator system	
Direct costs	**Cost (base case)**		**% of Base**	**Cost**	**% of Base**
Equipment	$14146,000	$14699,000	104	$18105,000	128
Facility	$ 1560,000	$ 1842,000	118	$ 1159,000	74
Total	$15706,000	$16542,000	105	$19264,000	123

Conveyor-Based Approach

In the conveyor-based approach, the automated loading and unloading system consists of a conveyor, with a load/unload module associated with each lyophilizer. Filled, partially stoppered vials will leave the filling machine on a conveyor and travel to the load/unload mechanism connected to the lyophilizer chamber being loaded. The Grade A zone over each lyophilizer slot door will be supplied with dehumidified air. As the vials enter this loader, they will be lined up in long rows and pushed row by row onto a lyophilizer shelf. This process is repeated until all shelves in the lyophilizer are loaded. The vials remain in the lyophilizer for the duration of the lyophilization cycle.

When the lyophilization cycle is completed, the load/unload mechanism at the front of the lyophilizer is reconfigured to singularize vials and transfer them to a conveyor. The pack of vials on the shelf is pushed from the back of the lyophilizer onto the unload mechanism. These vials are then conveyed using the unloading mechanism, moving in the same direction along the face of other lyophilizers, and are fed to a dedicated capper for sealing.

Conveyor-Based System in Conventional Clean Room

In the conventional clean room design option, the conveyor will have an integrated unidirectional HEPA-filtered airflow module, providing a Grade A area to protect the partially stoppered vials. The lyophilizer aisle is designed as a Grade B room, with Grade A zones over specific areas. The Grade A zone is provided by terminal, ceiling mounted HEPA filter modules (Fig. 9).

Automated lyophilizer loading and unloading within a Grade A/B area requires full aseptic gowning of the operators as well as sterilization of components and product contact parts.

Conveyor-Based System in RABS

The RABS unit case is very similar to the conventional clean room option, except that the critical clean zone of the operation is provided by a series of HEPA-filtered unidirectional airflow units integrated with the conveyor and load/unload mechanisms. This series of level 3 RABS

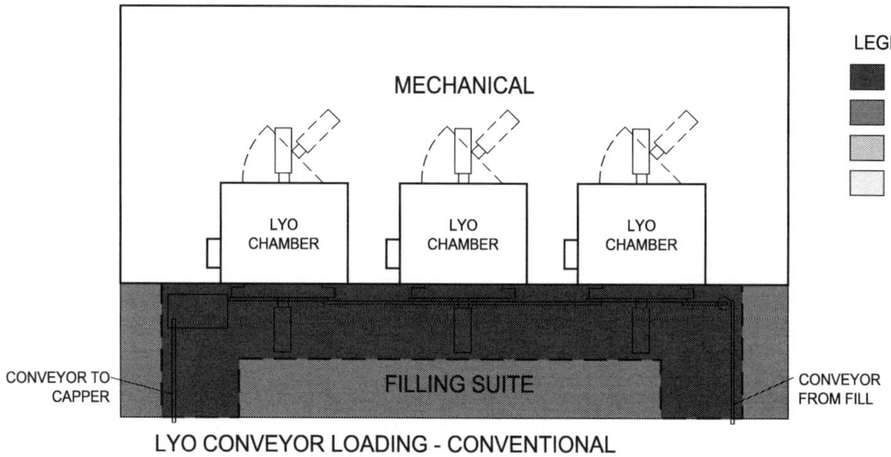

Figure 9 Lyo conveyor loading, conventional technology.

units provides a more rigorous separation of the clean zone from the background environment. Figure 10 shows a schematic layout of the area. The clean zone is protected by solid panels or doors to minimize interaction with the background room. Gloveports and RTP ports may be used to further limit the affect of the background area with the clean zone.

The lyophilizer aisle is designed as a Grade B zone, with Grade A zones over specific areas. Although the RABS units provide a measure of separation for the operators from the aseptic zone, process upsets may lead to closer interactions of the operators with the clean zone. Barrier doors are intended to be closed during operation, as per ISPE guideline. Proper equipment design should minimize the need for intervention during a fill batch. If the RABS barrier must be breached, it must be done under strict controls with the required safeguards built into the facility or the equipment. As the lyophilizer aisle is designed as a Grade B room, with Grade A level 3 RABS only over the conveyor, any interventions requiring door openings must be planned for.

Conveyor-Based System in Isolator

In the isolator option, filled, partially stoppered vials will leave the isolated filling machine on an isolated conveyor and be conveyed to the lyophilizer being loaded, which is equipped with an integrated isolator over the slot door. The vials are pushed into the lyophilizer row by-row, until the entire batch is loaded.

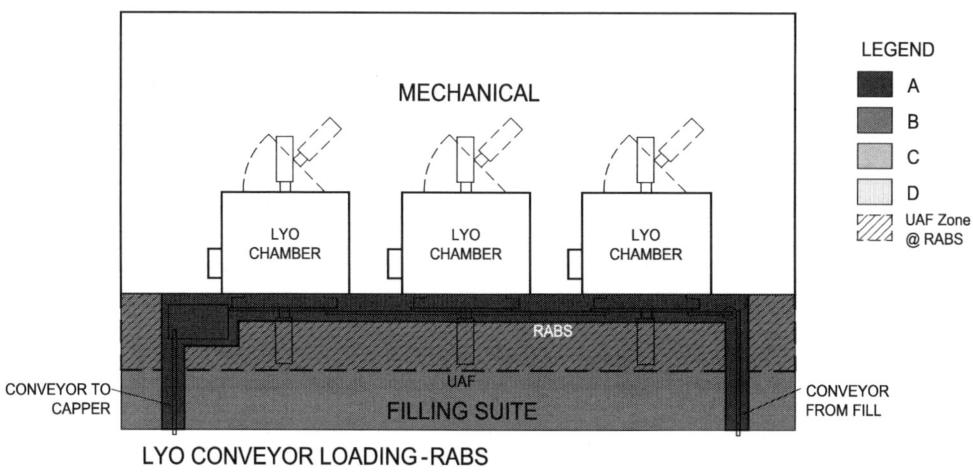

Figure 10 Lyo conveyor loading, RABS technology.

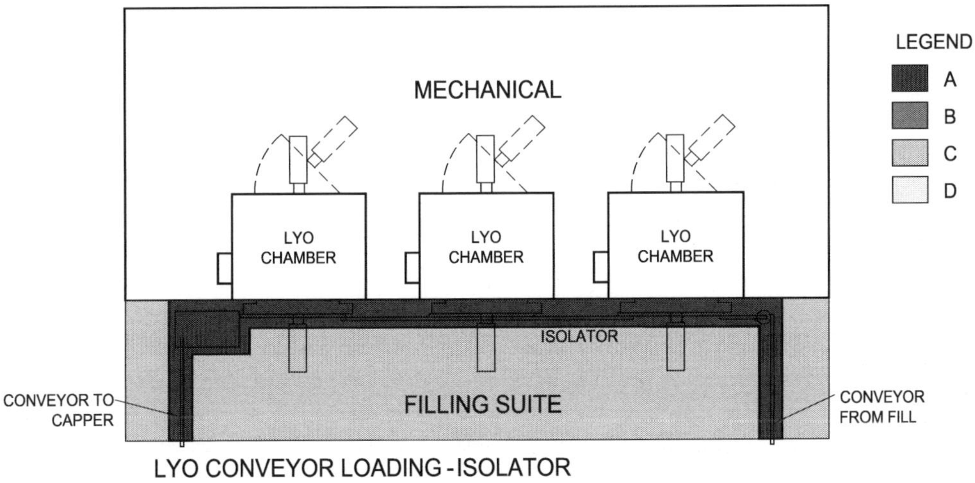

Figure 11 Lyo conveyor loading, isolation technology.

When the lyophilization cycle is completed, the lyophilized vials are unloaded back onto the conveyor, by pushing on the pack from the rear of the chamber. The unload mechanism is fitted with a descrambling device, either by working through gloves or by opening the isolator and re-decontaminating the enclosure. Vials are singularized, exit the unloading mechanism, and are conveyed through isolators to a dedicated capper for sealing.

The loading and unloading system features several integrated isolators that are located in a Grade C area. The conveyor is typically cleaned by manual wipe down, either through gloves, or by opening the barrier doors. Figure 11 shows a schematic layout of the filling and lyophilizer loading and unloading areas.

Operators are gowned appropriately for a Grade C area, which is less restrictive gowning than required for a Grade A/B area. Most items introduced or removed from the isolators contained within RTP canisters or some other form of transfer device. The isolator and gloves provide the means to separate the operators from the aseptic filling process.

Comparison of Cost

The relative core facility sizes for each technology selection are included in Table 7.

Table 7 Conveyor-Based Lyophilizer Loading and Unloading Area

	Clean room	RABS		Isolator system	
Area classification	**Size (base case)**	**Size**	**% of Base**	**Size**	**% of Base**
A (Class 100)	410 ft^2	via RABS unit	NA	via isolator	NA
B (Class 10,000)	290 ft^2	700 ft^2	241	0 ft^2	0
C (Class 100,000)	0 ft^2	0 ft^2	NA	700 ft^2	NA
D (Class 100,000 at rest)	0 ft^2	0 ft^2	NA	0 ft^2	NA
UAF (not included in subtotal)	0 ft^2	390 ft^2	NA	0 ft^2	NA
Total	700 ft^2	700 ft^2	100	700 ft^2	100

Comparison Between Cart-Based and Conveyor-Based Loading Systems

The use of either type of isolated loading system represents an increase in the SAL, although this comes at a significant increase in capital cost. The RABS system provides a measure of improvement over the conventional aseptic clean room case, at a lower increase in capital cost than the isolator system (Tables 5–8).

When comparing the two loading system technologies, it is important to note the relative sizes of the machinery, and therefore, the relative costs. Traditionally, the breakpoint in

Table 8 Conveyor-Based Lyophilizer Loading and Unloading

	Clean room	RABS		Isolator system	
Direct costs	**Cost (base case)**		**% of Base**	**Cost**	**% of Base**
Equipment	$17394,000	$19026,000	109	$23706,000	136
Facility	$ 700,000	$ 934,000	133	$ 584,000	83
Total	$18094,000	$19960,000	110	$24289,000	134

Table 9 Comparison Between Conveyor and Cart-Based Loading and Unloading

	Clean room		RABS		Isolator system	
Direct costs	**Cost (base case)**	**% of Base**		**% of Base**	**Cost**	**% of Base**
Cart-based	$15706,000		$16542,000		$19264,000	
Conveyor-based	$18094,000		$19960,000		$24289,000	
Delta	$ 2388,000	115	$ 3418,000	121	$ 5025,000	126

capital cost between the two technologies occurs once more than two lyophilizer chambers are installed, as more fixed equipment is required for each lyophilizer in the conveyor-based option (Table 9).

It should be noted that in an isolator environment, conveyor systems have enjoyed more popularity, although they require additional capital cost as compared to the cart-based system. Although the cart-based system requires less capital, less isolator volume, and less glove maintenance, potential concerns regarding the isolator docking mechanism require users to carefully define requirements to avoid issues during validation.

SYRINGE FILLING

Basis for Evaluation

Aseptic filling must take place in a Grade A or Class 100 environment to protect the product from particulate and microbiological contamination. This critical, clean environment may be provided in several ways. In the first option, this clean environment is provided by means of a Grade A/B clean room with its associated system of airlocks for entry and exit. In the second option, the clean environment is provided by means of a Grade A level 3 RABS unit with a Grade B background room. In the third option, this environment is miniaturized and provided as an integrated part of the filling system, in the form of an isolator.

An integrated filling line, running at approximately 300 units/min on nested 1 mL presterilized syringes, will be used as the basis for this evaluation, as this is a common application. Plungers are supplied in bags as RTS. Once autoclaved, the bags of sterilized components are transferred to the filling line. It is assumed that wetted path components are cleaned and sterilized out of place.

It is assumed that the syringes will be received presterilized by γ-rays, ready to use (RTU), inside packed tubs (100 syringes/tub). The syringes will be supplied on in-house pallets with all exterior particulate generating packaging (cardboard) removed prior to entering classified space. After external pallet wrapping is removed, syringe tubs in bags will be placed onto racks, and manually transferred into the airlock for the Grade C area. Syringe tubs will then be loaded onto the filling line, via different technologies.

Once loaded onto the filling machine, and opened, the syringe nests will be lifted out of the tubs, to perform the filling and plunger insertion process. The tubs will follow along the path of the syringe nest, underneath the nest. The filling machine receives the nest of syringes, delivers the dose of product and inserts the plunger into the syringe, and is located under Grade A. Filled syringes, in tubs, exit the facility. Operations occurring downstream, such as inspection or palletizing, are outside the scope of this exercise.

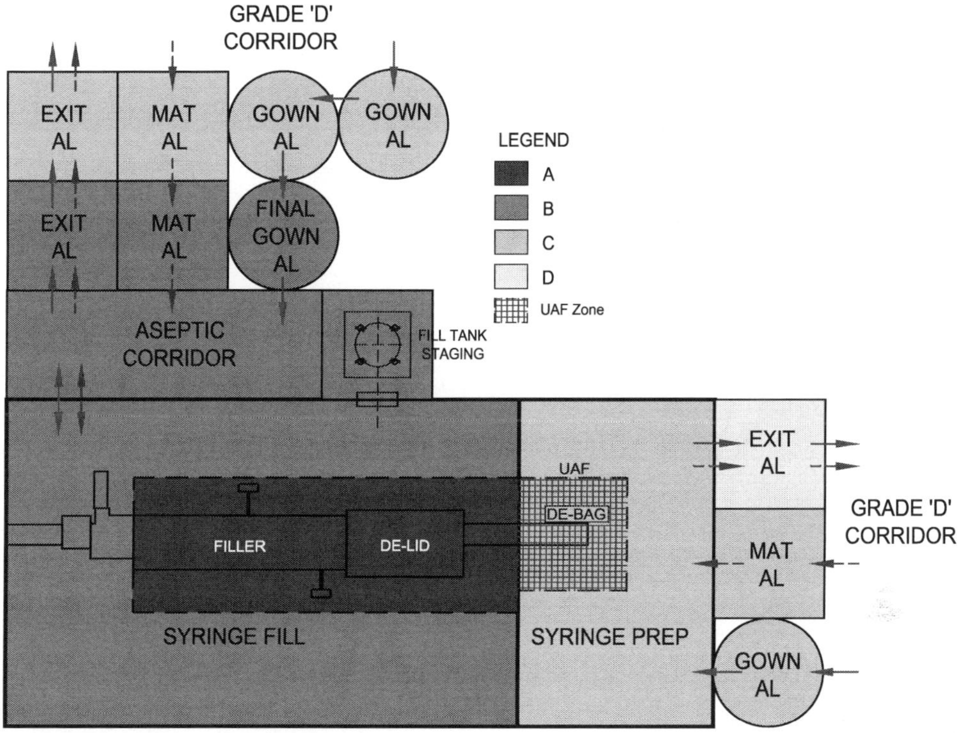

Figure 12 Syringe filling suite, conventional technology.

Syringe Filling in Conventional Clean Room

Racks of presterilized syringes enter from Grade D, into a Grade C material staging room. Outer bags are wiped down, removed using aseptic technique under HEPA filtration, and the tubs are placed onto gravity conveyors. The conveyors transfer the tubs, with final plastic bag, into the Grade B fill room, with the filler mounted under a Grade A zone. The Grade A zone is provided by terminal, ceiling mounted HEPA filter modules (Fig. 12). Once inside the Grade A area, the bag is removed via aseptic technique. As the tub is placed into the filling line, the lid and liner are manually peeled back and discarded into a waste receptacle.

Syringe filling within a Grade A/B area requires full aseptic gowning of the operators as well as sterilization of components and product contact parts. Operators will set up the filler, and supply plungers to the fill line under Grade A conditions. These operations require the operators to be in close proximity to the aseptic filling process while maintaining good aseptic practice throughout the fill.

Syringe Filling in RABS

The syringe filling line in this option consists of a syringe tub feeding system, e-beam sterilizer, manual de-lidding, and a filling and plunger insertion machine (with automatic check weigh). The syringe filler is located in a Grade B room.

Syringe tubs are debagged in a Grade C room, and placed in an e-beam sterilizer, which is designed to perform surface sterilization of the tubs. At the exit of the e-beam sterilizer, the syringe tubs enter the level 3 RABS enclosure for the filler, a Grade A environment that is provided by a HEPA-filtered unidirectional airflow unit integrated with the filling machine (Fig. 13). The RABS unit provides a more rigorous separation of the clean zone from the background environment. The clean zone is protected by solid panels or doors to minimize interaction with the background room. Gloveports and RTP ports may be used to further limit the effect of the background area on the clean zone.

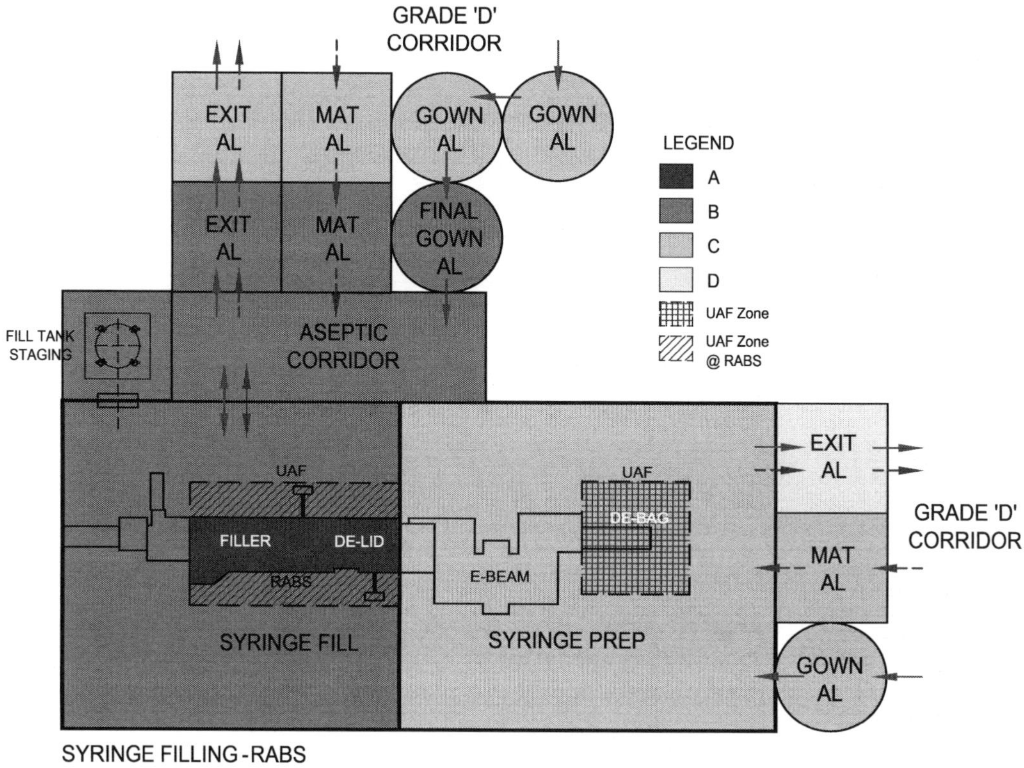

Figure 13 Syringe filling suite, RABS technology.

After entering the RABS, the lids and liners of the tubs will be manually removed through gloves, before the syringes can enter the filling/closing machine. The lids and liners will exit the RABS through a mousehole in the baseplate of the chamber, into a waste container. Inside the RABS, product syringes are filled, plungers inserted, and then the nests are replaced into the tubs. The tubs then exit through a mousehole to the Grade C room outside the facility.

RTP bags containing presterilized plungers are docked to the RABS enclosure for the plunger feed hopper. After docking, the bags will be lifted to allow for the plungers to be manually dumped into the hopper.

Operators will set up the filler and supply plungers to the fill line under Grade A conditions, through the RABS. The RABS units provide a measure of separation for the operators from the aseptic zone. However, process upsets may lead to closer interactions of the operators with the clean zone.

Doors are intended to be closed during operation, as per ISPE guideline. The need for intervention during a fill batch should be minimized. If the barrier system of the RABS must be breached, it must be done under strict controls with the required safeguards built into the facility or the equipment. As the filling room is designed as a Grade B room, with Grade A level 3 RABS only over machine, any interventions requiring door openings must be planned for. Grade A areas will also be required over certain door swings to maintain the SAL during for intervention.

Syringe Filling in Isolator

The syringe filling line in this option consists of a syringe tub feeding system, e-beam sterilizer, automatic de-lidding, and a filling and stoppering machine (with automatic check weigh). The syringe filler is located in a Grade C room (Fig. 14).

Syringe tubs are debagged in a Grade C room and placed in an e-beam sterilizer, which is designed to perform surface sterilization of the tubs. At the exit of the e-beam sterilizer, the

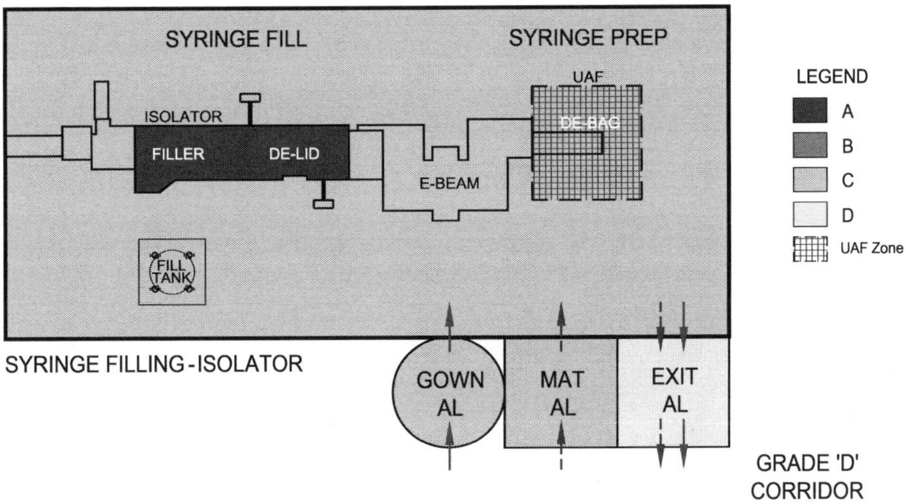

Figure 14 Syringe filling suite, isolation technology.

syringe tubs enter the isolator enclosure for the filler, which provides a Grade A environment that is segregated from the operators.

After entering the isolator, the lids and liners of the tubs will be automatically removed, before the syringes can enter the filling/closing machine. The lids and liners will exit the isolator through a mousehole in the baseplate of the isolator chamber, into a waste container. Inside the isolator, product syringes are filled, plungers inserted, and then the nests are replaced into the tubs. The tubs then exit through a mousehole to the Grade C room outside the facility.

RTP bags containing presterilized plungers are docked to the isolator enclosure for the plunger feed hopper. After docking, the bags will be lifted to allow for the plungers to be manually dumped into the hopper (Table 10).

Comparison of Cost

The relative core facility sizes for each technology selection are included in Table 10.

The facility costs for these core classified areas are estimated in Table 11 along with the associated equipment costs (including FAT).

Table 10 Syringe Filling Area

	Clean room	RABS		Isolator system	
Area classification	**Size (base case)**	**Size**	**% of Base**	**Size**	**% of Base**
A (Class 100)	430 ft^2	via RABS unit	NA	via isolator	NA
B (Class 10,000)	1840 ft^2	1590 ft^2	86	0 ft^2	0
C (Class 100,000)	1210 ft^2	1680 ft^2	139	2190 ft^2	181
D (Class 100,000 at rest)	100 ft^2	100 ft^2	100	100 ft^2	100
UAF (not included in subtotal)	100 ft^2	320 ft^2	320	100 ft^2	100
Total	3580 ft^2	3370 ft^2	94	2290 ft^2	64

Table 11 Syringe Filling Cost

	Clean room	RABS		Isolator system	
Direct costs	**Cost (base case)**	**Cost**	**% of Base**	**Cost**	**% of Base**
Equipment	$3421,000	$6646,000	194	$7907,000	231
Facility	$3395,000	$3238,000	95	$1941,000	57
Total	$6816,000	$9884,000	145	$9848,000	144

FACILITY IMPACT

Stopper/Plunger Handling

For small batches, RTP bags containing components are sterilized in a passthrough autoclave. Component processors are recommended for large lot size and would have to be added to the design. Components, including stoppers, plungers, and caps, can be washed, siliconized, sterilized, and dried in the processor, and transferred to RTP vessels for component delivery to the filling line. Use of component processors permits the size of autoclaves to be reduced. Component processors and the RTP vessels are considered in the scope of this exercise, as they would be used in all options and would not provide any differentiation.

Purchase of components as RTU is also possible and is recommended for small campaigns. RTU components do not require in-house sterilization, and therefore permit autoclave sizes to be reduced. This is also not included in the scope of this exercise, as no differentiation would be provided.

Cap Handling

It is assumed that caps are presterilized. This permits the caps to be used in a Grade A environment. The bags must be decontaminated and wiped down as they are transferred from Grade D into the capping room. An alternate method of decontaminating the exterior of the bags requires the use of a VPHP chamber. This equipment is outside the scope of the exercise.

Cleaning and Preparation of Filler-Wetted Path Components

It is assumed that the wetted path components need to be removed from the filling room for cleaning, wrapping, and sterilization. Depending on the filling technology employed, different equipment will be required to accomplish this task.

In a conventional installation, the components are washed, wrapped under HEPA coverage, and autoclaved. The passthrough autoclave exits into a Grade A space, with a Grade B background. The components are overwrapped and transferred to the filling room. There the parts are unwrapped under Grade A and manually installed. Figure 15 shows a schematic layout of the area.

In a RABS installation, the parts are washed and wrapped in much the same way as the conventional line. However, for parts that must be installed after the RABS doors have been closed, RTPs must be used to sterilize and transfer the parts.

In an isolator installation, all components must exit the autoclave in an RTP or a sealed autoclave bag. This permits the classification of the autoclave unload area to be downgraded to Grade C, without any need for a unidirectional hood (Fig. 16). In addition, it is possible to sterilize components in a transfer isolator by VPHP, and store them until required in the isolator. In this case, components can be transferred as needed to the isolator using an RTP container. This equipment is not in the scope of this exercise.

In this exercise, it is assumed that stoppers and plungers will be autoclaved on-site. Because this operation is critical to ongoing operation of the facility, use of multiple autoclaves is assumed, to provide limited redundancy.

RTP Canister Handling

RTP canisters containing wetted path components, if designed in stainless steel, can be ergonomically difficult to handle. Therefore, a system of transfer carts and lifts will typically be required for this purpose. Specialized carts capable of holding the canister will be supplied. When docking the canister to the filler, or loading it into the washer or autoclave, lifts are required. The lifts at the filler will permit the canister to be rotated into locking position or it will be required to install automatically rotating locking devices at the docking station.

Impact to Utility Systems

As the isolator system requires less Grade A/B space, less chilled water and plant steam are required for the facility. In addition, less electricity will be required to operate fans. UPS power can be limited to the isolator fans to maintain positive pressurization. Based on the differences

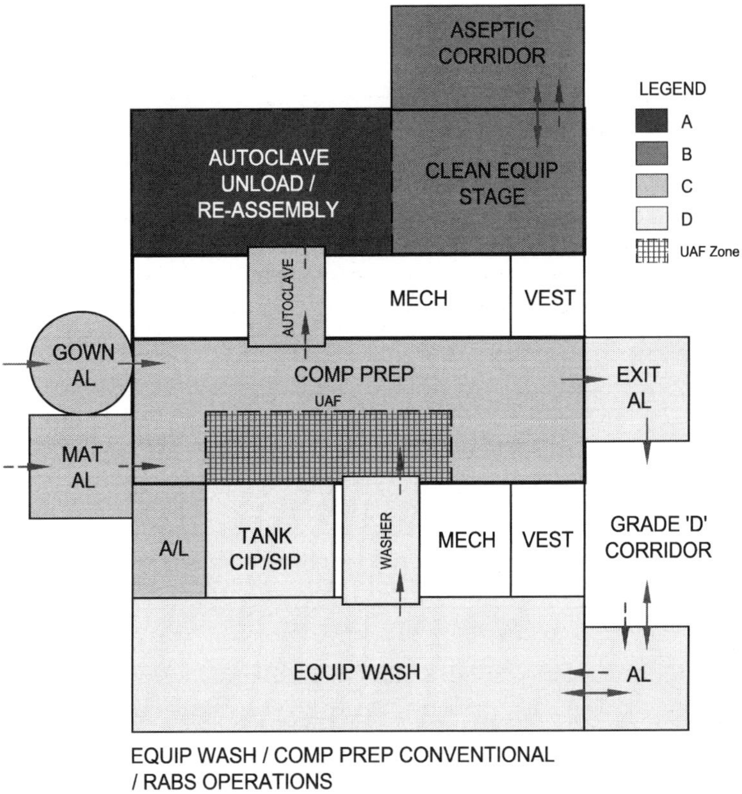

Figure 15 Component preparation suite, conventional/RABS technology.

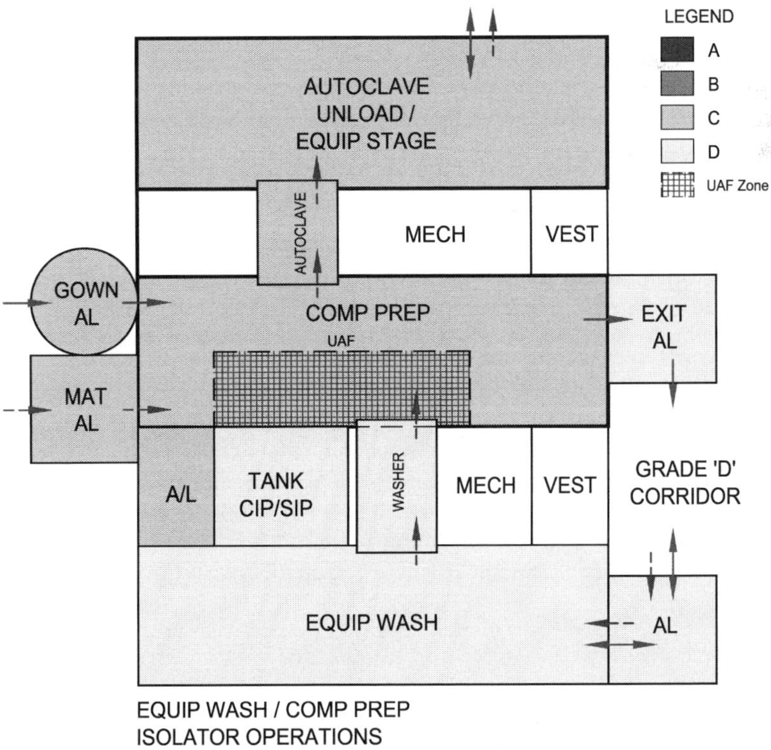

Figure 16 Component preparation suite, isolation technology.

in the layouts for each option, estimates for the impact to initial capital and operating costs can be generated.

Facility Impact Cost Analysis

The relative core facility sizes for each technology selection are included in Table 12.

The facility costs for these core classified areas are estimated in Table 13 along with the associated equipment costs (including FAT).

The use of an isolated filling line represents an increase in the level of assurance of sterility. Although the filling line equipment carries a higher capital cost, the costs for related support facilities are reduced. The capital cost of the RABS system is lower when compared to the isolator, but requires essentially the same support facilities as a conventional clean room.

Table 12 Equipment Wash/Preparation Area

	Clean room	RABS		Isolator system	
Area classification	**Size (base case)**	**Size**	**% of Base**	**Size**	**% of Base**
A (Class 100)	350 ft^2	350 ft^2	100	0 ft^2	100
B (Class 10,000)	440 ft^2	440 ft^2	100	0 ft^2	0
C (Class 100,000)	930 ft^2	930 ft^2	100	1530 ft^2	165
D (Class 100,000 at rest)	930 ft^2	930 ft^2	100	930 ft^2	100
UAF (not included in subtotal)	160 ft^2	160 ft^2	100	160 ft^2	100
Total	2650 ft^2	2650 ft^2	100	2460 ft^2	92

Table 13 Facility Cost

	Clean room	RABS		Isolator system	
Direct costs	**Cost (base case)**	**Cost**	**% of Base**	**Cost**	**% of Base**
Equipment	$2888,000	$2622,000	91	$2998,000	104
Facility	$2178,000	$2178,000	100	$1888,000	87
Total	$5066,000	$4800,000	95	$4896,000	97

INITIAL VALIDATION IMPACT

From the time an order is placed for a filling line, the technology selection influences the validation cost and schedule. As fillers requiring RABS and isolation technology are more complex, and possess more machinery, the systems require additional testing at the factory during the FAT, and once installed, during the Site Acceptance Tests (SAT).

Once acceptance testing is complete, the commissioning and validation phases are also impacted by the technology selection. As the requirements for testing and qualification at the filler increase, the facility qualification requirements decrease, as the sterile zone is reduced.

Conventional

When conventional clean room technology is selected, the basic functionality, such as fill accuracy, software sequence of operation and alarm generation are checked at the factory, and verified at site. As all other aspects of the operation are manual, a robust program must be developed for equipment cleaning and sanitization, including development of standard operating procedures (SOPs), test protocols for qualification, and training programs for the operation staff.

As the filling room is required to meet Grade A/B classification, a complete environmental monitoring program is required to satisfy validation requirements and demonstrate compliance, requiring continuous monitoring of all Grade A and B environments, in addition to areas where aseptic operations are taking place. All HEPA filters must be certified. It is also required to develop a robust program for routine facility cleaning and sanitization, including development of SOPs, test protocols for qualification, and training programs for the operation staff.

RABS

In equipment employing RABS technology, slightly more testing is required to demonstrate utility of glove ports and to prove that port locations are suitable to perform all operations while accounting for ergonomic limitations. Additional studies are required to demonstrate effectiveness of sanitization of the RABS, making use of the gloveports. In addition, SOPs are required for nonroutine interventions, which occur when the barrier doors need to be opened. Additional training is required to provide operators with an understanding of the different requirements for operations of this type.

As a RABS facility is designed to meet the same environmental classifications as a conventional clean room, the testing and qualification requirements can be considered to be the same.

Isolator

As the isolator is supplied with separate air handling equipment and is designed to be automatically decontaminated, this functionality must be tested and qualified. It is typical to provide a mock-up of the isolator in the factory to confirm compliance with ergonomic requirements. Tests on the air system functionality, including pressure control temperature control, air distribution, and leak tightness must be conducted. Smoke testing needs to be conducted as a part of this protocol.

A protocol for testing and qualifying the VPHP delivery system must also be generated. This includes development of an optimized cycle, to account for gas distribution, as well as aeration to eliminate residual peroxide prior to restarting operation. Gas distribution is proven through the use of chemical indicators, which are strategically placed throughout the isolator. To prove effectiveness of the decontamination cycle, a reliable set of biological indicators, generating reproducible data, needs to be used.

Comparison of Cost

To calculate the relative validation cost, information was used from Edwards and Chester, presented at ISPE 2006 (2). As qualification of baseline equipment and facility remains the same, the differential was used to determine the relative cost impact of technology selection (Table 14).

Table 14 Validation Cost Impact (2)

	Clean room	RABS		Isolator system	
Direct costs	**Cost (base case)**	**Cost**	**% of Base**	**Cost**	**% of Base**
IQ/OQ					
Isolator/decontamination system	$0	$0	NA	$150,000	NA
PQ					
Decontamination	$0	$0	NA	$300,000	NA
Facility qualification	$200,000	$200,000	100	$0	0
Total cost	$200,000	$200,000	100	$450,000	225

OPERATING IMPACT

Even after the facility has been successfully placed into operation, the technology selection affects the operating cost, in areas such as utility usage, gowning, testing and revalidation, and maintenance.

Conventional

In a conventional filling facility, operating cost and productivity are impacted by the aseptic garb required to work in a Grade B fill room. Each time operators enter the suite, it is assumed that new, disposable apparel is used. Over the course of a year, the costs associated with gowning can become significant. In addition, each gowning step consumes time and reduces the overall productivity of the operation.

As the facility is maintained as a Grade A/B room, continuous environmental monitoring of the rooms are required for particulate and viables during all production operations, in addition to monitoring of the critical zones on the filling line. Each operator is required to be routinely tested to demonstrate compliance with gowning procedures. In addition, routine monitoring is required for the surrounding Grade C areas.

When cleaning and sanitizing the equipment, aseptic technique is required. All components used in the wetted path are assumed to be autoclaved, and assembled under Grade A conditions, by operators in sterile garb, all resulting in decreased productivity for operators.

In the conventional facility, more air is required to be supplied to the Grade A/B room. This drives up the annual cost of utilities required for power, heating, cooling, and humidification of the space. When compared to the operation of a Grade C room, this annual cost can become significant.

RABS

When RABS technology is used, the equipment and facility operating costs are similar to that of conventional clean rooms, with one primary difference. As Grade A protection is only required outside the boundary of the filling line to protect doors that must be opened during interventions. This results in less Grade A space and a lower utility cost. However, as glove ports are used to perform manipulations without opening the barrier, costs for routine testing, sanitization, and replacement of gloves must be accounted for in RABS facilities.

Isolator

In a facility employing isolation technology, the operating costs associated with gowning can be drastically reduced due to the use of a Grade C fill room. As operators do not have to routinely don aseptic garb to enter the fill room, more time is spent on productive activities, resulting in an increased level of productivity. To achieve this savings, however, greater reliance upon isolator gloves is required. Routine glove testing, and the implementation of a regular glove change procedure, adds to the operating cost.

Cleaning of the isolator can be accomplished with the doors open, without special requirements to maintain aseptic technique, resulting in a more efficient operation. In addition, as the isolator relies upon VPHP decontamination, the complicated and labor-intensive sanitization procedure required for RABS facilities can be avoided, resulting in a more effective process, with a higher sterility assurance level. However, the automated decontamination process must be revalidated annually, in addition to any media challenges for the filler wetted-path.

As there is more machinery associated with the isolator, the annual cost for maintenance is slightly higher.

Utility Requirements

As the use of technology increases, total facility space and the need for higher environmental classifications are both reduced. In turn, this reduces the requirements for utilities such as chilled water and plant steam. See Table 15 for calculated utility requirements.

To calculate the annual cost for the utility systems, costs for chilled water ($0.25/ton) and steam ($0.02/lb) were calculated, based on an assumption that the utility systems, and HVAC systems are not taken off-line during the year. Annual results are included in Table 16. It should be noted, that in this comparison, it is assumed that conditioned air is supplied to the RABS and isolation equipment from the surrounding room. It can be observed that as the use of technology increases, the cost of utilities required to maintain the facility decreases proportionately.

Table 15 Facility Utility Requirements

	Clean room		RABS			Isolator system		
Utility	Load (base case)		Load		% of Base	Load		% of Base
Chilled water	349	Tons	240	Tons	69	130	Tons	37
Plant steam	2340	lb/hr	2250	Lb/hr	96	1300	Lb/hr	56
Air flow	339,000	CFM	137,000	CFM	40	58,000	CFM	17

Table 16 Annual Facility Utility Cost

	Clean room	RABS		Isolator system	
Utility	**Cost (base case)**	**Cost**	**% of Base**	**Cost**	**% of Base**
Chilled water	$ 762,000	$524,000	69	$284,000	37
Plant steam	$ 409,000	$393,000	96	$227,000	56
Total cost	$1171,000	$917,000	78	$511,000	44

Comparison of Cost

To calculate the operating cost, information was used from Edwards and Chester, presented at ISPE 2006 (2). For this analysis, the operating model includes representative costs for gowning, testing, revalidation, and utilities. To perform the calculations, it was assumed that two filling lines were operated in a single-shift operation, 5 days/week, for 45 weeks. The utilities for maintaining the environment are required year round. The calculations do not account for gowning of supervisors or cleaning staff. For testing of gloves, it is assumed that weekly glove replacement and leak testing would be required, for both RABS and isolator installations. For this analysis, it is assumed that a total of 36 gloves will need to be maintained (Table 17).

Once the annual operating cost has been determined, the data is used to calculate the total operating cost for a conservative ten year facility life. See Table 18 for the total operating cost.

RESULTS AND CONCLUSION

In an effort to compare the overall cost impact due to technology selection, a facility comprised of formulation, vial filling, lyophilization with cart-based loading, and syringe filling can be studied. Costs for support areas, initial validation, and operating costs over a 10-year life are also included. As indicated in previous sections, the overall area required for operation decreases as the level of technology increases, as demonstrated in Table 19.

Furthermore, the area class, and therefore the cost, is reduced as the use of technology is increased (Table 20).

From information developed earlier in the chapter, the overall capital cost for the facility can be calculated from individual costs for equipment and facility components. The results, contained in Table 21, indicate that the overall cost premium for RABS technology is 14% and rises to 24% when isolation technology is used.

Table 17 Annual Operating Cost

	Clean room	RABS		Isolator system	
Direct costs	**Cost (base case)**	**Cost**	**% of Base**	**Cost**	**% of Base**
Aseptic gowning	$ 300,000	$ 300,000	100	$0	0
Glove testing	$0	$ 150,000	NA	$ 150,000	NA
Annual revalidation					
HEPA recertification	$ 25,000	$ 25,000	100	$0	0
Gas system	$0	$0		$ 30,000	
Environmental monitor	$2700,000	$2700,000	100	$1400,000	52
Utility cost	$1171,000	$ 917,000	78	$ 511,000	44
Total	$4196,000	$4092,000	98	$2091,000	50

Table 18 Operating Cost Impact over 10 Years

	Clean room	RABS		Isolator system	
Direct costs	**Cost (base case)**	**Cost**	**% of Base**	**Cost**	**% of Base**
	$41960,000	$40920,000	98	$20910,000	50

Table 19 Overall Facility Area (by Function)

	Clean room	RABS		Isolator system	
Total area	**Area (base case)**	**Area**	**% of Base**	**Area**	**% of Base**
Formulation	1370 ft^2	1370 ft^2	100	1010 ft^2	74
Vial filling	3360 ft^2	3360 ft^2	100	2360 ft^2	70
Lyo load with cart	1560 ft^2	1560 ft^2	100	1390 ft^2	89
Syringe filling	3580 ft^2	3370 ft^2	94	2290 ft^2	64
Support area	2650 ft^2	2650 ft^2	100	2460 ft^2	93
Total	12520 ft^2	12310 ft^2	98	9510 ft^2	76

Table 20 Overall Facility Area (by Class)

	Clean room	RABS		Isolator system	
Total area	**Area (base case)**	**Area**	**% of Base**	**Area**	**% of Base**
Grade A (class 100)	2660 ft^2	440 ft^2	16	0 ft^2	0
Grade B (class 10,000)	4530 ft^2	6070 ft^2	134	0 ft^2	0
Grade C (class 100,000)	3900 ft^2	4370 ft^2	112	7980 ft^2	205
Grade D (class 100,000 at rest)	1430 ft^2	1430 ft^2	100	1530 ft^2	107
UAF (not included in subtotal)	360 ft^2	1180 ft^2	328	260 ft^2	72
Total	12520 ft^2	12310 ft^2	98	9510 ft^2	76

Table 21 Overall Facility Capital Cost (by Function)

	Clean room		RABS		Isolator System	
Total area	**Equipment (base case)**	**Facility (base case)**	**Equipment**	**Facility**	**Equipment**	**Facility**
Formulation	$ 751,000	$ 1299,000	$ 751,000	$ 1299,000	$ 1157,000	$ 814,000
Vial Filling	$ 4051,000	$ 3021,000	$ 5255,000	$ 3159,000	$ 7747,000	$ 1856,000
Lyo load with cart	$14146,000	$ 1560,000	$14699,000	$ 1842,000	$18105,000	$ 1159,000
Syringe filling	$ 3421,000	$ 3395,000	$ 6646,000	$ 3238,000	$ 7907,000	$ 1941,000
Support area	$ 2888,000	$ 2178,000	$ 2622,000	$ 2178,000	$ 2998,000	$ 1888,000
Subtotal	$25257,000	$11453,000	$29973,000	$11716,000	$37914,000	$ 7658,000
Percent of base	100%	100%	119%	102%	150%	67%
Total cost	$36710,000		$41689,000		$45572,000	
Percent of base	100%		114%		124%	

Table 22 Overall Cost Impact After 10 Years of Operation

	Clean room	RABS		Isolator system	
Direct costs	**Cost (base case)**	**Cost**	**% of Base**	**Cost**	**% of Base**
Formulation	$ 2050,000	$ 2050,000	100	$ 1971,000	96
Vial filling	$ 7072,000	$ 8414,000	119	$ 9603,000	136
Lyo load with cart	$15706,000	$16542,000	105	$19264,000	123
Syringe filling	$ 6816,000	$ 9884,000	145	$ 9848,000	144
Support area	$ 5066,000	$ 4800,000	95	$ 4896,000	97
Initial validation cost	$ 200,000	$ 200,000	100	$ 450,000	225
Operating Cost 10 yr	$41960,000	$40920,000	98	$20910,000	50
Total	$78870,000	$82710,000	105	$66942,000	85

Table 23 Summary (Formulation, Liquid Filling and Cart-Based Lyophilized Products)

	Clean room	RABS	Isolator system
Direct costs	**Cost (base case)**	**Multiplier from base case**	**Multiplier from base case**
Equipment	1.0	1.19	1.50
Facility	1.0	1.02	0.67
Initial validation	1.0	1.00	2.25
Operating cost (10 yr)	1.0	0.98	0.50
Total cost	1.0	1.05	0.85

When the overall operating cost is added to the analysis, the results change significantly. The facility employing isolation technology moves from the most costly to the least costly approach, as the results indicate it is 15% more cost effective than a conventional clean room. However, the RABS facility does not share the same result. As it has many of the same concerns as the conventional clean room, it contains much of the same cost, and for this reason, carries a 5% premium, as compared with the conventional clean room (Table 22).

The use of an isolated filling line represents an increase in the level of assurance of sterility, although this comes at a significant increase in the initial capital cost. The RABS system provides some measure of improvement over the conventional aseptic clean room case, at a slightly lower increase in capital cost than the isolator system, provided it is operated under strict procedural controls. However, when the cost for initial validation and operating costs over 10 years of facility usage are considered, the cost premium encountered for isolation technology is more than offset by the associated operating cost savings, when compared against conventional technology. In addition, when the full impact of capital and operating cost is considered, the use of RABS technology becomes more costly than that of a conventional clean room. Table 23 details the results of the cost comparison, relative to the base case of clean room processing.

These results demonstrate that isolation technology becomes favorable when the life cycle cost of the facility is taken into account. Although the use of RABS can offer improved sterility assurance, it can also be observed that the life cycle cost of a facility using RABS technology exceeds that of the conventional filling facility.

As there is an increased capital cost required to implement isolation technology, it becomes a more desirable option if additional project drivers are present. If the products require containment, an isolator is recommended for operator safety. If the facility is producing high volumes of a few products, it may be possible to run these products on a campaign basis on the isolated lines and increase the batch sizes. The decrease in number of batches coupled with increased output and lower testing costs can be used to offset the increased capital costs associated with the isolator lines. Conversely, small runs of many different products typically do not favor an isolator solution, unless there are other strong drivers present.

In the absence of drivers for the isolation solution, the RABS solution represents an improvement in SAL over clean room technology, at a modest increase in capital cost.

It has been demonstrated that the use of isolators represents a technical advance over conventional aseptic processing in a clean room. However, selection of the appropriate technology comes with a price that requires careful consideration for each application.

REFERENCES

1. ISPE. Definition of Isolator and RABS. www.ispe.org. Accessed 2004.
2. Edwards L, Chester J. Isolators and RABS: Evolution, Devolution and Revolution. Presented at ISPE Barrier Isolator Technology Meeting, Arlington, VA, June 2006.

13 Risk assessment and mitigation in aseptic processing

James Agalloco and James Akers

INTRODUCTION

Sterile products are frequently administered to patients through the dermal layer to attain rapid therapeutic response and accurate dosing. Delivery in this manner intentionally circumvents the body's protective mechanisms, and mandates that the product be largely free of infectious microorganisms and endotoxin. These concerns are heightened when the drug is delivered to patients whose health is already compromised as is common in clinical settings. Awareness of the patient has prompted regulatory preference for the use of terminal sterilization (1,2). Although the use of lethal processes on finished formulations in their final container is favored because of their lethality, material considerations have limited their application such that an estimated 85% of all sterile products are manufactured by aseptic processing, which are less abusive of essential material and container properties.[1]

Aseptic processing customarily use a variety of sterilization procedures for the individual components of the formulated product, container, and product contact parts enabling the sterilizing process to be chosen for preservation of the key quality attributes of the materials. The core aseptic process assembles the sterilized items into the final dosage form in an environment specifically designed for that purpose. Because product containers are closed after the individual sterilization processes are carried out, the potential for contamination ingress is ever present during aseptic processing. In the belief that knowledge of the conditions under which the aseptic process is carried out would be valuable in determining the acceptability of the resulting product, environmental monitoring has historically been considered essential. Microbial sampling of air and surfaces, as well as personnel gloves and gown within the aseptic environment were instituted as a means of environmental monitoring, which ultimately evolved into a program thought to provide critical information regarding sterility assurance. When monitoring was first instituted, the environmental conditions and gowning systems were markedly less capable than those presently in use. As a consequence, performance expectations and demonstrated performance were understood to be nonabsolute. Nevertheless, it was certainly understood that improvement in contamination control performance was both desirable and attainable. The gradual refinements in aseptic processing technology and performance expectations took place over a period of some 50 years and resulted in the advanced aseptic processing technologies that are described in this book.[2]

THE MYTH OF STERILITY

The manufacture of sterile products is closely associated with expectations for sterility of the finished dosage form. This is customarily defined by the probability of a nonsterile unit (PNSU) or sterility assurance level (SAL).[3] The minimum expectation for PNSU in terminally sterilized products is that it be no greater than one nonsterile unit in one million units or 1×10^{-6}. The origins of this target lie in the food industry as it was initially developed for canned foods where the concern was the avoidance of *Clostridium botulinum*, an anaerobic spore former. The goal was not sterility of the canned foods but an acceptable level of safety for the consumer. In actuality, it defines a maximum level of risk that a consumer might be exposed to in the consumption of the sterilized material. This approach is essentially the same as that employed for the terminal sterilization of pharmaceutical products, which although stated as a PNSU, is really a statement

[1] This is estimated as a percentage of products, and not as a percentage of the number of containers.

[2] See Chapter 1 for a brief history of aseptic processing.

[3] The current preference is for the use of PNSU rather that SAL, because PNSU is a far easier concept for the novice to interpret.

of the level of material safety (or risk minimization). Aseptic processing relies on the component and material sterilization methods for success, but differs in that calculation of a PNSU (or SAL) is impossible, there being no directly lethal element of the aseptic manufacturing process. Aseptic processing performance is evaluated using process simulation studies in which the maximum contamination rate in the exercise demonstrates the capability of the overall aseptic process during that exercise and that exercise alone. Suggestions that the success in a process simulation defines the sterility assurance capability of an aseptic process are entirely fallacious. The process simulation is a singular event comprising a number of individual sterilization, manual decontamination, and manipulations that cannot support the ability of those practices under different circumstance. The simulation demonstrates potential capability in a limited manner, but there are no means to extend the results to the same aseptic procedures in a separate event.

There is a common belief that the environmental monitoring performed in conjunction with every aseptic process provides a means for extension of the simulation performance to production operations. The limitations of microbial recovery from environmental samples in present-day manned clean rooms are that such claims are certainly spurious. Extension of this thinking to advanced aseptic processing technologies is similarly inappropriate. What has been demonstrated for every aseptic processing is can be most realistically described as safety. Aseptic processes are essentially considered safe because the patient outcomes are successful and contamination in aseptically filled products has only infrequently been linked to known product contamination derived from the aseptic process. Our industry's ability to detect contamination in aseptic processes through any form of environment monitoring is extremely limited both in terms of analytical limit of detection and sampling statistics. The monitoring sample sizes are too small to afford any meaningful evaluation of the conditions and the cultural methods employed do not have a limit of detection approaching zero. The sterility test is of such limited value in assessing process efficacy that it could be more aptly termed "the test for gross microbial contamination." FDAs recalls of aseptically produced products are rarely the result of demonstrated contamination in the finished product, but rather an absence of appropriate conditions or inadequate documentation during the production operations. What has been attained with aseptic processing is more properly described as "safety." "Sterility" of aseptically filled products is completely un-provable, as it would require the evaluation of an infinite sample size with analytical method capable of detecting *any* contamination present. This is simply impossible, so realistically proving sterility in aseptic processing is not simply a matter of being willing to make a greater effort in terms of sampling intensity.

The improvements in aseptic processing were instituted to effect greater control over the environment, as influenced by its basic design, decontamination method, and operator involvement with a singular goal of reducing the contamination potential. The true objective has always been reduction of risk to the patient receiving the aseptically produced product. Aseptic processing systems in their most evolved forms have reached the point where the monitoring methods to establish their acceptability are no longer adequate to provide any meaningful indication of performance.

As the processing capability evolved, closely followed (or at times preceded) by regulatory expectations, a critical component of the monitoring system remained unchanged. With each refinement of aseptic processing technology the microbial sampling methods were increasingly taxed. In today's advanced aseptic processing systems, the environmental monitoring is being asked to prove an absolute negative—that no microorganisms are present anywhere in either the processing environment or in the product. Although particularly true of isolators; restricted access barrier systems (RABS) and many newer conventional aseptic facilities suffer the same limitations. This presents industry with a substantial conundrum of some magnitude with respect to the evaluation, selection and, ongoing control of aseptic processing technologies.

RISK ASSESSMENT

We first noted the limitations of monitoring programs nearly 20 years ago when new facilities began to exhibit environmental control capabilities that challenged the sensitivity and resolution of monitoring methods then available. When contamination was detected in these environments, it was increasingly associated with personnel. This was consistent with the long-standing understanding across the industry and regulators that personnel are responsible for the majority of contamination in an aseptic process (3,4). Deceased former FDA Inspector Hank Avallone had expressed this exact belief in direct manner during the 1980s, "It is useful to assume that the operator is always contaminated while operating in the aseptic area. If the procedures are viewed from this perspective, those practices which are exposing the product to contamination are more easily identified" (5). Actually, from experience and published research, we need not merely assume that an operator is a source of contamination; rather we can take it as an absolute certainty that clean room personnel function as mobile contamination generators. The idea that it is possible to have "sterile" clean rooms or "sterile" gowned operators has in fact been completely debunked.

In late 2004, when we began the development of our risk analysis method, we drew heavily on the concept that the release of contamination by operators was not merely possible but rather inevitable. With this simple truth in mind, we focused our method on the human actions that are central to any aseptic process (6,7). The Agalloco-Akers (A–A) methods attribute risk almost exclusively to human activity within the aseptic process. The closer, longer, and more invasive the personnel intervention the greater the risk is for contamination introduction. In taking this tact we discounted the more traditional approaches to risk assessment that endeavored to associate risk with contamination transfer to open containers from the air or surfaces (8,9). Although we agree with the basic premises of these methods; the calculations required to calculate a risk value include values for which there is no reliable input data. It is our belief that because these methods use microbial recovery determination as a fundamental factor in the determination of the contamination ingress potential (and thus risk), they are inherently limited where the background microbial levels are largely devoid of recoverable microorganisms. Also, it is clear given the variability of microbial analysis and the extremely limited sample size that it is not possible for monitoring to give us much insight regarding patient risk. It therefore follows that it is not possible to determine through monitoring that an appropriate level of "sterility assurance" has been attained or to assess anything but truly gross changes in environmental control.

After the publication of the A–A method it has been successfully used by several firms to evaluate and improve their aseptic processing operations (10). Katayama and his colleagues compared its application with other risk methods and concluded that the A–A method offered the closest correlation to the historical performance at several aseptic sites when compared to other aseptic risk methodologies (11). A more general means for risk assessment related to sterile products has been developed by Parenteral Drug Association (PDA) (12). Regardless of the risk assessment methodology employed, it is essential that firms consider how their designs, practices, and expectations impact the contamination potential. Assumptions about outcomes must be evaluated in a rigorous manner to provide the greater confidence in the eventual design. Not only is this sound scientifically, it is expected by regulators (13,14).

Discussion of aseptic processing risk, or truly any risk assessment should not end with completion of the assessment. It must be acknowledged that although risk assessment is an important task, it is not an end onto itself. It must be followed by a far more important activity risk mitigation. Consider the driver of an automobile who notices that it is beginning to rain. That is the risk assessment, and although necessary, does not effect any improvement in the driver's safety. Until the driver mitigates the risk in an effective manner then there is no real benefit. Until the driver adjusts their speed, turns on the wipers, and the lights there has been no reduction in their risk potential. The assessment of risk is only the first step that must be accomplished, and aseptic processing is no different.

RISK MITIGATION

Risk assessment alone however is not enough; if the fundamental concepts adopted are inadequate the resulting risk might be lowest for a specific design, but not the lowest possible. It would be far preferable to define, and use design principles that ultimately result in the best aseptic processing design for a specific application. In considering what criteria to use, we believe adherence to the core principles of advanced aseptic processing is most appropriate: *"An advanced aseptic process is one in which direct intervention with open product containers or exposed product contact surfaces by operators wearing conventional cleanroom garments is not required and never permitted"* (15).

Full consideration of this expectation can be used to define the elements of facility design, equipment selection, container/closure selection, product delivery, personnel, procedure definition, and environmental monitoring.

Facilities

The selection of an appropriate advanced aseptic technology is central to nearly all of the subsequent design choices. The choice is often between closed RABS and isolators; however, others have been included in this text and should be given due consideration. Once that basic choice has been made, there are options within those alternatives that should be considered as well to further define the technology to be implemented. The design process for an aseptic facility is a lengthy process: proceeding from conceptualization, preliminary and detailed design with a myriad of choices and decisions to be made throughout. Considering the core objective the following preferences can be defined:

- Design for ease of execution through the choice of construction materials, designing for ease of access and details elements that facilitate both cleaning and decontamination of the core environment.
- The material, personnel, and equipment flows should be defined to minimize mix-ups and contamination potential.
- The heating, ventilation and air conditioning (HVAC) system should provide adequate air quality, and pressurization to prevent the ingress of contamination.
- Air flow should be sufficient to provide high dilution rates particularly within the most risk-intensive locations within the environment.[4]
- Air systems should be supplied with HEPA filters that are periodically integrity tested.
- Differential pressures for the system should be controlled, monitored, and alarmed to support continuous integrity of the critical core area.
- Temperature and humidity should be controlled to maximize personnel comfort during operations consistent with product stability/safety requirements.
- Materials and personnel airlocks should be used to increase separation between environments of different classification.
- Facility and enclosure surfaces must be resistant to the potential corrosive action of sanitizing and decontamination agents, especially sporicidal agents because of their generally greater chemical activity.
- The core aseptic environment should be maintained in an "aseptic" condition when in an operational state and periodically sanitized or decontaminated. Isolators and closed RABS should be decontaminated with sporicidal agents on a periodic basis.
- Only a minimum of materials should be retained in the aseptic portion of the facility through the utilization of just-in-time delivery to the aseptic area.
- Subjective regulatory tenants of aseptic processing such as smoke studies, air velocity measurements, unidirectional air flow, absence of eddy's should be considered but not overly weighted in the definition of HVAC design details. The absence of turbulence in any aseptic production environment is not physically achievable, and there are no objective metrics to define acceptable or unacceptable conditions.
- The completion of operation of RABS should be possible in a "closed" mode. Open-door interventions during aseptic processing are never acceptable.

Equipment/Utensils

In advanced aseptic processing the processing equipment located within the enclosure is always critical to success with aseptic processes. The reliability of the equipment and the sophistication of its design are paramount in minimizing the need for interventions within the enclosure.

- All product contact surfaces should be sterilized using validated methods. Vibratory feed systems may be exempted from this requirement provided they are high-level decontaminated with a sporicidal agent in situ. Their installation following sterilization often entails

[4] The use of high air dilution rates in isolators has not been demonstrated to be of any meaningful benefit as it is with other aseptic processing designs.

substantial and lengthy interventions that can result in contamination risk. Even in separative technologies the need to curtail interventions persists.
- Sterilization-in-place and clean-in-place should be used wherever possible for product and gas delivery lines and filters. At the current state of technology sterilization-in-place is possible for all types of aseptic filling processes including powder fill.
- Equipment and utensils should be sterilized in hermetically sealed containers/wrapping. The container design should be supported by scientific proof of their integrity. In separative technologies decontaminating utensils in situ may be the best alternative.
- Equipment and utensils should remain within sterile containers/wraps until entry into the critical zone just prior to use to avoid contamination that would occur if they were exposed in the adjacent less clean environment.
- Equipment and utensils should be sterilized/depyrogenated using a just-in-time approach.
- Processing equipment should be selected for high reliability, ease of change over and remote adjustment. Wherever possible they should be self-clearing to eliminate the need for personnel intervention in the event of a miss-feed, jam, or other fault.
- Equipment change over from one format to another should be possible with a minimum of manual intervention.
- The process equipment should use process analytical technologies (PAT) and other feedback systems for ease of control, operation, and documentation. This can result in fewer interventions in both the critical and background environments.
- Non-product contact portions of the equipment should be easily decontaminated and non-invasive of the critical zone.
- Equipment and enclosure surfaces should be resistant to the potential corrosive action of sanitizing and decontamination agents.
- Equipment surfaces within closed RABS should be easily accessible for high-level decontamination, automatic decontamination systems in RABS should be favored over manual decontamination activities as they are inherently lower risk as they can be accomplished with the system in a fully closed configuration and without human contamination.

Containers/Closures/Components

The containers and closures necessary are perhaps the most important items in an aseptic process. The ease of their introduction, transfer, movement, placement, and closure must all be successfully accomplished by the equipment with a minimum of human intervention. It should be immediately evident that they need to consistently process throughout the system, and thus high-quality components, with extremely tight dimensional tolerances may be required when compared to what might be customary in a less advanced (and thus markedly less capable) processing system part. As more complex and multifaceted combination products and medical devices are aseptically produced the ability to sterilize, introduce, and feed components with complex shapes and special fitments have become an absolute requirement. Robotics, which can now withstand frequent exposure to agents such as vapor phase hydrogen peroxide (VPHP) can often handle complex parts and by using vision systems and laser guidance achieve levels of flexibility and precision that would be impossible by more conventional means.

- Containers/closures/components must be prepared and sterilized/depyrogenated using validated processes.
- Containers/closures/components should be introduced in a manner that retains at least one layer of sterilized container or hermetic wrapping until entry into the critical zone. It is important to remember that in advanced aseptic processing systems such as isolators the entire enclosure must be considered the critical zone. The container should have a defined level of integrity. An important rule in isolator systems or closed RABS is that nothing should ever be transferred into the enclosure that is not equal to or superior to the microbial quality of the internal environment. This necessitates the use of VPHP pass boxes, e-beam tunnels or pass through systems that can be validated using biological indicators or in the case of radiation, dosimetry. With proper design, execution and procedures RTPs can also serve as transfer devices which ensure that the objective of taking in objects of equal or better contamination control quality than the environment is met.

- Containers/closures/components should be selected for reliability of handling in the processing equipment to avoid the need for corrective interventions. Higher acceptable quality levels (AQLs) for defects can result in a reduction in the need for interventions.
- Containers/closures/components should be sterilized/depyrogenated using a just-in-time approach. Inventories of materials within the aseptic environment (especially the critical environment) should be minimized. In typical separative technology based aseptic processing, space does not allow for substantial accumulation of parts and they are typically transferred in on an as needed basis. However, if the materials are of equal or better contamination control quality than the enclosure environment, there is no reason to be concerned that such objects might become contaminated within the validated use or campaign period of an enclosure. Materials do not become less microbiologically clean over time in a well controlled, separative, and unmanned environment.

Product

Delivery of sterile product to the critical zone is easily accomplished with minimal risk using either directly piped connections or RTP connection systems.

- Production materials must be prepared and sterilized using validated methods.
- Liquid product delivery piping should be cleaned and sterilized in place. Gas delivery piping should be sterilized in place.
- Any product delivery and other aseptic connections (e.g., inert gas) should be made within the enclosure.
- Where product is supplied to the critical zone in sterile container (e.g., sterile powders) it should be introduced in a manner that retains at least one layer of sterilized protective covering or wrap until entry into the critical zone.

Personnel

The operating personnel must be diligent in the operation of the equipment and adherence to the core principles of aseptic processing technique at all times. Their use of permanent and thicker gloves on an enclosure must not be misinterpreted as permission to operate in violation of defined aseptic procedures.

- Personnel must receive initial and periodic formal training in current good manufacturing practices, aseptic processing, microbiology, aseptic gowning and job specific tasks they must perform.
- Where appropriate personnel should be initially and periodically thereafter assessed for their proficiency in aseptic gowning, of course in many advanced aseptic processing systems gowning is limited and nonaseptic and will require no real training as it is not a critical risk mitigation factor in isolators and potentially in closed RABS as well.
- Personnel should be initially and periodically thereafter assessed for their proficiency in aseptic technique. Specific training should also be provided for those individuals performing the initial set-up of the equipment prior to the aseptic process. Obviously, in highly automated systems that do not rely in personnel or gowned operators conventional clean room practices and traditions are not necessary.
- Personnel shall conform to the highest standards of aseptic technique at all times even when working with a closed RABS or isolator.
- Personnel should be periodically monitored when exiting from the aseptic core. Isolator or closed RABS gloves, however, need only be tested at the end of a production run or campaign. It is not desirable to leave media residues on gloves, and sleeve assemblies. Also, in separative technologies glove integrity is the key to risk mitigation. That which does not leak cannot pass microorganisms, therefore physical testing is generally a better solution.
- Gown materials should be cleaned, and sterilized using validated methods. It is not necessary to use sterile gowns in rooms surrounding isolators. Also, it is worth remembering that sterility is always a trade off between microbial "kill" and damage to materials. Thus, extreme overkill is unwarranted where gowning materials are concerned, damage to the gown's integrity is a far greater concern than achieving extreme sterilization lethality levels that are meaningless anyway.

- Gloves must never contact product contact surfaces within an enclosure. Also, the gloves when used to make adjustments must never be put at risk from punctures, tears, or pinching. Operators should also avoid stretching glove/sleeve assemblies in an attempt to reach something within an enclosure. Stretching beyond the initial point of resistance can lead to wear at the glove/sleeve junction and perhaps even a full blown separation. We cannot overemphasize the need for careful ergonomic design, and should flaws in ergonomics be found in operations they should be corrected immediately. It is possible in many enclosures to relocate gloves to better access positions.

Procedures

Interventions always increase the risk of contamination in an aseptic process even those using advanced technologies (however, the superior environmental control inherent in advanced aseptic technologies makes personal risk a far lower risk factor than in conventional clean rooms). The design of the facility, equipment, component, and product supply should serve to reduce the complexity, duration, and number of interventions. The "perfect" intervention is the one that is not necessary (16).

- Procedures should be critically reviewed to eliminate and/or simplify interventions throughout the aseptic processes.
- All interventions should be designed for minimal risk of contaminating sterile materials.
- Interventions performed during aseptic processing must be recognized as increasing the risk of contamination dissemination.
- All interventions should be performed using sterilized tools whenever possible.
- Defined procedures should be established in detail for all inherent interventions, and more broadly for expected corrective interventions (where some flexibility in execution is necessary due to their greater diversity).

Monitoring

The monitoring of an advanced aseptic processing system plays a substantially less important role than it does in ordinary manned aseptic clean rooms, and it is important to recognize that even in standard clean rooms monitoring has a point of diminished return. Its eventual elimination as an anachronism in these extremely clean environments can be expected at some future time. In the interim, any monitoring performed must be accomplished in as minimally invasive and disruptive manner possible.

- Monitoring of any type must not subject the product to increased risk of contamination. No monitoring is preferable to monitoring that increases the risk of contamination for sterile materials.
- Environmental monitoring activities must be recognized as interventional activities and subject to the similar constraints and expectations (including detailed procedures) as any other intervention.
- Monitoring must be recognized as subject to adventitious contamination pre- and post-sampling that is unrelated to the environment, material or surface being sampled. Methods to minimize that potential beyond what is incorporated into monitoring of conventional manned clean rooms may be necessary.
- Viable monitoring should not be considered an "in-process sterility test" regardless of whether the sample is taken in the enclosure or of a so called "critical" product contact surface.
- Environmental monitoring results should not be considered as "proof" of either sterility or nonsterility.
- It must be recognized that microbial monitoring cannot recover all microorganisms present in an environment or on a surface.
- The absence or presence of microorganisms in an environmental sample is not confirmation of asepsis nor is it uniformly indicative of process inadequacy.
- Significant excursions from the routine microbial prolife within the enclosure and background environments should be investigated.

- Detection of low numbers of microorganisms in manned clean rooms should be considered a rare, but not unusual event.
- Investigations into recoveries of low numbers of microorganisms in manned clean rooms should be recognized as predominantly make work exercises.
- Process simulation are indicators of process capability, but cannot definitely establish the sterility of material produced at another time.
- Process simulations in excess of 5 to 10,000 units are of relatively limited value; their greatest utility is in the evaluation of aseptic set-up practices.

CONCLUSION

What has been presented above represents a major departure from the established doctrine for aseptic processing control. The ever-increasing capabilities of aseptic processing technologies have dramatically reduced the utility of the classical monitoring tools that this industry has used for decades. If some future technology enables effective monitoring at the extremely sensitive levels that advanced aseptic processing systems presently provide, there may be justification in their use. We might postulate that by the time those systems become available future aseptic processing technologies demonstrating superior capabilities to those presently available might make those new monitoring tools moot as well. In the interim is clearly time to shift the paradigm for advanced aseptic processing systems away from monitoring and toward their design. Where monitoring is used, total particulate monitoring has significant advantages over microbiological monitoring. Total particulate monitoring provides a real-time indication of a major change in the physical performance of HEPA filters or a significant increase in particles produced by processing equipment, something that conventional microbiological monitoring cannot do.

Our industry has always sought to improve the sterility of aseptically produced products. For many years this was accomplished through measures that were more or less instinctive rather than reflective of real science and engineering. The adoption of risk-based approaches is a relatively new concept, but it is essential that the practitioner take the next step. Mitigation is of far greater importance in the overall effort, and provides a greater measure of safety to aseptic operations.

REFERENCES

1. FDA.Guideline on Sterile Drug Products Produced by Aseptic Processing, 2004.
2. Decision Trees for the Selection of Sterilization Methods (CPMP/QWP/155/96), 1999.
3. Agalloco J, Gordon B. Current practices in the use of media fills in the validation of aseptic processing. J Parenter Sci Technol 1987; 41(4):128–141.
4. PDA TR# 36. Current practices in the validation of aseptic processing—2001. PDA J Pharm Sci Technol 2002; 56(3 suppl).
5. Avallone H. FDA Field Investigator Training curriculum, circa 1985.
6. Agalloco J, Akers J. "Risk Analysis for Aseptic Processing: The Akers-Agalloco Method". J Pharm Technol 2005; 29(11):74–88.
7. Agalloco J, Akers J. "Simplified Risk Analysis for Aseptic Processing: The Akers-Agalloco Method". J Pharm Technol 2006; 30(7):60–76.
8. Whyte W, Eaton T. Microbiological contamination models for use in risk assessment during pharmaceutical production. Eur J Parenteral Pharm Sci 2004; 9(1):11–15.
9. Tidswell E, McGarvey B. Quantitative risk modeling in aseptic manufacture". PDA J Pharm Sci Technol 2006; 60(5):267–283.
10. Akers J, Agalloco J. Personal communications, 2005–2009.
11. Katayama H, Toda A, Tonkunaga Y, et al. Proposal for a new categorization of aseptic processing facilities based on risk assessment scores. PDA J Pharm Sci Technol 2008; 62(4):235–243.
12. PDA TR #44. Quality Risk Management for Aseptic Processes. PDA J Pharm Sci Technol 2008; 62(1):S-1.
13. FDA, Pharmaceutical cGMPs for the 21st Century: A Risk-Based Approach, 2002.
14. ICH, Q9, Quality Risk Management, 2005.
15. Akers J, Agalloco J, Madsen R. What is advanced aseptic processing?. Pharm Manufact 2006; 4(2):25–27.
16. Agalloco J, Akers J. The truth about interventions in aseptic processing". J Pharm Technol 2007; 31(5):S8–S11.

14 Sterile product manufacture using form fill seal technologies

Harold Baseman

Form fill and seal (FFS) is a process by which a container is formed, filled with product, and sealed in a continuous and uninterrupted manner. FFS is a process used to package sterile products including medical devices, injectable drugs, ophthalmic products, respiratory therapy products, biotechnology products, and topical products. By their nature most FFS packaging is plastic, although some foil packaging is done.

This chapter is not intended to present all aspects of FFS to the reader. Rather it is intended to present a basic understanding of the various technologies and the concepts that should be considered when using these technologies for the filling and packaging of sterile products. FFS is used to a larger extent for the manufacture of nonsterile products, including tablets, capsules, ointments, powders, etc. The use of FFS for the manufacture of sterile products is significant and is the focus of this chapter. There are several types of FFS packaging used for sterile products, including *blister pack filling, pouch filling, bag filling, cup filling, and blow fill seal* (BFS). Each of these technologies is discussed later in the chapter. The most significant usage of FFS technology for sterile product manufacture is BFS. It is the most complicated and is discussed in greater detail than the other technologies.

The primary function of FFS packaging or any technology for sterile product manufacture is to maintain the sterility of the package contents. These contents may be the drug substance itself or a syringe or other filled device, the outside of which must be kept sterile. An advantage of FFS is that it is by its nature an automated process. The automation largely removes the need for human intervention. This creates an effective means of packaging sterile liquid products. In conventional aseptic filling, people are often in close proximity to the process. People represent a significant source of microbiological contamination. Steps must then be taken to protect the product from that contamination. Eliminating the source of contamination makes the process more predictable, thus reducing uncertainty, and reducing risk. An automated process such as FFS, properly designed and performed, operating with minimal personnel intervention will eliminate or reduce the source of most contamination and result in a more predictable process.

BLISTER PACKAGING

The terminology may vary from manufacturer to manufacturer, but the concept is the same. Blister packaging is used primarily to package tablets and solid dosage products. Blister packaging is also used as a method of secondary packaging for prefilled drug containers and medical devices, as well as sterile ointments, and some ophthalmic products.

Process Description

Blister packaging is a process by which a sheet of material, usually plastic or foil, is transported on a plate. The plate has cavities recessed in the shape of the container. The sheet is pressed against the plate. A second plate with extended metal also in the shape of the container is placed on the sheet, pressing the sheet material into the cavities of the first plate. Heat may be used to help soften and form the material. Vacuum may also be used to help draw the material into the cavity. This results in the formation of a cavity in the sheet of plastic or foil material in the shape of the container. This is commonly referred to as a "blister."

The sheet is then transported on a conveyor or conveying system to a fill area. Sterile product is filled into the blister. This product may be powder, semisolid material such as ointments, creams, gels, a liquid, or a solid. It may also be a syringe or other device. From the fill area the filled blister is transported to the sealing area. At the seal area a cover is placed over the blister. The cover is usually made of plastic, Tyvek®, paper, laminated foil, or other sealable material. The lid is placed over the blister and pressed on to the edges of the blister to form a seal. The union of the blister and lid material can be sealed by heat or compression adhesive.

The sealed blister sheet is then transported to the area to be punched or die cut. From there the package is completely sealed and can exit the filling line. Some blister lines may also include integrated check weigh systems, volume checkers, or other devices to assure package quality and integrity.

Sterile Manufacturing Critical Process Steps

The formation of the blister must be free of pin holes and weak points that could puncture during transport and storage. It is also important that the channels are not formed in the sealing surface that could result in a leakage. Leakage through the seal or the blister itself may allow microbial ingress and loss of sterility. Likewise, the formation of the lid material should be free of pin-hole leaks, weak points in the sheet that could cause puncture and disrupted or inconsistent seal material, which could cause leakage.

Sterilization of Blister and Lid Material

The blister material must be decontaminated or sterilized prior to filling or must be sterilized subsequent to filling and sealing using a terminal sterilization process. Sterilizing the material prior to filling can be accomplished by sterilizing the sheet or web using gamma radiation, e-beam radiation, chemical treatment, or ethylene oxide. The web material once sterilized can be transferred to the forming and filling stations by using aseptic and protective techniques.

In some cases the web or sheet material is sterilized on the FFS line prior to either forming or just after forming but before filling. This may be done by submersion in a liquid chemical sterilant such as hydrogen peroxide, by fast exposure to high temperature, exposure to ultraviolet light, or by exposure to other sterilizing conditions.

The material of the web must be compatible to the sterilization method. The plastics and coating materials may absorb chemicals that can contaminate or otherwise affect the quality of the product in the blister. Plastic materials may not be able to withstand the temperature or conditions of sterilization. Plastic web and lid may change shape, causing inadequate seals, leakage, and contamination. Plastic materials may not be able to withstand gamma or e-beam radiation. Changes may result in the structure and bonding characteristics of the plastic material, again resulting in inadequate seals and contamination. Exposure to radiation can cause changes in the structure of the plastic web, releasing extractables or reducing barrier capabilities.

If the blister package is used as the secondary package to hold a glass container filled with product, for instance a prefilled syringe packaged in a FFS blister, then extractables and sterilant residue will not be as much of a factor. This should still be considered in developing and testing the package. Plastic materials may not provide adequate barriers to extractable, volatile substances and therefore allow those substances to permeate the package and contaminate the product. Respiratory therapy and ophthalmic products packaged in plastic containers, then placed in pouches or labeled with adhesive-bearing labels may be susceptible to this penetration effect. Care should be taken in selecting the primary and secondary packaging materials to avoid extractable and volatile substance contamination. All materials that could affect the quality of the product should be incorporated in product stability testing and evaluation.

The primary purpose of blister packaging is to maintain sterility of the exterior of the contents of the package, the device, or primary container. The critical attributes of this type of package, relevant to sterility of the contents, include the completeness of the seal, seal strength, and package integrity. Completeness of seal is defined as a seal without disruption, flaw, or defect, which could allow the ingress of microbial contamination. Sealing surfaces may be smooth or patterned. It is not essential that the seal be "air tight" although that would be recommended. A nonairtight seal must present a barrier sufficient to prevent the ingress of microbial contamination.

Seal strength and package integrity are critical attributes of the FFS blister package. Seal strength relates to the ability of the package to maintain sealed conditions throughout normal or anticipated usage, including storage, shipping, transport, and handling. The package should not be sealed to the extent that it is difficult or impossible to open without significant package damage or effort that could compromise sterility or aseptic handling. Seal strength is usually a function of temperature, force, placement, design, and material compatibility. Package integrity is the overall completeness of the package, including the lack of punctures or other sources of leakage. Leakage could be caused by pin-hole punctures in the web or lid material, weak spots caused during blister formation, cracks, slits, or other defects caused during processing or handling. Leakage can be caused prior to processing, subsequent to processing, or as a result of defective materials.

Validation

Many elements of validation of blister packaging operations are common to the qualification and validation of most types of FFS technology, and similar to the qualification and validation of conventional sterile product manufacturing. There are additional considerations for the qualification and validation of BFS, which are noted and addressed in that section of the chapter.

Installation Qualification

Prior to the qualification, the line should be properly commissioned. Commissioning includes confirmation that the line is properly designed, installed, and functional. A sound-commissioning program will provide assurance that qualification studies are completed efficiently and with a minimum of unexpected deviations.

During qualification the blister line should be checked to confirm that the design is appropriate for the process. Related specifically to sterility issues, the line should be able to fit and form the blister correctly. The web materials should not be at the edge of the range of process capabilities. This could cause imperfect blister formation, weak spots, cracking, and inadequate seal surfaces. The design of the web sterilization sections should be adequate for the process. Instrumentation should be in place for controlling, monitoring, and recording critical functions. Critical functions may include temperature of sterilant bath, temperature of blister forming section, temperature of molds, temperature of sealing plates, pressure of forming plates, pressure of sealing station, speed of conveyor and transport mechanism, air flow in critical areas, speed, and flow at filling station.

All filters should be appropriate to the intended use. Filters may include HEPA and ULPA air filters, hydrophobic filters for air or gases, in line filters for liquid product sterilization, vent and dust collection filters. If placed in a controlled environment, the critical portions of the line should be within the designated controlled areas. Critical areas include any area where sterile or sterilized material, product, or product contact surfaces will be exposed to the environment without subsequent decontamination processing.

Operational Qualification

The blister line should be checked to confirm that it is capable of consistently performing the intended process in a predictable manner, within specification and regulatory requirements. The line should be capable of performing the operations necessary to manufacture a product within quality specifications, especially those concerned with establishing and maintaining sterile conditions related to the package interior, product contact surfaces, and package and seal integrity.

The critical operational parameters include line speed; temperature at critical process steps—sterilant conditioning, drying, web-performing station, blister forming, and sealing; pressure at blister forming and sealing stations; vacuum assist and blister formation; die cut station alignment and function; and controlled environment airflow.

Automation

Automated systems relying on computer or programmable logic to establish, control, sequence, monitor, record, or archive critical line function must be qualified, specifically those functions related directly to establishing and maintaining sterility; these critical functions include process steps and function where the failure of the system may result in contamination to the package interior, product contact surfaces, or the sterile product itself. It also includes any functions or process steps, the failure of which would adversely affect the product quality, sterility, or package integrity.

Process Qualification

Filling

For a discussion on liquid filling, product circuit cleaning, and sterilization in place, refer to the "Blow Fill Seal" section.

If a device or solid product is placed and sealed into a FFS package, the device or solid product must not be too large or otherwise protrude at a point in the package. This can cause stress to the package and result in package leakage from stress induced during package sterilization, shipment, or handling. For example, care should be taken for a medical device placed in a formed blister and sealed with a Tyvek® lid. If the device is tightly placed in the package, and the package is placed in a steam sterilizer for terminal sterilization, the device may expand. The expansion can result in added stress to the package during heating. The stress will be relieved at the weakest points in the package, perhaps the seal area. The package starts to "open" itself by pulling away seal area. In the end this produces a weaker seal. This package may appear to be sealed as it exits the sterilizer, but may no longer be adequate to withstand shipment, storage, and handling.

A filling operation concern especially critical to BFS packaging is splashing at the seal area, as a result of foaming, excessive, or forceful fill. The seal is relatively fragile. The seal is a fusion of like or compatible materials. It involves compression, usually under high temperature. It is not a complete fusion as is the case with ampoules, where the glass is melted and reformed together. In the case of BFS, the plastic is already semicooled when it is compressed. In the case of pouch and blister filling, the seal material must be heated and compressed. A foreign element to the seal material, in the seal area will compromise the integrity of the seal. There are two causes for seal integrity failure. First, liquid may be splashed on the seal surface. This will absorb heat, decreasing the temperature to the point where it is no longer effective in joining the materials. Second, the splashed material may leave a solid residue that forms an imperfection to the seal surface when dried. This imperfection is a point where there essentially is no seal. The seal is made between similar plastic materials, not a plastic material and a salt crystal. The result is weak or incomplete seals.

POUCH FILLING

Another type of FFS is pouch packaging. Sterile products packaged in pouches include medical devices, semisolids, topicals, creams, ointments, gels, some solids, and liquids. The primary use however is medical device secondary packaging and the semisolids. Pouches are used as dispensers of sterile ointments and creams. In most cases pouched products are terminally sterilized by gamma radiation, ethylene oxide, or moist heat.

The formation of the pouch usually occurs in one of two ways. One way is for a single pouch material to be folded over and then sealed at the bottom and other side; thus forming a three sided container open at the top. This can be done on a horizontal or vertical forming machine. The product can be placed or dispensed into the open top and then the top is sealed. The sealing operation may involve heat, pressure, or adhesive; with heat and pressure being the more predominate method. The second method involves overlaying two sheets of pouch material with similar or compatible seal surface materials. These materials may be different, as in foil to paper or plastic. In this case, the pouch is sealed on three sides and filled from the top.

Typically, in pouch formation no blister is formed, so no molds, preheat stations, or blister forming dies are necessary. This reduces the amount of transport and handling, therefore there is less chance of leakage and puncture from formation, transport, and handling. Areas where sterility can be compromised include pin-hole leaks in the pouch material and inadequate seals. Inadequate seal may be a result of seal plate malfunction or damage, lack of pressure, misalignment of pouch and plates, or too little or too much heat. Many of the attributes and conditions for sterile product packaging in blister packs are relevant for pouches, including material to sterilizing method compatibility, machine alignment and function, cleanliness and sterility of product contact surfaces, airflow patterns, and personnel intervention.

CUP FILLING

Cup formation and filling are essentially the same as a blister packaging operation. The blister in this case is in the form of a cup. The lid is sealed by heat and pressure, or adhesive. Cups may be filled with liquids, semi-solids, or powders. Care should be taken to assure that fill product residue does not contaminate the cup seal surface. Alignment of the seal lid and cup is essential to package integrity. Cups and their contents are typically terminally sterilized by gamma radiation, ethylene oxide or moist heat. Special care should be taken when sterilizing aqueous liquid products with ethylene oxide. Ethylene oxide in the presence of water will form ethylene glycol and other relatively stable and difficult to remove residual materials. These may contaminate the product and render it unacceptable.

FLEXIBLE BAG FILLING

Another FFS package used commonly for the filling of sterile product is the flexible poly bag. This may be a mini bag or large volume parenteral bag. This type of packaging is used for diluents, water, dextrose, ringer's solution, antibiotics, and other types of IV-administered products. If heat stable, these products are typically terminally sterilized by moist heat.

Sterilization

When sterilizing flexible packaging, including most FFS packages by moist-heat exposure, special precautions must be taken to protect the package from damage during the sterilization cycle. As the package and contents are exposed to high temperatures, their contents increase in temperature and expand. This expansion produces an internal package pressure. The internal pressure is offset by an equal pressure on the exterior of the package, produced from the surrounding environment temperature, which at this point is equal to that of the interior. Therefore, there is no pressure differential and no stress to the package.

As the temperature of the sterilizer is decreased at the end of the cycle, this equilibrium is lost. The exterior environment will cool more rapidly as the steam is withdrawn. The contents of the package however will maintain temperature and pressure longer. The result is that there will be a higher pressure on the interior of the container than the exterior. This will cause stress on the container. The pressure will be relieved at the weakest point in the package, usually the seal. This may result in distortion of the package and it may result in a puncture and therefore a place where microbial contamination ingress.

This will also be the case for a rapid temperature increase during the start of the cycle. Here the reverse situation may occur, where the pressure on the exterior of the package is more than the cooler interior. Again, in either case, special precautions must be taken to regulate and control temperature and pressure throughout the cycle. It may be necessary to add compressed air to elevate the exterior pressure during cool down and provide a slow heat up cycle to allow for internal pressure to come up and match external pressure at the start of the cycle.

BLOW FILL SEAL

Background

BFS, in the context of this chapter, describes the process of extrusion blow mold forming of plastic containers, filling with liquid, and sealing, in one continuous operation. The BFS process uses a machine, which contains a resin hopper/dispenser, a plastic extruder, a container mold, a mold transport system, product transfer lines, and a filler assembly.

BFS technology was developed in the mid-1960s as an attempt to shorten long plastic bottle formation cycles. In conventional blow molding, containers are manufactured empty, then cleaned, filled, and capped in additional off-line operations. BFS sped up the conventional blow molding process by introducing a liquid inside the container to enhance cooling. This resulted in a faster cycle and enhanced machine productivity. Improvements over the years have resulted in a shift in BFS from a means of enhancing blow molding efficiency to an application for sterile product manufacture.

In the early years, the technology was used largely to package consumer products. Lotions, soaps, detergents, mustard, motor oil, and drink products were among the early items packaged using this technology, as well as health and beauty aid products, such as creams, lotions, feminine hygiene products, and phosphate enemas. These types of products did not require the same US Food and Drug Administration approval as do sterile pharmaceuticals and were lightly regulated. The emphasis of early BFS machines and processes was on productivity and container design.

It was soon realized that the technology was nearly ideal for sterile product manufacture. Filters could be placed in the lines and the product transfer lines could be steam sterilized in place. The resin reached sterilizing temperatures in the extruder. BFS automation significantly reduces the risk of microbiological contamination from operator intervention. As more companies considered BFS for the manufacture of sterile pharmaceuticals, the emphasis began to shift toward sanitary machine and support system design. Machines were placed in controlled environments or clean rooms. Validation techniques, such as temperature mapping of the product lines and media fills were conducted.

BFS technology has long been a popular method for packaging sterile ophthalmic and respiratory therapy products. Its popularity as a method of manufacturing sterile products was primarily the result of three factors. (*i*) BFS by its very nature is highly automated. The complexity of the equipment and need for continuous processing require almost complete automation. Automation reduces the risk of microbiological contamination by significantly reducing the need for people. People are the major source of microbiological contamination. (*ii*) The relatively short exposure time and small, localized critical exposure area reduce the opportunity and risk of contamination. The exposure space and time refers to the point at which product or product contact surfaces are exposed to the environment. In BFS, both the time and the area of exposure are minimal. The result is that products properly manufactured using BFS technology should have a lower likelihood of microbiological contamination and therefore a higher assurance of sterility when compared to conventional aseptic filling. Ljungqvist et al. reported that a comparison of BFS and industry aseptic processing media fill results indicated that BFS media fills failed at a rate of 10% of total media fills (1). (*iii*) BFS packaging design can be creative. Unlike blisters, cups, pouches, and bags, which are limited in the types of package configuration and shapes, BFS can mold a very wide range of container shapes.

BFS containers may be terminally sterilized by heat only if polypropylene or certain higher temperature resins are used. The resins are relatively poor vapor and gas barriers and are therefore not appropriate for ethylene oxide sterilization. Most BFS resins may also be affected by gamma radiation. For these reasons BFS manufacture of sterile products is predominately an aseptic process.

Products

Ophthalmics

Ophthalmic solutions were among the first sterile pharmaceutical products filled on BFS machines. They remain one of the most common products packaged on BFS equipment. Unit dose eye drops are manufactured using BFS. These containers typically contain 0.25 to 1.0 mL of solution, and are intended to dispense one or two drops into each eye, and then be discarded. The solutions are usually nonpreserved. The BFS container forming process is essentially particulate-free, eliminating a major concern for eye care products.

Larger volume ophthalmic solutions, including multidose therapeutic drops, eye wash, and contact lens solutions are manufactured on BFS lines. Size ranges of these products range from 5 mL to 32 fl. oz. The products may be preserved or nonpreserved. Nonpreserved sterile solutions are particularly well suited for BFS, due to the reduced risk of microbiological contamination.

Respiratory Therapy

The inhalation therapy market (respiratory or oxygen therapy) represents another significant BFS market. Small unit dose solutions and larger volume humidifiers are commonly manufactured by BFS process. The unique container design makes them ideally suited for this type of manufacture. These products require strict microbiological controls, as they often are used on patients with damaged breathing passages and in some cases with compromised immune systems.

Oral Electrolytic Rehydration Solutions

These solutions are a combination of electrolytes and simple sugars and are primarily administered to infants suffering from vomiting and diarrhea to keep them from becoming dehydrated. Although the market for these solutions is quite large in the United States, it is greater in other parts of the world, where pure water is in short supply. The solutions are presently packaged either in 1-L containers, which must be refrigerated after opening to maintain purity, or in 8 fl. oz. containers, which are for unit dose application.

Parenterals

The relatively low risk of microbiological contamination makes BFS a possible packaging method for small and larger volume parenterals. In the case of heat-sensitive products (or packages) such as biologics BFS may be a suitable alternative to terminal sterilization if the plastic container temperature does not adversely affect product stability. Parenterals require control of endotoxin contamination and primary packaging is typically depyrogenated by a heat or rinse process prior to filling. This remains a challenge for BFS as is discussed later in the chapter. Aseptic processing guidance from both the United States and Europe suggest Grade A or Class 100 environmental conditions in critical zones where product or product contact surfaces are exposed. This presents a machine design and process challenge for most BFS machines where open parisons are filled.

BFS Process

The expansion of BFS usage is dependent to a large degree on the progress of the technology. As companies consider BFS for more complicated and sensitive products, regulatory and industry scrutiny has increased. Advances in BFS machine design and construction have resulted in expansion of capabilities and product types. Years ago, it was not uncommon for BFS operators to claim that it was nearly impossible to contaminate the product. BFS was considered a very forgiving technology. It is now widely recognized and understood that although BFS represents a less risky method of aseptic manufacture, it is not foolproof. Poorly designed and operated systems can fail, resulting in loss of product sterility and loss of sterility assurance. The need for operational control, sound validation methodology, innovative system design, and control of interventions is necessary to identify, address, and eliminate limitations to the technology.

BFS Process Description

Most BFS machines are self-contained consisting of resin hopper, extruder, parison head, fill assembly, mold and mold transport, fill and compressed air lines, valving, filters, traps, vents, shrouds, exhausts, and control systems all mounted on the BFS machine. For sterile product applications, BFS machines are typically located in Class 10,000 (Grade C) or better clean room environments. The product exposure sections of the machine are located in the front of the machine. These include the parison head and filling station. These sections are often located in an area of higher control, physically separated by a wall from the back portion of the BFS machine, where the extruder motor and resin hopper are contained.

Extrusion

The BFS process usually begins with the transport of plastic resin beads from a central storage container. Low-density polyethylene, high-density polyethylene, polypropylene, or mixtures are often used as BFS resins. The resin beads are transported usually via vacuum to a hopper located on top of the BFS machine. Resin is often mixed or blended with colorant pellets to produce the desired pigment for the container. The resin hopper is located just above the extruder. The extruder is a mechanism that heats the plastic beads and pushes it down a barrel using a screw apparatus. The action of the screw, heat, and resulting pressure creates a semimolten plastic material which is fluid. The temperature of the resin varies depending on the plastic from approximately 145°C to 175°C. Resin may remain in the extruder for 5 to 30 minutes. The conditions of heat and pressure are sufficient to destroy spores and render the resin sterile.

At the end of the extruder there is a mixing tip that is designed to provide a uniform composition to the fluid resin. The extruder is connected to a parison head. The parison head is a block of metal with die and pin assemblies, which allows the resin to flow and separate into one or more tubes or parisons. The parison moves downward from the bottom of the parison head as a hollow tube of semimolten hot plastic. The shape, wall thickness, consistency of the wall thickness, and the speed/flow of the parison are critical to the formation of the container. The parison may take the forms of individual rounded tubes, each one corresponding to a cavity. This is the type of parison typically used for manufacturing bottles and larger containers. The parison may also take the form of a single oval tube, which will be formed into multiple cavities and containers. This type of parision is sometimes used for small, less complex ampoules, and tube-like container designs. Sterile compressed gas, usually air, flows through the parison tube. This maintains the shape of the parison and prevents the parison from collapsing.

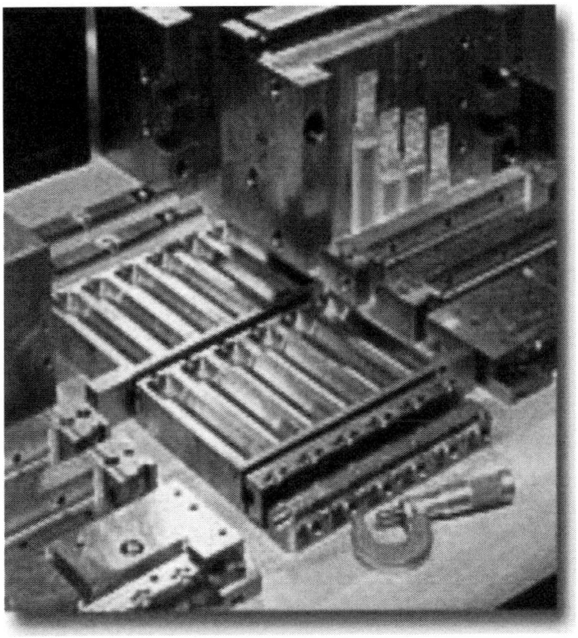

Figure 1 Bronze aluminum alloy mold disassembled.

Molding and Container Formation

Containers may be formed and filled using a relatively closed rotary type of system, using multiple sets of molds or an open parison system using a single-container mold set. In an open parison system, a container mold, usually in two halves, moves into place just under the exposed parison. The mold is typically made of stainless steel and bronze aluminum (Fig. 1). The mold has cooling lines and vacuum lines attached to all four sections. It is essential that these lines have secure, nonleaking connections. The cooling medium is not sterile and could become a source of microbial or chemical contamination if leaks at the cooling to mold connection occur during the container formation process. Leaks in the lines may also result in ineffective cooling and vacuum control and problems in container formation and sealing.

The two halves of the mold are positioned on either side of the parison. The mold closes on the parison. The mold consists of one or more cavities cut from the mold material. The number of mold cavities is equal to the number of units to be filled. As the mold closes, the parison is encased in a mold cavity. Typically there are four sections to a mold. There are two almost identical bottom halves, which include the cavities and form the container fill pocket. Then there are two almost identical top halves or sealing sections, which consist of the seal surface and top portion of the container. The seal sections remain in an open position until filling is complete—later in the process. Molds may also have sections or panels, which contain engraving, logo, text, and removable sections for insertion of lot numbers and expiration dates.

The mold, plastic parison, parison head assembly, and extruder are all connected. Then a mechanism cuts away the parison top from the parison in the mold cavity. At the same time the extruder lifts. This separates the extruder and parison head assembly from the parison and the mold. The mold then moves to the fill station. Most of the parison plastic is contained in the lower part of the mold however some of the plastic remains exposed at the top of the sealing section of the mold. This will remain hot and will not begin to form until after filling. The extruder continually processes and extrudes additional resin through the parison head as the plastic parison is cut away from the mold.

The cutting process is usually done with a hot, thin band of metal, known as a hot knife assembly. It may also be done with a swift moving cold knife assembly or other method. This cutting operation is a source of nonviable particulate generation as the parison plastic is burned or cut away. Although there is little evidence that the material produced during the cutting operation contaminates the interior of the BFS container or the filled product, those considering BFS as a method of packaging parenteral products and products where particulate contamination is a concern, should be aware of this condition.

As the mold moves to the fill station, the semimolten plastic that had been the parison is in contact with the walls of the mold cavity. These walls may have cool water flowing throw them, which begins the container formation process. For larger containers or more complex designs, vacuum may be used to pull the plastic more completely against the cavity walls. Air or other gas may be used to push the plastic against the walls as well. This is known as "blowing." Not all containers require vacuum or blowing to form. Many ampoule designs may be manufactured without assistance.

Filling

The mold moves to the filling station. The mold is usually positioned under a stainless steel horizontal filling assembly or tower. The fill tower consists of product transfer line and valving, compressed gas transfer lines and valving, and the fill dispensing mechanism. The fill tower may also include mechanisms for insertion of fitments and other components that are placed or inserted into the container during formation. Many BFS machines also include a fill shroud, air box, or other mechanism for protecting the product from the environment (Fig. 2).

The fill shroud is usually an encasement of some type, often constructed of stainless steel and Plexiglas (Fig. 3). The shroud defines and encases the area directly around the fill nozzles and open container top. Thus, the shroud forms a mini environment. Clean air from HEPA filters, hydrophobic filters, or other means may be blown into the shroud encasement. This provides a clean environment—equivalent to Grade A or Class 100—in proximity to the product and product contact surface exposure point. The shroud may also contain environmental monitoring and sampling ports and instruments.

The fill tower assemble contains the sterilization and clean in place assemblies. Steam and cleaning medium are transported through product contact lines and valving, through the fill dispensing mechanism, into nozzles and blow tubes. Typically there is a steam cup assembly that can be positioned over the nozzles. The assembly allows steam to pass through the interior of the fill nozzles and then pass over the exterior of the nozzles before leaving the assembly. This allows for moist heat exposure to all critical surfaces.

The fill assembly is connected to the product storage vessel by stainless steel or other nonreactive piping or tubing. Most aqueous solutions will travel through lines with sterilizing filters in housings placed in the lines and positioned on the BFS machine. Compressed air, which is used to blow-mold the containers, also passes through stainless steel lines with sterilizing filters and housings in place and positioned on then BFS machine. Automated valving is in place and the sequencing of the valves is essential to the formation, filling, and sealing of the

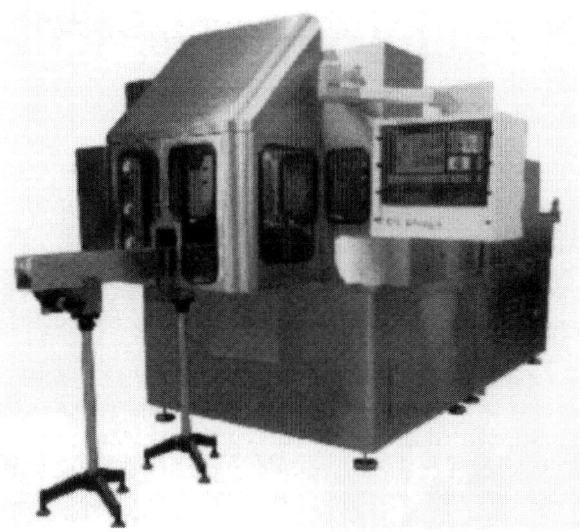

Figure 2 BFS machine with air shroud in place.

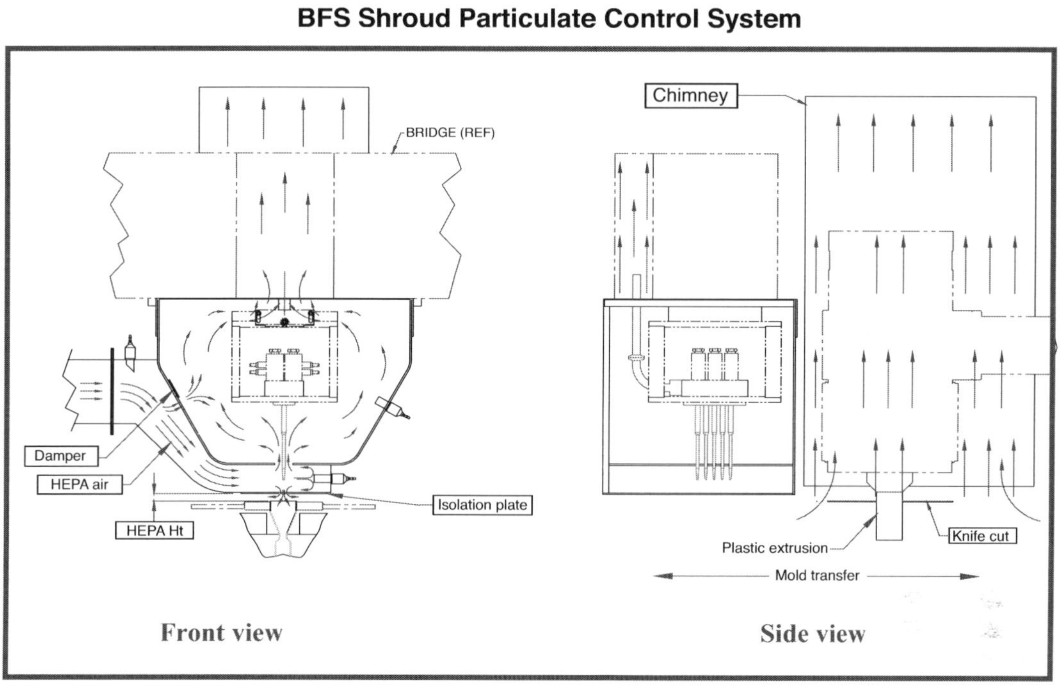

Figure 3 Air shroud diagram showing flow of HEPA filtered air protecting the critical fill zone.

container. The sequencing of the valves is essential to the line sterilization process, including the clearance of condensate and trapped air.

On most BFS machines, filling is accomplished using a time-and-pressure fill system. This typically involves opening and closing a preset orifice in the fill assembly for a set amount of time. Product is supplied at a relatively constant pressure. The result is a consistent flow from the fill assembly into the container, still housed in the bottom portions of the mold. As the mold is positioned under the fill tower assembly, the fill nozzles move downward, engaging the top of the mold. The nozzle pushes into the upper exposed plastic forming a seal of sorts around the nozzle. If air is to be used to blow form the container, this is the point at which it enters the cavity through an outer or inner tube assembly. Air is vented back up through the assembly. A second inner or outer nozzle dispenses the liquid or semisolid product. It is essential that the filling not overflow or foam excessively, causing product residue at the seal surface. Product residual should not collect on the exterior of the nozzle. This can become a potential cause of contamination at the seal surface. The design of the fill system and process should minimize foaming and splashing of product. Often bottom-up fill sequencing and nozzle tip designs are used to minimize foaming and splashing.

Sealing

At the completion of the filling process, the fill nozzle assembly retracts from the mold and moves back to its up position. If a fitment or a component is to be placed in the container, it is done at this time. The fitment may be a controlled dispensing tip, rubber septum, or other device. If this step is included in the process, special precautions should be taken to sterilize the fitment, transfer mechanism, and insertion mechanism. Procedures and equipment designs should be in place to transfer and place the sterilized fitments aseptically. Some BFS operations use isolator systems to protect sterilized fitments from microbiological contamination.

Fitments are typically made of dissimilar materials to the container resin. The sealing process is typically compression with fusion of material around the fitment. As such the seal may not be as good as that of the fused container and special precautions should be employed to assure that the seal is integral and withstands processing, storage, handling, and use without leakage.

The container is sealed by the closing of the upper portions of the mold. These are the sealing sections. As they come together, semimolten plastic remaining at the top of the mold is pushed together under pressure. The material fuses. Vacuum and cooling water may be supplied to the sealing section of the mold to assist with the fusion process. The alignment of the upper and lower mold sections, the sequencing of the mold closure and vacuum, the temperature of the mold, the pressure of the mold closing force, and the condition of the mold, assemblies, mechanisms, and seal surfaces are all critical to the proper formation and sealing of the container.

Continuous closed parison container formation and fill systems may be used for vial filling. Here units are filled and sealed prior to the cutting of plastic, therefore further reducing environmental exposure.

Deflashing

At this stage of process the container has been formed, product has been filled into the container, and the filled container has been sealed. The final step in the process is to trim away excess plastic material or flash. Flash is trimmed to give the container the proper aesthetic appearance and quality. It may also be necessary for the proper function of certain dispensing devices that are designed to fit into or with other devices or containers. Deflashing may occur on the BFS machine or outside of the clean room. Deflashing occurring at the BFS machine is automated and involves cutting the excess plastic away within a contained assembly.

Some of the deflashing may occur outside the clean room. This is done in an effort to remove all unnecessary steps from the clean room to protect those critical operations that must be performed in a clean room. As the deflashing is performed on a sealed container, it is usually no longer necessary to protect the product from the environment. The exception might be a product that requires a sterile exterior surface. But in most cases these types of products receive some type of terminal sterilization treatment.

Deflashing that occurs outside of the clean room may be performed manually or by a deflashing mechanism. The deflashing mechanism usually consists of a set of dies and punches that match the shape of the container. The deflashing is critical to the manufacture of the sterile product. A poorly deflashed container may result in punctures, leakage, or weakness in the seal or fused area. The alignment of the deflash components, dies, and punches, the positioning of the container, the sharpness and condition of the deflashing assembly, the speed of the transport, and the pressure and force of the mechanism are critical to the deflashing process.

Container Design and Formation

The container should be designed to allow for a filling process that does not compromise sterility. Containers should be large enough to contain the product with a minimum of splashing or liquid to seal area contact. The container opening should be adequate for fill nozzle insertion, allowing for venting and minimizing the potential for nozzle to seal area contact. The opening should also be as small as practical, given the usage requirements. The smaller the container opening, the lower the opportunity for microbiological organism ingress and contamination. The container opening feature should be robust enough to withstand processing, transport, storage, and handling without risk of leakage—yet be able to be opened without compromising sterility during usage. Inserts and fitments should be of compatible materials and not subject to leakage. If the production process includes terminal sterilization, the container material must be capable of withstanding sterilization process conditions without weakening or leakage. The temperature and sterilization conditions at which the container fails will vary according to resin type, container design, product, fill volume, and sterilization cycle. The manufacturer should determine feasibility of and specific conditions for terminal sterilization during process development.

If terminal sterilization is being considered, polypropylene is a BFS container material that can withstand temperatures in excess of 121.1°C for sterilization cycle duration. Polypropylene is more difficult to trim and to open and therefore may not be appropriate for all container designs. Certain low-density polyethylene plastics can withstand temperatures of 110°C for periods of time long enough to achieve sterilization conditions. Lower temperature, longer duration methods of sterilization in combination with aseptic processing steps have been used for sterile product–filled medical devices.

Container/Resin Sterilization

For the BFS process to be appropriate for aseptic product manufacturing, the product contact surfaces of the formed container must be sterile. There is no intermediate sterilization process between container formation and filling, as there would be with conventional container filling. Therefore, the method for providing a sterile container must be inherent in the BFS container formation process.

Aseptic process simulation studies, direct inoculation of resin studies, and extruder temperature evaluation indicate that the exposure of the resin to high temperature during the extrusion process is adequate to destroy spore and vegetative microbiological contamination to a level adequate to manufacture sterile product. Studies to challenge the resin sterilization process have been conducted and reported. These studies involved the controlled contamination of resin prior to processing. The contaminated resin was transported to the extruder on a standard BFS machine and used to form containers. The containers were filled with sterile media and incubated for a media fill study. At this point, it is accepted that the exposure of the resin to the temperature, pressures, and conditions in the extruder for the process time are adequate to destroy challenge organisms to a sufficient degree to assure sterility (2).

There are no process steps to sterilize the container subsequent to formation and prior to filling. If process steps and machine design are not adequate to maintain the sterile condition of the container, then contamination may be introduced after the container is formed. The container is vulnerable from the time the parison leaves the parison head until the filled container is sealed. The short exposure time and the small container opening minimize the risk of microbiological contamination during transport steps. Manufactures should take additional steps to provide as clean an environment as possible in this area. These steps include the elimination of interventions and the disposition of open units if interventions do occur. Air shrouds, exhaust systems, sterile compressed air-blow help to maintain these conditions.

The manufacture must keep these systems in place and in good working order. The BFS line, machines, and clean room should be kept clean and contamination free. Personnel should be trained and procedures should be in place to minimize the number and potential effect of interventions. Connections to the mold and machine that carry nonsterile fluids such as cooling water must be tight and leak proof. Finally, the operator must be aware of improper or unusual operating conditions and take steps to correct any problem that could compromise the sterility of the container or product.

BFS machines that use a closed parison system for filling and sealing the container do not expose the open container to the environment. These systems are used for some ampoule and small-container manufacture.

Endotoxins and Depyrogenation

Depyrogenation

Parenteral products and some ophthalmic applications are required to be pyrogen free. There are no steps for depyrogenating the container prior to filling, as might be the case with conventional container filling. The resin is exposed to 145°C to 175°C for a minimum of 5 minutes. This may not be enough to accomplish a 3log reduction in endotoxin as expected by regulatory agencies. However, the additional effect that extruder pressure has on the depyrogenation process is not clearly understood. It is possible that the combination of temperature and pressure results in a level of endotoxin deactivation. At this time the most effective means for assuring acceptable levels of endotoxin and endotoxin contamination is to maintain low levels of resin bioburden.

Resin is often stored in bulk containers; usually 1100 lb plastic lined corrugated boxes or gaylords. The boxes of resin may be stored for extended periods of time in uncontrolled environments. It is possible for plastic resin to become contaminated with endotoxin during storage, transport, or processing. If product endotoxin is a concern, then precautions should be used to minimize the opportunity for microbiological contamination of the resin during storage subsequent to manufacture. The use of resin storage silos, where large quantities of resin are stored for extended periods adds to the potential risk of contamination.

Resin itself should not support the growth of microbiological organisms. It is nonnutritive; if it is dry it could be stored for long periods. If proper precautions are used and the material tested, then there is little reason to believe that endotoxin will be present in the resin material prior to processing. Testing of incoming resin material for endotoxin levels and taking appropriate precautions to protect the material from contamination during storage, transport, and processing, then testing the finished product for endotoxin levels will reduce the risk of unacceptable endotoxin levels for BFS products that require endotoxin control.

Operations

The BFS line takes a significant amount of time to set up and start up. It is most efficient when run for long periods. It is not uncommon to run a BFS line for multiple shifts and multiple days before re-sterilization of the product transfer lines. This is a departure from conventional filling, where runs are typically conducted over a single or perhaps a double shift. Conventional filling processes may be affected by personnel activity, aseptic technique, and generation of personnel-borne contamination, which increase the risk of microbiological contamination.

Proper BFS operation is automated and better suited for extended runs. Because interventions occurring at the start of the run are usually the most impacting, it can be argued that the fewer start-ups, the fewer interventions and therefore the better the assurance of sterility. It may be better to set up the line and run for several days, rather than stop, break down, and restart the line several times.

BFS machines are typically designed for cleaning and sterilization of product contact surfaces in-place. These functions must be validated and closely monitored. Machine designs and sterilization processes may require modification for in-place cleaning and sterilization. Control and qualification of product hold time can reduce the risk of excessive bioburden and potential for microbiological contamination. The optimal duration of fill may be dependent on the product growth capability, intended use of the product, bioburden, method of sterilization, BFS machine design, contamination control features, facility history, experience of staff, intervention control policy, and process/product history and trends.

When compared with conventional aseptic filling, BFS processes are relatively complicated. Once properly set up, a well-maintained line will function without interruption. However, a hastily set-up line or a poorly maintained machine will require frequent interventions that compromise product quality and possibly even sterility. Each intervention or instance where personnel must enter the fill room or critical zone represents a risk to the process and increased potential for contamination. Automated processes require training and awareness. The increased assurance of sterility afforded by BFS is dependent of elimination of human intervention. Depending on the level of intervention, product may be quarantined, retested, or rejected. The response to the intervention depends on its category. The response may include documentation, product quarantine, product rejection, and line cleaning, sanitization, or sterilization.

Sterilization in Place and Cleaning in Place

Maintaining a sterile product pathway and transport system is essential to the sterility assurance. Product contact parts must be designed and fabricated to be cleanable and sterilizable. They must be made of materials that are compatible with the product and with the sterilization method. They must withstand leakage during assembly and operation. The BFS machine and system design should not have fittings and components that can harbor microbial contamination. Designs should avoid exposed grease fittings, exposed threads, absorbent materials, and openings that prevent adequate access for cleaning. Designs should not disrupt airflow or result in the spread of contamination.

To achieve the goal of reduction or elimination of human intervention and contact, filling systems or circuits should be sterilized in place. In FFS and BFS these circuits may include the compressed gas and air transport lines, the product transport line, the ballooning and blowing lines, the filter housings, valves, fill blocks, nozzles, steam cups, drain and vent lines.

Most sterilization in place (SIP) systems rely on steam for liquid product filling. Product contact circuits should be designed with proper drainage in place to avoid the pooling of condensate or collection of air. Condensate collection and air entrapment areas should be eliminated. These areas present places that will be difficult, if not impossible, to sterilize by reasonable methods. Some BFS product transfer and compressed gas circuits are lengthy and elaborate, condensing steam into condensate at a significant rate. Product and gas transport circuits typically incorporate filters and filter housings. These components are relatively difficult to sterilize. They are not designed for the free flow of steam. And the filter element itself will trap air. Special precautions must be taken to design and execute sterilization cycles on these circuits. Significant sterilization cycle development should be undertaken prior to qualification and validation.

The sequencing of valving in the gas and product circuit during sterilization is essential to clearing condensate and entrapped air. This sequencing may be a matter of evaluation, experience, common sense, trial, and error. The filling and compressed gas circuits are complicated, so it is important to conduct and document sterilization and cleaning cycle process development studies. Methods for clearing condensate and air from the circuit include the use of traps, valving, drains, vents, pitched lines, and properly insulated lines (a safety requirement), and the sequencing and timing of steam flow. It may also be necessary to open fill block valving fully to allow for adequate steam flow. These fill systems will have to be re-adjusted back to the proper settings before the start of filling.

Sterilization cycle development includes studies to determine the cold spots in the SIP circuit. Thermocouples and biological indicators are typically placed at the low points in the circuit, where condensate collects and at the high points in the circuit where air collects. These points will be more difficult to bring to temperature and sterilize.

Cleaning

Most BFS product contact lines and systems are designed to be CIP. The cleaning solution is usually transferred directly through the product transfer lines and out of the nozzles into a collection system. It is important to note that the complexity of BFS filling lines, the design of the fill block and valving, and the composition of the products often make it difficult to adequately perform CIP processes.

Manufacturers may choose to employ dedicated fill systems for specific products or product classes to minimize risk of contamination. The fill systems can then be removed and clean out of place. Gaskets, O-rings, and other elastic components should be changed on a routine basis. These components are difficult to clean and CIP should be considered only after diligent cycle development. Product transfer lines can be CIP, if properly designed and installed. Product filter housings cleaned prior to the placement of filter cartridges may present a challenge to the CIP process and warrant special attention to assure complete coverage of all housing surfaces during cleaning and rinsing.

Mechanical Operation and Personnel Intervention

It is common to place a BFS machine in a conventional clean room performing at Class 10,000 (Grade C) levels under static conditions and record counts over 100,000 during dynamic or operating conditions. The elevated level of particulates is notable, because although BFS is a barrier technology that isolates the critical product exposure zone, it is not a closed isolator. Although the environment around the BFS machine indicates high levels of particles, the environment directly in the area of the critical product exposure zone may remain free of contamination. This is due to the small exposure area and air flow near the critical zone.

BFS machines may employ exhaust mechanisms for the entrapment and venting of particle-laden air at the cutting and extruder areas, as well as shroud to protect the critical fill zone. The concern for most sterile products is protection from viable microbiological contamination. The contamination exhibited during the operation of the BFS line is primarily nonviable plastic particles and therefore may be of little consequence to the maintenance of aseptic manufacturing conditions. There is no conclusive evidence that particles generated by the cutting of the plastic parison adversely affect the product, and that they are able to enter the container or come in contact with the product.

To minimize the risk of microbiological contamination the BFS line should be operated in as automated a manner as possible, with little or no personnel intervention. Assuming that the fill room, machine surfaces, and environment have been properly decontaminated through sanitization, the personnel use proper aseptic technique during interventions, the BFS line is properly operated and maintained to minimize interventions, and procedures are taken to remove product during and directly subsequent to interventions; there should be relatively low risk of microbial contamination significant enough to contaminate product. The benefit of minimization of personnel interaction inherent in BFS manufacturing will outweigh the risk of potential adverse effect from the high levels of particles present during operation.

Environmental Monitoring

Continuous nonviable particulate monitoring by using a remote collection system is recommended. Particulate monitoring in the critical fill zone and shroud is recommended. Particulate level trends should be evaluated for the surrounding area and clean room. Active air sampling for viable contamination should be performed in the parison transport zone. Surface sampling for viable contamination should be performed in the critical fill zone at the end of the manufacturing process. Microbiological monitoring of personnel entering the clean room or involved in sampling or interventions should be routinely performed, as would be the case with conventional filling operations.

Additional BFS-Operating Points to Consider

- Resin transport is typically accomplished via a vacuum system. Lines should be cleanable. The resin delivery pathway should be easily purged and changed.
- Compressed air or nitrogen is used to form the parison and container. These gases contact product surfaces and must be sterile and contaminant free. Compressed gas venting should be piped out of the clean room. Air is vented at several steps during the container formation and filling process. Although this vented air may be clean, it can cause disruptions in airflow and turbulence resulting in contamination from floor and nonsterile portions of the line.
- Slight changes in the shape and configuration of the plastic parison can cause defects in the containers, including weak walls, leakers, and opening malfunctions.
- Fill accuracy is dependent on the condition of seals, O-rings, diaphragms and gaskets, which must be changed frequently. O-rings and gaskets may absorb product and media. They should be changed after production campaigns and media fills.
- The sealing is largely dependent on the quality of the mold, its condition, set-up, and adjustment.
- Trimming or "deflashing" is accomplished both in the clean room and directly outside of the room. Excess flash must be conveyed from the clean room in a manner that minimizes the opportunity for contamination. Wherever possible operations that can be accomplished outside of the clean room should be, including trim, leak testing, inspection, pouching, cartoning, labeling, etc. The conveyor belt that takes the filled units from the BFS machine out of the clean room should not re-enter the clean room. A second conveyor with a transfer plate should be used. The containers must be able to cross that plate. The conveyor re-entering the clean room and traveling to the BFS machine will pose a potential contamination threat.
- Condensate and excess product drained and removed from the lines must be transferred from the clean room or stored until the end of the run. It is not recommended that the condensate drain lines be attached to process drains in the clean room, or to lines that are later attached to process drains outside of the clean room. Drains should not be present in BFS clean rooms. It is possible for contaminated air or fluids to be drawn back up through these lines at the end of the steaming process as drain lines cool and create negative pressure. As these lines are connected directly to product or air transfer lines, there may be a potential for product contamination. Avoid dependence solely on valves and other mechanical devices to protect the lines. These devices fail at times, especially during the stress of sterilization, and it is difficult to determine when and where they have failed.
- The extruder surface is hot. This may create convection currents that can be disruptive to unidirectional airflow in the clean room. Take this into consideration when positioning HEPA coverage around the BFS machine.
- The connections between the cooling line and the mold segments are subject to leakage. These connections are in almost constant, jolting movement. The connections are typically threaded and should have a gasket or O-ring seal. Small leaks may not be readily apparent, but could cause contamination. This is especially of concern given the close proximity of the connection to the open container area.

- The space between the parison head and the fill system shroud is an area where the container interior is exposed to the environment as the mold is transported from parison to fill station. Although the risk of microbiological contamination entering the container during this exposure is relatively low, due to the exposure time, small opening size, and lack of personnel activity, attention should be given to the condition of this environment and design of this section of the machine.

Inspection and Leak Detection

One hundred percent inspection of filled containers for particulates is complicated by the level of clarity of the container. BFS resins are not as clear as glass. Gross levels of particulate contamination may be seen with visual inspection under strong light. Firms may rely on validation studies that consistently show acceptable levels of product particulate. This is combined with a statistical sampling for destructive analysis of container content.

Leak Detection

A critical product attribute for any flexible material container is the absence of leakage. The plastics used to form the BFS container are relatively soft and subject to puncture. Leakage in the BFS container may be immediately apparent after processing, or may develop during subsequent finished product storage and handling. The BFS process creates the potential for leakage during improper container formation fusion and sealing. Leakage typically appears at fusion points including the container side wall seals and the seal area. Poor handling of the filled containers can result in leakage from punctures to the walls of the container. Thin walls resulting from improper alignment of the parison head mechanism can be a weak point subject to puncture and leakage. Improperly designed engraving characters can also be an area of puncture and leakage. Precautions should be taken to properly design the process and containers to minimize the potential for leakage.

It is recommended to inspect all BFS containers for leakage. Inspections can be performed after any one of a number of postsealing manufacturing steps; however, it is recommended that a final inspection be performed after the last step that could affect leakage. If the product is terminally sterilized, then an inspection for leakage should be performed after that step.

Inspection techniques should be consistent and effective. Inspections techniques can generally be grouped into two categories; manual and automated. Manual methods involve using the human eye to detect leakage. Most manual methods involve some type of pressure applied to the container. This squeezing action is designed to push fluid through a hole in the container. The inspector can then detect the moisture on a contrasting element—like a blue towel material. These techniques vary in levels of automation. Higher automated manual methods involve a constant source of pressure applied to the container. More manual methods involve the inspector squeezing the container. The key to effective manual inspection is providing a constant pressure over a constant period of time, as well as being able to visually detect the leakage—which may be minute. This technique is difficult to validate and is subject to variable effectiveness. For that reason, it is recommended that the process qualification of the BFS machine include an extensive review of the container formation and sealing process. The study should be designed to provide a high degree of assurance that the process consistently results in leak free containers. With that validation completed a manufacturer can have confidence in a manual method of inspection of 100% of the containers, combined with a periodic check of samples using an automated method.

Automated methods of leak inspection involve a nonvisual method of detection. These include in-line methods such as pressure decay, pressure hold, moisture detection, and electronic current changes, as well as off-line methods such as dye and microbiological ingress. Pressure decay and vacuum decay involve placing the filled BFS container in a sealed holder. Vacuum or air pressure is applied to the holder. If there is a leak the vacuum will change as air leaves the BFS container and enters the holder. If pressure is applied a similar, but opposite effect occurs as air leaves the holder and enters the BFS container. The change in pressure is detected and the unit is rejected.

Moisture leak detection involves placing the BFS container in a holder. Vacuum is applied and the inspection machine detects moisture, which will pass from the filled BFS container through any puncture or leak. It is important that the exterior of the containers be dry for this to work. Obviously moisture detection will only work with aqueous-based products. Moisture, vacuum, and pressure detection systems allow for the inspection of the entire BFS container at once, regardless of where the leak occurs.

Electronic current change detection has been used for inspection of leakage on glass ampoules as well as BFS plastic containers. Here an electrical current is passed over an area on the BFS container. If a leak is present the current will be disrupted as it passes through the product. This method works best when the product is aqueous, conductive, and in contact with the puncture. If the BFS container is situated so that air is in contact with the puncture, the inspection effectiveness will be affected. Electrical systems are localized in the area that they can detect leakage. Electrodes must be placed where leaks are anticipated. On most, but not all BFS containers this can be predicted. Usually it is in the seal area. However, if there is another area of high incidence of leakers, a second set of electrodes may be needed. Electronic systems are sensitive to moisture contamination. Containers with gross leakage will tend to spread moisture onto the inspection machine and could cause malfunction.

Off-line methods are used for validation, process development, audits, and quality checks. They may be destructive and time consuming, and therefore are not used to inspect 100% of the containers. Dye testing involves placing a sample of filled BFS containers in a vessel with a dye, usually methylene blue. The containers are then subjected to pressure or vacuum that forces dye in through any leaks. At the end of the process, the containers are removed rinsed and the contents are inspected for evidence of dye. This is an easy to perform and common test to be performed off line to confirm that the in line inspection technique is working. This is especially useful when manual inspection methods are used as the primary inspection technique.

Microbiological ingress testing is more complicated and time consuming than dye testing. It involves filling BFS containers with a growth medium. The filled containers are placed in a bath or environment contaminated with an indicator microorganism. The containers stay in this environment for a period of time. The containers are then removed and incubated. The containers are later inspected for evidence of microbial contamination. Containers are set aside as controls and not subjected to the contamination. Microbiological ingress may not be efficient but it is the only method that directly addresses the potential for contamination of product.

A concern with the use of any of the methods, with the exception of microbiological ingress, is the definition of a leak, or the size of the container hole that will result in microbiological ingress and contamination. A 0.2 μm hole in a container might be considered as a place to start, because it is accepted as standard for sterile product filtration. However, a 0.2 μm hole in the side of a BFS container extending from the interior to the exterior is roughly equivalent to a 1 inch diameter pipe 1.5 miles long. How likely is it that a microorganism travels through that length? And how much force is necessary to overcome the surface tension to push product through that hole to detect the leak? How do we create such a leak to be able to validate our inspection method? The ideal standard may be 0.2 μm, but it is impractical in BFS leak detection. And it is doubtful that preventing that size hole has relevance to the quality of the product.

Correlation between levels of microbiological ingress and the size of the hole would confirm the appropriate size. A more practical standard for BFS containers might be a 5 μm diameter hole. Steps should not be taken to eliminate all leakage at any level. Any and all leakage detected on BFS containers should be thoroughly investigated and addressed. Leakage on a BFS container is indicative of other problems with container design, material compatibility, impurities in the extrusion process, misalignment of the forming and sealing mechanisms, mold damage, sequencing issues, product contacts, and other concerns that may have other adverse effects on the quality of the product.

Lasers and mechanical methods can be used to drill holes in BFS containers at 1 to 5 μm. Placement of these holes should be in areas that are close to the areas where actual leakers may become apparent. A 5 μm hole placed in the center of a smooth container wall may react differently to detection methods than a 5 μm hole that develops at a seam in the seal area at the top of the container. Artificially created holes have a finite useful "life" relevant to studies. Holes may become smaller over time or larger. Holes may change shape. These changes will affect the detection method ability and performance. It is important to understand the characteristics and performance life of the standard samples and change them when needed.

Although there are methods to detect BFS container leakers, the most effective way to assure leak free containers remains good container design and process control.

Validation

Qualification and validation of BFS machines, processes, and products are similar in many ways to the qualification and validation of conventional types of sterile product manufacture. This section of the chapter concentrates on some of the unique aspects of BFS technology validation that impact sterile product manufacturing. Filter qualification, fill system performance, SIP, clean in place, environmental and machine sanitization, personnel training and performance, line decontamination, and component sterilization and transfer are all critical to the manufacture of sterile products by using BFS technology, but are not unique to BFS technology. Validation of these processes should be undertaken using approaches used for conventional filling operations. Leak detection, container formation, and resin decontamination are somewhat unique to BFS and FFS, but they have been addressed earlier in the chapter and are not discussed further.

A summary of some of the validation activities and studies associated with the qualification of the BFS line include the following:

- Installation and operational qualification of the BFS equipment, the product transport system, clean room and associated HVAC, support utilities, deflashing and packaging equipment, and the resin-conveying system.
- Active air profile determination using smoke studies or other means to determine the flow of air from clean room to adjacent spaces, around machines, effects of extruder temperature on air flow, air flow in and around critical parison and mold transport zones, air flow in an around air shroud, and critical fill zone.
- Qualification of mold and container design, formation, and function; including wall thickness determination, seal characteristics, opening feature, functionality, and leakage.
- Validation of the sterilization process, including the compressed gas transport circuit, the fill system, filters, the localized controlled environment, and fitment conveying equipment.
- Validation of the sanitization process for the filling room and service rooms.
- Validation of the sterilization process for the fitments and any "off" sterilized equipment and/or components.
- Filter/product compatibility studies.
- Product/container temperature exposure studies.
- Validation of the cleaning processes, both those operated in place and those requiring disassembly of equipment, including the extruder.
- Seal integrity challenge studies for filled and deflashed product containers.
- Validation of the bottle forming process, including wall thickness consistency.
- Validation of automated/computer controlled or monitored processes.
- The successful completion of not less than three aseptic process simulation runs or media fills, using all aspects of the operation which could adversely affect product sterility, including shift changes, routine adjustments, product sampling in the room, environmental monitoring, and room sanitization. The BFS equipment is designed to operate without the presence of people, any procedure that involves people entering the environment should be challenged as part of the media fill. Because the operation of the BFS line is usually fully automated and often involves the filling of nonpreserved product, it may not be acceptable to allow any contamination during the fills. Zero contamination levels should be attainable with a properly designed and operated system. Media fills should include all routine interventions and periodically include non-routine interventions.

BFS operations rely on various support systems and critical utilities. A sound validation program will include the qualification of these systems. Some of the critical support systems, utilities, and equipment include the following:

- Purified water and water for injection for cleaning and rinsing of system.
- Central vacuum for forming bottles and transporting resin.

- Resin storage and transport system.
- Resin collection, regrind, and blending (pigment blending).
- Compressed air and drying.
- Clean steam system.
- Tempered or chilled water system.
- Building automation and/or facility monitoring systems.
- Leak testing apparatus.
- Clean room HVAC system.

Process and Intervention Simulation (Media Fills)

Special emphasis should be placed on the inclusion of inherent and anticipated personnel interventions. These interventions can be grouped as inherent and corrective. Examples of inherent intervention are environmental monitoring or the addition of a component. A corrective intervention may be a fill or parison adjustment, or reaction to a machine malfunction.

Interventions can further be grouped according to their potential impact on the quality of the product: low impact, moderate impact, major impact, or critical impact. Low impact may be an intervention which requires the operator to enter the clean room but not come in contact with the BFS machine, for example, to retrieve fallen containers. A moderate impact intervention may involve an operator contacting the BFS machine, but not in the critical fill zone area, for example, an adjustment to the extruder instrumentation, environmental monitoring, or room sanitization. A major impact intervention may involve activity near the critical fill exposure zone. This may involve fill volume adjustments. Critical impact interventions include any activity which by definition would have a high probability of affecting the sterility of the product, for example, removing or changing of filled nozzles. Note that critical impact interventions may require additional documentation, sterilization, or contamination control processes. The process simulation study should include as many intervention types as practical. The duration and quantity of each type of intervention should be similar to that of the intervention under actual operating conditions.

Many BFS runs occur over extended periods of time. It is necessary to simulate as closely as possible the effect of that duration on the process. It is not practical to fill media for multiple days, but thought should be given to capturing the most critical aspects of the fill run. It is recommended that at least one of the three media runs include the start-up of the BFS line (when interventions may be at their highest level) and one of the media fills capture each of the other production shifts. It is not essential that the media fills be conducted at the end of the multiple day fill run, especially if the environmental monitoring indicates that the clean room has maintained acceptable conditions.

If multiple product sizes and configurations are to be qualified on the BFS line, it is possible to bracket the containers for the media fills. Worst case should be included in the bracket. However, worst case may not be readily apparent. Smaller size containers may have smaller openings, allowing less potential for microbiological organism ingress, but they may also run at faster speeds which could result in more air flow turbulence and back draft form less clean parts of the line. It is not possible to change the speeds of the machine for purposes of media fills, as line speed greatly affects the ability to form the container. If the most challenging container configuration is not apparent, it is best to run them all.

BFS is almost fully automated. The risk of microbiological contamination is reduced, therefore if a contaminated media fill unit is found it is probably an indication of a larger problem. Airborne microbial contamination is expected to a certain extent on conventional fill lines. And a single contaminated unit, while requiring investigation and explanation, is of limited concern. However, a single failed unit on a BFS line will be harder to explain. It may indicate a problem with the BFS machine, connections, SIP circuits, etc. Caution and diligence are recommended when investigating this occurrence.

Risk assessment techniques may be used to determine media fill study design, including run duration, types and number of interventions included, and container configuration tested.

CONCLUSION

FFS and BFS offer interesting alternatives to the manufacture and packaging of sterile products. The technology has many inherent benefits in the sterile pharmaceutical field. It has undergone considerable scientific analysis in recent years, and proven to be an effective aseptic packaging technology. The technology and the process can be improved, and that should open the way to the packaging of more sophisticated and critical categories of products, especially biopharmaceutical products and small volume injectable drugs. Many of the issues discussed in this chapter are at the forefront of the FFS at the present time. As the technology is considered for more complicated and sensitive products, the need for continued improvement will drive the industry toward better manufacturing systems.

REFERENCES

1. Ljungqvist B, Reinmüller B, Löfgren A, et al. Current practice in the operation and validation of aseptic blow-fill-seal processes. PDA J Pharm Sci Technol 2006; 60(4):254–258.
2. Lindboe WG Jr. Validation of container preparation processes. In: Agalloco JP, Carleton FJ, eds. Validation of Pharmaceutical Processes. 3rd ed. New York: Informa, 2008; 376.

15 Genesis of the closed vial technology

Daniel Py and Angela Turner

INTRODUCTION

Aseptic processing requires "A strict design regime, not only on the process area, but on the interactions with surrounding areas and the movement of people, materials and equipment so as not to compromise the aseptic conditions" (1).

The Intact^{TM} containers are closed and stay Intact^{TM}, from the point of assembly, through radiation sterilization and aseptic filling, and ultimately until delivery to the patient. As a result, the product, when needle filled through a proprietary re-sealable stopper, is never exposed to the environment from within the sterile formulation tank to the body of the patient. The "compliance" has been engineered by the Intact^{TM} technology. Intact^{TM} is aimed to overcome the Food and Drug Administration (FDA) concerns with aseptic processing:

> .... it is critical that containers be filled and sealed in an extremely high-quality environment.... glass containers have been subjected to dry heat; rubber closures to moist heat; and liquid dosage forms to filtration... each of these manufacturing processes requiring validation and control. Each process could introduce an error that ultimately could lead to the distribution of a contaminated product... (2).

The essential difficulties in traditional aseptic technologies are in the assembly processes that follow the sterilization steps for the individual components. Table 1 shows the human factors and risk involved in this process (3).

With the Intact^{TM} technology, needle filling and sterile-closed containers, the container itself is the controlled environment and its own isolator, from sealing to filling.

Overall, the problem with aseptic technology is the high risks associated with open containers, exposed closures, and operator contact. These interventions will always mean an increase risk to the patient and because there is no truly safe intervention, the "perfect" intervention is one that does not happen (4).

The Solution: Intact^{TM} Technology

In the mid-1990s, closed systems were identified as superior to open systems in the aseptic processing of sterile active pharmaceutical ingredients (5). This Parenteral Drug Association (PDA) document was developed without mention of a risk assessment; nevertheless, it had a profound effect on Intact^{TM} technology. Intact^{TM} technology was conceived at Medical Instill Technologies, Inc., to address the need for a closed container that can behave as mobile isolator, keeping "Intact^{TM}" the inner surface sterile from sterilization through needle filling and laser resealing.

The materials used for the Intact^{TM} container were specifically designed for compatibility with parenteral solutions and also to minimize the potential for particle generation during the penetration of the needle into the container (Fig. 1).

- *Plastic vial body*—Cyclic Olefin Copolymer (COC) medical grade, United States Pharmacopeia (USP) Class VI, high purity, high transparency, gamma sterilization resistant, best combination of low permeability coefficients. These are sourced from Ticona and Zeon. Many other medical-grade plastics have been used since.
- *Stopper*—Thermoplastic elastomer (TPE) of a special formulation, developed with a large polymer compounding company, meets USP class VI. Other non-TPE materials have since been developed.
- *Needle*—Specially designed and treated stainless steel for low friction forces during penetration/withdrawal, which combined with the special stopper limit the size and number of particles to much lower levels than with traditional vulcanized stoppers.
- *Intact filling machine*—The machine is extremely simple, only two key mobile parts, the vial conveyor and the rack of needles. No assembly occurs in the machine. As a consequence the

Table 1 Aseptic Processing Risk Assessment: The Simplified Akers–Agalloco Method

Task	Ease of validation	Personnel sensitivity	Associated risk
Sterilization	Easy	Low	Low
Room design	Not applicable	Not applicable	Moderate
Monitoring	Moderate	Variable	High
Sanitization	Difficult	High	High
Gowning	Difficult	Very high	Very high
Material transfer	Difficult	High	High
Aseptic technique	Difficult	Very high	Very high
Aseptic assembly	Difficult	Very high	Very high

downtime is significantly reduced. The product is never in contact with the environment, from the sterile formulation tank to the inside of the sterile vial. The vials can be needle prefilled with nitrogen or other inert gas, with the same machine. Because the container is always sealed, the machine is nearly perfectly clean after operation, there are no splashing or broken containers, and CIP implementation is simplified.

The Intact™ filling technology was invented and developed in synergy with the stopper material of the closed containers. Noncoring needles, low-energy lasers for sealing the needle's path on the self-resealable stopper, special pigments to convert coherent radiation into heat enabling more efficient sealing, and IR sensors are used to assure that the melting temperature of the stopper material has been reached as a 100% quality control check. The Intact™ process offers several significant advantages over conventional aseptic filling that use glass containers, stoppers, and seals (Fig. 2).

- One supplier manufactures and assembles the complete container providing greater consistency and assured seal reliability.
- The assembly process is completed prior to sterilization essentially eliminating exposure during the process.
- The closure (the stopper itself) may be assembled and sealed within the molding machine and the closure integrity is 100% controlled, so that the inner surface of the closed intact vials/containers in general are never exposed to the environment (viables and nonviables).
- The sterilization process is performed on a sealed container eliminating potential for microbial ingress post-process.
- The inner surface of the closed vials are in contact with nothing but the liquid itself which is needle filled into the closed and sterile vials. Container product contact surfaces are never exposed even in the filling environment.

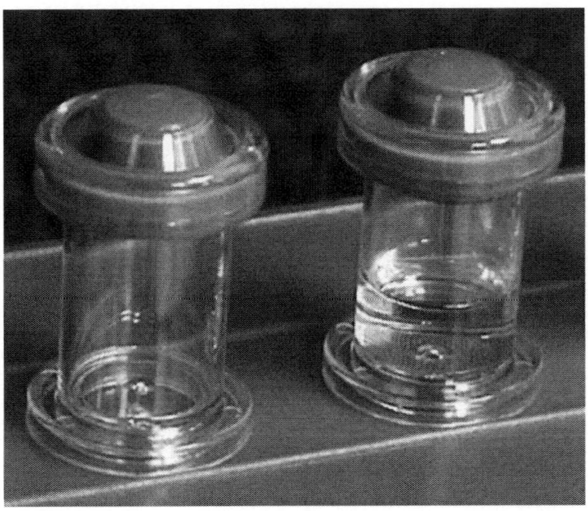

Figure 1 Early-stage Intact™ container.

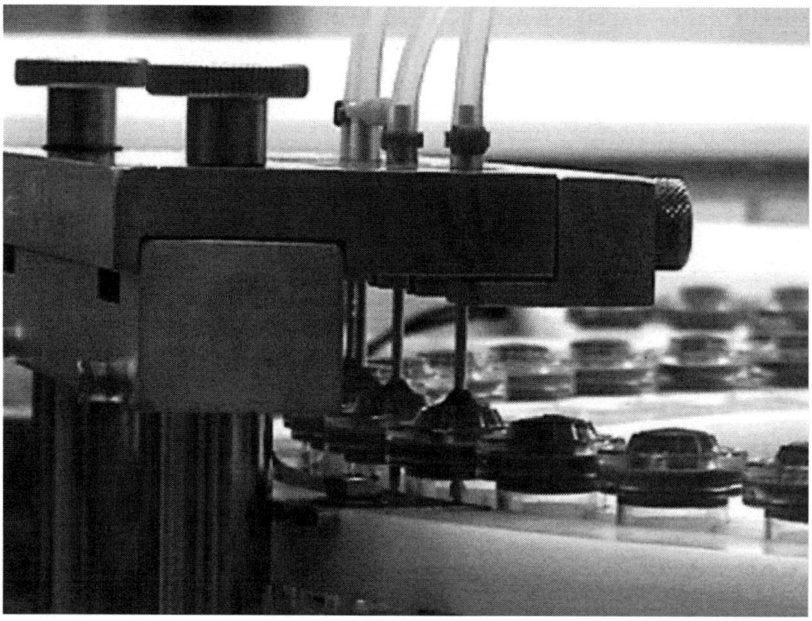

Figure 2 Rotary Intact™ filler: Laser sealing station.

- The Intact™ self re-sealable septum is laser resealed within seconds after needle removal.
- The pin hole sealing process of the pierceable stopper is verified for each container.

A traditional aseptic performance validation of the first prototype Intact™ filler was completed at the PDA in August 2003 by way of three consecutive media fill runs at 10,000 Intact™ vials each (6). A summary of the runs are as follows:

- Intact™ vials were filled with sterile filtered soy-based nutrient.
- The two primary operators of the Intact™ filler had no previous aseptic processing experience and carried out all interventions.
- No advanced aseptic processing techniques or barriers were used (mere laminar flow hood).
- Three filling-needle changes were made and other nonroutine and high-risk manipulations were purposely conducted during the three tests.
- All filled Intact™ vials, totaling 31,500 units were incubated at 25°C for 7 days (molds and yeast) and 35°C for 7 days (aerobic bacteria) for a total of 14 days.
- Four hundred Intact™ vials were purposely filled and not laser resealed to characterize the safety factor of the self-resealing property of the stopper itself before laser resealing. These nonlaser resealed units remained sterile for more than 3 months until they were discarded.

Table 2 identifies the results of the media fills.

Table 2 PDA-TRI Media Fill Results

Media fill run	1	2	3
Date	August 9, 2003	August 11, 2003	August 13, 2003
Units	10,377	10,730	10,645
Incubation	14 days		
# of Positives[a]	0	0	0
% Pass	100%	100%	100%
Microchallenge			

[a]Including the 400 nonlaser-resealed Intact™ vials.

A sample set of laser-resealed Intact™ vials were subjected to physical tests to assess the container integrity microbial ingress challenge and burst testing. The Intact™ vials were placed into a biobath of log7 concentration of *Brevundimonas diminuta* (ATCC# 19146) and successfully passed a 24-hour submersion and incubation. Finally, a USP <788> particulates test was performed on all Intact™ media fill vials with the following successful results (Table 3).

Table 3 PDA-TRI Media Fill USP <788> Particulates Test Results

Particulate size	Limits	Test results/per vial
25 μm	600	3
10 μm	6000	31

The conclusion of the media fills performed identified that

- Closed vial filling systems proved robust where interventions and operator training represented worst-case operating conditions.
- Sterile preassembled containers significantly reduce the number of processing operations.
- A substantial reduction in system and process complexity was successfully demonstrated.
- Rapid system installation and validation.

To further advance the capabilities of the Intact™ filling process several enhancements have been made in newer fill systems to further improve upon the aseptic capabilities of the technology.

- The filling of Intact™ containers is performed in a hydrogen peroxide decontaminated isolator that operates without gloves. All internal movements are accomplished through mechanical or robotic systems. No human interventions are necessary during Intact™ filling.
- For extra safety precaution, the outer surface of the Intact™ container's septum are sterilized with hydrogen peroxide on-line upon entering the decontaminated aseptic fill zone. A characterization study for a log6 reduction of *Bacillus subtilis spp. niger* (ATCC 9732) was performed on a lot of 100 containers and determined to be met with minimal hydrogen peroxide concentration (7). This vapor hydrogen peroxide (VHP) station replaces advantageously any sterile transfer port.
- The integrity of each laser seal is supported by individual confirmation of temperature at the point of the seal (the laser melts the closure to reseal the opening).
- Linear filling platform replaces the first rotary platform.

These differences serve to enhance the reliability of the Intact™ filling relative to the risk of microbial contamination (Fig. 3).

In December 2003, an invitation from Dr. Peter Cooney and Dr. David Hussong of the Office of Pharmaceutical Sciences, CDER, FDA was given to Dr. Daniel Py to discuss the Intact™ technology based on the media fill performance at the PDA-TRI (Training and Research Institute) aseptic fill suite. Upon review of the data and discussion of the technology, Dr. Peter Cooney stated that "this is the paradigm shift in sterile filling technology" and praised the "engineered compliance" provided with Medical Instill Technologies.

ULTIMATE CHALLENGE TEST: MICROBIOLOGIC AEROSOL IN THE FILLER ITSELF

Although the risk for the closed vial to be contaminated is already essentially negligible as confirmed by multiple media fills under laminar flow, further experimentation has been undertaken in noncontrolled environments, to further determine the safety of the Intact™ filling process. One of the primary compliance expectations that are required with aseptic processing is continuous environmental monitoring to provide evidence that both viable and nonviable particulates have not breached the aseptic zone area. With Intact™ technology the risk of contamination is so low that several experiments were carried out to challenge both the closed vial and the Intact™ filler in a "dirty" environment worse than "filling in a parking lot," without

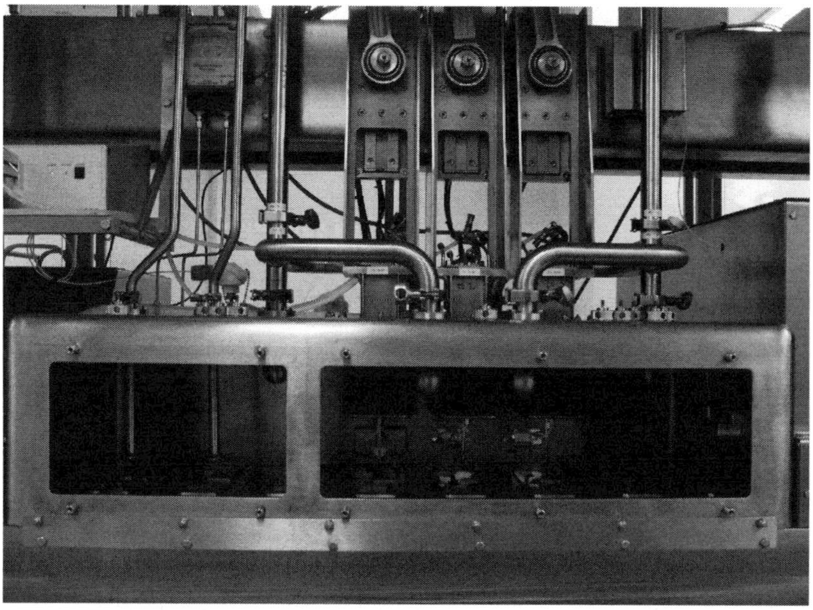

Figure 3 Linear Intact™ filling (Universal Filler).

laminar flow or VHP on the stopper, as if the manipulator had forgotten the HEPA filters and the H_2O_2 vapor on the stopper.

To create such a condition, a nebulizer, fan, and containment unit were used to place the filler and containers into a "dirty" environment. Both wet and dry aerosol microbial challenge tests were conducted with a log3 concentration of *Bacillus subtilis spp. niger* (ATCC 9732). The goal was to determine if Intact™ filling with a closed container in a "dirty" environment without controls could allow the filling of a closed container with sterile tryptic soy broth. To further challenge the Intact™ technology, several units were filled and not laser re-sealed to further ensure the safety of the filling process. Figure 4 shows for the chamber and test system with a clinical Intact™ filler used during testing.

Before running the nebulizer with either a dry or wet microbial aerosol, two negative controls were filled via Intact™ filling without environmental control. Additional environmental monitoring to confirm the level of microbial aerosol was conducted throughout the run. After the test samples were ran, a 30 to 300 CFU/mL of *Bacillus subtilis spp. niger* (ATCC 9372) was added to two closed containers to establish positive controls. After 20 closed containers were Intact™ filled in a dry aerosol (concentration of 1.3×10^3 CFU/1000 m^3) and 10 closed containers were filled in a wet aerosol (concentration of 4.2×1010^3 CFU/1000 m^3) the samples were incubated for 14 days at 30°C with evidence of no growth (8). Further evaluations at increased *Bacillus subtilis spp. niger* (ATCC 9372) concentrations are under way to establish an edge of failure value. With this information larger sample size studies at this log3 concentration will be established.

Process Benefits

An additional advantage beyond the added compliance using intact™ filling is attained by reductions in both labor and time. The Intact™ process eliminates the extended exposure of sterile/depyrogenated containers and closures to the operating environment. Intact™ containers are supplied sterile and sealed, such that contamination ingress is eliminated. In addition, concerns for sterilization of product contact surfaces for the closure system at the fill site are also eliminated. The only concerns with the Intact™ process are the sterility of the closure surface at the point of penetration, the integrity of the re-sealed container, and maintaining sterility of the fill needles over the duration of the filling process.

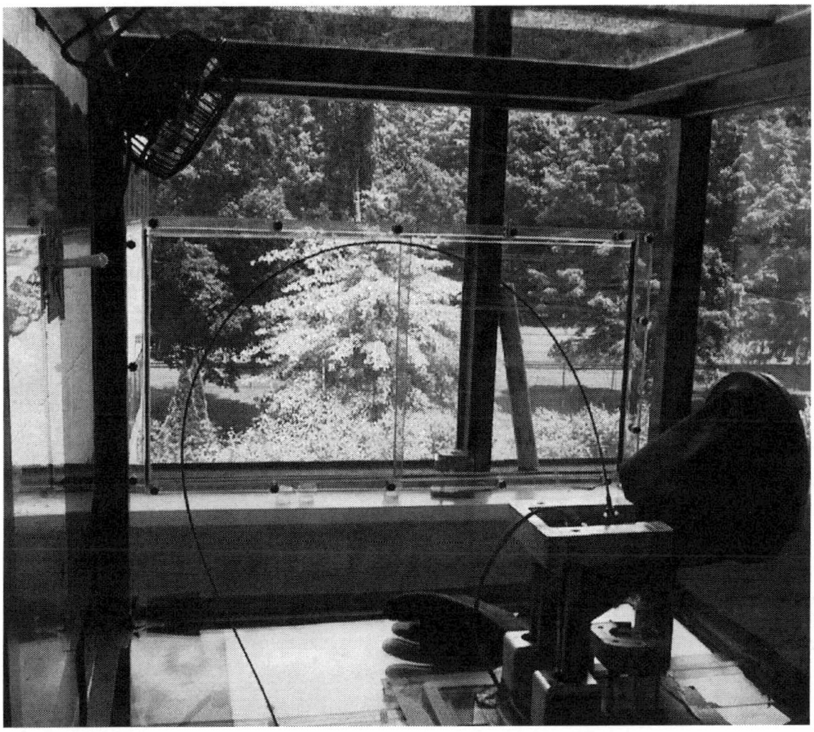

Figure 4 Aerosol microbial challenge testing chamber unit

Moreover, the Intact™ filling eliminates several of the major cost areas associated with filling of glass containers by aseptic processing regardless of the specific technology: conventional, RABS, or isolator-used. Water for injection requirements are dramatically reduced as the only requirement for water is that required in the formulation. Washing of stoppers and glass containers prior to sterilization is eliminated as well. Sterilization of stoppers and fill parts by steam are eliminated as well as depyrogenation by heat of the glass containers. The expense of the equipment and the utility costs to operate these systems is thus averted as well. Figures 5 and 6 shows a cost comparison of current aseptic technology and Intact™ technology (9).

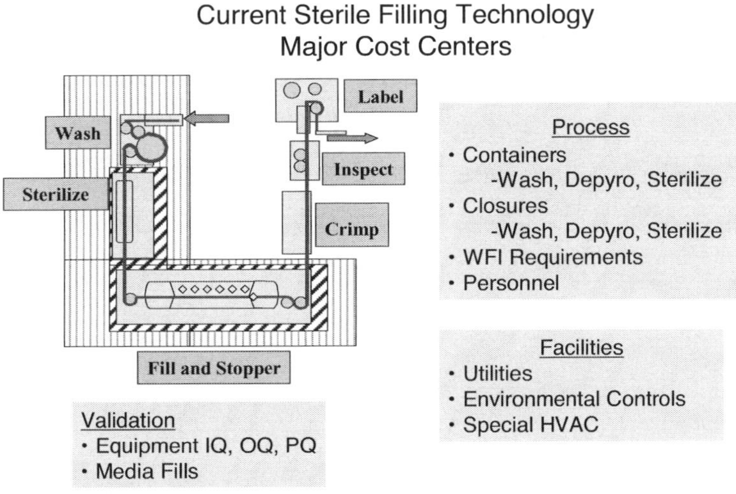

Figure 5 Operational cost for current aseptic technology.

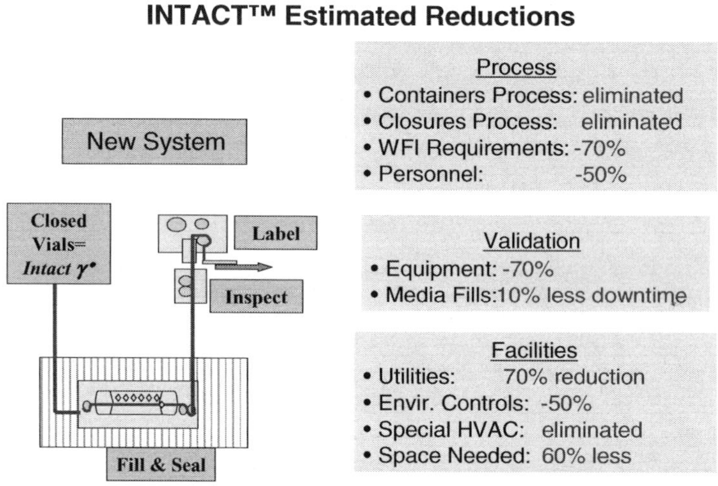

Figure 6 Operational cost for INTACT™ technology.

All the traditional operations and controls for sterile washing, sterile drying, sterile transfers, and as a result, are obsolete due to the "engineered compliance" resulting from transfers and filling of the Intact™ closed vials. The estimated saving on the operation cost is about 65% and this does not take into account the dramatic improvement of the downtime, and of the consecutive elimination of the numerous media fills and quarantines usually needed with aseptic filling of the traditional open vials.

APPLICATIONS OF THE INTACT™ FILLING TECHNOLOGY TO NONPRESERVED PRODUCTS

The Intact™ vial for a nonpreserved vaccine was the first application of the Intact™ filling technology. In 2004, Intact™ filling and Intact™ "Diablo" vials were licensed by Medical Instill Technologies, Inc., to GSK and Aseptic Technologies (a subsidiary of GlaxoSmithKline) for filling nonpreserved vaccines and nonpreserved injectables (chapter 40 of this book outlines the related capabilities and experience of Aseptic Technologies, the GSK-owned company to which we licensed the Intact™ vials and filling technology mentioned above for vaccines and pharmaceutical injectables and that they now make available for commercialization in that field of use under the "Crystal™" brand).

Infant bottle (with teat) nonpreserved infant formula was the second application of the Intact™ filling technology. In 2005, Medical Instill Technologies, Inc., invented and developed an infant bottle to be Intact™ filled, and licensed it to a leader in the nutrition field for an unmatched safety level provided with infant formula. A focus of this application is premature infants who have yet to develop their immune system. In addition to the Intact™ baby bottle for single use, an Intact™ multiple-dose noncontamination bulk dispensing package for infant formula also was licensed to the same leading nutrition company for use in ambient conditions. This technology expands to allow for the use of sterile dispensing (Intact™ valve) from first to last dose in nonrefrigerated conditions for over a month of sterile use.

The PureDose® Valve

The application of the Intact™ valve evolved into the PureDose™ valve for dispensing solutions, suspensions, gels, and creams in pharmaceutical and medical device applications. The PureDose™ valve is a one-way viscoelastic valve that performs as a mechanical barrier to bacterial ingress, over multiple doses. This concept allows for the elimination of preservatives, now shown to be associated with numerous topical and systemic side effects. In addition, this allows for an increase in stability through the prevention of oxidation and no microbial ingress. The viscoelastic valve was designed based on a coronary artery that is itself a pump, using stress differential to eject residual volume. It can be described as the valve behaving by "squeezing a cherry pit" or product from the container to prevent any microbial ingress.

A line of containers for various topical and systemic administrations are in the development process. Approximately 600,000 microbiological challenge tests have been successfully carried out with the PureDose™ valve.

Next-Generation Intact Products

Further applications of Intact™ technology with the PureDose valve™ have lead to new concepts in the areas of sterile powder filling, sterile connectors, lyophilization processing, and a second generation of Intact™ vials for multiple dosing. Modifications to the container and filler can accommodate both lyophilization and dry powder filling.

The sterile connector allows for the immunocompromised patient, either at home or a hospital, to prevent contamination of viable particulates into their bodies when either feeding or receiving pharmaceuticals.

A **needleless transfer container** has also been developed to sterile transfer any liquid product into another sterile closed container. The first application is the transfer of a complementary nutrition product into another nutrition product container. The same container will then be used for sterile transfer of pharmaceuticals without a needle.

A sterile powder filling machine using the Intact™ technology will be available for filling closed vials with sterile powder milk before the year end. The same system will be usable for sterile filling pharmaceutical powders. There are two main advantages of such a system:

- The absence of powder projection in the filling machine, and as a consequence, a very low-maintenance filler is provided;
- It allows for reconstitution of the product with sterile water through the needleless transfer feature into another closed sterile container.

This new series of Intact™ devices is aimed at preventing any contact with a nonsterile environment during the reconstitution of the product, during the needleless transfer, and/or multiple dose delivery. As a consequence, Intact™ devices will significantly contribute to the reduction of nosocomial infections and associated costs.

CONCLUSION

The Intact™ filling and nontontamination valve technologies, validated in vaccines and nutrition products, has generated a "paradigm shift" to reach the epitome of sterile filling through the elimination of the multiple interventions that had previously made aseptic filling operations increasingly complex. As a consequence, with the Intact™ technology, the increasingly complex compliance has been "purely" engineered as Dr. David Hussong of FDA has said. The elimination of the open container and of the separate stopper reduces the contamination potential to levels believed unattainable by other means.

It is also a stepping stone for filling and reconstitution of powder products and a variety of noncontamination multidose delivery devices. The Dr. Py Institute is the technology leader in developing these sterile filling and nonpreserved dispensing devices. The Intact™ technology prevents contact between the products and the environment from within the sterile formulation tank to the bodies of the patients. The scope of this technology has been proven in medical devices, pharmaceutical, nutritional, and skin care products. It has been proven to also reduce manufacturing cost and to simplify operations, especially for emergency supply in much less controlled environments. It is now aimed at reducing significantly the incidence nosocomial infections.

REFERENCES

1. ISPE Sterile Manufacturing Facilities Guide. Volume 3. January 1999.
2. FDA. Guideline to Sterile Drug Products Produced by Aseptic Processing. 2004.
3. Agalloco J, Akers J. Simplified risk analysis for aseptic processing: the Akers–Agalloco method. Pharm Technol 2006; 30(7):60–76.

4. Agalloco J, Akers J. The truth about interventions in aseptic processing. Pharm Technol 2007; 31(5): S8–S11.
5. PDA. Process Simulation Testing for Sterile Bulk Pharmaceutical Chemicals. PDA Technical Report #28, PDA J Pharm Sci Technol 1998; 52(4 suppl):9.
6. MEDInstill internal document, PDA-TRI, Media Fill (PQ) Report, August 2003.
7. MEDInstill internal document 00055400R0701.00, May 5, 2009.
8. MEDInstill internal document 00055400R0902.00, June 10, 2009.
9. Myers R. Presentation to PDA Annual Scientific Meeting, March, 2004.

16 Aseptic containment

Julian Wilkins

INTRODUCTION

Why is containment an issue? The reason is that drug substances can pose a hazard to those handling it, the environment, where cross contamination occurs to other products and ultimately the patient, recipient of the contaminated drug.

In the aseptic world, handling high hazard substances ($<10\ \mu g/m^3/8$ hours) (1) requires the protection of the product from people and the environment and the protection of the environment and people from the product.

Exposure to the drug substance can cause a wide range of reactions ranging from short-term reversible nonthreatening effects to long-term irreversible and life-threatening effects and even death. Exposure of patient populations can be more catastrophic due to age, gender, and health. Once solely a health and safety concern high hazard compounds are now clearly in the regulatory domain (2).

Why high hazard rather than "highly potent?" Potency refers to the pharmaceutical efficiency of the compound. A highly potent (low dose/effect) compound is not necessarily highly hazardous.

At the time this chapter was written, the International Society for Pharmaceutical Engineering (ISPE) had submitted a baseline guide for a science- and risk-based approach to the manufacture of pharmaceutical products (RiskMaPP) to the worldwide regulatory body. The main objective is to prevent regulation enforcing segregation and dedication based solely on product/compound classification. So a chapter on containment that is relevant to quality, regulatory, operations, environmental, health, and safety is provided. Containment is no longer an annoying cost of doing business, but is essential to the avoidance of regulator observation and worse. Data in this chapter are likely to change rapidly.

Objectives of a Risk-Based Approach

The objectives of a science- and risk-based approach to handling compounds of varying degrees of hazard are the following:

1. To base decisions on science and risk assessments rather than emotional responses for patient and operator safety.
2. To use the allowable daily exposure (ADE) as the yardstick of performance in cleaning and in cross contamination based on the understanding that there is no such thing as zero cross contamination or zero exposure. Using therapeutic dosages or parts per million as indices is not scientifically sound.
3. Risk is a product of hazard and exposure. Exposure can be controlled, hazard is inherent in the molecule and risk should be consistent throughout the industry. There is difference in the risk a patient can be expected to tolerate because of the potential benefits of a drug. Where cross contamination occurs there is no such benefit to outweigh the risk and so a much stricter definition of risk is required (3).
4. Only where compliance with the scientifically determined limits for retention and exposure is not possible should segregation/dedication be required unless the manufacturer wishes to use segregation/dedication for other reasons.
5. Reference to potent, cytotoxic, cytostatic, etc. should no longer be made. These terms illicit emotional reactions in some areas including the regulators. There is a continuum of hazard from the least to the most hazardous.

CONTAINMENT

Containment has been used as a catch all phrase to cover the control of operator exposure to hazard. The hazard is based on the risk a compound poses to health. Compounds such as cytotoxins, cytostatins, hormones, and sensitizers are seen as being highly hazardous in many cases unjustifiably. Regulators and industry have been seen to react in a nonscientific way to these hazards. The boundary between "potent" and "nonpotent" has been arbitrarily set at 10 mcg/m^3/8 hours, but hazard data is a not bright line. It is likely that industry will move to a continuum approach where all pharmaceutical compounds are subjected to a scientific risk assessment. One of the drivers for this change is the regulatory concern about cross contamination and the suggestion by some of the single molecule hazard for cytotoxins and cytostatins. This theory is unsupported by science.

Protection of Operator and Environment (Industrial Hygiene, Health and Safety Versus Protection of the Patient (cGMP, current Good Manufacturing Practice)

Industrial hygiene monitoring for worker safety has been practiced to protect the operator from exposure to hazard. Worldwide regulators who have no mandate for operator safety have been concerned by the effects of cross contamination by another drug substance. Currently there is confusion in regulation worldwide. The risk is that regulators will revert to the "penicillin/beta lactam" model and insist on dedication and/or segregation. The cost implications for clinical and nonblockbuster drugs are in the billions of dollars and will significantly impact the cost of drug manufacture.

Some of the terms used have resulted in regulatory responses that are not consistent with science. Cytotoxics and cytostatics and many hormones evince a reaction that does not equate to the formula.

$$\text{Risk} = \text{Hazard} \times \text{Exposure}$$

Many of the other descriptors such as teratogenic, mutagenic, and carcinogenic also do little to help. There is now a move to eliminate these descriptors and to look at hazard as a continuum between the low and highly hazardous.

Because industrial toxicology has set limits for operators and regulators have seen no method to review the risk to the patient they have latched onto the occupational toxicology data to indicate the risk of cross contamination. Up to now industrial hygiene (IH) data and monitoring, except for very few regulated actives and intermediates, have been at the company's discretion and fall outside the regulatory review. Instances have occurred where regulatory comment based on IH data and equally surrogate testing has been included as part of the installation qualification and operational qualification and as so falls under regulatory scrutiny. This is a very dangerous situation because uninformed review of IH data is highly vulnerable to misinterpretation and as Figure 1 (I) shows the mechanism for operator exposure is different to that of cross contamination.

There are two current initiatives that may impact this issue:

1. The European Medicines Agency is writing guidance that is reputed to be moving in the segregated/dedicated direction for the substances quoted as "certain" in 3.6 of the Orange Guide. The EMEA issued a letter in December 2009 stating that a risk-based approach could be used to support multiproduct facilities.
2. ISPE has written guidance for industry based on good science, the use of the ADE and risk management to demonstrate acceptable risk in the handling of pharmaceutical compounds. This will be on a case-by-case basis and covers all active drug substances. The document was reviewed by the US Food and Drug Administration (FDA).
3. ICH Q9 is now widely adopted and it provides a simple roadmap to risk management. Figure 1 (4) shows the structure of the document. This chapter covers risk assessment and risk control and describes some tools that can be used in risk assessment.

The inevitable conclusion is that data on the presence of drug substance outside the production boundary are going to come within regulatory scrutiny because of the patient.

The next section covers hazard and exposure in greater detail. It is important to have an understanding of how occupational toxicologists set safe levels for operator protection. The exposure section covers the engineering controls. Because nothing can be done to change the hazard as it is inherent in the molecule, it is clear that the risk goal can only be changed by

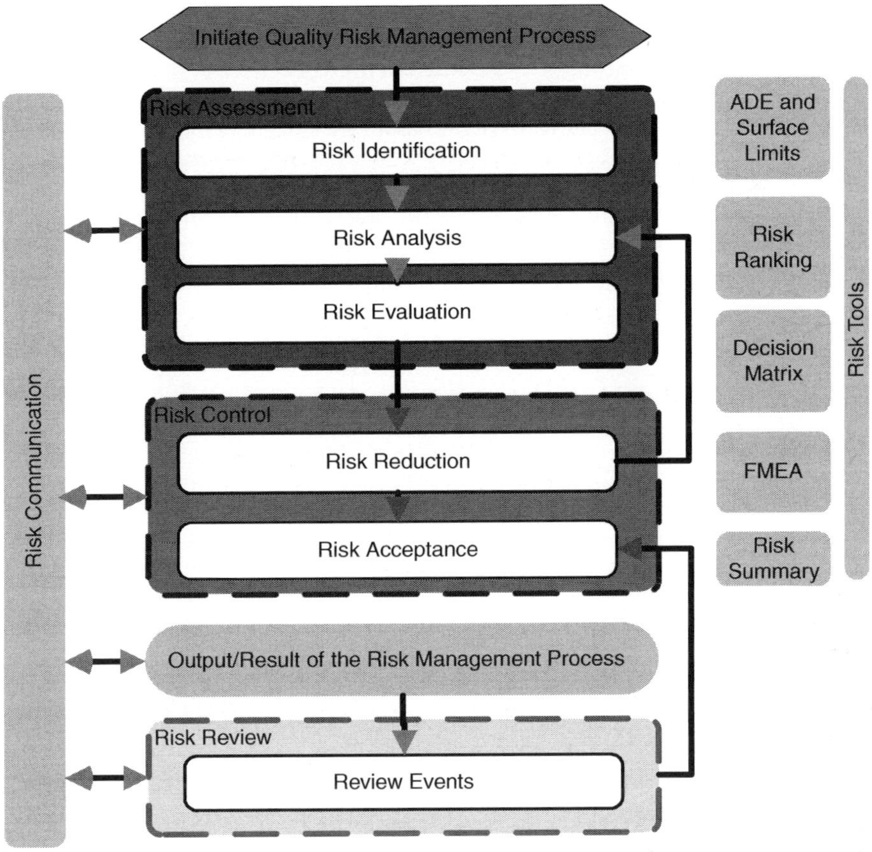

Figure 1

controlling exposure. To achieve an acceptable level of risk there must be interaction between these groups of specialists and without it there is significant risk of failure:

- Drug Metabolism
- Pharmocokinetics
- Toxicologists
- EHS/SHE environmental health and safety/safety health and environment
- Cleaning specialists
- Quality/Regulatory
- Engineering
- Production
- Operators

It has to be a holistic approach and the traditional compartmentalization has to be broken down.

The Good Manufacturing Practices Connection

Aseptic processing is about protecting the product from personnel and the environment, whereas containment seems to be all about protecting the operator from the product. Conventionally this has been achieved by closing up the process as far as practical and then applying positive pressure for aseptic environments and negative pressure for containment to overcome the leakage in the process and the "mouseholes" created for continuous transfer in the aseptic environment. Containment and asepsis seem to be mutually exclusive.

By creating small high-quality highly engineered enclosures, containment systems create highly controlled microenvironments, more importantly it is an environment in which people are excluded by a contiguous boundary. The result is a product environment uncontaminated by people and the environment, and people and the environment are protected from the product. It is clear that these environments provide for higher assurance than can be created by other means. The FDA now readily accepts that an isolated aseptic environment correctly conceived provides a better good manufacturing practices (GMP) environment than that provided by conventional systems. By minimizing the volume and area requiring decontamination and cleaning, faster and better turnaround can be achieved. As more contained processing systems are installed it is clear that the regulators will quickly realize the improvements that can be achieved.

Key Concepts

The concern of containment is to prevent exposure to the hazard in the aseptic world it is also about exposure to the environment. This section discusses health risk to the operator rather than the risk to the patient.

Containment is all about segregating the product boundary from the rest of the world. To get the highest performance, there must be no way for the active pharmaceutical ingredient (API) to escape into the environment. This is difficult to achieve and with high hazard materials the permissible levels are expressed in thousand millionths of a gram in cubic meter of air over 8 hours, when it is realized that visible dust occurs at about 100 $\mu g/m^3$ over 8 hours orders of magnitude more than the limit for many drug substances.

Containment systems leak; some more than others, some use air movement to capture escaped particles. These systems cannot and do not perform as well as closed systems. To overcome this and because of concerns over operator safety the way forward in the past was to wrap the operator in appropriate personal protective equipment (PPE) and hope that a few doors and pressure cascades would protect the environment.

PPE has limitations and in many cases the protection factor of the PPE is severely challenged. Starting in Europe and now accepted in the United States, PPE cannot be the primary line of protection. This means that other engineering controls have to be in place with PPE as the final line of defense. These controls over the last 20 years have developed in a number of forms, which are discussed later. There is also a belief that the more effective the containment the greater the cost. With the increasingly stringent requirements for cleaning validation, the cost of losing high-value product from the process and the costs of implementing facility heating, ventilating and air conditioning (HVAC) and room improvements, it is no longer true to say that containment to the highest levels costs money; in fact, in many cases it has been shown to save money.

GENERAL PRINCIPLES

$$\text{Risk} = \text{Hazard} \times \text{Exposure}$$

Risk

Risk is the likelihood of harm occurring to people and patient. The term "people" includes any person other than the patient. They could be operators in the pharmaceutical plant, pharmacists, care givers, nurses, or anyone, anywhere who could become exposed to a hazard. Because we all live in the environment, this too is covered by the term "people," because the environment directly impacts us all.

The patient is the recipient by some form of dosage delivery of the pharmaceutical compound. The patient by definition (unless undergoing an elective procedure) is unwell and has reduced resistance. The safety of the drug is determined from toxicological data. As has been previously mentioned, risk and benefit have to be balanced.

The dosage is set by the physician so that the patient can derive benefit at an acceptable level of risk. At the same time the patient must be protected from contamination, cross contamination by other pharmaceutical compounds and mix up.

Hazard

Hazard is the effect that is created by the pharmaceutical compound, the intermediates used in its manufacture and the chemicals used to process the compound. These latter items may be more hazardous than the pharmaceutical compound itself. The hazard for a pharmaceutical compound is normally defined by its ADE. The hazard for a compound does not vary, by for instance dilution; however, varying process steps may increase or decrease the risk of exposure. The limit for exposure to the operator is expressed conventionally in the form occupational exposure level (OEL), or other company-specific descriptor such as occupational exposure guideline. It is uniformly expressed as micrograms per meter cube per 8 hours ($\mu g/m^3/8$ hours). This is the safe limit at which a person may be exposed for 8 hours a day, 5 days per week for 40 years and is based on inhalation. The ADE is the ADE for 40 years with no observable adverse effect. It is typically 10 times the OEL, which is based on a human consuming 10 m^3 air a day. The ADE for patient protection may be different due to route of exposure and the differences of age, health, and monitoring.

The effects of pharmaceutical compounds and to a far lesser extent intermediates are assessed by a variety of methods, the chief of which is a full in vivo toxicological study. This takes at least 2 years and on the order of US $5 million to undertake. Major blockbuster drugs will have undergone this review, but many early-stage compounds have not undergone this level of scrutiny, their review is based on similar substances and on the use of correction factors. One of the significant areas of current concern is cytotoxic and cytostatic compounds. The argument is that they are designed to cause harm and how do we know that a single molecule does not cause harm?

Much has been made of potent compounds and various authorities have taken a starting point for potent compounds at 10 $\mu g/m^3/8$ hours. Therefore a pharmaceutical compound with an OEL of 11 $\mu g/m^3/8$ hours is treated differently to one of 9 $\mu g/m^3/8$ hours. This is patently nonsense, particularly bearing in mind the variability factors used in the calculations. The truth is that there are no bright lines of demarcation, merely a continuum of hazard from compounds with low activity and no undesirable "gens" (mutagen, teratagen, carcinogen, etc.) to those with higher activity and some "gens"/sensitization.

Most companies have adopted a method of characterization, initiated in the early 1990s. These characterizations were meant to reflect performances of various exposure control technologies, which led to some significant anomalies. Today a base 10 approach is almost universally adopted. The diagram below indicates commonly adopted bandings or characterizations.

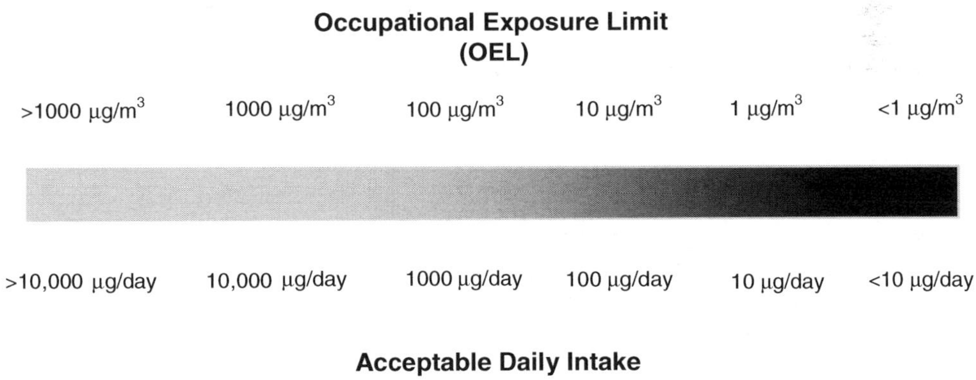

Such bandings are useful as a shorthand description of a compound. For instance a Category 5 indicates the highest level of activity and requires fully contained processing.

In many cases, such as contract manufacturing organizations and generic manufacturers, the only data on the toxicological effects of a compound are derived from material safety data sheets (MSDS). The data contained in a MSDS is at best insufficient and at worst useless. MSDSs are written in such a way as to absolve the producer of the MSDS from liability. They are peppered with meaningless phrases such as "not known" and "seek medical help." Any one handling high hazard compounds should seek the advice of a qualified occupational toxicologist, who will be able to conduct a literature search and set an ADE and OEL.

Exposure

Exposure occurs as a result of an emission caused by energy being imparted into the hazard, which can be a simple act of moving a container, up to the effects of high-speed milling. An emission becomes an exposure when it becomes available to a person or product, other than the hazard. Not all emissions are exposures, but all exposures are the result of an emission. Exposure is controllable and is the release of pharmaceutical compounds from its process boundary, making it potentially available to people and by cross contamination to patients.

Contamination is product adulteration by environmental contaminants including particulates derived from the operators. Cross contamination is caused by one pharmaceutical compound entering another product through one of three mechanisms:

1. Airborne entrainment. Here intermediates or pharmaceutical compounds in suspension are entrained into another product; this requires the aerosol, because it may be atomized liquids to settle into the other product.
2. Mechanical transfer where the cross contaminant is deposited on surfaces or equipment that is used to process or transfer materials into the pharmaceutical substance.
3. Retention, where equipment are used for multiple products and cleaning is not within limits the cross contaminant can directly enter the subsequent products.

It is possible to set safe levels by risk assessment for each type of contamination.
There is no such thing as zero risk.

Mix Up

The most effective means of adulteration is the use of the incorrect pharmaceutical compound or an incorrect concentration or at different potency. The old adage, normally used as an excuse, is that mistakes will occur. It is essential to provide the correct checks and balances to ensure adherence to formula. Containment and automation can help. Containment provides a highly controlled access to the containment boundary and automation can be used to verify critical ingredients at the point of entry into a contained system.

There is no magic formula that provides a matrix of hazard and exposure from which a suitable engineering control can be selected. The actual hazard of the compounds of interest may be less stringent, but the truth is that less than 10 $\mu g/m^3/8$ hours there is no difference in how a system is contained, total containment is essential.

Each compound must be evaluated on a case-by-case basis and a risk assessment as part of an overall risk management document should be produced prior to processing so that they are available for regulatory review.

The use of "cookie cutter" decisions on containment is extremely dangerous. Careful evaluation of the process, set up, operation, interventions, sampling, upset, recover, clean up, and maintenance must be done. Those with sufficient knowledge to safely use an engineering control matrix also know enough to use it as a rough and ready guide. Such material in the wrong or inexperienced hands is **extremely dangerous**.

Hazard Setting the Limit

Effective and efficient hazard communication concerning the relative degree of toxicity and/or pharmacological activity of APIs, intermediates, purchased (e.g., excipients and solvents), and other chemicals are an important component in assuring employees' health and safety. Use of occupational exposure bands (OEBs), typically in four or five bands, in conjunction with additional designations (i.e., R, S, or C) provides a common and understandable "language" to accomplish this communication, as clearly stated in ICH Q9. As there is no clear consensus in the industry, it is that much more important to understand the principles.

OEBs are established qualitatively (as will be explained in more detail later in this chapter) and quantitatively based upon the resulting OEL (if one exists). OELs are the airborne limit concentrations of compounds that are believed to be protective of the health of employees. Industrial hygienists conduct monitoring to assess employees' exposures relative to these levels. Many functions, including occupational health, engineering, and management use the results to make important decisions to assure on-going protection of employee health and the prevention of cross contamination.

Typical Banding

Variously based on a base 10 principle, some companies have bandings based on perceived performances by varying engineering controls. There are significant risks with this approach (5).

A typical base 10 banding system is illustrated here

OEB	Range of OEL (μg/m³)	Toxicological/pharmacological properties
OEB 1	1000–5000	Harmful, and/or low pharmacological activity
OEB 2	100–1000	Harmful, and/or moderate pharmacological activity
OEB 3	10–100	Moderate toxic and/or high pharmacological activity
OEB 4	1–10	Toxic and/or very high pharmacological activity
OEB 5	<1	Extremely toxic and/or extremely high pharmacological activity

Occupational Exposure Band Assignments for APIs

Default OEB Assignments—Exploratory Studies and Candidate Identification Stage

During the early discovery phase, limited data are available for a compound. During this period, research compounds are assigned to a default category, unless a structure–activity relationship analysis of the molecular structure or other indicators (such as therapeutic class or compound class) suggest potential for high to extremely high toxicity or pharmacological activity. Especially of concern are mutagenicity and/or carcinogenicity (6).

Preliminary OEB and Preliminary OEL

The active chemistry gives an overview regarding structural characteristics and possible implications on physicochemical and biological properties. They also provide possible toxicity and predicted pharmacokinetics and metabolism characteristics.

Pharmacology data are reviewed comparing the degree of activity with related drug products for which an OEL already exists. However, the results from in vivo studies should be considered as more suitable for evaluation.

Both acute and subchronic data are considered. To assess the potential acute effects, both the toxicity and pharmacological activity of the compound are evaluated. The type of pharmacological effect(s) expected, the mechanism of action and the dose required to produce these pharmacological effects are important considerations. The severity of acute (life threatening) effects is assessed. An important aspect of the assessment is a determination of whether emergency medical intervention might be required and how rapid the response must be if an occupational overexposure occurs. Compounds with a high order of acute toxicity and poor or delayed warning properties are of greater concern.

Assigning OEBs for Isolated Intermediates

In addition to the decision points for active ingredient development, chemical and process development have their development timeline, which includes transfers from research to pilot and then to production. During the first development phases, the isolated intermediates that are presumably active and have not yet been investigated are assigned a default OEB.

Factors Considered in Assigning OEBs (OELs and OEGs)

APIs are intended for administration in human patients through oral or parenteral routes. Normally, sterile products are restricted to parenteral, inhalation, and ocular products. Consequently, experimental toxicological data are developed in laboratory animal species using these routes of administration. However, the important routes of exposure for humans during production and manufacturing are inhalation and dermal/mucosal contact to aerosols.

For dusts, particle size is an important consideration. In general, small particles penetrate deeper into the bronchial system, which enhances the opportunity for absorption.

When an OEL (or equivalent) is available, this would drive the OEB. However, when this is not the case, especially in the early development phases, the OEB should be assigned after considering the data available.

Allowable Daily Exposure

The ADE evaluated generally by the formula

$$\text{ADE (mg/day)} = \text{NOAEL (mg/kg/day)} \times \text{BW (kg) UF} \times \text{MF}$$

where UF is the uncertainty factors, MF is the modifying factors, NOAEL is no observable adverse effect level, and BW is body weight

This is the factor of choice in determining safe levels of exposure for patients and people.

Acute Warning Properties (Odor, Irritation, Etc.)

Acute warning properties are of particular importance when a compound has significant potential to harm health. Irritation is a good warning property and is also considered as a toxic effect. When possible, the odor threshold (the concentration at which there is perceptible odor) should be expressed in relation to toxicological properties and NOELs.

Sensitization

To be sensitized requires two stages. In the first induction phase the person is exposed to concentrations that trigger a response, once sensitized re-exposure results in a reaction. Occupational exposure to sensitizers may induce respiratory and/or dermal sensitization. Lack of sensitization after oral and parenteral administration does not necessarily mean that dermal/mucosal or respiratory sensitization will not occur.

For compounds that are sensitizers, it is important to consider the degree and type of sensitization. There is general agreement about the following:

- It is not possible to establish an airborne concentration of a compound that is protective of health for the individual who is already allergic to the material in question.
- Minimizing dermal exposure and lowering the airborne concentration of strong sensitizers reduces the potential of sensitizing employees in the first place.

Carcinogens

Carcinogenic effects detected in animals, which cannot be explained by nongenotoxic properties, play a key role in OEB assignment.

Reproductive/Developmental Effects

Effects on male and female fertility are an integral point of the evaluation and the determination of the OEB and OEL. APIs that can adversely impact any aspect of the human reproductive process (e.g. libido, fertility, conception, spontaneous abortion, fetal development and growth, parturition, and breast feeding) are identified as having reproductive/developmental effects.

Cumulative Effects

Cumulative effects refer to accumulated effects following repeated administration with or without toxicological manifestation. For the extrapolation of animal data to humans the different kinetic/metabolic behavior is of importance, because the clearance of a chemical in animals is, in general, faster.

Likelihood of Chronic Effects

These criteria have significant impact on the assignment of the OEB and determination of the OEL, based on the severity of effects and whether they may have disabling consequences or the potential to cause early death. A very important consideration is whether effects are reversible or irreversible.

Effects Are/Are Not Medically Treatable
A judgment is made whether adverse effects are medically treatable and the ultimate impact on the quality of life of an individual.

Effects Do/Do Not Require Emergency Medical Intervention
Overexposure to some compounds at levels, which could be encountered in the occupational environment, may cause immediate life-threatening effects and may require emergency medical intervention. An example is an extremely potent hypertensive agent that with minor exposure can induce an immediate and significant decrease in blood pressure.

Finalizing Occupational Exposure Levels

When a compound nears regulatory approval, the results of chronic animal and human pharmacokinetic studies are generally available.

They reassess the OEB assignment that was made at earlier stages of development and modify, if necessary, based on new data and experience that have become available. They also apply all relevant data to discuss and derive an OEL. Exceptions, where OELs are not derived, are those compounds for which no safe exposure level can be defined (e.g., genotoxic carcinogens).

Only a qualified person can make the determination that has been briefly described above and is presented here merely to assist other disciplines in understanding the hazards assessment process.

EXPOSURE

In a perfect world all pharmaceutical processes would be closed so that the product boundary and the rest of the world would be completely separate. At the other end of the spectrum is the open process where operators openly handle pharmaceutical product. In aseptic processing, conventional filling and lyophilizing can fall into this category. Exposure is how much compound is released to people and product. Controlling the mechanism that causes emission reduces exposure and therefore risk.

Routes of Exposure

This diagram illustrates how pharmaceutical compounds and intermediates can enter the body. By far the most common evaluation of exposure is done using airborne concentrations expressed as weight/m^3/8 hours, typically in micrograms.

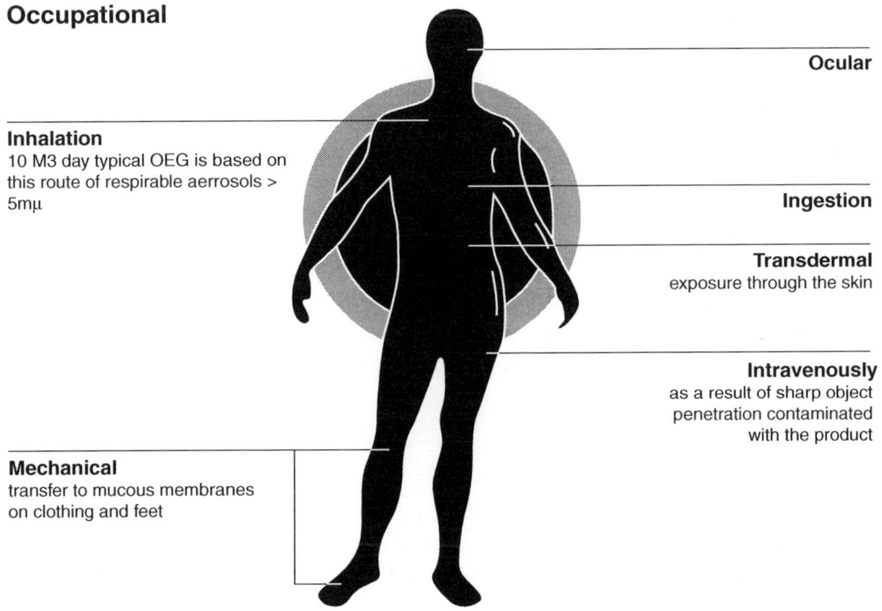

For this reason the standard is based on the operator breathing a standard 10 m^3 of air a day. Inhalation is not the only way of ingestion. There are significant risks from transdermal and mechanical transfer routes. In mechanical transfer, the active is carried on packaging, equipment, clothing to be liberated at another time and place of dosing, not necessarily, the operator, but whoever is unfortunate enough to be present. Note micrograms should be used universally; there are far too many chances to mistake milli- and micrograms and it is easy to get lost in nanograms. It is also important to use "mcg" to describe a microgram for fear that it is thought to be milligrams and because text transfers using "μ" can default to m making micrograms milligrams.

Dermal transfer with certain solvents is very fast and effective so dermal protection is very important. Mechanical transfer is also a major issue. Watch any meeting and take a count of those with their hands on or close to the mouth, it is normally 20% to 30% at any one time. It would be a mistake to think that this behavior never occurs in the presence of exposed pharmaceutical compounds. Hence, gowning is part of the protection of the patient by reduction of contamination and part, people protection by reduction in dermal, ingestible, and mucosal transfers caused by normally involuntary human behavior (just observe what people do with their hands in a completely voluntary way; the hands are placed on the face constantly to rub, scratch, or as a comfort and every time this happens exposure is risked.)

It is no good believing that training will eliminate these behaviors. In one instance continuous video recording was in place and the staff was fully aware of this. To gain a full understanding of the processes and interventions required a day was taken at random and the tape played at high speed then stopped at each intervention and reviewed in real time. There were innumerable infractions of aseptic behavior. Not because of poor training, but because the operators were unaware of what they were doing.

Applying the Performance Requirement to an Actual Process

Actual performance has to be proven for any system, a wide range of variables makes it impossible for a generic or parametric performance to be stated and a case-by-case performance validation and monitoring is therefore required.

Actual performance as opposed to the exposure level (the not to be exceeded limit) is expressed as a time weighted average (TWA). It has to take account of the following challenges to the system.

- Material characteristics
    - Specific gravity
    - Particle size distribution
    - Electrostatic properties
    - Flow characteristic
- Equipment issues
    - Late in the maintenance cycle
    - Equipment wear and damage
    - Distortion of high accuracy components
    - Equipment malfunction
    - Operability
    - Ergonomics
- Iterations
    - How many tasks are performed in a shift
    - What type of task is performed at each iteration
- Operators
    - Operator fatigue
    - Operator technique
    - Operator error
- Utility failure

Because each active liberating event is subject to so many factors the actual liberation at each event will vary.

This graph shows the liberation levels of active material from a containment system over a sequence of repeated events. As can be predicted, the results vary over a range of exposures. The exposure control system must consider the worst-case liberation. It also shows how important constant monitoring and proper evaluation is. Most systems are challenged tested with inappropriate materials with too little iteration under ideal circumstances. This cannot truly reflect real, not to be exceeded, performance.

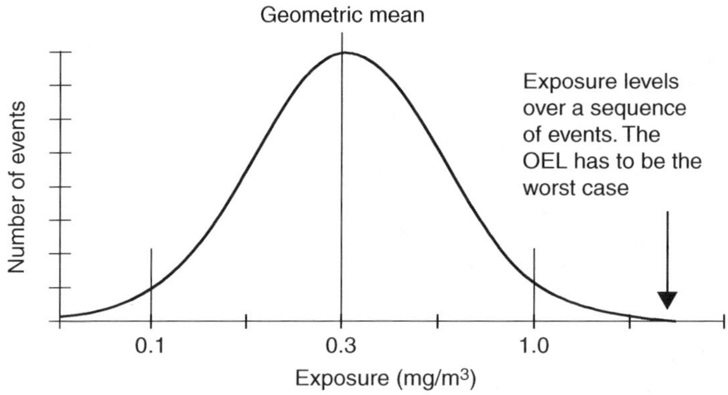

Emissions and therefore possible exposure will vary from iteration to iteration and from operator to operator. The greater the dependence on technique and air entrainment as the mechanism of exposure control, the greater the maximum exposure and the variability (Table 1).

A fully contained system where issues of energy, pressure, and technique have been holistically addressed provides one surprising and one obvious effect. Concentrations inside fully contained processes appear to be significantly lower than the open process concentrations. Although figures up to 32,000 $\mu g/m^3$ over the event duration are seen for open operations, such as scoop and dump, only 6000 $\mu g/m^3$/event (60 + minutes) has been seen on the same open operations inside an isolator and this figure reduces to 1000 $\mu g/m^3$/event in very low airflow glove bags. The reason is simple—control—isolator environments are controlled within very precise parameters; the airflow inside an isolator is simply not intended to support aerosols whereas that is exactly what open processing requires conveying emissions to the nearest boundary filters.

Table 1 Table Showing Factors That Effect Exposure

Wet	Dry size
Large > 100 micron particle	Small < 10 micron
Dense	Light
Closed	Open
No energy / velocity	High energy / velocity
No technique required	Highly technique dependent
Low Δp	High Δp
No transfer	Multiple transfer
Well maintained	Poorly maintained
No explosion risk	High explosion risk
One iteration	Multiple iterations

Pressure

There is another major factor and that is the differential pressure between the contained environment and its surroundings. To protect people a negative pressure is desirable, where protection of the patient is the concern, then the pressure gradient should be reversed, or so goes the current wisdom. Most failures of isolators and transfer valves are directly attributable to over pressurization. This can be as simple as a powder mass descending during blending imposing a piston effect and therefore pressurization. The over pressure can result in significant emission through imperfect seals.

Actual Performance Testing

It is usually difficult to test a system using the active; often the active is too expensive or does not exist in sufficient quantities for repetitive testing, or the test location will not and cannot handle pharmaceutical actives, but surrogate testing has its challenges too. The criteria that have to be considered in developing a testing protocol are the following:

- Surrogate or API handling
  - The test environment has to be checked for the presence of the compound before any test is performed.
  - Personnel handling the target compound can have no part in the operation recovery or testing of the surrogate.
  - The surrogate must have similar specific gravity and size distribution to the active so as to ensure that the dwell time in the air is similar to and similar in concentration to the active.
  - The surrogate must be easily detected in the concentrations encountered and be in the mid-range of detection for the equipment.
- Iterations
  - The worst case number of shift iterations must be taken into account to ensure statistical relevance.
- Operators
  - The operators should as far as possible try to ensure a reasonable level of poor technique performance, which is best done by giving minimal training to the operators before testing.
  - The operators should have minimal training so that real-world conditions are induced. There is little benefit in using highly skilled operators as no account will be taken of suboptimal events which will inevitably occur in use.
- Equipment
  - Should undergo a number of repetitive uses to represent end of maintenance cycle conditions.
  - Where malfunctions can be predicted they should be induced on some of the cycles.
- Cycles
  - The whole test sequence has to be repeated a number of times.
  - A range of operator skill and dexterity models should be applied.
- Air Sampling
  - Both long duration, preferably over 1 hour and short term 15 minutes should be used, the former to give a sound basis for TWA calculations and the latter to identify the emission event, to allow it to be reviewed and improved.
  - The results expressed as weight per cubic meters for the duration. It is also possible to extrapolate this to a TWA so long as the residual exposure for the rest of the day is known and where repetitive events occur, how many events would make up a worst case day?
  - The results should be below the action level set for the active.

In designing the system, it has to be expected that suboptimal conditions can prevail. The *ISPE Good Practice Guide: Assessing the Particulate Containment Performance of Pharmaceutical Equipment* provides a standard methodology for performance testing; as of writing it is being revised to broaden its scope.

Real-Time Monitoring

Though real-time detection of API is possible using ion mobility detection, similar to that used in airport snuffers, it has not been adopted in the pharmaceutical industry due to issues with calibration, sensitivity, and cost.

Ion mobility detectors offer the ability to detect a library of compounds at very low concentrations (1 ng/m^3) using a sampler through which a known volume of air has passed. This is then tested with results in about 1 minute. The same system can be used to detect the presence of the compound in rinse water streams ongoing in about 1 minute. Such real-time monitoring is likely to become more widely used.

Parametric Real-Time Monitoring

By measuring and alarming airflow, pressure, etc. in isolators, fume hoods, etc., many believe that they have an indication of performance. In all the data we have reviewed there is no correlation. In the past, the use of particulate counters has been seen; typically these systems are good for gross containment systems where the liberation of particulates from the process is significantly greater than the background levels of particulate. When dealing with OELs in single-digit micrograms and nanograms the problem is that a critical liberation is insignificant when compared with the background.

	Particle size		ADE (μg)		10
API	1	Volume (μm^3)	OEL (μg/m^3)		1
μm	0.1	$V = 4/3\ \pi r^3$	Particles	Actual(μg/m^3)	Total OEL
0.1	0.05	0.000524	1	0.000523599	1910
0.2	0.10	0.004189	1	0.004188790	239
0.3	0.15	0.014137	1	0.014137167	71
0.5	0.25	0.065450	1	0.065449847	15
1	0.50	0.523599	1	0.523598776	2
5	2.50	65.449847	1	65.449846958	0

Note: Number of particles of varying sizes that could be present for the OELs stated with a density of 1.

The table shows the size and weight of particles at the size shown and the number of particles at each size that could be present in 1 m^3 of air and below the OEL for the compound, in this case 1 μg/m^3/8 hours.

Transfer Systems

Without question the most important containment concern is the way in which the actives are connected to the various items of process equipment and are moved around the plant. The key challenge to any containment system is the make and breaks that occur as transactions between processes and equipment.

Where a containment system can be shown to provide robust performance below the action level, typically 50% of the OEL, consistently then full dermal protective equipment can be dispensed with (a disposable uniform is still suggested to maintain a disciplined approach to handling high-hazard substances). However disposable single-use gloves should always be worn for the duration of critical events such as bag out, RTP transfers, and wiping. Aseptic technique should be used to prevent cross contamination. Using real-time monitoring enables operators to escape in the event of a significant fugitive emission without risk. In an aseptic environment transfer has to protect both product and operator. The key to successful containment is to keep the inner product contaminated layer separate to the outer environmental contact layer. This may seem simple, but is very complex and difficult in reality. This section discusses and reviews the options. The key elements of a transfer system are that it provides robust containment and is easily handled.

Transfer Technique Matrix

Technique	Issues	Comments	Suitability
Open scoop and dump	Powder plumes Mechanical transfer Risk of cross contamination	Not really acceptable at any level	Inappropriate
Wipe down/pass in pass out, no airlock via a door in an isolator	Impossible to prove decontamination High risk of mechanical transfer and air borne concentration	Requires the containment device to be clean	Inappropriate
Pass in pass out via airlock on an isolator	As above, the lock chamber becomes more contaminated Very prone to operator issues	Requires decontamination in the airlock Must have differential pressure, interlocks and a dwell period to have any effect	Inappropriate
Pass in only Air lock with bag out to an isolator	Less risk than above, but the air lock can still be contaminated when opened to the contaminated chamber	Requires decontamination in the airlock Must have differential pressure, interlocks and a dwell period to have any effect	Can be considered for + 1 μg OEL materials Aseptic risk on pass in unless in ISO 5 environment
RTPs Central Research ACE IDC LaCalhene	Indications of seal contamination abound. Must use a seal protector where powder handling is concerned. No direct powder transfer is possible	Dock by rotation and requires an isolator, clear pathway. Sizes 450, 350, 270, 190 and 105 mm nominal clear diameter Variety of manufacturers, but LaCalhene is the leader Very wide range of devices available	Can be considered down to 0.1 μg/event Acknowledged as suitable for aseptic transfer
Split Butterfly Valves Buck Glatt LB Bohle Matcon PSL	Transfer at seals, over pressure leakage, malfunction Beware leakage of wash agents into product Some available for aseptic operation	Some have air sparge some have washing Results vary Buck and Glatt are the main suppliers Restricted pathway	Can be considered Not proven for aseptic transfer
Cut and Crimp Panduit – PharmaConsult US method ILC Dover Inflatable head liners Stott Howorth HECHT	Technique results dependent on how close and how tight the crimp is. HECHT is a different system.	Preformed or layflat tube is used to create bags that are disconnected using twin crimps Can be irradiated on RTP Passive	Can give the best results of all but would have to be sterilized in place for pass out, could not be used for pass in

ASEPTIC PROCESSES AND EXPOSURE RISK

The following table shows the operations typically associated with aseptic processing and indicates the types of exposure risk that exists. Though this varies from compound to compound, the table reflects the consensus view. There is no substitute to gathering and reviewing data, however the overwhelming evidence is that handling the API in dry powder form is unquestionably the biggest risk and once in liquid form the risk diminishes significantly.

Positive Versus Negative Pressure

Negative pressure should be used for all powder manipulations so long as they are not aseptic. If they are aseptic then the isolator should be run at the lowest feasible positive pressure +25 Pa and should be pressure hold tested to the equivalent of approximately 0.5% volume per hour and with a test pressure of +50 Pa. The very low differential operating pressure means that outward leak is much lower than the test.

Surrogate or performance monitoring would verify the external concentrations. Note the isolator has to be robust and mouseholes, etc. cannot be present in positive (or negative) powder-handling isolators.

Aseptic Process Risk Table

Process	Exposure	Comments	Solution
Weighing	Open handling of the active	Highest risk	Isolator, negative pressure
QA Sampling Nonsterile	Open handling of the active Contamination of the packaging by the active	Second highest risk of exposure Operator risk	Isolator and re-package before returning to quarantine or storage
Sterile	Handling of active Contamination of the packaging by the active	Normally only where sterilization by filtration is not possible. Issue is the pass in of the material and surface decontamination	Isolator with integrated vessel for solution or suspension. All steam/autoclave sterilized
Formulation Hygienic/sterile weighing	Handling of active	Can be two-stage hygienic for powder to solution or aseptic powder for suspension then filter chamber for solution sterilization by filtration then aseptic connection to fill vessel	Isolator for formulation
Sterile	Handling of active	Single-stage decontamination on pass in	Isolator requires decontamination plus decontamination of all passed in items. Can be gamma or heat sterilized in RTPs or VPHP decontaminated on pass in or spray and pray or rip and pray
Filling	Aerosols—very low risk if: • Peristaltic • No foaming • Bottom up filling Data showing detectable concentration very rare	Avoid piston pumps where aerosols can be generated. Or locally exhaust/HEPA filter. Avoid foaming and incorrect velocity and needle size that can cause aerosols	The use of an isolator is discretionary. IH monitoring must be undertaken to ensure that aerosols are not being generated. Spills must be wiped up immediately using protocols to prevent Dermal exposure and mechanical transfer
Lyophilization	Sublimination can allow contamination and liberated powder. Depends on how the cake forms, the risk is light fluffy electrostatic finely divided particulates	IH monitoring is essential to determine the exposure where unknown. Veer towards isolator loading and unloading. Other issues are vial burst, stopper hang and thermocouple insertion	Isolator if hazard is unknown (i.e. development/clinical), multipurpose otherwise base on IH data. Incorrect parameters can cause significant Sublimination

(Continued)

Aseptic Process Risk Table (*Continued*)

Process	Exposure	Comments	Solution
Capping	External vial contamination Vial burst due to capping	Not necessary for liquid fills	Should be in an isolator or engineering control for Category 3, 4, and 5 compounds
Vial Decontamination	Mechanical transfer from packaging	Can only be partial	NIOSH issue Carry over of active on crimp
Postcapping handling of lyophilized product	Breakage, needle stick (broken glass) Surface contamination	IH monitoring and swabbing greater than the ADE on a 4″ × 4″ nominal area (10 × OEL) would indicate concern. Inspection Labeling Packaging All issues where vial contamination is an issue Consider blister packing as soon as possible or overwrap	Consider airflow, operator screens and dermal protection. All procedures should require gloves. Consider face masks to avoid hand/face contact.

Abbreviations: RTP, rapid transfer port; VPHP, vapor phase hydrogen peroxide.

RISK

There is in general a very low risk associated with the filling of parenteral medicines due to the inherently low potential for cross-contamination. Among the reasons for this inherently low risk are:

- Formulation vessels may be dedicated to a single product, subject to a validated cleaning method, or rely on disposable materials.
- Risk in the product filling process, which have a small surface area product contact pathway, can be reduced by the use of disposable tubing and fill reservoirs, avoidance of piston pump fill systems, or the use of dedicated equipment.
- Filling needles or nozzles have an extremely small surface area, can be readily cleaned to the ADE, and may also either be dedicated or disposable.
- Where parenteral products require lyophilization in general the risk is easily controlled and modern lyophilizers can be cleaned and sterilized in place where user requirement specifications so dictate.

COST

Containment projects are normally custom-made; there are really no "off the shelf" solutions. It is therefore essential to competitively bid each project. As work ebb and flows manufacturers change their pricing policy. Equally in the aseptic world there are few vendors who truly understand containment issues. Always ask for and take up references, try to use at least four. Try to find others that may have had a less than stellar experience with the vendor and try to understand the real issues that caused concern. Sometimes it is the client and not the vendor.

It is important to fully define what you need. Too often the design is left to the vendor and what you get is often not what you need. Equally be careful of creating requirements without input from containment specialists. Often the client document includes impractical requirements.

Quality

Not all containment providers are created equal; make sure you choose a reputable vendor. Equally, be aware that the more "features" on the equipment, the greater the risk of failures. Keep it simple. Also choose an appropriate quality; there is little point in spending money on cosmetic improvements.

SCHEDULE

When scheduling a project bear the following in mind:

- It takes longer than you think to fully agree what is required.
- You can be certain that people who will have a lot of input when it is too late will not have the time or inclination to provide input at the onset. QA, validation, calibration, operations, technical transfer, and others tend not to make the necessary input at the right time and create variation cost and controversy later. Make sure they get involved early.
- Allow sufficient time for de-bugging as systems are custom, it is almost inevitable that there will be bugs, particularly where interfacing with existing equipment is concerned.
- Make sure that "owners" are allocated who are responsible for every aspect of the equipment.
- Get the stakeholders involved at the onset; make sure all the sterile gurus are on board.
- The finished product requires ownership by the users.
- Always mock up the line in detail.
- The devil is always in the detail.
- Set cut off dates for stakeholder inputs so that they have their say at the beginning, fully buy into the URS and are not allowed to slow down, create change orders, or re-invent the wheel during the implementation phase of the project.
- Start planning qualification and validation on day one. Only qualify and validate what you have to.

TRENDS, FUTURE DEVELOPMENTS, AND THINGS TO CONSIDER

Containment is still an art and not yet a science; however, as more and more actual performance data are gathered and shared, more science can be applied and many myths exploded. The pharmaceutical industry is littered by containment systems that do not meet expectations. The main reason is that containment is thought to be all about boxes with gloves. Actually it is all about the process, transfers, interventions, and function. The smallest detail will make an expensive system fail. To have a successful project requires a team effort with the following:

- The owner understanding when they need professional help.
- The engineers understanding that getting it right is very difficult and is not done by attending a few lectures or relying solely on the vendors.
- The vendors do not have access to a great deal of performance data and then only on some of their projects. Clients tend not to tell vendors of failure.
- The operators, who are rarely trained in containment and who are rarely told why a system is the way it is.
- Get professional help and bring all the parties together to make a team.
- Ensure you have excellent project management.

What are the yardsticks by which a project can be judged? The following are a few bullet points. Successful containment should be the following:

- Protect the patient.
- Provide a safe working environment for the operator and the outside world.
- Provide product protection from the environment and other drug substance.
- Provide redundant protection when systems fail.
- Allow safe escape, local containment, and safer recovery in the event of a cataclysmic failure.
- Provide real-time indication of safe operation.

In addition any project must do the following:

- Do all the tasks required easily, safely, ergonomically, and functionally.
- Provide economy of operation when compared to open operations by
  - reducing clean up time, providing a validatable, repeatable clean
  - reducing product loss, minimized waste disposal costs, and high-value product cost
  - reducing facility costs by robustly containing the process.

17 Points to consider in the design of a filling isolator

Valerie Welter

This chapter focuses on a few of the advanced technologies available for consideration in the design and installation of an isolated filling machine. The points presented are primarily applications associated with small-volume parenteral installations, but the concepts can be broadly applied to any isolated filling installation. As described in previous chapters, design is a very important element in the lifecycle of an advanced processing technology application. If the desire is to get past installation, and into operation with an isolated filler, design is critical. Not so many years ago it was fairly typical to piece together a washer, a tunnel, and a filling machine with a few turntables and some conveyors and assemble a filling line. With today's advanced isolated technologies inclusive of integrated programmable controls and feedback loops this is no longer possible. From the conceptual design, through factory acceptance test (FAT), installation, and validation, every aspect of what is required for the *users* must be defined before the first piece of what will become the integrated filling train is fabricated. It is important to note the word "users" in the previous sentence, this it meant to emphasize that not only operations personnel, but also maintenance, engineering, environmental control, validation, certification, literally anyone who will have a function to perform within the isolator or supporting the isolated environment needs to have a level of involvement in the design. It is important to remember support groups such as materials planning. The planning group needs to fully understand the criticality in defining all product configurations that will be, or are planned to be running on the installation under design. Once a small-vial isolator is in place changing it over to run a 100-mL vial is probably not going to be possible without a significant reinvestment. All it takes is a visit to the mezzanine or that corner of the basement in the facility, to see at least a cage full of equipment where inadequate time in design resulted in a shiny piece ready for the scrap yard shortly after receipt. Isolated filling applications are not simply putting a box over the top of a traditional aseptic filling line and running it as usual. There will be issues that can only be visualized once the design is complete and a fully integrated mock-up is constructed. Only then can it be determined that the mechanics cannot reach the filling pumps or that a nonviable particulate horn is needed where there is a sidewall. So the first technology that is critical in the design of an isolated filler is not a technology at all. It can be foam board or plywood or any structural material set up as a complete and integrated mock-up of the proposed design. This relatively simple process will assure that the investment allocated on technologies supporting the isolated filler will not have to be redesigned, or worse designed out of the application, simply because they will not fit or are not appropriate as determined after installation.

Aseptic filling within isolated environments requires the same general principals as traditional aseptic filling within a clean room. Fill volume checks, headspace analysis, commodity loading, interventions, environmental monitoring, maintenance, and cleaning all will need to be performed within the confines of a rigid structure. As the pharmaceutical industry has moved toward elimination of direct human intervention in filling processes there has been an expansion in the support technologies available and today there are many technologies available designed specifically for installation and use within an isolator.

With the publishing of US Food and Drug Administration's Pharmaceutical GMPs for the Twenty First Century—A Risk-Based Approach (1) and the process analytical technology (PAT) movement that ensued, there is no shortage of equipment and instrumentation out there with every bell and whistle imaginable. It is important to realize that with advanced technologies the investment is often significant in complexity. Keeping the installation as simple as possible will not only save in the short run, but also will allow the possibility of keeping the line running without calling in technical support from across the globe. For companies that are just embarking on a conversion to advanced aseptic technologies involving isolation of filling processes, it is important to document a strategy. This strategy will ensure that all personnel who may be involved with designing, engineering, qualifying, or ultimately using these technologies understand the overall approach and desired state the company has for new installations as well as addressing the continued compliance of legacy installations. It is important to understand and characterize the risks and the benefits of investing in isolated filling. For example putting an isolated filler on the back end of a legacy process may not result in significantly improved compliance of the overall process as compared with a RABS installation that would provide an incremental improvement. The driver for investments must be based on an overall compliance strategy. The strategy document can also provide a bridge for regulatory presentation of legacy installations installed next to advanced technologies and define the company's continuum for improvement.

CONSIDERATIONS FOR COMMODITIES

By purchasing an isolated filler, the firm is also signing up to purchase, install, and validate isolated commodity processing equipment. As discussed earlier, piecing in isolated filling is not the best option available. Minimally there is a need to design a process for introduction of sterile commodities into the isolator. For glass, this is relatively straightforward as long as there is an integrated depyrogenation tunnel. Air pressure dynamics associated with the temperature fluctuations across the tunnel/isolator interface will need to be characterized to assure a proper balance is maintained. If batch processing of glass is provided through an oven, then special consideration will need to be designed into the transfer and unloading of depyrogenated trayed glass into the isolator, and do not forget to provide a mechanism for handling trays and lids as the glass is unloaded. Each transfer into or out of the isolated filling environment is a potential contamination event. Linking these activities to media fill challenge and intervention profiles will provide data supporting that the intervention can be accomplished without negatively affecting the aseptic process. However, just like in traditional aseptic processing, designing out interventions where possible and limiting those interventions that must occur is the desired practice.

Technologies available today for the processing of rubber commodities assure an isolated environment from washing all the way through application to the final container. Traditional commodity processors can be outfitted with rapid transfer ports such as alpha beta ports technologies to facilitate docking of transfer vessels or bags without breaching the sterile barrier. More advanced technologies for one-pot processing of rubber commodities are also available with fully integrated wash–sterilization–depyrogenation cycle control. Containers can be sized to contain all of the commodities needed for a single-processing run, further reducing the risk of multiple isolator dockings. Programmable logic controller (PLC) interfaces provide for added control by assuring that cycles meet required parameters, and track commodities from initial processing through use. PLC interfaces on the isolator-docking station are available that verify that the appropriate commodity within its allowable processing time is being docked to the isolator before allowing docking to be completed.

For commodities that are received sterile ready-to-use, containers will need to be specified specific to the docking technologies designed into the isolator. Where presterilized commodities are required to be used without sterile transfer docking devices, material transfer chambers with self-contained vapor phase hydrogen peroxide (VPHP) decontamination cycles can be designed into the isolator. These transfer chambers are designed such that commodities or other items can be loaded into the chamber and subjected to a decontamination process independent and isolated from the main isolator. Where large volumes of commodities are needed to keep the line running, consideration for downtime due to the batch sterilization process through the material transfer chamber should be determined.

CONSIDERATIONS FOR ROUTINE PROCESS INTERVENTIONS

Today's isolated fillers are typically designed with integrated PLC control. The fully integrated installation provides for continuous control and monitoring of the entire process inclusive of commodity loading, filling, overgassing as appropriate, sampling and testing, stopper placement, and capping. For installations supporting lyophilization, vials with stoppers partially inserted are indexed for loading either in the more traditional tray/ring configuration or via the more advanced auto shelf-loading indexing table. These advanced installations are designed to remove operators from the process as much as possible as robotics has replaced many of the manually intensive processes of traditional aseptic filling and transfer. With the benefits of removing people from the process comes the downside of removing people from the process. Robots and PLCs are not the common human eyes that can see or even predict when vials are indexing incorrectly, or a tip-over in the middle of a shelf. These advanced applications although programmable are not yet intelligent. Engineering design, especially in transfer points is critical or the number and complexity of interventions associated with isolated processes will exceed those within traditional lines.

There have been significant advancements in technologies required to support aseptic isolated filling. Technology integrating a check weighing system eliminates the need for manual volume checks and provides for a feedback loop to the filling pump system. As volumes drift, the feedback control loop adjusts the appropriate pump and filling is only interrupted should an out of specification event be documented. Individual units with out of specification volumes are tracked by the integrated PLC and automatically rejected. All volume readings are collected via the PLC and are constituents of the electronic record associated with the batch run. Integrated feedback control loops such as this allow for the process to be defined under continuous verification and lessen the reliance on process validation and batch testing.

Further advancement in technologies such as nuclear magnetic spectroscopy (NMS) has been applied as an in-line fill volume determination instrument. NMS subjects a filled vial to a magnetic field followed by application of radio waves at a predefined frequency and duration resulting in a determination of fill volume on 100% of vials passed through the field. Integration of the NMS with the filling system provides for closed loop feedback control of fill volume. This type of advanced technology requires significant development and validation efforts in the creation of a library associated with the defined characteristics of each solution to be subjected to the technology. However, once the library is created the process provides for a 100% verification of every vial filled for appropriate volume.

If volume checks must be determined manually then a mousehole and integrated sampling conveyor system should be designed into the isolator. In all cases opening of the isolated environment to collect samples should be avoided and in cases such as these samples are always destructive. The effect of any opening on the overall balance of the isolated environment must be fully characterized. Having penetrations in the isolated environment such as a mousehole can be acceptable; however, consideration and expectations for environmental control and monitoring of the surrounding environment are heightened and typically continuous monitoring for overpressure at these locations is expected.

The science, operation, and maintenance of certain advanced technologies will pose a significant change to the operation. Procedures and the associated training must be specific, detailed, and robust for operating within the isolated environment. One of the biggest myths associated with isolated environments is that aseptic practice and behavior are not as critical. Being lax with aseptic discipline will result in investigations and potentially sterility events. All interventions from a vial tip-over, to the change out of a filling pump must be performed with the same attention to aseptic discipline as would be incurred in a traditional aseptic filling operation. Gloves should not contact anything but sterile tools, not the isolator and not each other.

CONSIDERATIONS FOR ENVIRONMENTAL MONITORING

Determination of an environmental risk profile is a valuable tool not only for initial qualification of an isolated environment but also in the event that an investigation is necessary when in operation. During initial qualification attention should be given to all transfer points and to areas where manipulation or intervention will be required. Air flow patterns in a contained isolated environment should be rigorously mapped and the effect of temperature and pressure gradients associated with routine operations need to be characterized dynamically as well as statically. In certain climates, seasonal variation may need to be characterized as wide fluctuations in temperature and/or humidity may affect the decontamination process. Every required intrusion into the isolated environment is a pathway for contamination and must be either determined not to be a potential concern or routinely monitored. The principal authors and editors of this text Akers and Agalloco have outlined an approach to determination of risk associated with aseptic processing as published in *Pharmaceutical Technology*, in November 2005 (2), which provides for logical scientific determination of risk. By deciding to invest in isolated aseptic technologies overall risk is being mitigated as compared to traditional aseptic filling. However, an isolator will not provide protection against improper technique or bad practices. Each process that will be required to interface with or be performed within the confines of the isolated environment should be reviewed for associated risk.

Once risk has been determined there are many options available for performing monitoring in isolated environments. As the tenant of isolated filling is removal of direct contact by personnel, it has already greatly reduced the sample load. However, a sound program for monitoring the gloves of personnel working in isolated filling environments is suggested. Specifically the gloves in the interior of the isolator where contact with product surfaces is probable should be routinely monitored. This baseline of monitoring data can be used to support investigational activity associated with equipment or environmental events potentially affecting sterility of the isolated environment and provides an ongoing data set demonstrating control.

Continuous nonviable particulate monitoring is an expectation for aseptic filling applications, with our without an isolated environment. As with traditional filling lines, sample collection horns should be located on the basis of risk to open containers/product and be based upon the environmental qualification/mapping already described. Viable monitoring provides for another opportunity in transferring of materials into and out of the sterile environment. Although promising designs have been proposed and the bulk of equipment can be remotely located, viable monitoring still routinely requires media to be transferred into and out of the isolated environment pre- and postsample collection. As already discussed for commodities, a transfer chamber is a mechanism that will lower the overall risk associated with required introduction of materials into the isolator and the transfer of samples out of the isolator. Advanced technologies available for both continuous nonviable and viable monitoring allow for minimal intrusion into the isolated environment with most of the hardware and associated software for sample collection located outside of the filling cabinet. The key to success in monitoring of an isolated environment is planning. As first discussed, the design phase of the isolation project must include monitoring personnel such that a plan is designed into the isolator for staging of monitoring materials, dynamic sampling, and the transfer of materials into and out of the enclosure. Monitoring personnel will need to have access to a range of areas within the enclosure that are not necessarily the same areas where operational personnel will spend the majority of time. Glove placement, accessibility to corners, enclosure floors, and sample placement fixtures need to be considered in the initial design.

CONSIDERATIONS FOR QUALIFICATION AND VALIDATION OF ISOLATED FILLERS

This body of work contains several chapters associated with qualification of advanced aseptic processing installations. Aseptic fillers require the same rigorous design, installation, operational, and performance qualification expected to support traditional aseptic lines, with the addition of sterility assurance as provided within the enclosure. It is recommended that the design qualification be performed once the line is fully integrated such that all design considerations can be covered in one document. Operational tests specific to the isolator include the following:

- Dynamic smoke testing covering all interventions and planned transfers, Note that smoke stick residues are typically not compatible with hydrogen peroxide. Dry ice or liquid hydrogen should be used.
- Glove breach tests and determination of positive pressure allowances
- Operating pressure differentials. Static pressure differentials as well as mapping of opening and closing any isolator access doors/transfer devices.
- Isolator leak testing, inclusive of all seams, penetrations and the determination of a pressure decay rate.

Typically isolated filling equipment is designed with an integrated clean in place/sterilize in place (CIP/SIP) loop allowing for the installed equipment train to be cleaned following a run and sterilized in place prior to the subsequent run. The cleaning validation program must specify the order of operations and take into consideration any cleaning agent as well as process residues that may be carried over. For isolators using a sterilant that is affected by moisture, consideration to a qualified drying time should be documented and qualified.

In an isolated environment particularly if campaign filling is planned, the cleaning program needs to consider the possibility of process residues being visually apparent on the floor of the isolator. The validation program and the routine operating procedures should reflect the process requirements for spills and other potential cleaning events outside of the CIP pathway.

In advanced technology installations, CIP/SIP cycles are automated through feedback control loops so that cycles are dependent on reaching predetermined and validated processing parameters. Real-time data and feedback control afford these types of installations to be defined as PAT and the reliance on traditional process validation and revalidation is significantly less.

The sanitization method chosen for the isolated environment will need to be supported through process validation achieving a 10^3- to 10^6-spore log reduction and total kill of all biological indicators placed in the product zone. It is very important to consider all "potential" product zones and to provide a documented rationale for the spore log reduction and kill required for all areas and surfaces within the isolator. There has been much discussion among industry and regulators concerning the requirements for, and the definitions associated with, sterility requirements within advanced isolator technologies. Without question the process by which equipment and instrumentation is installed and then subjected to a sanitization cycle within an isolator is inherently less risky than the off-line sterilization of equipment and instrumentation followed by transfer and aseptic assembly onto a traditional open Class 5 filling line. The primary consideration and responsibility is with the firm to assure that the sterility assurance program reflects a sound rationale supported by scientific evidence. Documents should clearly define the application of sanitized versus sterilized surfaces.

Considerations specific to isolated environments include taking care to assure that all surfaces intended to be sterile have exposure to the sterilizing medium and that any wrapped previously sterilized materials are not penetrated. For example, change parts that are intended to be staged on the sidewall, need to be in full contact with the sterilizing medium or they may not be sterile. Items that are sterilized off-line and then staged within the isolator, for example tools or media, must be demonstrated to not be affected by penetration of the sterilant.

Advanced technologies for monitoring the VPHP concentration during sanitization cycles are available and provide for real-time data associated with concentration of the sterilant within the isolator. These integrated chromatographic instruments provide for automated feedback control of the VPHP sanitization cycle assuring that the cycle is optimized; this can be significant when compared with historical half cycle approaches. It is important that probe location is defined during initial mapping studies and that the instrument is routinely calibrated.

Isolators are often designed with integrated alarm features. As with all alarms it is critical to consider and define alarms that are actionable versus those alarms that are notifications. The following alarms are typical and should be verified during qualification testing:

- Power/electrical interruption
- Enclosure open door
- High/low temperature
- High/low pressure
- High/low Humidity
- Low sterilant supply and low sterilant flow

As defined earlier during design is when alarms and conditions need to be defined. Advanced equipment can be manufactured with seemingly endless possibilities. Defining what the process requires and validating to those requirements will simplify the qualification effort.

CONSIDERATIONS FOR VALIDATION OF AN ISOLATED ASEPTIC FILLING PROCESS

As is discussed in detail within the qualification and validation chapters of this book, considerations for a detailed and defined validation plan are critical for the successful validation of any process, inclusive of an isolated filling process. Worst-case parameters should be determined cautiously to avoid reaching failure points and considerations for each aspect of the advanced technology supporting the installation should be used in support of the overall process. The validation plan is the document to spell out the integrated approach to processing based on risk and the ongoing ability to demonstrate a state of control.

Isolated filling equipment is critical processing equipment and a rationale and schedule for periodic review and resulting requalification requirements should be documented. Considerations of the level of control provided for by the isolation technology allow for schedules beyond the historical 6-month schedule. Firms must be willing to challenge historical requirements based on the real-time process control that advanced technologies can provide or there is a significantly diminished return on the investment.

CONSIDERATIONS PRIOR TO INVESTING IN A FILLING ISOLATOR

Advanced technologies inclusive of isolated filling technologies need to be designed and installed with a common understanding across the organization of what they provide and what they will not provide. The following are discussion points to consider within the organization prior to determining the investment path.

- Design is absolutely critical—Isolators and other advanced technologies are expensive and very difficult to reverse engineer.
- Changeover within isolated environments should be minimized; changeovers add risk and are often difficult.
- Invest in turn-key engineering—Do not retrofit.
- Working in an isolator is a learned skill—Training is critical.
- Maintain a rigorous preventive maintenance schedule, gloves and sleeves tear.
- VPHP sterilizes everything it directly comes in contact, as long as contact time, temperature, humidity are controlled.
- The surrounding environment is your first protective barrier—Control it.
- Media fills will fail without aseptic discipline.

THE STATE OF ADVANCEMENT IN ISOLATED FILLING

At trade shows in the last couple of years we have seen the future of advanced aseptic processing:

- Plastics containers with integrated closure systems eliminating the need for both rubber closures and glass vials.
- Container closure systems that are sterilized, introduced into an isolator, and then filled through a piercing needle.
- The concepts of blow-fill-seal introduced in ways that eliminate commodity preparation and transfer risks, in the space of a tabletop incubator.
- Isolated commodity preparation integrated with isolated filling further integrated with isolated transfer to lyophilizers.
- Robotics replacing human intervention and integrated feedback control loops providing real-time process intervention.

Although technologically on the forefront of engineering, each of these advancements comes at a significant price. The balance between what is possible and what is required has never been more critical. This chapter has provided some points to consider or at a minimum some challenges to avoid, for the design, installation, and use of advanced isolated filling environments. Determining the appropriate combination of technologies that will provide the desired state of control, that is defining the "user-s" requirements, will go a long way toward installing an advanced isolated filler that can actually be used.

REFERENCES

1. FDA. Pharmaceutical CGMPs for the Twenty-First Century—A Risk-Based Approach. Rockville, MD: FDA, 2004.
2. Akers J, Agalloco J. Risk analysis for aseptic processing: The Akers–Agalloco method. Pharm Technol 2005; 29(11):74–88.

18 Sterility test isolators—a user's perspective

Robert J. Keller

ISOLATORS VERSUS TRADITIONAL CLEAN ROOMS

With the high cost of most new parenterals and the restrictions by the US Food and Drug Administration on sterility retests, many companies are choosing isolators over conventional clean rooms for sterility testing because of the greater environmental control. Unlike a conventional clean room, in an isolator, highly toxic surface sterilants, that is, vapor phase hydrogen peroxide (VPHP) or chlorine dioxide, can be used easily and effectively to control the microbial levels.

Moreover, once an isolator is disinfected, the highest source of contamination, the test personnel, no longer has direct contact with the test environment. With a conventional clean room, no matter how well disinfected, the sterility test environment is still at risk of contamination by the test personnel.

There are many considerations to keep in mind when planning to use isolator technology for sterility testing. The first consideration is the cost of isolators versus a conventional clean room. The actual cost of a particular sterility test clean room or isolator will vary depending on a number of factors. The following comparisons are just a guideline. A simple sterility test isolator set up using a two or three glove isolator (Fig. 1) and a VPHP generator will cost approximately half that of a conventional clean room. A larger isolator system that includes a two half suit workstation isolator (Fig. 2), half suit autoclave interface, double-door autoclave, transfer isolator, and VPHP generator can initially cost twice as much as a conventional clean room. Thus, the initial cost of the sterility test isolator system can vary from half to twice the cost of a conventional sterility test clean room.

In addition to the potential savings, isolators have the following advantages over the conventional clean room. First, isolators can easily be relocated. As a company grows, it may be necessary to move the sterility testing laboratory to another floor or another building. With a conventional clean room, this would mean constructing a completely new facility. In marked contrast, relocation of an isolator requires a reduced requalification of the isolator. If the isolators were validated as a portable piece of equipment and are reinstalled in a room under the same temperature and humidity conditions, no revalidation may be required.

Second, with isolators the test environment can easily be increased in capacity by adding new isolators. Increasing the space in an existing clean room requires demolition, construction, and revalidation. During the expansion of a clean room, all sterility testing must be stopped. Unlike a clean room, sterility testing can continue in the validated isolator whereas the new isolator is validated. Once the new isolator is validated, it can be docked to the existing isolator using the alpha and beta flanges.

Third and most important, the number of false positives is greatly reduced in a sterility test isolator over a conventional clean room. In a conventional clean room using laminar flow hoods most companies have sterility failure rates that are trended. A failure rate of "not to exceed 2%" (1) is considered acceptable in a conventional clean room. In a sterility test isolator, the false-positive failure rate approaches zero. The cost of sterility test failures to a company can easily justify purchasing sterility test isolators over a conventional clean room. Most users see a significant decrease in false positives. However, some companies do report having occasional false-positive tests in isolators. Therefore, it is important to remember that although isolators provide a better testing environment than clean rooms, they are not a substitute for proper aseptic technique. For all the above-mentioned reasons, isolators are becoming the standard for sterility testing. For a company just starting sterility testing, it is wise to start with isolators and save the cost of converting from a clean room.

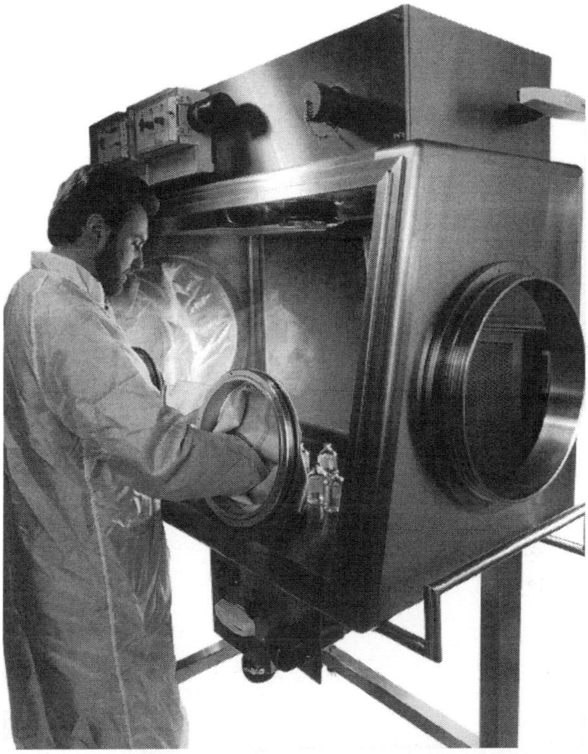

Figure 1 Rigid-walled two glove isolator. *Source*: From La Calhene, Rush City, MN.

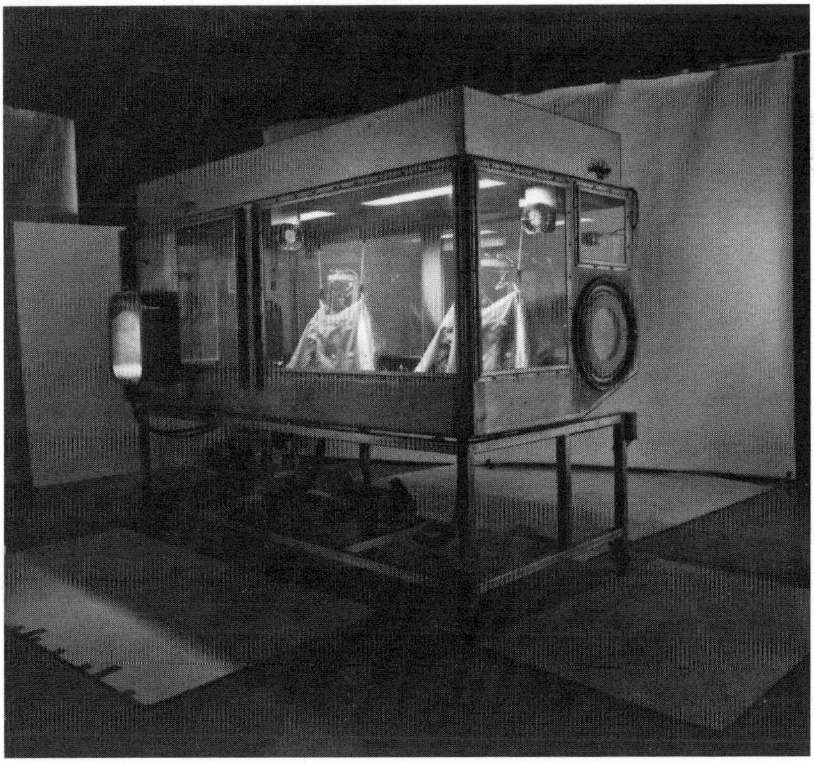

Figure 2 Rigid-walled two half suit isolator. *Source*: From La Calhene, Rush City, MN.

ISOLATOR ROOM REQUIREMENTS

Ventilation

The ventilation of the room that contains the isolators should have a minimum of 10 air exchanges per hour. A high number of air exchanges, usually 18 to 20 air exchanges per hour are recommended to help remove any residual sterilant that may enter the work environment through diffusion or a breach in the isolator during a decontamination cycle. The average laboratory air handling system is usually designed with 18 to 20 air exchanges per hour. (D. Eddington, Metal and Plastic, personal communication, 2009).

Because the isolators are a barrier to the room environment and are operated under positive pressure, the sterility test isolator room pressure in relation to the adjacent rooms and hallways is irrelevant.

From a safety perspective it makes sense to design the sterility test room with negative pressure to adjacent rooms. If a breach in the isolator were to occur during a decontamination cycle, having the sterility test isolator room negative to the adjacent rooms would prevent the sterilant from entering other areas of the building.

Moreover, sterilants like VPHP cannot be seen or easily smelled. It is detected as an irritation to the eyes, skin and mucous membranes (2). Chlorine dioxide, another type of sterilant, is visible but more irritating to eyes, skin, and mucous membranes (see "Chloride dioxide decontamination/sterilization," Chapter 28). Ammonia hydroxide used in leak testing isolators is also very irritating to the eyes and mucous membranes (3). Because exposure to these chemicals can cause adverse health consequences, operation of the isolators in a negatively pressured room with high air exchanges is ideal.

The VPHP decontamination systems have many standard safety features to help prevent injecting sterilant into a breached isolator. Although these features significantly reduce the chances of a breach, a breach can still occur. The two most common types of breech are either from an undetected hole in a glove, canopy, hose, etc., or an improperly assembled isolator. Isolators must be carefully inspected prior to each run from damage to components. Most isolators for sterility testing have motors that compensate for small leaks. This will allow the isolator to remain operational with a leak large enough to allow the VPHP to reach irritation levels in the room. Also, fittings that are not properly closed, for example, a pinched or missing gasket, can also allow high levels of VPHP to leak out of the isolator during a decontamination cycle. In both cases, the operator merely needs to leave the room and allow the room to aerate. An extra exhaust blower can be added to the room that can be switched on after a breech to remove the VPHP more quickly. Wall-mounted sensors (Fig. 3) are available to detect low levels of VPHP (4). A hand-held pump and detector tubes sensitive to hydrogen peroxide (Fig. 4) can also be used to detect the levels of the VPHP from 0.1 to 3 ppm (5).

Some companies have chosen to make their sterility test laboratories positive to the adjacent rooms. They argue that a sterility test isolator room that is positive to the adjacent rooms may give an added safety assurance to the sterility test isolator environment. This goes against the principles of the isolators as a barrier environment. If the isolators are maintained under positive pressure, the external environment should not matter. Some companies have set up their sterility test isolators in rooms that are negative to the adjacent rooms or hallways. Even with a sterility test suite in a negatively pressured, there is no impact to the sterility testing in a properly maintained isolator.

To provide extra safety, an anteroom can be added between the isolator sterility test and the adjoining room. The anteroom would be negative to the adjacent laboratory and the sterility testing room. In the event of a sterilant leak, the vapor would only enter the anteroom and not the adjacent laboratory. If a company is converting a former sterility test suite to use with isolators, an anteroom is already available and would only require air balancing to make it negative to the sterility test laboratory and the adjacent laboratory. Adding a negatively pressured anteroom would be expensive and probably excessive based on industry experience with sterility test isolators.

Whether the isolators are placed in a positive or negative pressure environment, it is important to include in the isolator standard operating procedures what steps should be taken if a breach were to occur.

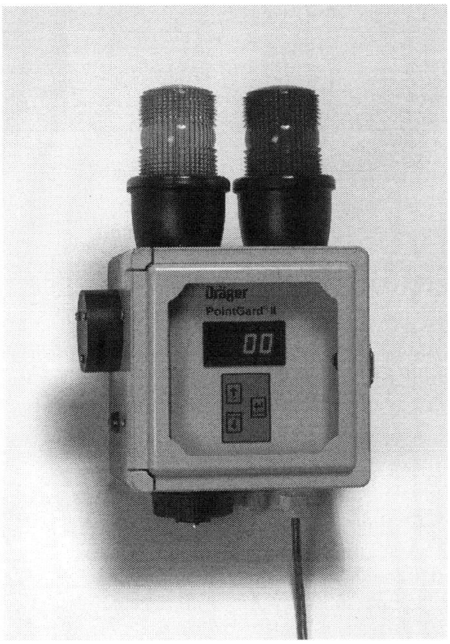

Figure 3 Wall-mounted hydrogen peroxide sensor. *Source*: Dräger Sicherheitstechnik GmbH, Lübeck, Germany.

The ventilation system on the exterior of the building should also include ducting directly to the isolators and VPHP generator to allow for 100% external aeration. The sterilant exhaust should not be ducted into a facility air handling system the recirculates within the building. This could introduce the sterilant exhaust to other areas of the building.

Electrical

Electrical connections must allow for the isolators and VPHP generator to be moved to make decontamination connections, perform leak testing, etc., and still remain running. Electrical connections can be made from under the isolators but generally laboratories are constructed with solid concrete slab floors that make floor outlets impractical. Also, when the isolators or VPHP generator is moved, a plug in a floor outlet can become a trip hazard.

Electrical connections from the ceiling allow the greatest mobility of the isolators and VPHP generator. The equipment can be moved around the room without the electrical cords being a trip hazard. If electrical connections are made from the ceiling, twist-locking plugs with stress reduction electrical cords are recommended. Excess electrical cord can be suspended from hooks installed in the ceiling to prevent trip hazards. Electrical cords can also be installed on spring loaded take up reels—such as the air hoses at gas stations—these allow the electrical

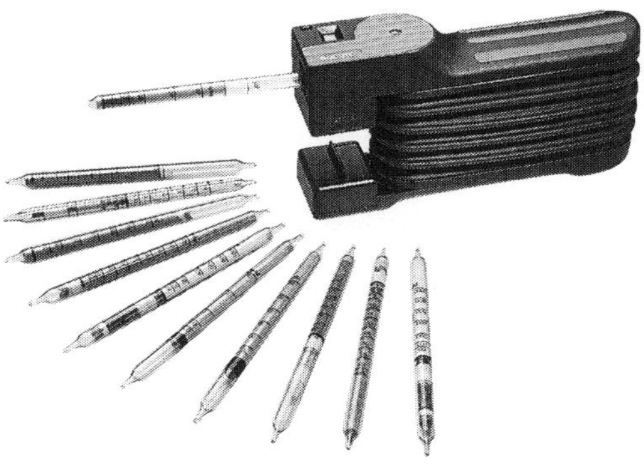

Figure 4 Accuro Dräger hand-held pump. *Source*: Dräger Sicherheitstechnik GmbH, Lübeck, Germany.

cord length to be adjusted as needed. Wall plugs can also be used with the ceiling hooks to keep the electrical cords off the floor when moving equipment.

The isolators and VPHP generator will each need dedicated 20 A circuits, preferably with backup power. An autoclave, if used, will generally need to have dedicated 120 and 220 or 440 V service.

Humidity and Temperature Control

The temperature and humidity of the sterility test isolator room are very important. In general, the room temperature should not vary by more that $\pm 5°C$. It is better to validate the decontamination cycles at the lower end of the room temperature range to prevent condensation under routine use. A room humidity between 40% and 60% works well with VPHP. If the room humidity varies a lot, the dehumidification step in the VPHP cycle may not be able to bring the isolator down to the same level of humidity for each cycle. This can affect the concentration level in the isolator. During the decontamination cycle, the temperature and humidity must be similar to those during validation. If the humidity of the room is too high or the temperature of the room is too low, the sterilant may condense during the decontamination cycle. If the VPHP condenses, the decontamination cycle may be less as effective and the condensing peroxide can be damaging to equipment. The sterility isolator test room should have good temperature control and the isolators should not be installed directly under the inlets or outlet ducts for the room ventilation. The humidity should also be monitored and if the humidity varies enough to effect the decontamination cycle, that is, condensation is observed during a routine decontamination cycle, the room humidity will need to be controlled. The room should have independent temperature control with the thermostat located where it will be unaffected by any process equipment.

Restricted Assess

The proper operation of sterility test isolators is dependent on the integrity of the isolators. Because untrained personnel can compromise the isolators' sterility, it is recommended that the isolators be placed in a room with restricted access. Only trained personnel should be allowed into the sterility test isolator room. Access can be restricted by the use of card key locks. If the cost of a card key reader is too expensive, combination door locks or a simple pad lock may be used. If a pad lock is used, it is important to train personnel to secure the lock in the latch when the room is in use to prevent being locked in.

A system must be developed to ensure that decontaminated isolators are not opened and nondecontaminated isolators are not used for testing. An easy solution is to tag the isolators when they are decontaminated and remove the label when they are opened. Another alternative is to document in the isolator equipment logbooks every time the isolator is decontaminated or opened. The advantage of using the equipment logbooks is that they are already required for each piece of equipment to document use, preventative maintenance, calibration, etc. Adding the decontamination and opening information to the equipment log will keep all the equipment information in one location. The equipment logbooks are considered as permanent records.

When choosing a location for the sterility test isolators, it is best if the room is free of personnel when the decontamination cycles are being run. The sterilant can diffuse through the gloves, half suits, and flexible isolator walls. If the room access cannot be restricted during decontamination cycles, a sensor should be installed in the room to monitor the sterilant levels during decontamination. The time weighed average (TWA) exposure for VPHP is 1 ppm for 8 hours (2).

If the isolators are installed in a laboratory where other testing is performed, it is important to remember that the isolator noise levels can be 70 to 75 dB. Although this may not be loud for a manufacturing environment, it will seem very loud in a laboratory environment. Hearing and talking in a room with several isolators in operation can be difficult.

The entry doors to the room where VPHP is used should be clearly posted with a sign to warn those that enter when VPHP is in use. The warning sign should also contain the names, phone number, and pager numbers of contact personnel.

CHOOSING A STERILITY TEST ISOLATOR

Flexible versus Rigid

When choosing a sterility test isolator the first decision that must be made is whether to purchase flexible- (Fig. 5) or rigid-walled isolators. Flexible-walled isolators have the following advantages.

First, the initial cost of flexible-walled isolators is about 75% of rigid-walled isolators. If the budget for the sterility isolator project is limited, flexible-walled isolators can keep the initial cost of the equipment down.

Second, flexible-walled isolators are much lighter and easier to move than rigid-walled isolators are. This is important to consider if the isolators will have to be moved frequently.

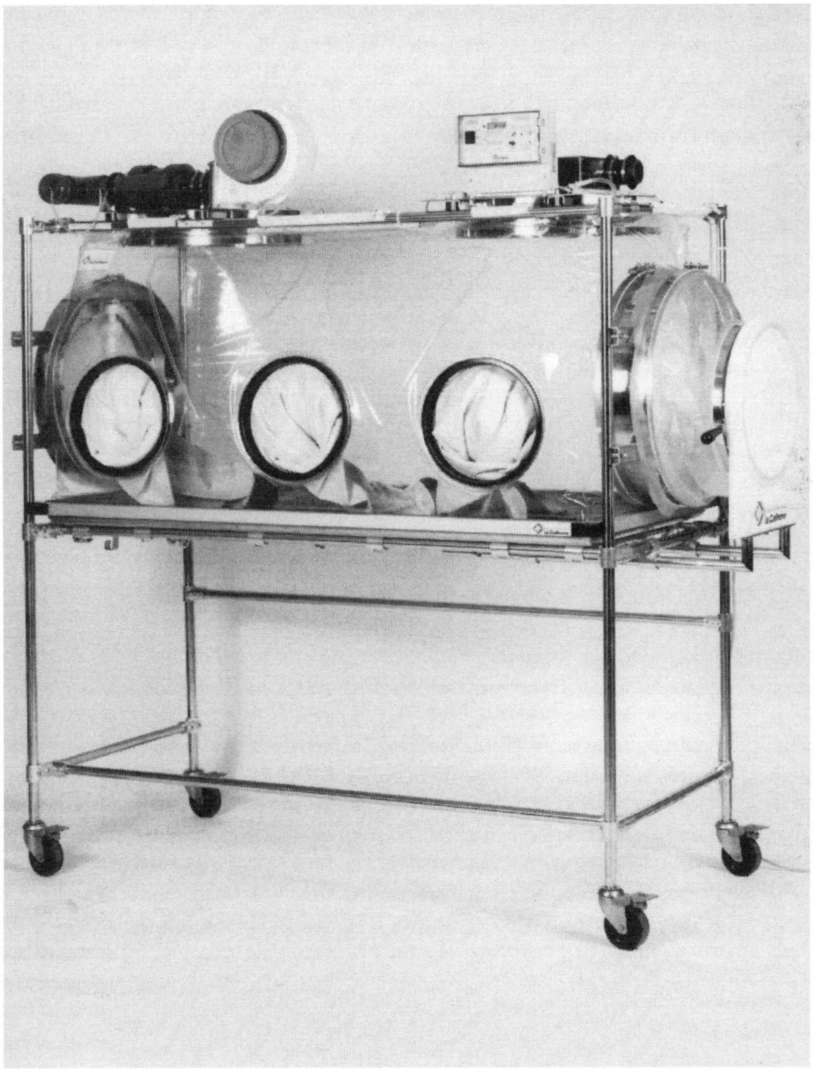

Figure 5 Flexible-walled two glove isolator. *Source*: From La Calhene, Rush City, MN.

A flexible-walled transfer isolator weighs about 40% less than a comparable rigid-walled isolator.

Because of the added weight, rigid-walled isolators can require two or more people to move.

Third, the flexible-walled isolators have the advantage of being easily assembled on site. Rigid-walled isolators are usually shipped fully assembled. The size of the isolators can make them difficult to manipulate down existing hallways and through standard doorways. With rigid-walled isolators it is not uncommon to have to widen doorways and knockout walls to bring them into an existing laboratory. Using flexible-walled isolators in an existing facility can save considerable construction costs.

Although the flexible-walled isolator may have the above-mentioned advantages, the trend in the industry is to use rigid-walled isolators for the following reasons:

First, the rigid-walled isolator is more durable. The rigid-walled isolator is made of stainless steel and glass or Lexan™ windows whereas the flexible-walled isolator is made of a PVC canopy on stainless steel frame. It is much harder for an operator to damage a rigid-walled isolator than a flexible-walled isolator. Sharp tools and supplies if mishandled can easily puncture the PVC canopy of flexible-walled isolators.

Second, the rigid-walled isolator has fewer areas that can leak. Only the window seals, gloves, half suits, transfer ports, and fittings need to be tested. On the flexible-walled isolator, the entire canopy needs to be tested in addition to the parts mentioned on the rigid-walled isolator. This makes leak testing of the rigid-walled isolators much faster than the flexible-walled isolators. Depending on the frequency of leak testing, this can be a significant savings in time.

Third, PVC will degrade overtime from exposure to VPHP. The lifespan of a PVC canopy will vary depending on the number of times it is exposed to VPHP, the manufacturer claims an average life span of 5 years. With proper care, the canopies of flexible-walled transfer isolators that are decontaminated a few times a week have been able to last 7 to 10 years. Because the canopy of the flexible-walled isolator will periodically need to be replaced, the cost of the flexible-walled isolator will eventually exceed the cost of the rigid-walled isolator. The other parts of the rigid and flexible isolators will need to be changed on the same frequency.

Fourth, there are many more manufacturers of rigid-walled isolators than there are for flexible-walled isolators. The competition allows the end user to pick the manufacturer that offers the best equipment for their needs at the most reasonable price.

Once the decision of flexible- or rigid-walled isolator has been made, check with the manufacturer's on the lead-time. Most isolators are not fabricated until they are ordered and depending on the number of orders that a manufacturer has received the lead-time can be 12 to 14 weeks or more.

Attached or Remote Autoclave

If the sterility test requires the use of materials that can only be sterilized in an autoclave, then either an attached double door or remote autoclave must be used. An attached double door autoclave is an autoclave that is connected to an isolator and allows materials to be steam sterilized in the autoclave and brought directly into the isolator. Remote autoclaves are not connected to an isolator and the sterilized materials must be brought into the isolator by alternate methods. The attached double door autoclave has five major advantages.

First, media sterilized in an attached autoclave can be brought directly into the sterility test isolator without the need for container closure studies against VPHP.

Second, an attached autoclave only requires that the material be sterilized once and then it can be brought directly into the isolator. A remote isolator can require up to two steps—the contents are steam sterilized in containers and then the surfaces of the containers are decontaminated with VPHP in the isolator.

Third, an attached autoclave gives you the flexibility to bring in any size container into the isolator. The door sizes of most isolators are limited and with shelving installed movement of large tubes and bottles can be difficult in smaller isolators.

Fourth, the attached autoclave allows items to be steam sterilized and brought into the isolator on the same day. If a remote autoclave were used, the materials require additional handling that can add as much as another day of preparation for a sterility test.

Fifth, large volumes of waste can be brought out through the autoclave. For products that contain heat-sensitive potent compounds, the waste can be denatured by passing it into the autoclave and running a steam decontamination cycle before removing it.

If a remote autoclave is the only option for your application the following are examples of how to bring materials into the isolator.

Materials can be autoclaved in a rapid transfer port (RTP). The RTP container is then docked to the test isolator's alpha port and the contents brought into the test environment. The RTP containers can be expensive depending on the size and number needed to bring in the autoclaved materials.

Materials sensitive to VPHP can be autoclaved in a remote autoclave in dual peel pouches. After autoclaving, each side of the pouch is then covered with foil tape. The foil tape is a heavy gauge aluminum strip with adhesive on one side. The foil tape covered pouch can then be surface decontaminated in the isolator using VPHP. This technique is useful when only small amounts of autoclaved materials need to be brought into the sterility test isolator; however, the taping process is very time consuming. Also, it is important to remember that the surfaces between the tape and the pouch are not sterile and care must be used when opening the pouches to prevent exposing these surfaces. Care also must be used when handling foil-taped packages as the edges of the tape can be very sharp and can cut through isolator gloves.

Gloves Versus Half Suits

The choice between gloves and half suits is a strong area of debate. Many operators who have not used isolators before are afraid of the half suits and prefer to work with gloves. Operators need to try the half suits and gloves while performing manipulations that are unique to their sterile products. The range of motion in glove ports is greatly restricted in comparison to the range of motion in half suits. The depth of a single sided isolator, an isolator with glove ports on one side, must generally be no deeper than the length of the operator's arms to allow full access to the interior of the isolator. A half suit isolator can generally be made a few feet deeper and a foot taller than a glove port isolator because the operator's torso is actually inside the isolator.

Half suits are designed to fit a large number of sizes and shapes of personnel. This means that the half suits for most people are on the large side. Getting in and out of the suits takes practice. To help increase the range of motion while in the half suit, electric lifts can be purchased from the isolator manufacturers to bring the operator's waist up to the base of the half suit. Shorter operators can also stand on adjustable aerobic benches to bring their waist up to the base of the half suits. The aerobic benches or lifts raise the operators up high enough to bend freely at the waist in the isolator.

In a half suit, the operator can sit or assume a natural standing position, which is important for long testing periods. In a glove isolator, the operator's hands are unnaturally extended in front of the body. Over extensive testing periods, this can cause muscle strain in the shoulders, neck, and back. It is important when using glove isolators that the operators take frequent breaks to prevent muscle strain. If a lot of hand manipulations are required, as in direct sterility testing, half suits are often a better choice.

Operator comfort is greater in the half suit. The half suits are supplied with HEPA-filtered air to keep the operator cool. Some models even are equipped with air-conditioned air into the half suits. The glove ports do not have air circulating through them and if the operator is performing multiple tests their arms can become very sweaty. When working in half suits or glove ports it is a good idea to wear long sleeves to prevent the operator's arms from sticking to the plastic sleeves. Gloves or glove liners should also be worn in the half suits and glove ports to facilitate the removal of the operator's hands. Also without gloves or liners the operator would shed large numbers of microorganisms directly into the isolator gloves. Because the isolator's gloves are the most easily breeched portion of the isolator and have the closest contact with the product being tested, it makes sense to take any and all precautions to prevent a high bioburden in the gloves. Although not required, wearing sterile gloves inside the isolator gloves help keep the bioburden in the gloves even lower.

Gloves

Whether choosing half suits or glove port isolators, both types of isolators require the use of gloves. Hypalon-coated gloves have a longer use life than neoprene gloves. The neoprene gloves can react with the VPHP and deteriorate at different rates. Neoprene gloves can deteriorate after only one exposure to the VPHP and tear when used. The hypalon-coated gloves resist degradation by VPHP better than the neoprene gloves. The hypalon-coated gloves, however, are thicker than the neoprene gloves causing the operator to have less dexterity. All types and sizes of gloves should be evaluated by the end users before the isolator is purchased, as more than one operator will be using the isolators.

The gloves that best suit the most operators and the test application should be installed on the isolator. Changing gloves during a sterility test or between decontamination cycles is not recommended. Aseptically changing gloves on an isolator is very difficult and it is almost impossible to determine if a breech occurred during the glove change. To ensure proper isolator integrity, leak testing should be performed after every glove change and a decontamination cycle run.

Determining Isolator Size and Quantity

If a company is installing sterility testing isolators into existing laboratory space, the space is usually very limited. The size of the isolators, ancillary equipment, and supplies require a significant amount of space. Careful consideration should be taken to maximize the workspace in the sterility test isolator and still allow easy access around the equipment.

After determining whether to use glove or half suit isolators, one can then determine the size of the isolator needed to perform sterility testing. The isolator dimensions can be customized to specific needs. For sterility testing using a glove transfer isolator or a half suit isolator, the work surface in front of the operator should be at least 3 feet deep. The back 12 inches of the isolator are usually occupied by shelving to hold all the supplies needed for testing. This will leave a work surface of approximately 24 inches deep. An effective work area must be at least 12 to 24 inches deep depending on the manipulations performed.

When determining the width of the work surface needed to perform sterility testing, remember to consider the location of the shelving and supplies. Because each testing application is different, the operator should collect all the supplies needed to perform a test and lay them out on a surface to simulate the isolator work surface and shelving. This will allow the operator to determine the amount of space needed and the best material flow. This is very important when only one isolator is being used for testing. Most isolator manufacturers will provide a mock up isolator, a plywood shell, to confirm dimensions and material placement. However, it is still helpful to do some estimation prior to the generation of the mock up.

The frequency samples are received is also important to consider, as isolators require several hours to aerate. This usually allows for only one sterility session per shift. Additional isolators may be needed if the frequency of testing is more than once per shift. Some companies turn isolators around faster by running sterility tests with VPHP well above 1 ppm. When performing sterility testing in isolators with high levels of VPHP, it is extremely important to perform the bacteriostasis and fungistasis (B/F) with samples under the same conditions. Testing at high VPHP levels can allow peroxide into open containers and inhibit the sterility test. This is of particular concern for direct sterility testing. Membrane filtration testing with a closed system such as the Steritest limits the contact of test materials to VPHP.

Maximizing the Work Surface

The work surface can easily be increased by the addition of another isolator for supply storage. However, an additional isolator may not be cost effective and other cheaper options are available. An aseptic bagging device (Fig. 6), available from la Calhene, attaches by a beta flange to the alpha flange on the isolator and allows materials to be removed and bagged out from the isolator without breaching containment. RTP canisters can be used to bring in or remove material from

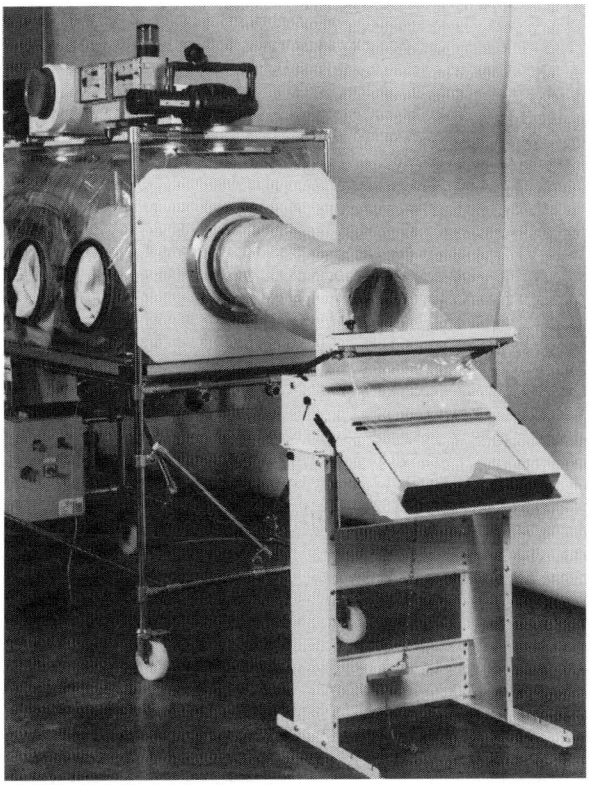

Figure 6 Beta-tubing system for sterile bagging of materials out of an isolator. *Source*: From La Calhene, Rush City, MN.

the isolator during testing. Keep extra empty wire baskets in the isolator to store waste generated during testing. The wire baskets can be stacked to keep waste off of the work surface.

Shelving and Containers

To surface decontaminate supplies in an isolator it is important to minimize surface contact points. Wire shelving, wire baskets, wire test tube racks, and hooks are often used to suspend test materials. Wire baskets and wire test tube racks are available through most scientific supply catalogues.

Because the shelving must be compatible with VPHP, the preferred shelving material is stainless steel. Most isolator manufacturers upon request will provide the shelving with the isolator.

The shelving can be supported in a variety of ways. The shelving can be mounted to brackets on the isolator back wall; this is best done at the isolator manufacturer. Mounting the shelves to the back isolator wall eliminates the need for front legs. Wall mounted shelving can also be cantilevered to lift out of the way when not in use. The only drawback to this type of shelving is that it cannot support as much weigh as compared to shelving with legs. Media bottles and test supplies can be very heavy and their weight must be considered when choosing shelving.

If shelving with support legs is used, sealed support legs are better than support legs with slits in the leg to hold shelving brackets. The slit legs have small openings exposing the interior of the legs to the isolator environment. These openings are too small to allow VPHP to penetrate but could be a source of bacterial contamination. The chance of contamination arising from these openings is very small but it is better to avoid the potential problem, if possible. Once the ideal shelving location and shelf height are determined they should not be changed. A different shelving configuration will require additional VPHP cycle validation.

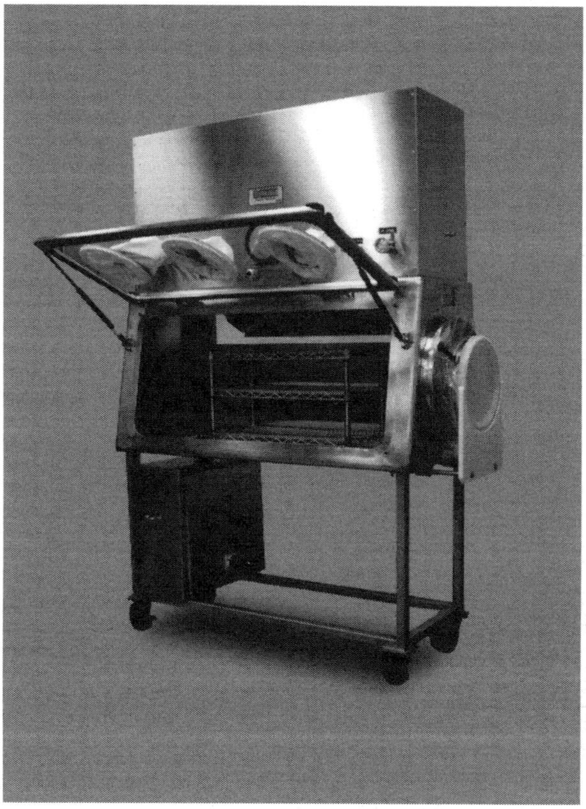

Figure 7 Isolator with flip-up glass front. *Source*: From Carlise Walker, New Lisbon, WI.

Flip-Up Glass

To make the set up and clean up easier, isolators can be constructed with front glass panels that flip up (Fig. 7). These panels allow samples and equipment to be easily placed inside the isolator; instead of handling them using the gloveports. Samples in baskets can easily be knocked over when placed in an isolator. A-flip up front glass allows easy access to stand the sample containers upright again. The only disadvantage of flip-up glass panels is that they are more prone to leaking than fixed glass panels.

Direct Versus Membrane Filtration

Direct sterility testing requires more isolator space than membrane filtration because of the additional media requirements. A direct sterility test will use 20 to 40 containers of media per test whereas the membrane filtration test requires only five containers: two containers of test media and three rinse containers. When performing direct sterility tests, it is important to have a large isolator to store the additional media.

Membrane filtration can be done a number of ways. If only membrane filtration sterility testing is going to be performed in a sterility test isolator, one should consider the Steritest Integral 316II and III pumps from Millipore (Fig. 8). The unit is specifically designed to be used in an isolator. The unit is stainless steel and mounts to the work surface of the isolator. Because the unit requires that a hole be drilled in the work surface of the isolator, it should be installed at the isolator manufacturer. The motor and electronics of this unit are outside of the isolator. The sterilant will not contact them. The exterior motor allows for the motor to be replaced without re-decontamination of the isolator. This can be very important when large numbers of sterility tests are performed and testing cannot be delayed for isolator re-decontamination.

If the work surface space is limited and both membrane filtration and direct sterility testing are performed, a better choice would be a filtration manifold or a portable Steritest unit.

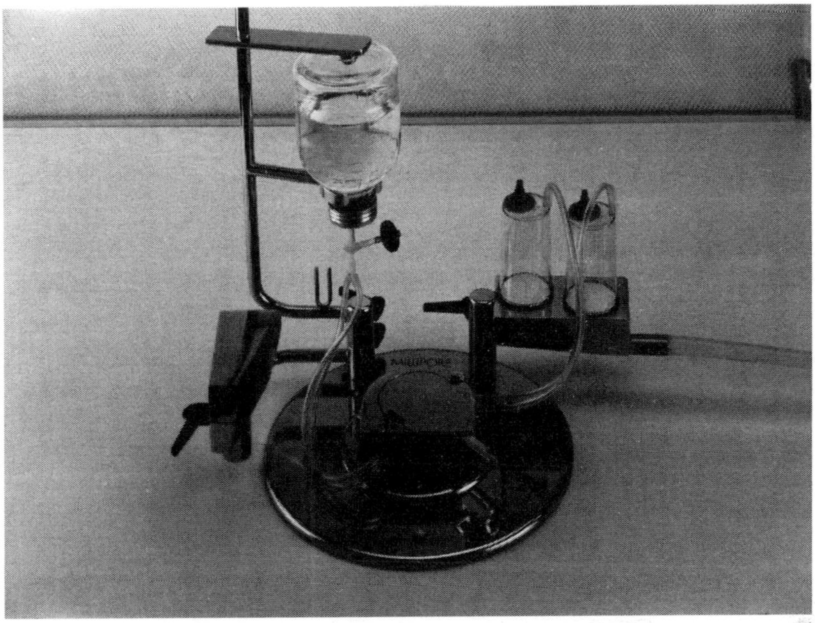

Figure 8 Steritest Integral 316II and III pumps. *Source*: From Millipore Corporation, Bedford, MA.

Both of these units can be moved out of the way when not in use or even removed from the isolator.

DETERMINING UTILITY NEEDS INSIDE THE ISOLATOR

Electrical

Electrical outlets should not be installed inside a sterility test isolator as they cannot be fully decontaminated with VPHP. The VPHP is an oxidizer and can corrode electrical connections. It is better to run all electrical cords out of the isolators through compression fittings to electrical outlets.

Gases

If gases are needed to perform specific sterility tests, access must be provided through the exterior of the isolator. Utility panels are a good place to add these outlets. Utility panels are stainless steel plates bolted over openings in the exterior of the isolators. The utility panel can easily be removed and sent to a machine shop or back to the isolator manufacturer to have additional compression fittings or sanitary fittings added. Utility panels add flexibility to the isolator, as sterility testing needs change. It is difficult to modify an isolator wall to add ports after the isolator is installed at your facility.

Drainage

If membrane filtration is used, a drainage system is required. For low volumes of liquids the effluent can be collected in the isolator. For most application, however, a drainage system to the exterior of the isolator must be installed. An exterior drainage system allows unlimited volumes of effluent to be removed from the isolator.

The drainage system must be able to be closed to the outside of the isolator when not in use. Sanitary valves and sanitary check valves work well for this application. The sanitary check valve has the added benefit of closing when pressure is not being applied. This prevents back flow into the isolator. A peristaltic pump on the drainage tubing of a sanitary valve will also prevent back flow. If the exterior drain port is higher than the drain tubing in the isolator then a pump will be needed to draw the effluent out of the isolator.

When collecting the effluent from membrane filtration it is important that the collection vessels consist of a primary vessel and an overflow vessel. The collection vessels should also be visible to the operator when performing the sterility testing to help minimize the potential for a spill. The collection vessels should be drained after each test and disinfected as needed. As an extra precaution, the operator should calculate the volume of effluent that will be generated for each sterility test session and plan to change the collection vessels accordingly.

ISOLATOR STERILANT/EQUIPMENT

There are several different sterilants that are available that can be used with isolators. These sterilants include, VPHP, peracetic acid and chlorine dioxide to name a few. VPHP generators have been available for about 18 years (C. Fritz, Steris Corporation, personal communication, 2009). The effectiveness of VPHP as a sterilant is well established in the industry. The Steris VHP^{TM} 1000 ED biodecontamination system (Fig. 9) is one of the currently used decontamination methods for isolators. Chlorine dioxide is also available as a sterilant for isolators (see "Chloride dioxide decontamination/sterilization," Chapter 28, for more details). Before choosing a sterilant for your isolators compare the pros and cons of the sterilants that are available and the materials that you will be sterility testing. Aeration times, material compatibility, sterilant toxicity, sterilant corrosiveness, and sterilant cost are just a few of the factors that should be considered.

STERILITY VALIDATION IN AN ISOLATOR

Container closure

Container closure evaluation of finished product containers should be performed before the B/F test is performed. Container closure testing can be performed in a number of different ways. It is up to the sterility testing group with the input of the validation and quality assurance department to determine the extent of container closure testing that will be performed.

The easiest way to perform container closure testing is to obtain media fill vials from production. Four containers are needed for each microorganism that will be tested. Select the test microorganisms on the basis of their sensitivity to the sterilant being used and the type of contaminants expected from the environment. For example, *Staphylococcus* species have been shown to be very sensitive to VPHP and are regularly isolated from most aseptic production areas due to personnel shedding.

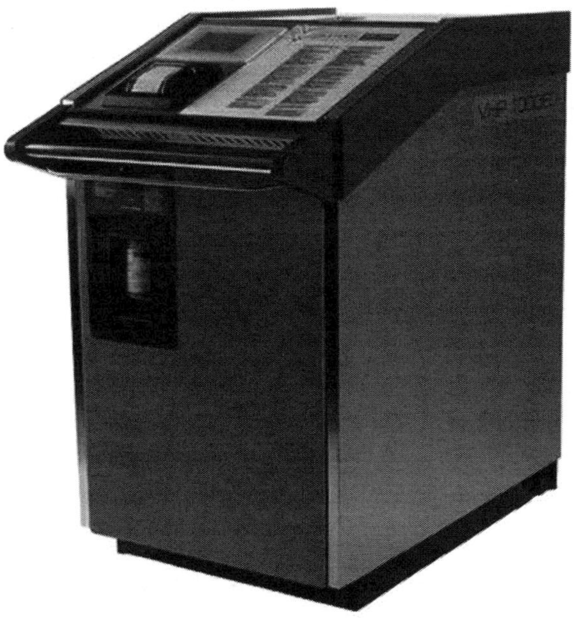

Figure 9 VHP^{TM} 1000 ED biodecontamination system. *Source*: From Steris Corporation, Mentor, OH.

The 6 recommended B/F microorganisms are also a good spectrum of microorganisms to include in container closure testing (6). Using all of the B/F microorganisms gives you additional information when evaluating the container closure results.

Label the four containers with the name of the test microorganism. Label two of the containers "exposed" and two "unexposed." Place the containers labeled "exposed" into the isolator and perform a decontamination cycle. After VPHP exposure inoculate less than 100 CFU of the test microorganisms into each of the two "exposed" and "unexposed" containers. Two additional containers that have not been inoculated or exposed to the sterilant will serve as negative controls. Perform plate counts to verify the inoculum. Incubate all the containers at 20°C to 25°C. Comparable growth should occur in both the exposed and the unexposed containers within 7 days.

In addition, four product containers can be filled with water. Two are exposed to the decontamination cycle and two serve as negative controls. The levels of the hydrogen peroxide in the containers are compared to the unexposed controls using a chemical indicator, that is, EM Quant^{TM} Peroxide Test, mfg. EM Science.

Subculturing

For samples that require subculturing, that is, opaque products, two methods of subculturing can be used. The simplest but more expensive option is to incubate the test samples in a transfer isolator or a canister with a RTP that can dock directly with the sterility test isolator. When the test samples need to be subcultured the transfer isolator or canister can be aseptically docked to the sterility test isolator and the subculturing performed. After subculturing, the test containers are returned to the incubator. Once the subculturing is performed the samples no longer need to be kept in a contained environment.

If a canister is used to incubate the samples in the incubator the internal temperature of the canister must be shown to meet the test incubation temperature range. If the samples are incubated in an isolator a thermocouple can be installed to constantly monitor the temperature.

The second option is to place the samples that need to be subcultured back into the isolator and expose them to VPHP prior to the subculture. To ensure that VPHP has not entered the test containers, container closure testing should to be performed on the media container. The container closure testing must be performed after the test media containers have been processed like an actual test

Bacteriostasis and Fungistasis

All materials that are used to perform the B/F testing must be exposed to the decontamination cycle that they were validated in. For example, if the product containers, test media, rinse fluids, and filtration units are surface decontaminated by VPHP then they must all be exposed prior to the B/F test. The B/F test does not need to be performed in the isolator. The inoculation and testing can be performed in a laminar flow hood or other suitable test environment. It probably is not wise to bring spore formers like *Aspergillus niger* and *Bacillus subtilis* into the sterility test isolator.

Membrane filtration testing requires that information of the filter compatibility with the sterilant also be evaluated. Some filter suppliers like Millipore have already done studies to show that their filters are not adversely affected by sterilants like VPHP.

STERILITY TESTING IN AN ISOLATOR

Environmental Monitoring

Environmental monitoring media should be tested to confirm it will support the types of organisms that you will be looking for from the environment.

Some companies use only one type of media, soybean casein digest broth (TSB), that they have shown can support the growth of bacteria, yeasts, and molds. For isolators with attached autoclave, the TSB is sterilized in the autoclave and brought directly into the isolator.

It is also acceptable to use two different types of media for the isolation of bacteria, yeasts, and molds, that is soybean casein digest agar (SCDA) for bacteria and sabouraud dextrose agar (SDA) for yeasts and molds. Using two different media makes the incubation of plates easier.

There is no need to transfer plates from one temperature to another. SCDA media is incubated at 32.5 ± 2.5°C and SDA is incubated at 22.5 ± 2.5°C. Because the media packaging can be affected by shipping and handling, it is recommended that each time environmental monitoring is performed; additional plates are exposed to the sterilant. Low-level growth promotion is performed on these plates to confirm package integrity. VPHP and other sterilants can be absorbed into the media if the package integrity has been compromised. Inhibition can range from 50% to as much as a few logs.

When performing low-level growth promotion, the growth on VPHP exposed media is compared with inoculum counts on non exposed media. Recovery counts should agree within 70% of the inoculum counts (7).

With any environmental monitoring program, in addition to establishing a reasonable monitoring program, it is important to set meaningful alert and action limits. The bioburden in sterility test isolators is very low but with large volume sampling it may be possible to isolate microorganisms. Alert and action limits of 1 cfu or more should be justified based on trending data. Just because microorganisms are isolated in a sterility test isolator does not mean they will jeopardize a sterility test result. Validated isolator decontamination cycles and aseptic technique should prevent any low bioburden if present in the isolator from affecting the sterility test. The most critical areas to monitor are those at the sterility testing area. Environmental monitoring in an isolator is very similar to environmental monitoring in a traditional clean room. In a sterility test isolator, air and surface monitoring need to be performed. There are many different techniques available to perform each type of monitoring.

Air Monitoring

Passive air monitoring can be performed using settling plates exposed during the testing. Settling plates are easy to validate and use. During validation, the container closure integrity of the packaging needs to be confirmed, if the plates are surfaced decontaminated with VPHP. Currently, there are several manufacturers of specially packaged media that are resistant to penetration of VPHP, that is, PML Microbiologicals, BBL, and Biotest. Any manufacturer's claims should be confirmed in-house using specific decontamination cycle and load configuration.

Wide-mouth containers filled with broth media can also be used to passively monitor the air quality. If the media-filled containers are sterilized by steam in an attached double-door autoclave and then brought directly into the isolator no VPHP container closure validation is required. Of course, the media sterilization cycle must be validated.

Active air monitoring can be performed with systems like the Sartorius MD8 Air Sampler (Fig. 10). These systems, unlike passive air monitoring, have the advantage of being able to monitor large volumes of isolator air. These systems need to be installed in the isolator prior to the isolator validation.

Surface Monitoring

The isolator surfaces can be monitored using contact plates. If contact plates are used to monitor surfaces, it is important that the residual media be wiped up using sterile towels and sterile water or sterile 70/30 isopropyl alcohol/water. The residual media can prevent the proper decontamination of surfaces by providing a barrier to the VPHP.

Isolator surfaces can also be monitored using swabs moistened with a diluent. The swab is then placed in a nutrient broth for a qualitative result. Alternately, the swab can after sampling be vortexed in a diluent and membrane filtered for a quantitative result.

The surface of gloves should be monitored. The gloves can be monitored with either a swab or contact plate, dipping in a broth or buffer, or by leak testing. The leak testing equipment is expensive but it allows the operator to integrity test the gloves before and after each test.

Operator Qualification

All operators before sterility testing in an isolator should be trained in proper aseptic technique. Although the isolators have been proven to be effective barriers this does not mean that the operators should deviate from the aseptic techniques that are used in traditional clean rooms

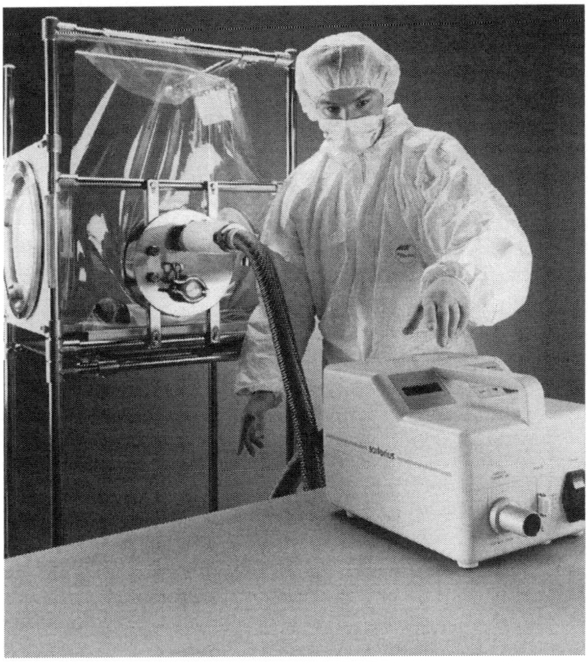

Figure 10 Sartorius MD8 air-monitoring system. *Source*: From Sartorius Corporation, Goettingen, Germany.

for sterility testing. The operator should avoid touching work surfaces, generating a lot of turbulence in the isolator or reaching over open containers. The operator should use slow and precise movements.

Once the operator has reviewed proper aseptic technique and been trained on all the required procedures, the operator should perform a "qualification" sterility test in the isolator. The qualification of the operator is to verify that they are capable of performing all of the test manipulations without contaminating the test. The easiest way to qualify an operator is to use media fill containers from the production facility. The container closure systems are the same as the final product and they contain media that will support microbial growth. The media-filled containers should be processed in the same manner a sterility test samples. The operator should perform the sterility test as outlined in the internal sterility testing procedure (6) including performing environmental monitoring during the test. To pass qualification, the operator's sterility test samples must not show growth after 14 days of incubation and the environmental monitoring must be below the alert and action limits.

Sample Incubation

Samples are usually removed from the isolator for incubation. Remote incubation works well for most samples. If subculturing is required, see the suggestions mentioned in the subculturing section. Extreme care should be used when handling the environmental monitoring samples after removal from the isolator to prevent accidental contamination.

PREVENTATIVE MAINTENANCE AND CALIBRATION

The preventative maintenance and calibration schedules should be determined prior to purchasing isolators and support equipment. Preventative maintenance and calibration agreements should be arranged for the isolators, autoclave, and VPHP generator. Because these service agreements can be very expensive and are a recurring expense, the cost should be determined before purchasing the equipment.

It is important that the preventive maintenance and calibration service contract is signed in advance or training arranged for internal personnel. Establishing preventive maintenance and calibration requirements early will greatly reduce the time required to qualify the sterility test isolators. Be sure to check references to make sure the service contract provider is reliable. Timely preventative maintenance and calibration of isolator equipment are usually critical to avoid delaying the sterility test and the release of product.

Sterility isolators have pressure gauges, pressure alarms, and chart recorders that are calibrated on a quarterly or semiannual basis. The calibrations usually require the isolator to be down for a day but the isolator can be re-decontaminated for use the next day.

Other parts like gloves, gaskets, bands, and O-rings can be changed by the users. The preventative maintenance schedule will vary depending on the decontamination and use frequency of the isolators. Document when all parts are changed in the equipment log. This log will be helpful in determining the replacement interval of most parts. Lubrication of the RTP should be done on a regular basis, once a month for most users is generally adequate. If the docking of two isolators is difficult, lubricate the gaskets.

Gloves should be leak tested on a regular basis. Depending on the amount of usage the gloves may need to be leak tested more frequently. At a minimum the gloves should be tested each time the isolator is breached to certify the HEPA filters, usually every 6 months. Glove leak testers are available to test glove integrity in place (Fig. 11). The gloves can also be removed from the isolator and tested for leaks by inflating them and dipping them in water to looking for bubbles. Alternately, the gloves can be coated with a soap solution and inflated to look for bubbles.

Although it may be possible to aseptically change the gloves in a sterility test isolator, it is very difficult to check for leaks between the gloves and sleeve cuffs after installation without performing a leak test. Because the sterility of the isolator is critical in maintaining low failure rates, leak testing should be performed with every glove change to ensure that the gloves have been properly installed.

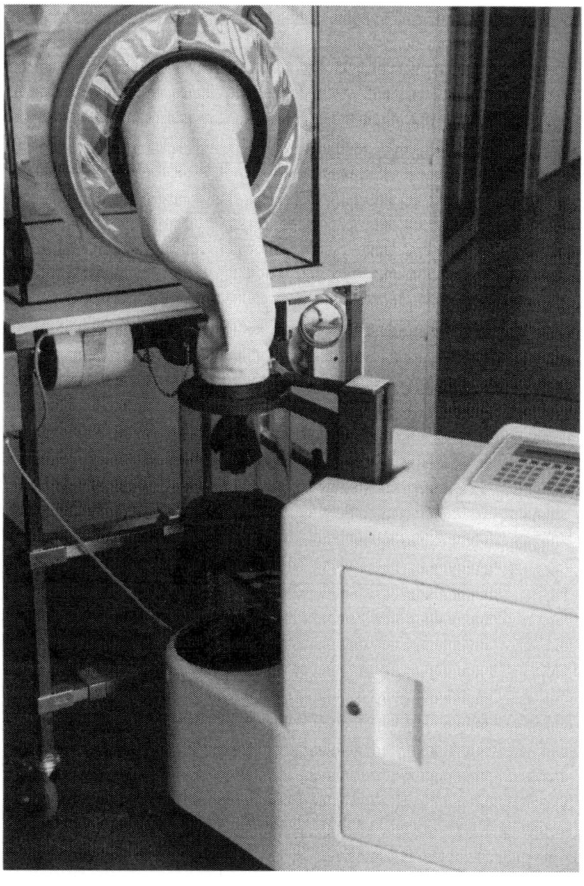

Figure 11 Glove-integrity tester. *Source*: From La Calhene, Rush City, MN.

The isolator HEPAs are generally qualified every 6 months and require the integrity of the sterility test environment to be compromised. The HEPA test ports are opened and the face velocity readings require a probe be introduced into the testing environment. The isolator should be leak tested after every HEPA certification. If an ammonia leak test is performed, the isolator will be down for a few days. Half a day to perform the HEPA testing, half a day to perform the leak test and aerate the isolator, and 1 day to decontaminate the isolator. Note that if the testing isolator is decontaminated with every new test then only 1 day of testing is lost during HEPA recertification.

The VPHP generator's preventative maintenance and calibration is usually performed on a quarterly basis.

The autoclave generally has preventative maintenance every other month and calibration on a quarterly basis.

As with most laboratory equipment, if satisfactory calibration results are consistently obtained the time between calibrations can be increased.

TYPICAL PROBLEMS AND SOLUTIONS

A. Contacts
   1. Learn which companies are using isolators with similar applications to share information. Possible resources for contacts include the PDA's Isolation Technology Interest Group, isolator conferences/seminars, isolator manufacturers, and the VPHP suppliers.
   2. Learn which companies are near you that use the same isolator equipment. They might be a good source for a spare part or hydrogen peroxide when you are in urgent need.

B. Extending the life of isolator parts
   1. Extend the life of the elastic half suit supports by keeping the half suits elevated on support frames when not in use. Support frames are usually used to fully extend the half suit or gloves when decontaminating the isolator.
   2. Keep gasket lubricated with silicone spray avoid tearing and maintain easy operation.
   3. Purchase a repair kit for flexible isolators. The patches can repair a hole in a PVC sleeve or half suit.

C. Hydrogen peroxide
   1. Always keeps at least a 2 months supply of hydrogen peroxide in house. Hydrogen peroxide must be shipped by ground and takes 4 to 6 weeks for delivery.

D. Leaks
   1. Often the HEPA test port bolts/caps are not properly installed after HEPA recertification. The Teflon tape round the threads should be replaced every time the bolts are removed.
   2. Check the glove cuffs and half suit bands for leaks. Make sure there are no pinches in the gloves at the cuff or in the half suit at the band.
   3. For flexible-walled isolators, leaks often occur around the door bonnets and for rigid-walled isolators the seals around the windows and doors. Keep extra door bonnets, bands on hand and silicone sealant, respectively to correct these leaks.

E. Leak testing
   1. Use only concentrated ammonia to perform the ammonia leak test and use approximately 50 mL/100 square feet of isolator. The more concentrated the ammonia the easier to detect a leak.
   2. Do not reuse the ammonia solution. Discard after every use to prevent low ammonia levels in the isolator.
   3. For rigid-walled isolators cut the ammonia detection cloth into long strips to make testing connections and seams easier. For flexible-walled isolators cut the detector cloth in large blocks to measure large portions of the canopy at one time.
   4. Keep the ammonia detector cloth in an airtight container in the dark.
   5. Never touch the ammonia detector cloth with your bare hands. The cloth will react with the oils in your hands.

F. Software upgrades
   1. Equipment with computerized controllers like the VHP™ 1000 ED and most steam sterilizers will have periodic software upgrades. Most manufacturers provide the upgrades

for free but it is up to the individual user to determine if revalidation is required. In some cases, the end user may choose not to or wait to install a software upgrade because of the revalidation required.

G. Sterility testing
    1. Always take in extra samples and supplies. This helps prevent having to abort a test when a sample is accidentally dropped, a filtration unit leaks, a tube of media breaks, etc.
    2. When working with ampoules, place a sterile wipe over the work surface to capture any shards of glass. Discard the wipe after the test to prevent the chance of damaging a glove from a shard of glass on the work surface.

H. Supplies
    1. Keep sterilized wipes in the isolator to clean up spills.
    2. Bring small vials or tubes filled with sterile water into the isolator for cleaning. Use the container once then discard.

REFERENCES

1. <1211> Sterilization and Sterility Assurance. The United States Pharmocopeia. 32 ed. The United States Pharmocopeial Convention, Inc, 2009:724.
2. Material Safety Data Sheet. Hydrogen Peroxide, Steris Corporation, 1992.
3. Material Safety Data Sheet. Ammonia Solution, Strong, J. T. Baker, 2008.
4. Wall Mounted Sensor. Product Information Sheet, Drager SicherheittechniK GmgH.
5. Accuro Gas Detection System, package insert. Drager SicherheittechniK GmgH.
6. <71> Sterility Test. The United States Pharmocopeia. 32 ed. The United States Pharmocopeial Convention, Inc, 2009:80–86.
7. <1227> Validation of Microbial Recovery. The United States Pharmocopeia. 32 ed. The United States Pharmocopeial Convention, Inc, 2009:738–739.

19 Advanced aseptic processing fill finish trends: options to consider, restricted access barrier systems, and/or isolators

Jack Lysfjord

INTRODUCTION

The question of what technology to use for a renovated or new aseptic processing area or processing line is asked with an eye to the regulators who prefer a risk-based approach. The overall objective is to produce an aseptic environment that will be under control at all times and reduce risk to the product and patient. The author has been involved with the transition from conventional clean room technology to isolators and restricted access barrier systems (RABS) since the 1980s, and has chaired and cochaired conferences and spoken globally on barriers and isolators. In the 1996–1997 timeframe it was common to ask about what was being done at pharmaceutical companies with respect to the implementation of isolators (isolators having preceded RABS). In 1998, a concise two-page survey on the use of isolators for automated aseptic fill finish applications was conducted. The survey continued on even numbered years. The results outlined industry trends relative to isolator technology implementation. A RABS survey was begun in 2005 and continued on the odd years. The resulting data is typically presented at ISPE (International Society for Pharmaceutical Engineering) barrier isolator conferences and published in the ISPE magazine, Pharmaceutical Engineering. This chapter reviews the results from both the 2007 RABS survey (1) and the 2008 isolator survey (2).

BACKGROUND AND CLARIFICATION OF TERMS

The collection and evaluation of survey data first requires that participants use the same definitions and terms. US Food and Drug Administration (FDA) compliance officers have frequently found that RABS installations are defined and operated differently by different companies. To obtain good data, the following definitions were used to help better clarify the questions being asked. The most critical issue is the degree of separation of operators from the critical zone where the aseptic filling and closing occurs. ISO 14644-7 contains a chart that looks at the various levels of separation and product risk (Fig. 1) (3).

The text blocks in the lower left corner represent processing performed in a conventional open clean room (Figs. 2 and 3). RABS would be in the lower range to midrange depending on how such systems are used. Isolators provide the greatest degree of separation and are in the upper right corner location yielding the greatest product protection. The diagrams and example photos follow the progression of conventional clean room processing to containment isolators. Moving upwards on the chart in Figure 1, RABS can be found near the center. The RABS surveys covered three different types of RABS: passive, active, and closed.

- A passive RABS is supplied with air from the classified room in which it is located and is the simplest of all designs (Fig. 4). Note that the airflow at the top of the barrier walls must be the same inside and out. If the velocity is higher inside, a venturi effect could draw in contamination from the surrounding environment, which is a lower air quality classification.
- Active RABS have their own air supply system that allows for the independent selection of the internal air velocity eliminating one of the negative concerns associated with passive RABS designs. Depending on the extent of integration of active RABS into the facility, the air system could be either positioned below the ceiling of the classified room, or installed flush with that ceiling (Figs. 5–7).
- Closed RABS closely resemble isolators with the difference being manual biodecontamination with closed RABS instead of H_2O_2 vapor as is used in isolators; surrounding room classification (ISO 7 minimum in operation) and appropriate gowning of personnel (Fig. 8).

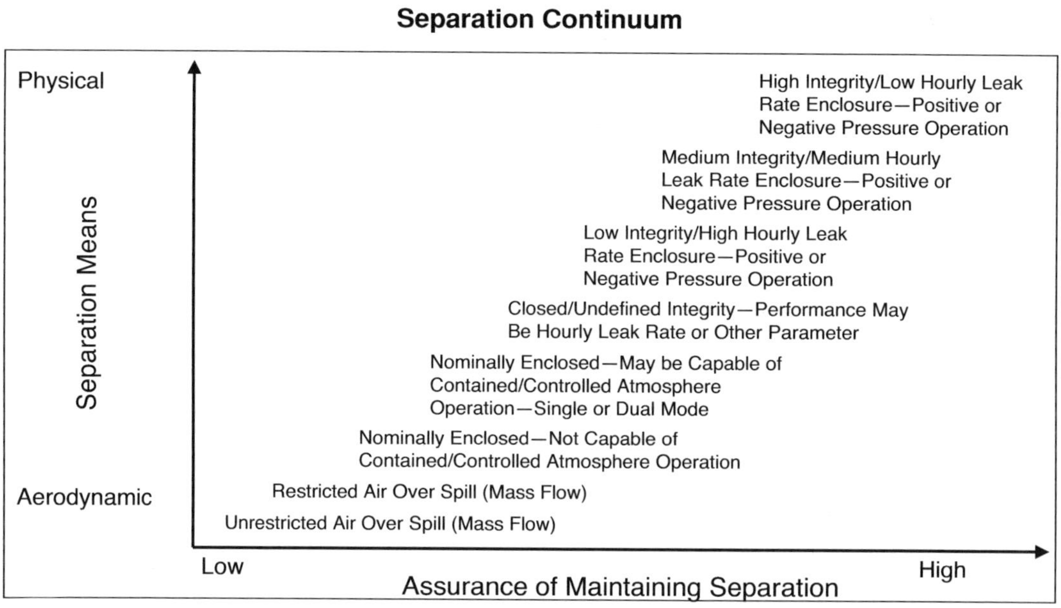

Figure 1 Chart from ISO 14644 showing degree of separation and product risk. *Source*: From ISO 14644.

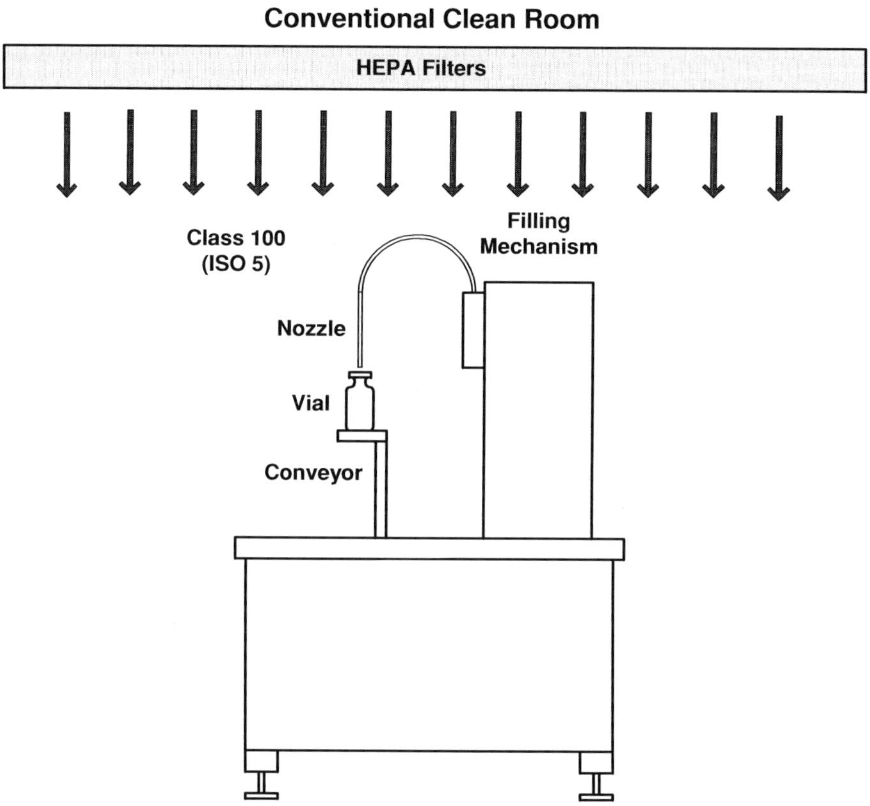

Figure 2 Conventional clean room aseptic fill finish processing section view. *Source*: From Bosch Packaging Technology.

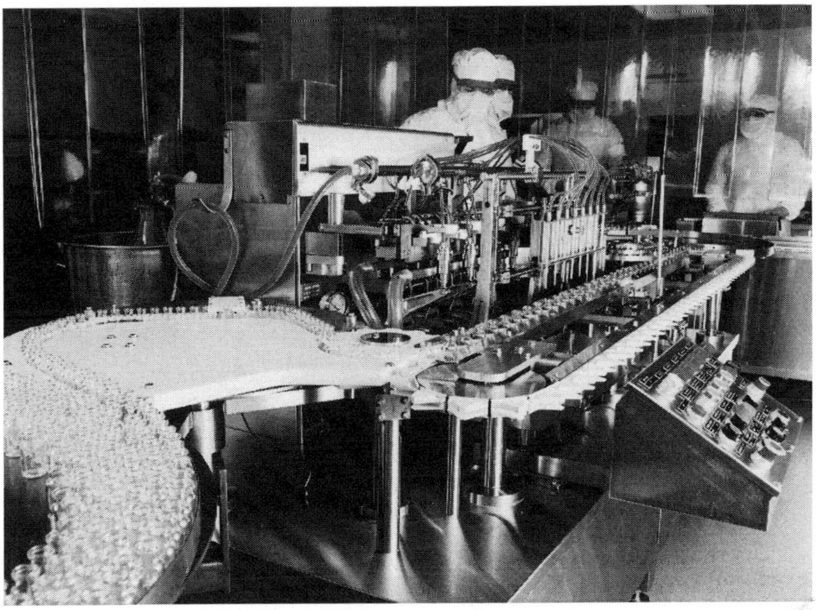

Figure 3 Photo of a conventional clean room fill finish application. *Source*: From Bosch Packaging Technology.

- A barrier to prevent human intervention.
- Air flow provided by ceiling HEPAs to critical zone.
- Bottom of enclosure is open for air outlet.
- Glove ports and transfer ports used for manipulations and commodity additions.
- Manual high level disinfection.

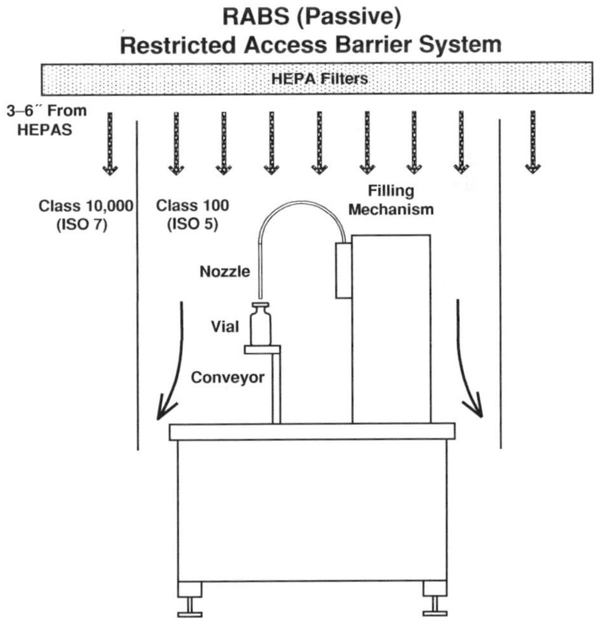

Figure 4 Diagram of a passive RABS. Note that the air flow at the top of the barrier walls must be the same inside and out. If velocity is higher inside, a venturi effect could draw in contamination from the surrounding room that is a lower classification. *Source*: From Bosch Packaging Technology.

- Similar to passive RABS but with integral HEPA/HVAC air supply to critical zone.
- Easiest way to have flow from critical area to room in case of open door intervention.
- Manual high level disinfection.

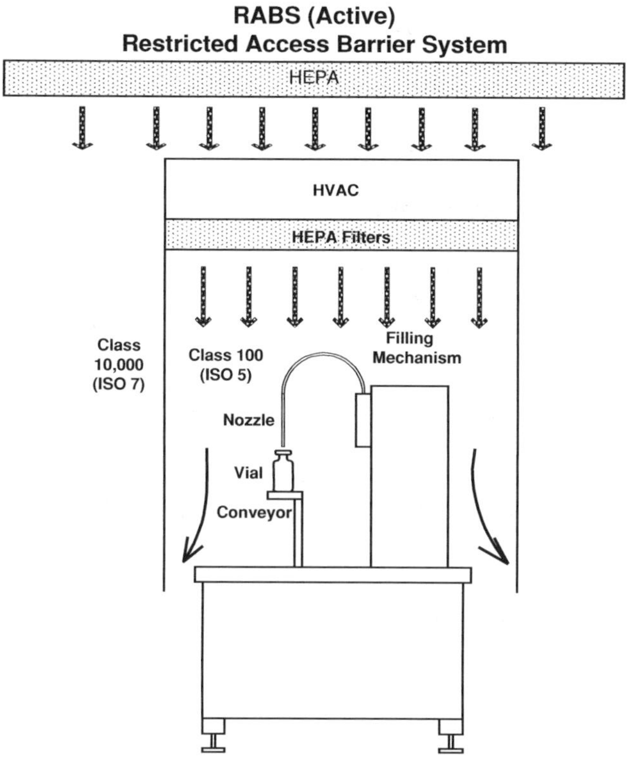

Figure 5 Diagram of an active RABS in a clean room. Here there is a dedicated HVAC system with HEPA filters for ISO 5 critical process zone. *Source*: From Bosch Packaging Technology.

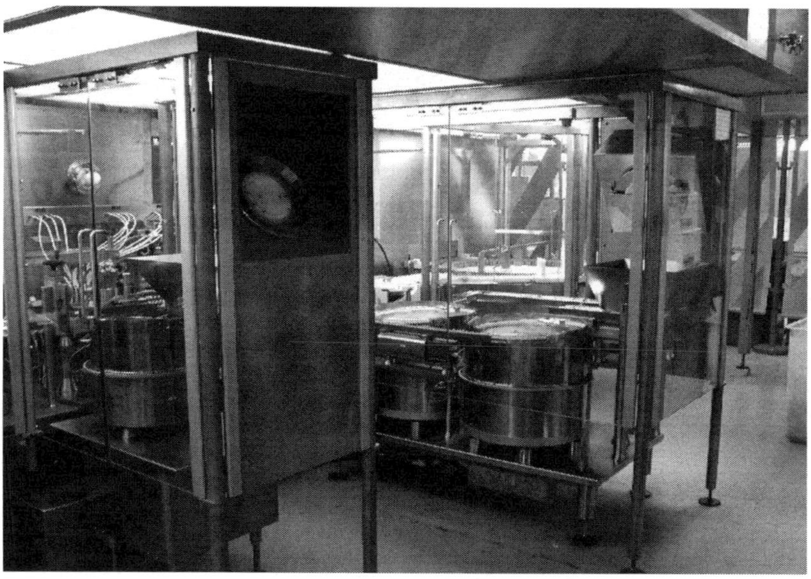

Figure 6 An active RABS example with a barrier and air flow for separation. *Source*: From Bosch Packaging Technology.

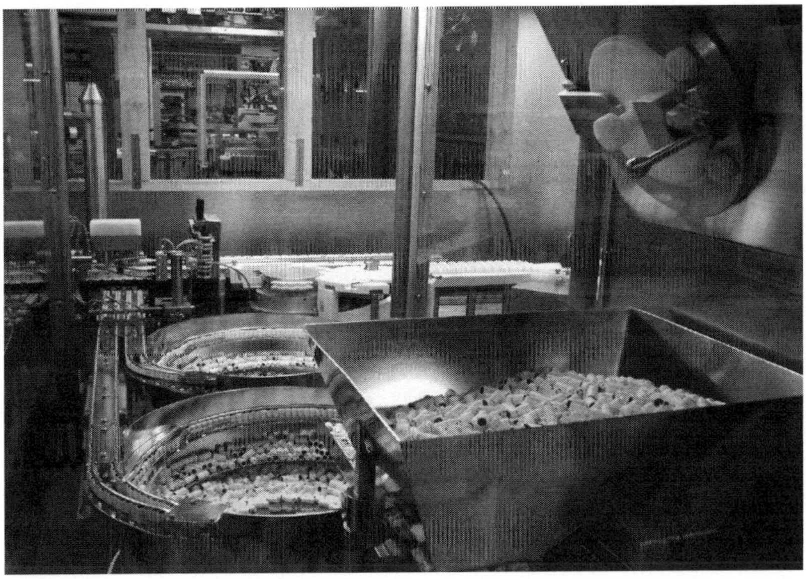

Figure 7 Another view of the same application as Figure 6, showing the rapid transfer port (RTP) for transfer of components. *Source*: From Bosch Packaging Technology.

- Similar to an isolator without vapor biodecontamination.
- Manual high level disinfection.
- Can be used for containment applications

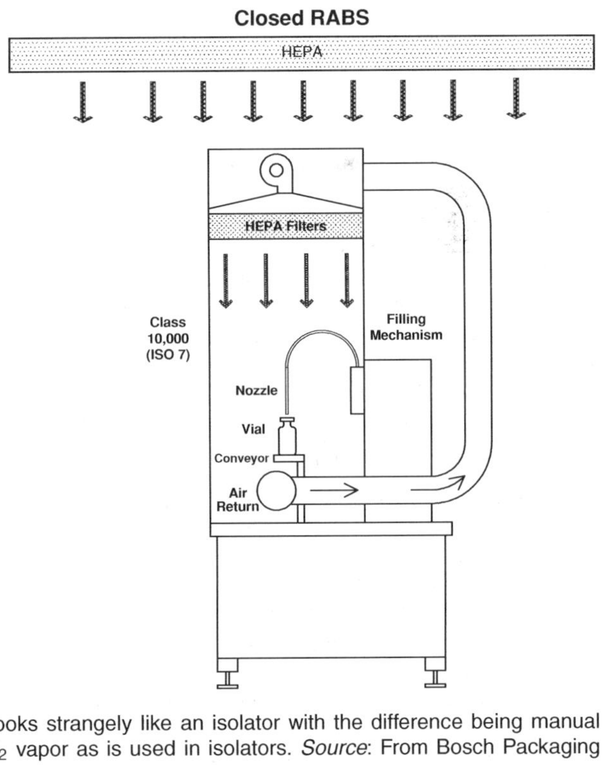

Figure 8 Diagram of a closed RABS which looks strangely like an isolator with the difference being manual biodecontamination with RABS instead of H_2O_2 vapor as is used in isolators. *Source*: From Bosch Packaging Technology.

RABS is an acronym for restricted access barrier system. If personnel access is restricted, they are kept, to varying degrees as defined by user requirements, out of the critical environment. The barrier is the enclosure that uses air flow to keep contamination out. In this definition, "system" is the word that is abused at many companies. They have an enclosure that they believe is magic in some way and therefore consider it acceptable to open the doors frequently in operation. **This is not true!** The FDA accepts RABS if the doors remain closed. Companies have been cited in FDA 483s for frequent door opening with RABS installations.

A RABS design needs the following for the system to be under adequate control.

- Management oversight (keeping the patient's safety in mind)
- A effective quality system (that has power to stop production when appropriate to protect the product)
- Proper surrounding room design
    - Additional ISO 5 areas outside RABS if open-door interventions are allowed
- Proper aseptic gowning of personnel
- Proper current good manufacturing practices training
- Initial high-level disinfection with a sporicidal agent
- Properly designed equipment
- Proper standard operating procedures (SOPs) for defined rare interventions
- **If** open-door interventions are allowed (a policy decision is required dictating under what circumstances open-door utilization is acceptable, under what circumstances and how to do it with SOPs.)
    - Proper and appropriate disinfection for product requirements (nonsporicidal)
    - Appropriate line clearance
    - Documentation of the event

Companies with RABS that have a policy of never opening the doors achieve media fill results equivalent to what is found in isolated filling lines. When doors are frequently opened, the firm has an accessible system with an occasional barrier and that system is likely to be worse in product protection that the conventional clean room processing. Regulators strongly prefer installations that keep the doors closed at all times during the production cycle.

Moving further upwards on the chart in Figure 1, aseptic and containment isolators are found. Aseptic isolators are like closed RABS in appearance, but use a sporicidal vapor as the biodecontamination agent with a barrier, usually, continuous positive pressure differential between the internal and external environments, surrounding room of lower classification (ISO 8 in operation) and appropriate gowning (Figs. 9–12). Containment applications may require wash down for product inactivation, HEPA filters on the air return and perhaps negative pressure to protect operators. Air handling gets more complex with the use of pressure cascades and positive or negative pressure annexes to prevent escape of toxic products through depyrogenation tunnels or mouseholes (Figs. 13–15).

Application of the Advanced Aseptic Technology

What is interesting is that there are many companies who have not started to look at these technologies. This may be result of an inherent fear of change. But, there are many pharmaceutical industry drivers that will impact how aseptic fill finish will be done in the future that push for using RABS and isolators:

- Regulatory harmonization with quality by design, process analytical technology, and use of a risk-based approach.
- Products are shifting to large molecule biologics (biotech) without preservatives (which means they are more prone to allow growth of contaminants), and that are very expensive to produce (business risk).
- EU GMP annex 1 changes for overcapping requiring Grade A air to be provided until the cap is crimped.
- Both RABS and isolators can provide efficiencies when well-designed campaign strategy is used.

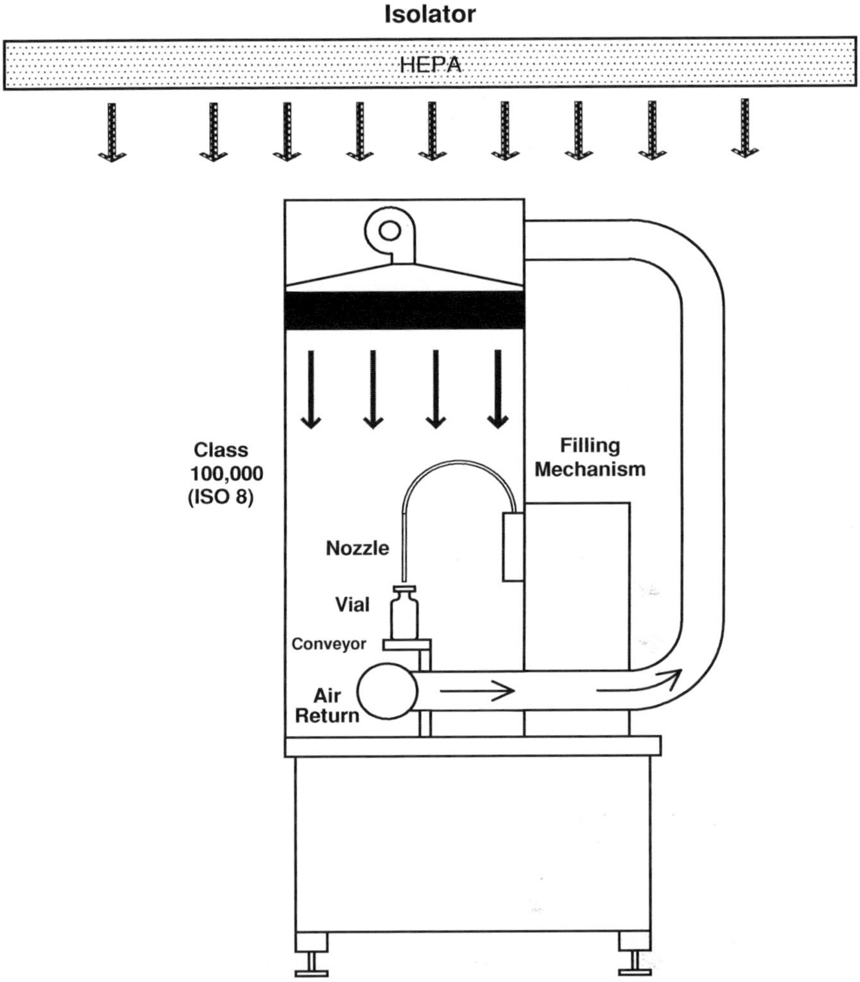

Figure 9 Diagram of an isolator. *Source*: From Bosch Packaging Technology.

- An increasing number of future products are expected to have a containment need to protect the operators.
- There is often a requirement for clinical manufacture before completion of safety/toxicity data is available necessitating worker protection.
- People are still the most important source of contamination in the fill finish process.
- An engineering approach that provides the most control over the environmental conditions.

MAJOR CONSIDERATIONS

The following information is derived from periodic surveys the author has conducted with Mr. Michael Porter of Merck & Co. The answers to the questions reveal some interesting insights into how industry has evaluated their operational requirements and made selections of equipment and defined procedures to best fit those requirements.

Gloves on these systems are always an area of concern because of their potential vulnerability to failure. Usage is almost equally split between one- and two-piece gloves/sleeves. Smooth sleeves are generally preferred to pleated sleeves large because of cleaning and sterilization or decontamination considerations. The preferred test method for gloves is visual inspection with pressure decay test. Glove life varies from a change out with each batch to a service time as long as 6 months; however, the most common replacement period is defined as "as needed."

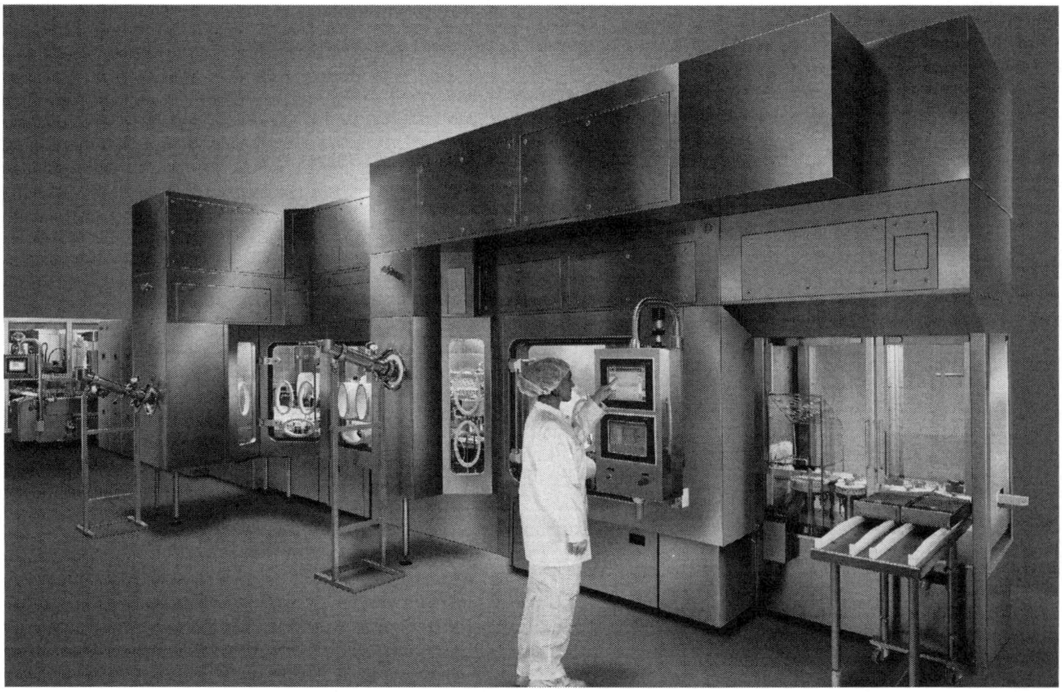

Figure 10 Photo of an isolator line installed. *Source*: From Bosch Packaging Technology.

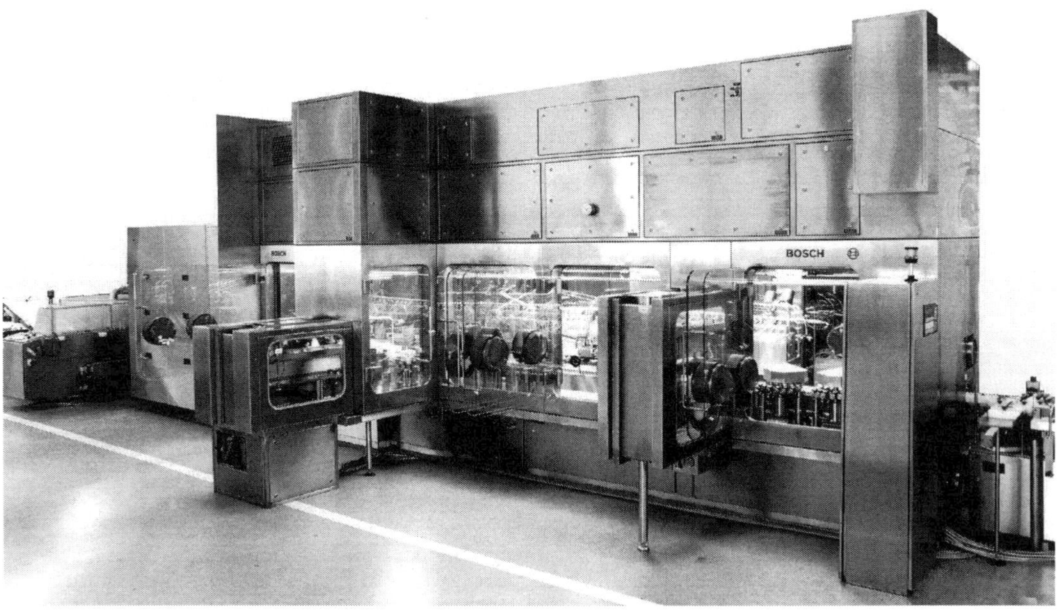

Figure 11 Another example of and installed isolator line. *Source*: From Bosch Packaging Technology.

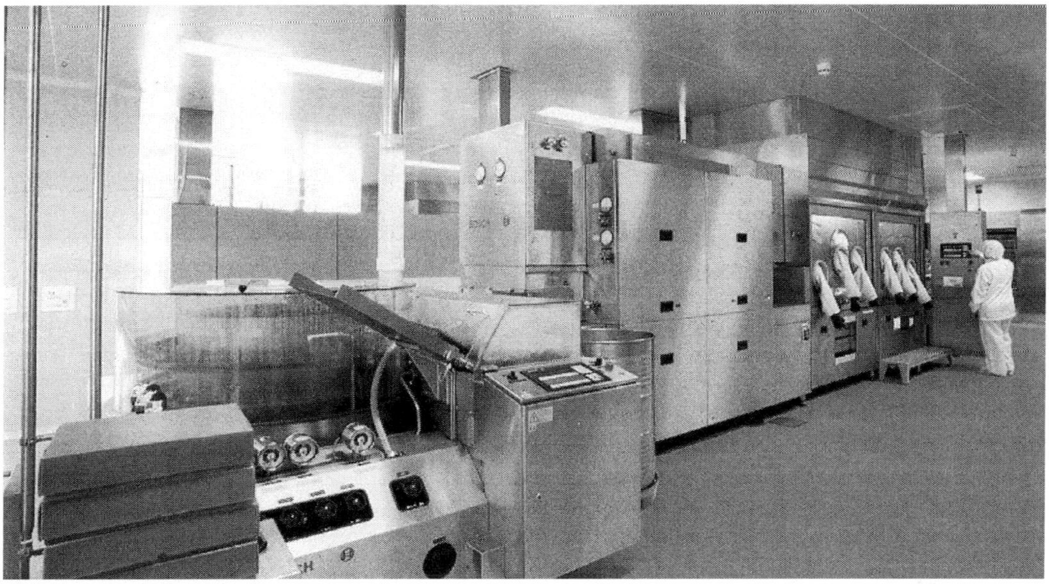

Figure 12 Another isolator installation. *Source*: From Bosch Packaging Technology.

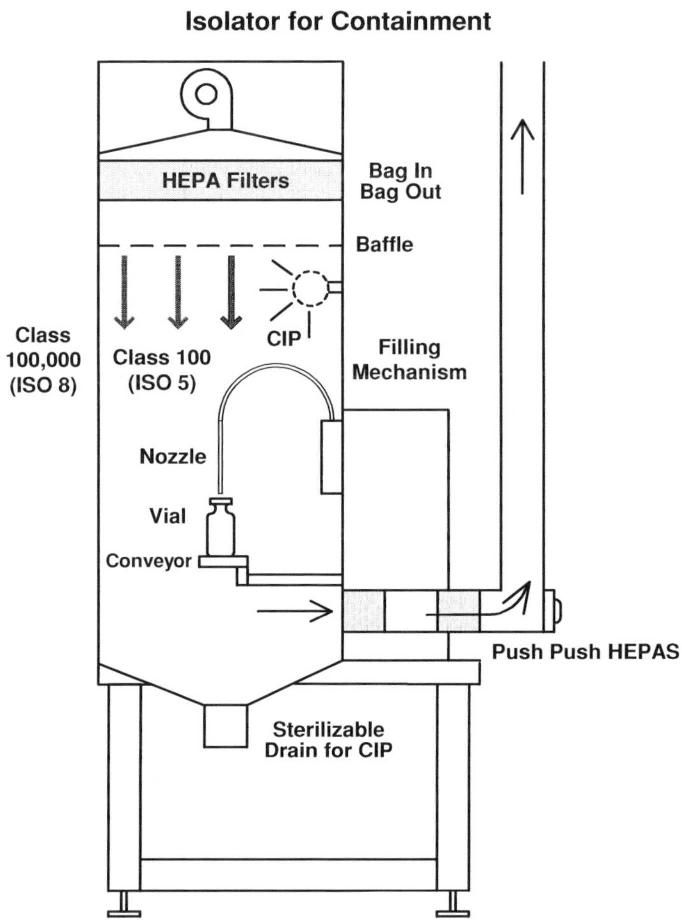

Figure 13 Diagram of a containment isolator. *Source*: From Bosch Packaging Technology.

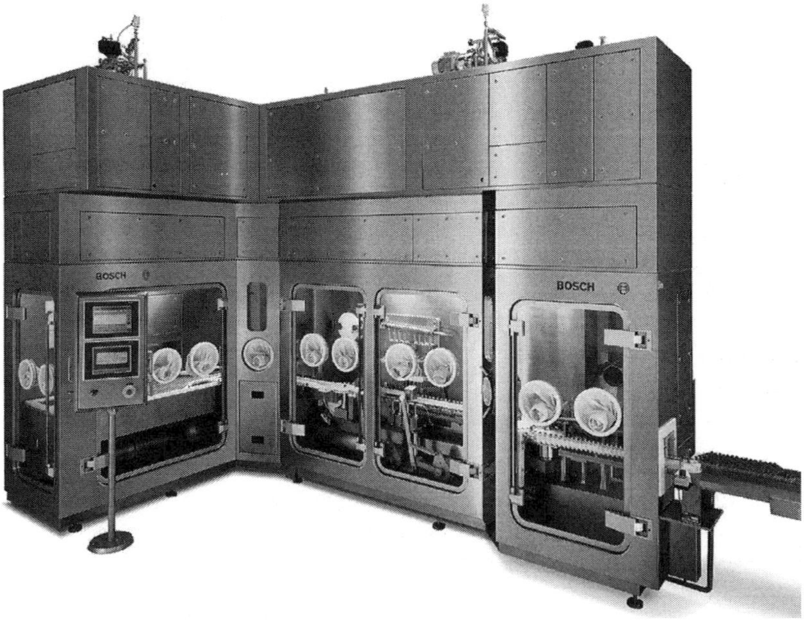

Figure 14 Photo of a containment isolator capable of being washed down before doors are opened for changeover. *Source*: From Bosch Packaging Technology.

Products that require containment are increasing and this may shift the choice of technology toward isolators. Nearly half of early isolator installations indicated a containment need as a part of the reason for their installation, 100% of lines with isolators added between 2006 and 2008 had a containment need! With RABS lines only six new production lines indicated a containment need in 2007.

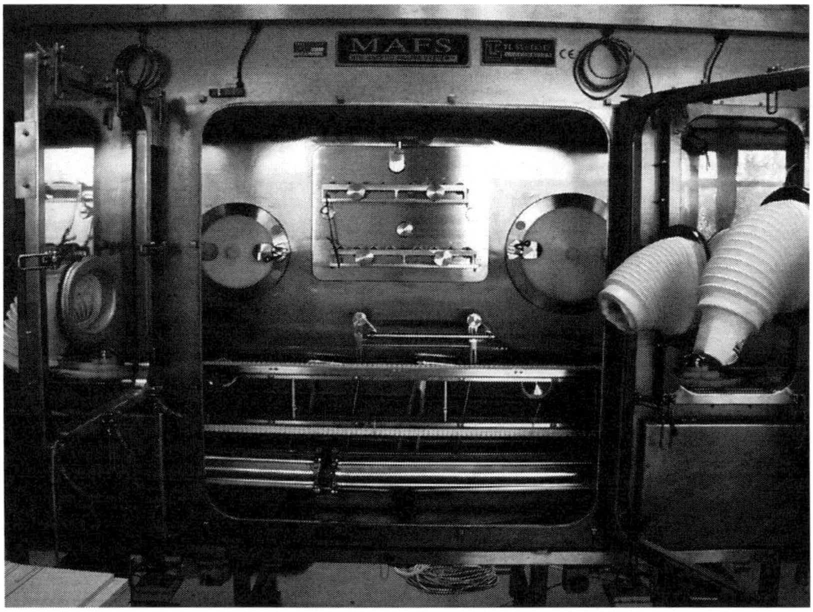

Figure 15 Photo of the filling location of a containment isolator with wash down capability. *Source*: From Bosch Packaging Technology.

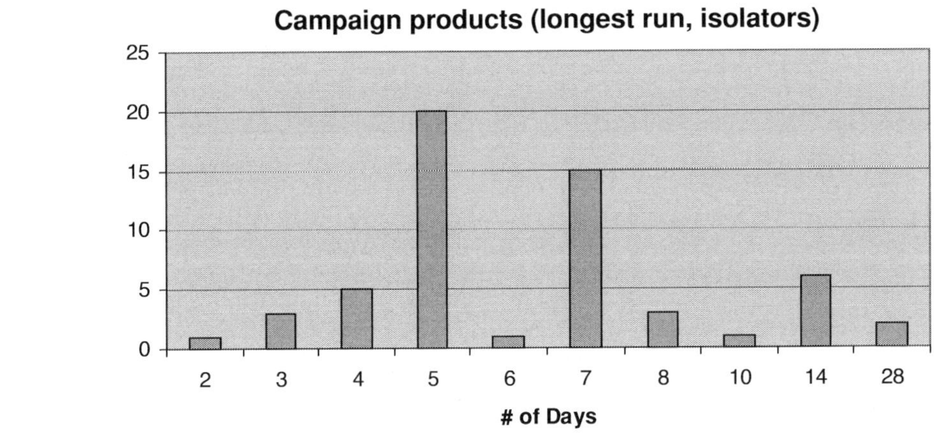

Figure 16 Isolator line campaign length. *Source*: From Lysfjord/Porter 2008 Barrier Isolator Survey.

Campaigning or running several days between biodecontamination cycles to gain efficiency is increasingly popular as experience with these technologies has grown. Figures 16 and 17 indicate campaign days versus how many lines at that frequency for isolators and RABS lines.

INTERPRETATION OF INDUSTRY TRENDS

There are certain trends that are evident in the results of these surveys:

- Isolator lines for aseptic automated fill finish applications have increased at 27.5 lines/year on the basis of the data from 2004 to 2008.
- RABS lines for aseptic automated fill finish applications are increasing at a slower 16 lines/year on the basis of 4-year data from 2003 to 2007.

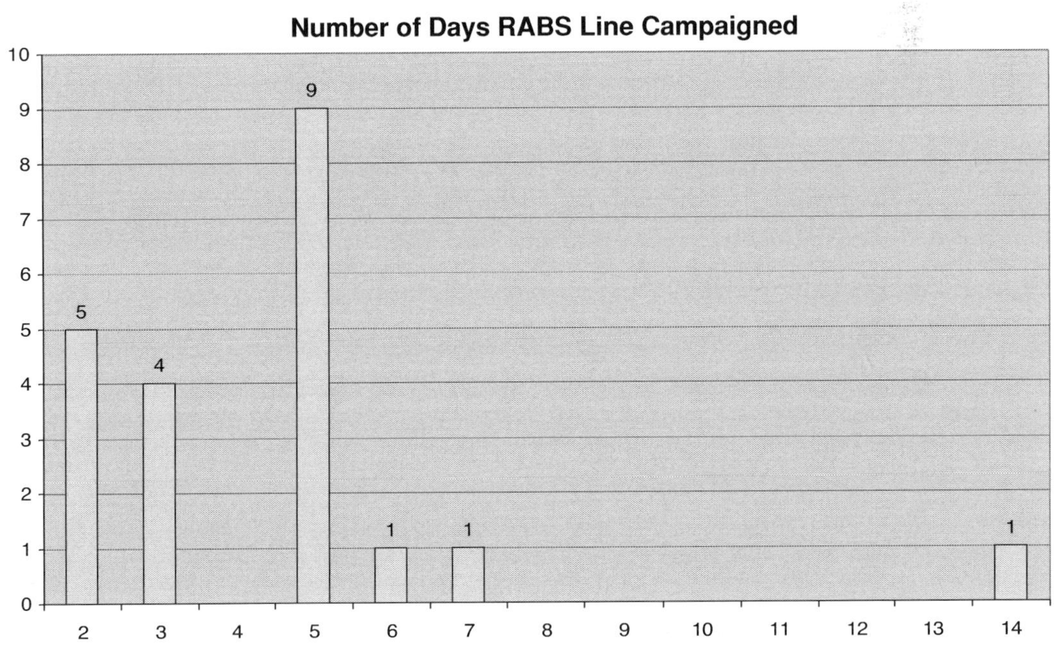

Figure 17 RABS line campaign length. *Source*: From Lysfjord/Porter 2007 RABS Survey.

- Syringe processing in presterilized tubs is rapidly increasing in Europe and could overtake vial lines soon.
- Containment needs are increasing with 100% of isolator lines needing containment in past 2 years.
- Isolator biodecontamination is accomplished using H_2O_2 in 92% of all reported applications.
- Campaigning is increasing with 59% of companies answering the question for isolator lines doing campaigning for up to 28 days. RABS has campaign length of up to 14 days.
- RABS use presents a difficult situation with stopper feed components being a product contact part and requiring a 6 log reduction in bioburden. Autoclaving and remounting is more difficult with RABS while still maintaining the sterility of components. Companies in Europe (Bioquell), North America (Steris), and Japan (Shibuya, Airex, and JGC) make equipment for room gassing with H_2O_2 that includes the RABS interior and stopper components. This works but results in much longer cycle times.
- More and more often closed RABS are being biodecontaminated with H_2O_2, with ISO 7 surrounding room (and ISO 5 annexes for door-open situation) instead of isolator in ISO 8, with Grade C or D surrounding room. This provides a RABS system that is really an isolator situated in a higher classification room with full gowning that could have situations where the door is opened. This approach would be opposite to the position of the FDA!
- The biggest issue with RABS is that 14% are opened frequently and this will result in regulatory issues due to added product risk.

CONCLUSION

A frequently asked question is "Which technology should we use, RABS or isolator technology?" My answer is "It depends on the product and application needs. Both are tools that work if used properly. Cars and guns are also tools and improper use of them causes large problems. The same is true for RABS and Isolators. The data from surveys is always interesting and each survey paints a better picture of what is going on currently with advanced aseptic processing."

REFERENCES

1. Lysfjord JP, Porter M. Restricted access barrier system (RABS)—2007 final data. Pharm Eng 2009;29(3): 56–59.
2. Lysfjord JP, Porter M. 2009 Barrier isolator history and trends—2008 final data. Pharm Eng 2009;29(3): 50–55.
3. International Standards Organization, ISO 14644-1,2,3,4,5,6,7. Cleanroom Classification and Separative Enclosures.

20 Process simulation for advanced aseptic processing

James Agalloco and James Akers

INTRODUCTION

Aseptic processing is acknowledged as one of the most, if not "the most" critical process challenge within the global healthcare industry. Technological improvements in this area have raised performance capabilities substantially over the years (1). Significant improvements in aseptic processing capability had already occurred prior to the introduction of the latest technologies for aseptic processing such as isolators, restricted access barrier systems (RABS), closed transfer systems for aseptic connection, and closed vial technology. The wider adoption of these technologies will improve the safety of aseptically produced materials to levels unattainable in the past. The traditional means for evaluation of an aseptic process is the process simulation test or media fill. These tests are conducted periodically to demonstrate the capabilities of the aseptic practices, and controls. This chapter reviews methods for the assessment of performance where the newer technologies available are employed.

The preparation of products labeled sterile often requires that firms use aseptic processing, as there are many formulations, devices or delivery systems where terminal sterilization is incompatible with the finished product. The inherent and largely unavoidable risks associated with the use of aseptic processing are widely recognized; regulators and practitioners across the globe acknowledge that aseptic processing should only be used where lethal treatments are not possible, or where a labile product delivery system offers safety advantages at the point of administration. A lethal process directed at final containers is always preferable to one that relies on the uncertain exclusion of microorganism as a final product is assembled from a number of previously sterilized materials. As aseptic processing ordinarily requires activities be performed by personnel, there is the additional concern for introduction of human-borne microbial contamination. The regulatory preference for terminal sterilization has been formalized by both US Food and Drug Administration (FDA) and European Medicines Agency (EMA) (2–4). Regrettably, although the expectation and intent is that terminal sterilization will be used wherever possible, there are a variety of materials where aseptic processing is currently the only possible means for preparation, that is, sterile bulk antibiotics, freeze-dried formulations, most (but not all) biological products, and materials without sufficient unbound moisture (a minimum of approximately 3%).[1] For the production of these types of products, aseptic processing is the only current methodology available.

Manufacturers and regulators must recognize that aseptic processing cannot be evaluated parametrically. No amount of physical measurements, microbial, or particle monitoring can definitively establish whether an aseptic process is suitable. This fundamental limitation has greatest significance in the "validation" of aseptic processing. As there is no means to directly establish the successful outcome of any aseptic process, it cannot be "validated" in the sense that an autoclave can. The literature may be ripe with references to "validation of aseptic processing" however, all that has ever been demonstrated by a satisfactory media fill is the capability for successful operation at that point in time. A media fill with zero contaminated units does not prove sterility of the test articles to say nothing of production lots made the day before (or the day after). Although rarely discussed, the sensitivity of a media fill test is unknown but certainly unlikely to be one microorganism even if we were to consider only the organisms that could grow in the broad spectrum media used. So, although sometimes considered as a means of measuring sterility assurance, in reality media fills do nothing of the kind.

[1] The authors' personal experience supports this level; however, it must be determined on an individual formulation basis for moist heat terminal sterilization. Terminal sterilization by radiation or gas does not have a comparable limitation on moisture content.

Aseptic processing has historically been a rather uncertain method, subtle variations in operator practice can profoundly affect the result, and yet there are no ready means to detect, or eliminate those variations. Nevertheless, firms endeavour to "validate" aseptic processing on a regular basis. Awareness is growing that process simulations demonstrate little more than the capability of the firm's facility, practices, operating procedures, and personnel on that day. That "validation" of the aseptic process is expected represents a misinterpretation of the information that a process simulation or any of the data obtained from the process can provide. The advanced aseptic processing technologies described in this book will reduce (and in the future virtually eliminate) the uncertainty that has been a feature of manned clean room aseptic processing. However, these advances will not make measurement of performance easier, quite to the contrary they will further strain the already insufficient sensitivity and limits of detection of available process control and monitoring methodology.

SCOPE

The focus of this chapter is on the unique considerations associated with aseptic processing for finished pharmaceuticals including process design and process simulation with emphasis on various advanced aseptic processing technologies. The reader should consult the more extensive treatment provided elsewhere on the many background considerations in support of aseptic processing (5).

BUILDINGS AND FACILITIES

The aseptic production of sterile products is performed in classified environments supplied with HEPA-filtered air. The classification of the environments used for aseptic processing varies with the criticality of the specific activity being performed. Any assembly of sterile materials should be conducted in ISO 5 environments that have been treated to essentially eliminate the background microbial count. Although manned clean rooms, RABS and isolators all incorporate theoretically identical ISO 5 environments, from a microbial contamination control perspective their capabilities are different. EMA and FDA have adopted Grade A/B approach on top of ISO 5 that may actually add confusion rather than clarification. Given the limitations of microbial recovery and growth methodology in any of the present day ISO 5 aseptic processing environments, we are loath to consider microbial levels as a meaningful means for discrimination.[2] Less critical activities such as washing and component preassembly are carried out in ISO 7 environments where microbial control expectations are more relaxed. The microbial requirements for the various classifications are addressed later in this chapter.

Critical Area

The most important activities are carried out under ISO 5 environments in which environmental control measures have been taken to effectively control microbial contamination. This expectation encompasses every location where sterilized and/or depyrogenated components are exposed to the environment. In manned clean rooms, this is accomplished by disinfection of room and equipment surfaces with antimicrobial agents. Aseptic processing isolators are fogged or gassed with similar agents to accomplish the same objective. Depending upon the specific design of the equipment and facility unidirectional air may be provided within the critical area (or zone). Expectations for unidirectional airflow were established years ago when manned clean rooms were predominant. The transition to isolator-based filling has resulted in some questioning of the need for unidirectional air. The very first aseptic isolators successfully employed turbulent air systems, and although many newer designs incorporate unidirectional air there is no definitive proof that it is necessary at all. Certainly, disinfection is critical but the user should know that by and large it will play a secondary role to the proper control of personnel-released contamination that experience has taught us is by a wide margin the most prominent cause of media fill positives.

The primary objective in the various advanced aseptic processing technologies has been to reduce, or to the extent possible (which is growing with each passing year) eliminate the impact on personnel within the critical zone to the maximum extent possible. The presence of personnel within or proximate to the critical zone is recognized as the primary source of

[2] Chapter 23 of this book addresses this subject in substantially greater detail.

microbial contamination. Aseptic processing technologies have always endeavored to reduce the impact of personnel through a variety of means:

- Separation of personnel—Separative approaches dominated industry practice for many years. Aseptic gowning and partial barriers systems were introduced in the 1950s when the availability of HEPA filters resulted in the first clean rooms for aseptic processing. The most evolved of the currently available separative technologies is the open isolator for aseptic filling.
- Limiting personnel interaction—This entails technologies where automated equipment and/or robots perform many of the activities customarily executed by gowned personnel. The first examples of this were blow-fill-seal (BFS) and form-fill-seal (FFS) for aseptic filling. Other examples can be found in lyophilizer loading/unloading and other conventionally manual tasks. RABS with open-door interventions would be a less automated system operating under the same principles.
- Removal of personnel—In these designs, the aseptic process is conducted without direct personnel exposure. The first of these to become widely available was the closed isolator for sterility testing. Newer examples include closed vial filling and aseptic connection systems,
- Combinations of the above—Many of the newer aseptic processing technologies being introduced incorporate multiple elements from each of the preceding categories.

Supportive Clean Area

In manned clean rooms the area immediately surrounding the critical zone is nearly as important. The personnel required for operation of the equipment are present in this environment at all times, and as they must occasionally access the critical zone, preventing contamination on them is essential. This extends to corridors and gown rooms used for access and are ordinarily classified as ISO 5 as well. Comparable activities in a RABS system are conducted with the same expectation as for manned aseptic clean rooms with ISO 5 required if the doors are to be opened. The background environment surrounding an isolator is of substantially less importance due to the more certain separation between the critical zone and the environment where the personnel are located. Current regulatory expectations are for ISO 8 externally, but there is little evidence that external classification of any type provides any further risk abatement beyond the enclosure itself in aseptic processing.

Environments for Component Preparation

Activities prior to the sterilization/depyrogenation of materials are conducted in a variety of classifications. Once they are washed, items are protected by ISO 5 quality air until they are either wrapped or enter a sterilization/depyrogenation process. The preparations area proper is commonly defined as ISO 8. The background environment for compounding is almost universally ISO 7, with localized ISO 5 if necessary.

PERSONNEL TRAINING, QUALIFICATION, AND MONITORING

Personnel performance must be the focus of attention in aseptic processing. The operator is often required to perform precision activities (e.g., set-up of filling equipment from individual component parts) without introducing microorganisms to any of the product contact parts. That this can be accomplished on a consistent basis is a tribute to the skill of these employees as the gowned human operator is universally acknowledged to be ***the only significant source*** of microbial contamination and therefore controlling operator derived contaminants is *the* critical risk modality. The routine accomplishment of such actions without shedding bacteria is accomplished through careful attention to the precepts of aseptic technique. Aseptic technique is a loose assembly of practices originally conceived for laboratory manipulations; however, the principles are fully adaptable to aseptic processing of pharmaceuticals. Among the typical aseptic techniques intended to protect sterile materials form contamination by personnel are the following:

- Every surface of the gowned person is considered nonsterile.
- Never touch a sterile object with a nonsterile object.
- Never place a gloved hand over an open sterile container.
- Use a tool for every activity wherever possible.

Additional principles can be found in various microbiology texts and must be recognized as suggestions rather than hard rules, and of course must be adapted to the specific circumstances of the equipment and materials being handled. The reader must understand that there is no such thing as a "sterile" room and that operators no matter how carefully they are qualified and supervised in gowning remain a consistent source of contamination. They are indeed best thought of as mobile contamination generators whose rate of release increases proportional to activity (6).

The operators who work in advanced aseptic processing must still be cognizant of the basic principles of microbiology, sterilization, disinfection, aseptic technique, gowning practices as well as details of their assigned tasks. Training of personnel should include both classroom session and practicums in which their ability to perform the required procedures or other similar tasks can be evaluated. Training should be near continuous and of course the media fill (process simulation) is perhaps the ultimate evaluation of the operators' proficiency. As with almost any activity in our industry, the aseptic training program should be well documented.

Personnel should be monitored upon exit from the aseptic core, as sampling during the process itself risks residual media on gown or glove surfaces that can prove disastrous to the aseptic process as they could aid the survival of microorganisms shed by the sampled individual. Sampling at the end of the process addresses the potentially weakened integrity of the gowning system after a lengthy and perhaps rigorous period in the aseptic core. However, the reader is cautioned that the recovery of microorganisms from an operator does not mean product was at risk and the recovery of no organisms in sampling does not mean that product is surely free of contamination risk. Monitoring results have real scientific meeting only when looked at over time so that patterns can (if present) emerge. Routine monitoring on exit typically focuses on the operator's gloves and forearms, as these are often closest to the sterile materials. Gowning certification is a usual prerequisite for entry into the aseptic core and ordinarily entails sampling of many more surfaces (7). Monitoring requirements for personnel in isolators is generally restricted to gloves impression taken at the conclusion of the process, as gown surfaces are not present.

Many advanced aseptic processing technologies are focused on either reduction of personnel participation or their complete elimination from the process. Because the safest intervention is the one that is avoided, automated systems are increasingly preferred. The goal of advanced aseptic process technologies is to eliminate direct contact between gowned personnel and sterile materials/surfaces

MATERIALS, COMPONENTS, AND CONTAINER/CLOSURES

The sterilization and/or depyrogenation of components and materials used in the aseptic process can be performed using any of the many methods available: steam, dry heat, radiation, gas, or filtration. With respect to the aseptic process, it is essential that whatever sterilization method is selected, that it be validated to attain a minimum probability of a non-sterile unit (PNSU) of 1×10^{-6}. An important consideration is the selection of a package configuration that allows for adequate sterilization, yet affords adequate protection of the sterilized materials until ready for use in the process. The maximum time interval between sterilization and production use of the materials (other than the process solution itself) is established in conjunction with the execution of the process simulation by using materials that have been held for the maximum specified time period.

TIME LIMITS

Time limits are imposed to minimize the duration of the aseptic process to reduce the risk of microbial contamination. Time is an important consideration for a variety of reasons:

- Operator fatigue could potentially result in poorer adherence to required technique. It should be noted that fatigue, to the extent that it plays a role in aseptic risk, is very well mitigated by the use of separative technologies that more directly eliminate human contamination risk.
- Extended use of gowning material can lead to their failure/compromise.
- Microbial counts in prefiltration solution can increase during hold periods resulting in either filtration issues and/or pyrogen concerns.

Process duration related to operator fatigue is easily factored into the aseptic process simulation (see the following section), whereas that associated with microbial growth in the formulation is product specific and must be addressed in the validation of the formulation. There is no evidence to support an increase in microbial population within an aseptic environment and given the absence of nutrients and moisture, the potential for microbial proliferation in these extremely clean locations should be considered minimal.

ASEPTIC PROCESS SIMULATION

There is a widespread misunderstanding that aseptic processing can be validated such that a defined sterility assurance level can be claimed. This belief is unsupportable. As aseptic processing ordinarily entails the participation of personnel to perform some portion of the process, variability in personnel performance limits the certainty with which the process can be considered. A successful media fill on a particular day affords no added confidence in the same procedure performed the next day during a production lot. Process simulations establish that the methods and practices are capable of success; they cannot support that materials produced using identical methods are sterile to the same extent under different circumstances. The oft-cited sterility assurance level (SAL) of 1×10^{-3} for aseptic processing is nothing of the sort, it is merely the established maximum projected contamination rate associated with the successful filling of 3000 media units (8). In the intervening years, firms have produced media fills in excess of 100,000 filed units. If such a large fill were devoid of contamination, the firm might be tempted to claim a SAL of greater than 1×10^{-5} for their operations. Any SAL claim for aseptic processing based upon media filling is without basis, all that is known is the contamination rate of the units filled that day.

The sole use of a media fill is to demonstrate that under the specific circumstances of an individual simulation that the facility is suitable for use in aseptic processing. The inability to consistently achieve the expected result—zero growth in any of the filled containers—is an indication that the process is perhaps overly risky (3,9). Nevertheless it must be recognized that a process simulations ordinarily represent "worst-case" challenges of the process in that the increase in interventional frequency associated with media fills and absence of process inherent characteristics (i.e., bacterial inhibition by the formulation) should increase the potential for microbial contamination in the media filled containers relative to a production batch. Industry surveys have established that nearly 10% of all media fills evidence some contamination (10). Provided that the level of contamination remains at low levels within the expected acceptance criteria it should not be considered problematic. The identification of a single positive in a media fill should only rarely trigger a full-blown investigation into the source of the contamination as the incidence rate is within expectations and absolute resolution of the contamination source is well nigh impossible.

Study Rationale and Design

Before embarking on an initial media fill program (and periodically thereafter) the firm should prepare a study rationale outlining how its program supports the capabilities of its aseptic operations. For a single-product facility, this can be quite easy to prepare as the permutations of lot size, fill volume, fill speed, container–closure, and other process details are likely to be rather limited. In those facilities where each filling line produces a variety of products, the possibilities can increase substantially. The study rationale should provide justification for each filling line indicating how the chosen process simulation studies performed support the product permutations filled on that line. The rationale should be reviewed periodically to insure its appropriateness consistent with any changes in products, components, practices, or equipment that could alter the circumstances. Provided below are some of the more common considerations and choices to be made in developing this rationale.

Media Sterilization

Although it may at first appear unusual the sterilization of the media is not a meaningful concern. The media due to its differing formulation from the product(s) being simulated may be more confidently sterilized by using a different means than the product(s). Provided that it is introduced into the sterilized system by using identical methods and equipment it can be presterilized by steam, alternative filters and even radiation. The intent of the process simulation is to confirm the acceptability of the processing procedures with sterilized equipment not to validate the sterilization of the product by the filtration system. Validation of the sterilizing filtration must be carried out for each formulation and the ability of the filtration system to sterilize the media is irrelevant to that product by product validation. At the same time, the media used in the simulation must be sterile for a valid challenge of the aseptic process, but proof of that sterilization is relevant only to the media process and nothing more.

Frequency and Number of Runs

The initial media fills for a facility are defined in the study rationale and is normally at least three trials per filling line. In larger facilities, making a variety of presentations the number of initial studies required may increase commensurably. Once the baseline capability has been established, a minimum of two fills per line per year is considered current good manufacturing practice (3,11). The conduct of additional media fills may be useful for a variety of reasons, that is, environmental contamination due to an unique event (power loss, water leakage, major breach of asepsis; substantial change in the equipment, processes, components, etc.; adverse environmental trend; or sterility test failure) (3).

Although it is certainly preferable to await definitive results from a 14-day incubation period (and satisfactory growth promotion), there is no obligation to do so (7). There are firms that conduct their media fills just prior to shutdowns as confirmation of capability at the end of a long operating period and take advantage of overlapping the incubation and shutdown periods. Other firms conduct their media fills immediately after their shutdown period as demonstration of renewed capability, including any minor changes to the facility or equipment. For those firms that conduct process simulation postshutdown practices also vary in relation to whether definitive results are awaited prior to the start of production operations.

It should be possible to reduce the frequency and sample size of process simulation studies for advanced aseptic processing systems that rely on automation/robotics for the critical activities. With proper calibration and maintenance, there is no reason to expect changes in proficiency as might be encountered with personnel over extended periods.

Duration of Runs

The seemingly best answer to the required minimum duration of a media fill is that it should exceed the duration of the longest routine filling process and this is oft cited by regulators (3). Although that approach may seem the soundest it presents some substantial problems for those firms making very large lot sizes. The most comprehensive advice on this subject is provided in the Parenteral Drug Association's (PDA) TR#22, where recommendations for the complete range of process batch sizes are provided. The latest PDA document on this subject is based on 5000 unit media fills, adjustment of that value upwards to suit more contemporary expectations is perhaps the only change required to adapt the approach (12).

Very Small Batches—1000 $> N$

For batches of this size, which are common in certain clinical and radiopharmaceutical operations, a process simulation test at the maximum batch size is recommended. Forcing the production of 5000 or even 1000 units may produce situations so different from the normal operation that the results may be meaningless. For simulation of these batch sizes, the process simulation test must evidence no growth in any of the filled containers to be acceptable.

Small Batches—5000 $> N >$ 1000

For this batch size, which might be common for a clinical batch or other developmental situation, the minimum process simulation batch size should be equal to the standard maximum batch size. Although this does not afford the level of statistical confidence frequently associated with full process simulation tests, it is a reasonable compromise, given the limitations of the small batch size.

Batch Sizes—$N > 5000$

For these very common production-scale process, the number of units to be filled with medium should be as needed to demonstrate proficiency of personnel in execution of the aseptic process. The number filled need not be substantially greater than 5000. Current practice is to produce somewhat larger media fills to accommodate the required interventions into the simulation (7). Filling substantially more than 5000 units is of limited utility in advanced aseptic processing systems where personnel involvement is minimal,

What is almost universal in simulation design is that the fill is truly representative of the production process. Larger production fills force the media fill to reflect a duration that is a realistic representation of the production process. A lengthy process can neither be supported by a simulation that is over in less than an hour, nor is there any merit to a 4-hour minimum simulation duration for what might be ordinarily be a 2-hour fill session.

Where automation predominates in the aseptic production process as is increasingly common with the newer advanced technologies, considerations relative to the length of the process simulation become less significant. Machines and robots do not suffer from fatigue within the short context of an aseptic process. Once demonstrated as initially successful following decontamination and set-up for processing simulation provides little value over extended periods.

In-Process Media Fills

The conduct of a simulation supporting the production of large batches can be accomplished by in part by the performance of a media fill immediately after the completion of the production fill. The filling line is cleared of the last containers of the production batch, the liquid line is flushed to remove any traces of the product, a vessel of sterile media is connected to the line, and filling restarted with media into the same components used for the production fill. Alternatively, the product contact parts used for the product can be replaced with a freshly sterilized set of parts. The other aspects of the simulation are essentially unchanged from the other practices described in this chapter. The results of the media fill must be considered in the lot release decision for the production lot.

In-process media fills are particularly useful in the support of large batches as their successful execution at the end of a long production batch can support that even under the adverse environmental conditions expected after the production that successful aseptic filling can occur. The use of in-process media fills as the sole means of supporting aseptic processing is uncertain, as the impact of the ordinarily highly manipulative system assembly is deemphasized by the time period between the initial set-up and the in-process fill execution. The potential for flush out or inhibition of any set-up related microorganisms by the product being filled must be considered as well.

Line Speed

Supporting the full capabilities of a filling line used for different containers is easily accomplished. Filling lines will often operate at a variety of speeds with smaller fill volumes associated with higher filling rates, a consequence of the smaller volume being dispensed into each container. One set of media fills for a line should use the smallest container operating at the highest speed as this may present the greatest handling difficulty the line may encounter. As handling difficulty is associated with an expected greater need for human intervention in either routine or corrective activity then this is an obvious "worst-case" selection for the process simulation program. The largest container filled at the slowest speed presents the greatest opportunity for airborne contamination to enter from above and is often selected as the other "worst-case" extreme for filling systems.

Container/Component Selection

The largest and smallest containers are often chosen as they represent the extremes of either exposure duration or handling difficulty, but other selections may be appropriate. Consider small vials of similar diameter such as 1-, 2-, and 3-mL units. The 3 mL due to its higher center of gravity may present more of a handling difficulty its smaller companions, and thus might be a more suitable choice for use in the process simulation. Similarly, the elastomeric closure chosen for use should be the one that presents similar handling concerns. Recognition that excessive handling represents the greatest contamination potential may result in a simulation regimen that includes more than the obvious choices of largest and smallest containers.

There have been regulatory recommendations to replace opaque containers with clear one to aid in the detection of contaminants postincubation (3). That is an accepted practice provided the removal of the coloring agent or wrapping does not alter the material handling characteristics of the container, in which case the opaque container is preferable despite the added inspectional difficulties (see later section).

The availability of closed vial technologies may dramatically alter concerns with respect to container/closure handling and reduce the number of trials and units to be filled. Similarly, neck-hold approaches and other automation may eliminate the component handling concerns associated with smaller containers.

Media Fill Volume

In the execution of a media fill, the amount of media filled in the container can be modified from that ordinarily filled. The media amount is ordinarily reduced to extend the duration of the fill with a limited media quantity (media quantity is sometimes limited by sterilization constraints on the media that can restrict the maximum amount available for use). There is no minimum media volume that need be used provided the following: there is adequate media to contact the entire sealing surface; there is sufficient media to allow for detection of growth; and there is sufficient media to pass growth promotion. In a few instances the volume filled in the container has been adjusted upwards by firms from that typically used in the container to address one or more of the concerns cited.

Media Selection

Selecting the test media to be used is at the core of the simulation process, and in the vast majority of cases is accomplished by the use of soybean casein digest medium (SCDM). This general purpose media is the usual choice because of its ability to support the growth of a variety of aerobic environmental and human-derived organisms. In only very limited instances is another media appropriate.

> A firm with persistent low level microbial contamination in its inventoried products never detected microbial contamination in media fills that utilized SCDM. When media fills were performed with media that resembled its product substrate were conducted the contamination source was identified. (J. Agalloco, personal communication, 1994)

Anaerobes/Inert Gassing

Expectations that media fills address anaerobic contamination are only appropriate in limited situations. True anaerobic conditions are not attainable in manned clean rooms even where inert gassing is used. Low percentages of oxygen are toxic to true anaerobes and thus anaerobic media fills using fluid thioglycollate media (FTM) are largely unnecessary.

In ordinary media fills, to facilitate microbial recovery air is often substituted for the inert gas on the filling line. This practice hopes to eliminate the potential microbial inhibition that the inert gas might impact aerobic organisms that might find there way into the gas distribution system during poststerilization assembly (7).

Typical headspace oxygen concentrations are in the range of 1% to 3%, which is perhaps all that is attainable in a clean room operation. When using an isolator, it is possible to attain much lower oxygen headspace concentrations. Closed isolators can be filled with the inert gas, allowing for attainment of essentially zero oxygen in the container headspace. In this type of a process, true anaerobes may be present, and media fills should be performed using FTM to detect the presence of these organisms. This differs from the practices in manned clean rooms where air replaces the inerting gas as true anaerobic conditions cannot be attained, and thus the use of FTM and an inert gas is inappropriate.

Manual Filling

In the preparation of small-scale lots there is often a heavy reliance on personnel to perform many of the functions provided by a filling line, that is, container movement, closure placement, seal administration, etc. The operator essentially replaces some or all of the filling equipment required for the process. In this instance, each operator assigned to this process should perform triplicate initial and semiannual repeat media fills to demonstrate their aseptic processing proficiency.

From an advanced aseptic processing technology perspective, the only acceptable modes for manual processing of any type would be those performed in an isolator setting.

Aseptic Assembly

The execution of an aseptic process will often necessitate some preparation steps to configure the equipment and materials. The most apparent task of this type is the set-up/assembly of the fill line from individually sterilized components into a complete line ready for the fill. Adjustment of conveyor, limit switches, vibratory feeders, and perhaps the fluid material pathway may all be a part of this activity. The aseptic process begins with these steps and they must be performed and evaluated with the same care devoted to the process itself. These activities are an inherent part of the process simulation, as the equipment must undergo the same preparatory steps, nevertheless observation of these activities, and environmental monitoring must be incorporated.

Environmental Monitoring

The aseptic processing environment used for the aseptic process should be monitored in accordance with the routine program used for the operation of the facility. The temptation to increase the monitoring during the media fill should be resisted as it may have an adverse affect on the results of the simulation. Environmental monitoring, especially microbial sampling must be recognized as an intervention in the aseptic core, and increasing above normal levels may result in the introduction of microbial contamination that might not otherwise be introduced. Expanded sampling of the surfaces postfilling may be useful in identifying/confirming that the appropriate locations are being used during monitoring of the production.[3] The conduct of environmental sampling must be recognized as an intervention, and there must be a balance between the desire to gather information about the conditions proximate to the sterile materials, and the potential introduction of microbial contamination as a consequence of the human presence required to obtain that information. There is "no free lunch"; the gathering of environmental data must not risk product sterility.

Product Contact

As media-filled units are removed from the fill line, they should be manipulated to ensure there is contact between the media and the container–closure seal surfaces. Physical contact between the media and the seal surfaces insure that those surfaces of the container that are more vulnerable to contamination during the process are properly assessed. For syringes and ampules, incubation of the media-filled containers can be performed in a random orientation to maximize the contact between media and the sealing surfaces. Vials are generally inverted briefly prior to incubation (and mid-way through the incubation period if there is a 7-day inspection of the units). Some firms have chosen to invert vials during incubation but that is not a universal practice (7).

New Facilities and Lines

The start of operations in an aseptic facility must be supported by initial simulation studies that establish the capability of the facility, equipment, procedures, and personnel to manufacture sterile products (3). Depending on the specific circumstances of the products being manufactured the number of required media fills may be as few as three; as line complexity/capability increases this may entail additional studies. These studies can ordinarily be matrixed to reduce the overall number; however, even if the facility has lines comprising identical components, each line must be evaluated independently of the others.

Suspensions and Aseptic Manufacturing

The process simulation should embrace all portions of the aseptic process from the point of sterilization through closure of the container. All of the interventions (sampling, filter integrity

[3] This practice has minimal utility in isolators and environments where personnel are excluded.

testing, etc.), which are a portion of the formulation process must be included in the simulation. The vessel used for the media fill should be identical to that used for commercial operations—the use of a carboy for the media fill where the commercial product uses a stainless steel vessel is inappropriate. This can prove more challenging where the formulation includes aseptic steps such as required in the preparation of suspensions, ointments, and other more complex products (3). These processes may require extensive sterilization in place (SIP) and complex equipment, and thus present some unique issues in the design of the simulation. The practices originally designed for sterile bulk can be adapted for use in these instances (13). In some instances, the simulation process may require the use of a sterile solid (generally a placebo material) in portions of the simulation (see following section).

In the preparation of suspensions and many less common aseptically produced sterile products and containers, overlapping simulations addressing the overall process may be appropriate with some portions of the simulation being largely conducted using a sterile powder and the remainder with a sterile liquid media. This is acceptable practice provided the entire process is covered by overlapping where one part of the simulation ends and another begins.

Sterile Powders

Sterile powder processing and filling presents a unique difficulty in the conduct of the simulation as the equipment used for powder processing cannot easily accommodate the liquid media ordinarily used for the simulation. In the majority of instances, execution of the process simulation will require the addition of both sterile liquid media and a sterile powder placebo to the container. The order of the additions and the extent to which the powder filling process is adapted to accommodate the liquid fill can make this one of the more difficult simulations to execute. PDA's TR #22 provides a description of the processing options. TR #28 also from PDA provides considerations in the selection and preparation of the sterile placebo powder (13). As liquid filling on a powder line is an infrequent event, some firms choose to fill a number of liquid only containers in conjunction with the powder fill to establish that this activity is not the cause of any detected contamination. As the sterilizing filtration for sterile powders may be conducted in a separate facility (or by a separate firm), simulation concerns at the filling site are generally restricted to the activities performed there including milling and blending as appropriate.

Other Aseptic Filled Dosage Forms and Formulations

Process simulation studies are required wherever aseptic processing is used for the manufacture of sterile drugs. The base case for all simulations is the solution fill and adaptations to that situation are added to accommodate the equipment and processes used for other products. Some of the modifications are quite simple, (the incorporation of a freeze dryer, or filling into a plastic tube) whereas others may introduce substantial complications (a multichambered syringe with a lyophilized powder with liquid diluent or a liposome formulation requiring extensive pre filling processing). The added complexity of these more intricate processes may entail modifications to permit simulation and thus increase the potential for failure. Nevertheless, their association with simple solution filling precludes the use of looser acceptance criteria reflecting the difficulties associated with the simulation. There are instances where process simulation of the types described here for pharmaceuticals have been adapted for the aseptic preparation of medical devices albeit sometimes with even greater modification to accommodate their rather different processing requirements.

Campaign Production

The campaign filling of a series of batches without intervening cleaning/sanitization (and in rare instances sterilization of all product contact equipment such as stoppers bowls) is a common practice for some large-volume sterile products. The use of campaigns in which a series of batches is produced following sterilization, with or without intermediate cleaning, is increasingly common with BFS/FFS and isolation technology. Typically for campaign operation only limited cleaning would be performed between lots of the campaign. Decontamination of the system environment and/or removal, cleaning, and sterilization of filling parts is not normally performed between batches. However, product pathway clean in place/sterilization in place (CIP/SIP) and filter changes may be performed between production lots.

In campaign modes the following situations may be possible and supportable in appropriately designed aseptic process simulations:

- Multiple product lots of the same formulation can be manufactured.
- Configuration/fill volume may change during the campaign.
- Campaign lengths substantially greater than one day are attainable.
- There is the potential to change the product formulation if cleaning and re-sterilization of delivery system can be performed aseptically.
- Production may not be continuous over the time period (days or shifts without production are possible.

Initial and periodic demonstration of campaign duration (total time or batches) should be based on an assessment of the operational elements. This is an appropriate activity to use risk-management approaches.

Interventions

The production of sterile products in either manned clean rooms or isolators relies on the execution of any number of manual tasks by the operator. These interventions are either inherent or corrective in nature. An inherent intervention is one that is either an integral part of the process (i.e., set-up of the equipment, initial supply/replenishment of components, etc.) or required procedurally (i.e., product sampling, environmental monitoring, fill weight adjustment, etc.) Corrective interventions are performed in response to errors or problems such as container–closure jams or missfeeds, or other mechanical problem with the equipment. The inclusion of inherent interventions in process simulations is relatively simple; by following the standard operating practices for the process they would be included at the same frequency, as they would occur during a production lot. Corrective interventions must be integrated into the media fill in the event they do not occur as a natural consequence of the process, and the frequency should match the incidence in the production process. As was noted earlier, the extent of the interventions required whether inherent or corrective is an important consideration in the selection of the appropriate components and process to be simulated. Practices for all intervention should be carefully defined to insure consistency between routine production and simulated operations (14).

The most importance aspect of interventions is their proper design and execution. First and foremost is the awareness that the best intervention is the one that is not performed at all. The aseptic process should be designed to eliminate interventions (inherent or corrective) of all kinds, or at the very least minimize the need for their execution. The premium paid for more uniform components, higher quality equipment, and preventive maintenance is well spent if it results in more reliable filling. Preassembly of components prior to sterilization, leave behind samples and careful attention of equipment design can eliminate interventions that can impact asepsis completely.

The use of isolators or RABS may require that human manipulations be performed using the gloves installed on the enclosure. These manipulations mimic those that are required in manned clean rooms and should be performed with the same considerations for aseptic technique that must be practiced in that environment. That the isolator or RABS has been decontaminated, and effectively removes the operator from the aseptic environment does not eliminate the need to operate in an aseptic manner. Although these technologies are highly capable, they should not be considered "perfect" and some small potential for residual contamination exists. As gloves may have minuscule leaks, the opportunity for contamination is ever present just as it is in any other aseptic process.

Aseptic interventions unique to isolators and RABS are those relating to the transfer systems used to connect an isolator or RABS to either an isolator or container. These connections are typically made to allow for the transfer of materials into the enclosure in conjunction with the execution of the aseptic process. Where the usage of the RTP system mimics that of routine operation, there is no need to augment the process simulation with additional transfers.

Automated systems and robotics are an increasingly common element in advanced aseptic processing designs. They offer the opportunity to dramatically reduce in number, if not completely eliminate all manned interventions, including those that are inherent as well as those that are corrective.

Execution of the Process Simulation

The process simulation should be performed following a defined procedure outlining the various requirements beginning with the sterilization of the media. The use of a batch record as least as detailed as that used for production filling is recommended; however, it may be necessary to supplement this to adequately document the interventions included during the process. The time of execution for the interventions should be recorded, and if possible correlated to a specific portion of the filled units for use in problem resolution. An observer positioned outside the critical area (and preferably outside the aseptic area) can provide a level of documentation well beyond that of the aseptic operator(s) without risking contamination. Firms have found the use of videotape beneficial in media fill execution as it can capture substantially more detail than an observer (the simultaneous use of videotape and an observer/supervisor has also been used); however, in some jurisdictions labor laws may preclude the recording of operators at their jobs.

Initial Inspection of Filled Containers

It is customary to inspect the media-filled units immediately after sealing and prior to incubation to remove nonintegral containers from the test units to be incubated. Nonintegral containers should not be incubated and their removal prior to incubation avoids the unanswerable and inevitable later question when a nonintegral container is found contaminated postincubation (15). The temptation to discount nonintegral contaminated units must be resisted, as there is no means to establish whether the container was originally nonintegral prior to incubation. Once a container has passed this initial inspection, any contamination detected must be counted against the simulation as these units are intended to represent materials that would be released for distribution. Integral containers that would otherwise be rejected for cosmetic defects (i.e., particle in solution, fibers, marks on container, etc.) are not culled in this preliminary inspection, as their removal in a postfill inspection is not certain and thus they represent potentially marketed units. The number of units placed into the incubator should be accurately determined.

Incubation Time and Temperature

At one time this was among the more controversial and variable practices were in effect at many firms (7,16). The approaches included incubation at multiple temperatures with transfer from one to another after 7 days of incubation. There was even confusion as to whether it was preferable to begin at a higher temperature (30–35°C) followed by a lower temperature (20–25°C) or begin the incubation at the lower temperature and then move to the higher one. Recognition that growth promotion is required regardless of the actual conditions selected, has led to a more broadly defined practice where the incubation temperature can range from 20°C to 35°C including a single temperature for the entire 14-day period (3). Provided the selected temperature is uniform (the usual range is ± 2.5°C) the use of a single-incubation temperature eases the execution of the media fill and coupled with satisfactory growth promotion results is appropriate. This practice allows for flexibility of approach thereby accommodating the greatest potential for microbial recovery.

Postincubation Examination of Media-Filled Units

After conclusion of the incubation (currently 14-day incubation is almost universal) the containers are carefully inspected to detect microbial contamination. This inspection can ordinarily be performed by trained personnel with a qualified microbiologist present to support the selection process. Microbiologists may be preferable for the entire inspection where the media must be removed from opaque containers, as might be the case with plastic tubes or other difficult to inspect items. Units that are suspected to be contaminated are counted and set aside for further evaluation. The total number of units inspected should be recorded.

A preliminary inspection is sometimes employed part way through the incubation period to allow for an early assessment and is used by some firms as support for the commencement of aseptic filling at risk pending the final results.

Growth Promotion

Upon conclusion of the incubation, sterile units are selected randomly from the filled units and individual units are inoculated with less than 100 cfu/container of selected microorganisms. The usual choices for these microorganisms are those identified in the United States Pharmacopiea/European Pharmacopiea (USP/EP) for the verification of media efficacy, plus some additional microorganism(s) of the firm's choice. Where microorganisms are added to the panel they are usually selected from common environmental isolators not already represented in the compendial panel or isolated in sterility test failures. The inoculated units are incubated at the same conditions as the test units and must demonstrate satisfactory growth in a limited timeframe, typically 2 to 3 days.

Firms would prefer to select units at random immediately after filling and use those in a concurrent growth promotion test in an effort to shorten the timeframe to obtain definitive results; however, regulators frown on this practice as potentially obscuring contamination that might be in the units randomly selected for the growth promotion. Given the low incidence of contaminated unit observed in contemporary media fills such caution hardly seems justified, nevertheless growth promotion is generally performed postincubation (7,11).

Microbial Identification

Where positive units are detected in the postincubation inspection they should be identified to the extent necessary for investigational purposes. Although the majority of any microbial contamination can be expected to be human derived, microbial identification can in some cases provide additional information that can be helpful in investigating media fill failures. Correlation of the microbial identification information to the environmental monitoring during the simulation can also prove useful, but given the low level of contamination seen in modern systems this is rarely the case. In advanced aseptic systems environmental monitoring/media fill correlation is unlikely to be of significance. Regardless of what information is gathered about the microorganism, the objective in the identification is to identify the source although generally such insights are limited and only of a general nature.

Accountability

The media fill endeavors to establish that the contamination rate for filled units is less than the firm's acceptance value. Counting the number of positives found postincubation is generally easy given the generally successful results observed. In a recent survey, nearly 90% of all media fills were reported as being devoid of contamination (10). Some aggressive FDA inspectors have raised concerns that unless the accountability of filled units is 100%; missing units must be considered as positives. That perspective seems overly conservative, and accountability for the media fill that is comparable to that of a similar sized production fill should be considered acceptable.

Acceptance Criteria

Selection of an acceptance criterion for process simulation is the province of the regulatory agency. For many years the standard of acceptance for media fill contamination rate was a criterion of not more than 0.1% (11,17). When the first written guidance was published no statistical treatment was provided (18). Over the years, aspects of statistical confidence following a Poisson distribution were added (19,20). Use of a Poisson distribution was considered appropriate as it was believed that microbial contamination in media fills was a random occurrence associated with a variety of possible causes. This expectation reached its zenith in publications that appeared at then end of last century in which the statistical treatment included alert and action levels for the evaluation of aseptic processes (21,22). This approach seemed inappropriate given the growing realization that environmental contamination recovered from aseptic clean rooms (and media fills as well) is predominantly derived from the human operator, and thus is likely to be associated with operator activities rather than a random source. This perspective was first voiced in PDA's TR#22, where the limitations of statistical treatment were addressed. The use of statistics allows a number of contaminated units (9 in 15,710) that is less than 0.1% of the number of units filled. Approached in this manner an aseptic process capable of slightly less than 0.1% contamination rate would be considered acceptable (under investigation certainly, but acceptable nevertheless). This realization led to changed expectations in newer regulatory guidance in which a target of zero contamination as the goal of every aseptic process as first defined by PDA is included (23,24). The latest regulatory word on acceptance criteria for aseptic processing is that provided by FDA in its Guideline on Sterile Drug Products Produced by Aseptic Processing that extends the most recent thinking and takes it a bit further (3). This guidance has a goal of zero contamination, but accepts no more than one contaminated unit in either 5000 or 10,000 units (the document can be interpreted to require either). The authors believe an acceptance criterion with a fixed low percentage of contaminated units (0.02% or NMT one in 5000 units, two in 10,000, etc.) might be more useful as it doesn't penalize firms that produce larger lots and consequently use larger media fills.

IMPLICATIONS OF RESULTS FOR ASEPTIC FILLING

When the results of the media fill are available, there is certainly no issue when all of the filled containers are free of microbial contamination. Given that microbial contamination is almost always human derived, contaminated units may provide insight into potential sources if they are associated with an intervention. In the absence of linkage to an intervention, any investigative effort is likely to be inconclusive. Nevertheless, an investigation is mandated when any contaminated units are detected, as it is a regulatory expectation (3,12). It has been common for correlations to be made between a media fill outcome and product manufactured prior to or after that fill. Actually, there is no scientific or statistical reason to believe that a media fill result above the acceptance criteria means that product made prior to or after the fill should be called into question any more than a contamination-free media fill means that contamination risk was zero in each lot produced. Historically, the view has been that each media fill is merely a snapshot in time and that in manned systems, contamination, although better controlled in modern systems, remains an ever-present possibility. Sometimes contamination is detected and other times it is not, but this may relate more to analytical sensitivity and variability than to process control. Advanced aseptic processes rarely result in process simulation growth as human contamination is so much better controlled.

Certainly, investigations should be done when a positive container is observed. However, such investigations may not result in a clear assignable cause. In fact, this is to be expected given the limited information available for investigation. It is important to be cautious in one's zeal to determine an assignable cause; it is quite easy to jump to a conclusion regarding cause. It does more harm to assign a flimsy cause with only the most tenuous link to performance than to merely accept that manned clean rooms are not sterile and that contamination can arise at any time and sometimes that contamination is detectable.

Placebo Materials

Where a placebo material is required in the process simulation as is necessary in suspension or bulk powder processes, a placebo is commonly used. The selection of the placebo is a compromise between a number of factors: that is, ease of sterilization, handling properties similar to the production materials, ease of clean-up, lack of microbial inhibition, etc. PDA's TR #28 provides useful information on the selection of the placebo material (13). Regardless of the placebo material chosen for the simulation, the material should be packaged in an identical fashion as the materials they are substituting for. The sterilization of the placebo must be validated to ensure that it does not become a source of contamination in the simulation.

ENVIRONMENTAL MONITORING

A properly conducted process simulation incorporates environmental monitoring as performed during the routine process. Although, it may seem appropriate to increase the level of monitoring during the simulation that practice can result in increased contamination potential. Environmental monitoring entails the manipulation of materials and equipment in proximity (or within) to the critical zone where sterile products (and media) are present. These activities can introduce microorganisms to the materials being processed and should not be increased above routine levels during the simulation. Postprocess monitoring in the form of increased surface or air samples may prove useful, and as the process is complete do not increase risk. Suggestions that routine monitoring be increased after detection of microorganisms in a media fill should be resisted for the same reason.

ADVANCED ASEPTIC PROCESSING TECHNOLOGY

The successful conduct of an aseptic process relies on a number of individual activities each of which could contribute microorganisms and thus induce process failure. Some of these activities relate to the sterilization of materials, others to the facility design whereas a larger number are associated with the activities of the personnel performing them. Table 1 lists a number of tasks associated with aseptic processing and defines the relative ease of validation, personnel sensitivity (the extent to which variations in operator performance can influence the outcome of the task) and the overall impact on sterility assurance in manned clean rooms.

Recognition that personnel are the primary source of microbial contamination in aseptic processing is one of the major reasons for the introduction of isolators. The lower half of Table 1 highlights those activities in which personnel play the largest role, and consequently have the greatest potential for the introduction of contamination. Not only is the microbial contamination potential greater with these activities, but the variability of performance from operator to operator increases as well; the variability with the same operator from day to day is even greater than with those elements not closely related to human activity. Tables 2 and 3 show the same tasks are evaluated when performed in a closed RABS or isolator environment, respectively. If a RABS is opened whether for set-up, decontamination, or midprocess intervention, then the system is not a true RABS and the relative weights assigned above should prevail as the system is functionally still a manned clean room (this would be the case even where the background environment surrounding the RABS is ISO 5).

With aseptic processing conducted in closed RABS or isolators the overall impact of personnel on the sterility assurance of the materials being produced is reduced by their removal from the environment. This leads to the expected superior performance of these technologies for aseptic processing.

The use of isolators (or other advanced aseptic processing technology) alters very little in the conduct of process simulations from the perspective of current regulatory policy. All of the aspects and rationale considerations cited earlier are applicable essentially unchanged. FDA has indicated that isolators (and perhaps other advanced technologies) by virtue of their superior performance potential may be demonstrated capable using media fills of shorter duration than in conventional clean rooms (3). No further details on this were provided by FDA, and firms will have to define their practices in the study rationale.

Table 1 Impact of Personnel on Sterility Assurance in Manned Clean Rooms[a]

Task	Ease of validation	Personnel sensitivity	Impact on sterility assurance
Component sterilization	Easy	Low	Low
Product sterilization	Easy	Low	Low
Depyrogenation	Easy	Low	Low
Room design	N/A	None	Moderate
Nonviable monitoring	Easy	None	Low
Viable monitoring	Moderate	High	High
Room sanitization	Difficult	High	High
Gowning	Difficult	Very high	Very high
Materials transfer	Difficult	High	High
Aseptic assembly[b]	Difficult	Very high	Very high
Aseptic technique[c]	Difficult	Very high	Very high

[a]RABS designs that require "open-door" interventions would be considered similarly.
[b]The set-up of the equipment required for the process from the individually sterilized/depyrogenated items.
[c]The operation of the equipment for the aseptic process including both inherent and corrective interventions.

Table 2 Impact of Personnel on Sterility Assurance in Closed RABS

Task	Ease of validation	Personnel sensitivity	Impact on sterility assurance
Component sterilization	Easy	Low	Low
Product sterilization	Easy	Low	Low
Depyrogenation	Easy	Low	Low
RABS design	N/A	None	Moderate
Nonviable monitoring	Easy	None	Low
Viable monitoring	Moderate	Low	Low
RABS decontamination	Difficult	High	High
Gloves	N/A	None	Moderate
Materials transfer	Difficult	Low	Moderate
Aseptic assembly[a]	Difficult	Low	Moderate
Aseptic technique[b]	Difficult	Low	Moderate

[a]The set-up of the equipment required for the process from the individually sterilized/depyrogenated items.
[b]The operation of the equipment for the aseptic process including inherent and corrective interventions.

Table 3 Impact of Personnel on Sterility Assurance in Isolators

Task	Ease of validation	Personnel sensitivity	Impact on sterility assurance
Component sterilization	Easy	Low	Low
Product sterilization	Easy	Low	Low
Depyrogenation	Easy	Low	Low
Isolator design	N/A	None	Moderate
Nonviable monitoring	Easy	None	Low
Viable monitoring	Moderate	Low	Low
Isolator decontamination	Moderate	Low	Moderate
Gloves/half suits	N/A	None	Low
Materials transfer	Difficult	Low	Moderate
Aseptic assembly[a]	Difficult	Low	Moderate
Aseptic technique[b]	Difficult	Low	Moderate

[a]The set-up of the equipment required for the process from the individually sterilized/depyrogenated items.
[b]The operation of the equipment for the aseptic process including inherent and corrective interventions.

The ability to process a lengthy campaign in an isolator is highly desirable. The validation of campaign length uses methods similar to that employed for very large batches provided earlier in this chapter. In-process media fills are another means for the establishment of campaign length in isolators. PDA's TR#28 provides some useful guidance in means for the establishment of isolator integrity over the campaign duration.

CONCLUSION

Demonstration of aseptic processing proficiency as provided by media fills (process simulations) is an integrated exercise incorporating every aspect of the process. It has been a prominent component of aseptic processing compliance beginning in the 1980s. When first introduced to the industry it may have served a meaningful purpose; however, performance in even manned clean rooms has evolved to the point where its utility as an evaluation tool has begun to diminish. Performance of process simulation for advanced aseptic processing was an early expectation given that the ultimate process objective, sterility of the filled product containers, was identical. Industry performance in aseptic process simulation has improved substantially over the past 20 years indicating continual improvement in the safety of sterile products produced aseptically (1,7,10). Advanced aseptic processing systems afford the ability to take this performance to levels that cannot be readily assessed with the media fill. The limited available data on process simulation in advanced aseptic processing systems is so overwhelmingly successful, there seems little point to the entire exercise. The growing experience base with advanced aseptic processing suggests that just as with environmental monitoring, the process simulation has little real value once basic proficiency has been demonstrated. Control over aseptic processing in these systems may devolve to some advanced technology yet to be discovered under the guise of process analytical technologies. In the interim, process simulations for advanced aseptic processing will likely continue, until it is understood by all that we have reached a point where the results are little more than a foregone conclusion.

REFERENCES

1. Agalloco J, Akers J, Madsen R. Aseptic processing: a review of current industry practice. Pharm Technol 2004; 28(10):126–150.
2. FDA.Guidance to Industry for the Submission Documentation for Sterilization Process Validation in Applications for Human and Veterinary Drug Products, 1994.
3. FDA, Guideline on Sterile Drug Products Produced by Aseptic Processing, 2004.
4. EMEA. Decision Trees for the Selection of Sterilisation Methods (CPMP/QWP/054/98), 1998.
5. Agalloco J, Carleton F. Validation of Pharmaceutical Processes. New York: Informa, 2007.
6. Avallone H. FDA Field Investigator Training curriculum, circa 1985.
7. Current practices in the validation of aseptic processing—2001. PDA Technical Report # 36. PDA J Pharm Sci Technol 2002; 56(3 suppl).
8. Agalloco J, Akers J, Letter to the editor—re: apples, oranges and additive assurance. J Parenteral Sci Technol 1992; 46(1):2–3.
9. Process simulation testing for aseptically filled products. PDA Technical Report # 22. PDA J Pharm Sci Technol 1996; 50(suppl S1).
10. PQRI Aseptic Processing Working Group—Final Report—2002. Available at www.pqri.org/aseptic/imagespdfs/finalreport.pdf. Accessed May 14, 2010.
11. EU GMP Regulations, Annex 1. Manufacture of Sterile Medicinal Products, 1998.
12. Process Simulation Testing for Aseptically Filled Products. PDA Technical Report # 22. In process of revision, 2010.
13. Process simulation testing for sterile bulk pharmaceutical chemicals. PDA Technical Report # 28. PDA J Pharm Sci Technol 1998; 52(4), supplement.
14. PDA TB# 2003—02. Incubation of Intervention Units in Aseptic Process Simulation Tests (Media Fills), 2003.
15. PDA TB# 2003—01. Damaged Containers in Aseptic Process Simulation Tests (Media Fills), 2003.
16. Agalloco J, Gordon B. Current practices in the use of media fills in the validation of aseptic processing. J Parenteral Sci Technol 1987; 41(4):128–141.
17. FDA.Guideline on Sterile Drug Products Produced by Aseptic Processing, 1987.
18. WHO. Sterility and Sterility Testing of Pharmaceutical Preparations and Biological Substances. WHO/PHARM/73.474, 1973.
19. Validation of Aseptic Filling for Solution Drug Products. PDA Technical Monograph # 2. PDA, 1980.
20. Validation of Aseptic Drug Powder Filling Processes. PDA Technical Report # 6. PDA, 1984.
21. The Use of Process Simulation Tests in the Evaluation of Processes for the Manufacture of Sterile Products. Technical Monograph #4. The Parenteral Society, 1993.
22. ISO 13408—1. Sterilization of health care products—Aseptic processing—Part 1: General Requirements. International Standards Organization, 1998.
23. CEN/TC 204WG 8 N 38—Recommendations on Validation of Aseptic Processes, 1998.
24. PIC/S PE002-1—Recommendations on Validation of Aseptic Processes, 1999.

21 Qualification/validation of aseptic processing environments, systems, and equipment

James Agalloco

Validation is an activity that has been an absolute requirement across the global healthcare industry since the late 1970s. As in the case with many process control activities within industry, validation has evolved into a far more complex activity than was originally envisaged. Although clearly the requirement to demonstrate both reliable equipment function and suitable process control is essential for the production of safe and effective products, individuals and firms have obsessed about it to the point where validation has been the proximate cause for delays in the implementation of numerous projects. Perhaps nowhere has this been more evident than where firms have endeavored to validate installations using new and advanced aseptic processing technologies, isolators serving as an excellent example.

Much of the pain associated with the validation of isolation technology has been self-inflicted. This chapter reviews the qualification and validation requirements associated with the validation of environments, systems, and equipment including isolators. The goal to clarify the subject as it relates to this equipment (and particularly isolators) to the point where it becomes an achievable reality rather than the dreaded and near-endless exercise it has become. The activity of validation has been defined by US Food and Drug Administration (FDA) as follows:

> Process validation is a documented program which provides a high degree of assurance that a specific process will consistently produce a product meeting its pre-determined specifications. (1)

Unfortunately, being the definitive statement on validation from the world's largest drug regulatory body, it leaves substantial room for interpretation. The one element of this definition that seems to create the most difficulty is establishing what "a high degree of assurance" actually is. For more established processes, such as steam sterilization or even cleaning validation the criteria for acceptance have been widely discussed and are thus largely consistent across the industry. Although it must be noted that even in sterilization, where engineering requirements and microbiological outcomes have been clearly defined for decades, what has been termed "regulatory creep" has occurred turning what were once straightforward validation requirements into convoluted, expensive, and often frustrating activities. Sadly, examples can be cited in which regulatory creep has added only expense and delay in return on investment, and has not added value with respect to either safety or efficacy of product or operational efficiencies.

As the focus of the FDA definition was on product and process, and initially on sterilization processes, the initial approaches to qualification of processes and equipment relating to isolator technology took a very extreme approach. The late 1980s and early 1990s witnessed approaches to equipment qualification that were excessive in the extreme, largely as a consequence of contract validation service firms that touted the need for more and more extensive documentation. One of these firms used the phrase, "Enough paperwork to bury the inspector" in their advertising, whereas others employing gallows humor talked of "validation by the pound" referring to the increasing tendency to confuse quality of work with mass of paper. Fortunately, not everyone agreed with the bloated approaches to qualification that continue to prevail in too many cases. There was substantial support for a refocusing of qualification efforts to more realistic and appropriate criterion. A means to accomplish this can be found in a more recent definition of validation that placed it within a larger context:

> Validation is a defined program which in combination with routine production methods and quality control techniques provides documented assurance that a system is performing as intended and/or that a product conforms to its pre-determined specifications. When

practiced in a "life cycle" model it incorporates design, development, evaluation, operational and maintenance considerations to provide both operational benefits and regulatory compliance. (2)

Where the acceptance criteria are derived from the operational needs of the process rather than arbitrary expectations they become more realistic, and substantially more likely to strike a better balance between level of effort and process control required. If this model is followed, rigorous criteria can still be established; however, those criteria are defined by satisfaction of real operating needs rather than arbitrary dictates. In the area of sterile product manufacturing using aseptic processing validation efforts have been further hamstrung by the rigid imposition of user requirement specifications (URS) that are actually technically impossible to prove. In aseptic processing, there has evolved the notion that no effort should be spared in proving with absolute certainty that each and every container is, without the slightest doubt, sterile. This does not seem unreasonable until one considers that the validation professional has no tools at their disposal that would actually enable them to achieve this objective. The approach taken to validation of isolators has too often been built around the notion that the existence of a negative absolute, the absence of microbial contamination could actually be proven by validation. Sadly, the fact that proving a negative absolute is impossible has only very slowly, if at all, reordered regulatory priorities or expectations.

The "life cycle" approach to validation provides for cradle-to-grave consideration of a system's compliance in a validated state. This model is appropriate for all types of systems, including both physical systems such as heating, ventilation and air conditioning (HVAC), and isolators, and computerized systems controlling process equipment. Discussion of this model is best considered in an essentially chronological order. The various stages of the model include user requirements; conceptual design and planning; detailed design and fabrication; installation and operational qualification; sterilization cycle development (if required); performance qualification, operational use of system and maintenance. When the "life cycle" approach is used, the initial requirements and design documents/drawings are kept current throughout the operational life of the system to facilitate its use and maintenance in a validated state. An appendix to this chapter provides extracts of installation qualification (IQ), operational qualification (OQ) and performance qualification (PQ) protocols for an aseptic fill isolator system (see Appendix I). Comparable documents for a RABS system would be a subset of the same document.

USER REQUIREMENTS SPECIFICATION

The user requirements specifications begin as something akin to a shopping list. They outline the desires of the firm for the intended facility, equipment, or system they are seeking. With infinite money, time, and skill, they could be fully realized as the "perfect system" for its intended purpose. More often, the realities of the project impose themselves and the user requirements become a more narrowly defined statement of the firm's objectives outlining such elements as capacity, range of products, extent of automation, project timing, etc. As it evolves, it becomes more sharply focused and may include substantial detail on such aspects as container sizes, fill volumes, line speeds, documentation requirements, air changes, etc. The level of detail must be adequate, so that those charged with delivering the completed system be they facility engineers, piping designers, equipment vendors, or software developers have a thorough understanding of what it is they are expected to provide. The final version of this document is formally approved and is considered the URS against which the system will be designed, engineered, built, and delivered.

CONCEPTUAL DESIGN AND PLANNING

The origin of any system begins with basic design that must focus on what it is intended to do. Questions to be answered include the what, where, when, and most importantly, the how. Implementation options are reviewed, discussed, refined, discarded, and resurrected as the design process proceeds. Ultimately a system design is developed which satisfies the firm's user requirements and capabilities. At this stage, the design incorporates decisions regarding: system configuration; expected capacity; location; classification of the surrounding environment; adaptation to existing equipment and facilities; and preliminary process description [use;

cleaning and decontamination (if required)]. This stage of the project is often iterative in nature as concepts are tried and evaluated against the requirements. Once the design is completed and accepted the project proceeds to detailed design and fabrication. Projects which are complex enough to require the development of validation plan can start the development of the plan at the completion of the conceptual design. In any aseptic processing project, this phase of the exercise must not be limited strictly to product throughput requirements. Because contamination control and associated risk management activities are so vital they should be completely integrated into the conceptual design process.

DETAILED DESIGN AND CONSTRUCTION/FABRICATION

At this point in there is a divergence of approach depending upon whether the system is one that is fabricated from individual components at the end users' site by contractors (e.g., HVAC system, clean-in-place (CIP) system, etc.); or constructed remotely at a vendors location (e.g., isolator, RABS, autoclave, etc.). Each differs with respect to the specific tasks involved, but the general principles are somewhat similar.

DETAILED DESIGN AND CONSTRUCTION FOR ASSEMBLED SYSTEMS

Systems that must be assembled on site such as HVAC and piping systems go through detailed design in a manner specific for each system. Once the conceptual design is approved, detailed designs for the individual system are developed drawing upon the firm (or their A&Es) expertise. For HVAC, this will start with the user requirements for the various environments in the facility, and the local temperature/humidity conditions that must be reconciled with process needs. For piping systems, the largest concern is the volume of fluid to be handled, which will dictate tank, line, and pump sizes, and in some ways the scale of the entire facility. In many instances, detailed design customarily draws on earlier projects with appropriate adaptations to suit the local conditions. As these systems are being developed in parallel, attention must be paid to their ultimate integration into the finished whole. Each design must be considered in relation to the others in the facility, as well as the process equipment to which it will be connected. Obviously piping runs must not pass through ductwork, and equipment that requires periodic maintenance not built into walls without providing suitable access panels.

The detailed design culminates in a set of drawings for the entire facility that will be used for the construction of the various systems. The final drawings and specifications are ordinarily submitted to the customer for approval before the start of construction of each system. Construction against the approved drawings proceeds on the site and may include a turnover of the system to the owner.

DETAILED DESIGN AND FABRICATION FOR PURCHASED EQUIPMENT

Early in detail design the system will be preliminarily sized for its intended use. For isolators/RABS that are custom designed for a specific purpose, it is common to build a mock-up of the enclosure to confirm that the intended design meets the end user needs. As many advanced aseptic processing systems rely upon operators to perform a variety of tasks, ergonomics can play an important role in the suitability of the final design. The mock-up is used to confirm that the operators can readily perform all of the required functions. It is beneficial to consider the full complement of operators who will use the system, and the effect fatigue may have on their ability to perform the necessary tasks. The time and expense associated with a mock-up evaluation is generally invaluable and can lead to an understanding of where automation may be applicable to solve difficult ergonomic situations that may result in greater aseptic process risk or operator safety issues. A substantial amount of useful information can be gleaned from a simple mock-up made of plywood. The extent of detailed design for "standard" enclosures used for some compounding, component transfer or product testing activities may be less demanding. Many isolator/RABS applications such as sterility testing or aseptic filling are performed in nearly identical fashion at multiple firms. In these instances, neither mock-ups nor detailed design with extensive interaction between the supplier and the customer may be necessary.

Where detailed design is performed it expands upon the conceptual design defining all of the specifics of the intended system. Detailed design culminates in a set of drawings that will be used for the construction and assembly of the equipment. Where the enclosure includes some measure of functionality (CIP, automatic purging of oxygen, system decontamination, etc.), these are defined in a written specifications for the systems operation. The final drawings and specifications are submitted to the customer for approval before fabrication of the system. At many vendors there are defined work rules that define how individual systems are designed, fabricated, and delivered to customers. The most evolved of these production systems result in documentation packages that satisfy essentially all customer questions regarding the delivered equipment.

Fabrication against the approved specifications is performed at the vendor's site and may include a factory acceptance testing or FAT. The FAT, which is often a part of the formal qualification of the system, is customarily performed in concert between the manufacturer and the purchaser's personnel prior to shipment. The original intent of the FAT was to confirm that the system was ready to be relocated from the vendor to the user; that is, there were no required modifications that had to be made by the vendor before it was relocated. In recent years, the factory acceptance test (FAT) has tended to become a first step in the qualification of the equipment, whereas still providing the important acceptance of the completed system prior to shipment. Many of the simple dimensional and construction checks that have traditionally been incorporated in the IQ are done during the FAT and need not be repeated after shipment and reassembly of the equipment at the purchaser's site.

SYSTEM AND EQUIPMENT INSTALLATION/COMMISSIONING

After acceptance from the contractor or supplier, the new owner (with or without the contractor's/supplier's assistance) will prepare the equipment for formal qualification. This activity is not considered a controlled activity in that it is usually not performed in accordance with a set of written procedures. The later portion of this activity is sometimes called commissioning or shakedown in which the equipment is informally checked for conformance to specifications. The commissioning serves to ensure that the system is ready for formal qualification. Although this activity may seem redundant, it makes little sense to institute qualification activities on a system where the vendor may have made some minor error of omission or commission. As is the case with the FAT, static test functions such as electrical supply verification, enrollment in maintenance or calibration programs or dimensional checks required for qualification can be done during commissioning; however, the formal qualification activities that are to be done with the equipment in operation should not begin until the commissioning activities are done and the machinery deemed ready for operation.

EQUIPMENT/SYSTEM QUALIFICATION

Qualification of equipment is a preliminary step in the overall validation that has been well described in the literature. Although it may be common in the industry to divide qualification into separate activities entitled installation qualification and operational qualification, there is in fact no reason to do so. FDA describes this activity as equipment qualification making no distinction between those activities that focus on the installation details relative to those which focus on the operation of the equipment. This separation is entirely artificial and cumbersome, and the reader is encouraged to execute this activity in a unified manner. Recent efforts with ASTM have developed a more practical approach to the activities that precede performance qualification of systems (3). The reader is encouraged to follow the precepts of that document which can help eliminate some of the bloated documentation practices previously prevalent.

The qualification is little more than confirmation that the system conforms to the user requirements specification approved for its design, fabrication, installation, and operation. This is accomplished through a protocol that confirms that the system is everything it is expected to be. The system specifications including drawings, schematics, and performance requirements are compared to the final delivered system to establish its conformity to expectations. Deviations to the design are noted and are either corrected through modification of the system, or by revision to the specifications if the system can be accepted although somewhat different from the intended design. There are no differences in the execution of qualification for any isolator or RABS from what is typical of other mechanical systems. The operational aspects of qualification for isolators and RABS include elements of equipment design similar to those of typical clean room qualification, but are otherwise comparable to what is typical for other process equipment.

AUTOMATED AND COMPUTERIZED SYSTEMS

Present-day pharmaceutical equipment and utility systems are almost always equipped with some form of automatic control. Automation brings a level of sophistication, reproducibility, and unprecedented documentation to system operation that makes its incorporation into system and equipment designs essential. Endeavoring to operate an advanced aseptic processing system in the present day without computerized systems is completely impractical. Thus equipment and system providers have incorporated computerized systems extensively to facilitate the operation of the system.

When computerized systems first became commonplace in the pharmaceutical industry, there was confusion regarding the means to qualify and validate their inclusion into current good manufacturing practices (CGMP) operations. The early effort of PMAs (now called PhRMA) Computerized Systems Validation Committee (CSVC) laid out some of the more basic concepts that have enabled industry to implement computerized systems (4). Earliest and most basic was describing the parallels between hardware as equipment and software as procedures. It must be recognized that the "life cycle model" recommended for pharmaceutical process validation is an adaptation of similar models used in the software development industry. The similarity was not accidental; it was adopted by the CSVC to assure that persons from the process or automation perspective would have a common understanding of the project objectives where a computerized system was used. The CSVCs efforts culminated in a document that laid out the principles for the validation of computerized systems. Later refinements were made to this under good automated manufacturing processes (GAMPs), but the basic tenets of this have not markedly changed (5). With time and now more than two decades of experience with automated, software-driven systems has also come the recognition, that computerized systems are not a significant source of process control risk in CGMP processing. The control systems provide a means to operate the equipment, whose effectiveness must be demonstrated independently of the hardware and software. In many ways, the perspective taken by the inspector is that "The ends justify the means," and that although the computerized system is important, it is not more important than the CGMP activity it is supporting.

PERFORMANCE QUALIFICATION CONCERNS

Following equipment qualification, production materials can be introduced into the system and its performance assessed by testing of the process/product executed in the equipment/system. These of course vary with the specific system and are the real focus of regulatory concern. Recent regulatory initiatives and publications have helped bring about appropriate changes in emphasis that assure a proper perspective is being taken (6–8). The typical performance qualification studies required to support aseptic processing include sterilization of components; sterilization of product contact surfaces; sterilization of the product; decontamination of the enclosure, sterilization/decontamination validation for any materials in-feed systems, process validation for the systems intended use (formulation, aseptic filling, subdivision of potent compounds, medical devise assembly, etc); cleaning validation; etc. The execution of these tasks is well described in the literature and undergoes no meaningful changes for implementation in an advanced aseptic process setting (9–11). In addition to these preliminary tasks, an environmental monitoring program must be implemented that addresses all of the classified environments including the background areas as well as the critical processing zone (12). Personnel skills in aseptic processing must always be addressed; however, the effects of aseptic technique will be far more profound in systems that allow personnel entry into the critical zone of aseptic processing as opposed to those that rely on truly advanced aseptic processing. The aseptic processing performed in the system must have their capability demonstrated in a process simulation study (13–15). Details on aseptic processing simulation are provided elsewhere in this volume, and will not be repeated here. Given the superior performance of the advanced technologies as described in this text, it should be recognized that regulatory expectations are out of synch. Current environmental monitoring and process simulations are inadequate to establish the suitability of these highly capable systems. Those practices do not "validate" the acceptability of an aseptic process, something that was heavily commented on in relation to FDAs 2008 revision of the 21 CFR 211 regulations.

ISOLATION TECHNOLOGY

When first introduced into the industry, it was believed that isolators represented some unique challenges as they combined elements of sterilization, aseptic processing, environmental control, clean rooms, and containment into a single system. Within the context of the multiple validation concerns that must be satisfied, and the expected superior performance of isolators (as contrasted to ordinary human-scale clean rooms for aseptic processing), well intentioned, but unfortunately inexperienced (at least with isolators) individuals, and firms suggested criteria for isolators that mandated perfection in all aspects. Their stated objective was an aseptic filling isolator capable of providing finished product containers equivalent in sterility assurance to terminally sterilized products! This is a patently unattainable goal; no technology that relies on exclusion of microorganisms from sterile materials can ever realize the same degree of sterility assurance as a terminal treatment that destroys their viability. Nevertheless, the damage was done. Isolators were portrayed as systems that must be capable of operating contamination free for extended periods to be acceptable. The unfortunate consequences of this expectation were requirements for absence of leaks, perfection in sterilization, complete absence of any internal microbial presence and others equally unattainable (16). Given such unrealizable goals, laudable as they might be, it is no wonder that the validation of isolator systems became for many an exercise in futility.

Less aggressive recommendations for acceptance criteria for isolation technology been articulated (17). In its guidance document the Parenteral Drug Association (PDA) addressed the subject of appropriate acceptance criteria by focusing on the definition of appropriate user requirements specifications. An isolator need not be perfect to fully satisfy operational requirements; it need only be suitable for the intended use (16).

USE OF ADVANCED ASEPTIC PROCESSING SYSTEMS

An aseptic processing system is built for a specific purpose, and its qualification/validation must support that purpose. The performance qualification efforts confirm the acceptability of the design and procedures that provide the desired functionality. Each of the primary standard operating procedures required for use with an enclosure: decontamination/sterilization, operation, and cleaning are usually the direct result of a supportive qualification study that demonstrates how the system performs in that procedure. In conjunction with supportive procedures such as instrument, leak testing, environmental monitoring, etc., these procedures define how the system will perform. The application of change control to the procedures and physical system ensures that changes are reviewed for their potential impact on the validated state of the final system. The only other aspect of the systems use which must be considered is training of operating personnel in the proper execution of these procedures to ensure their continued proper execution.

SYSTEM MAINTENANCE

As with any other piece of mechanical equipment, advanced aseptic processing equipment must be supported by a preventive maintenance program to ensure it operates reliably over time. Among the ongoing maintenance considerations are calibration of instruments, inspection/lubrication/replacement of seal surfaces, gloves and half suits, periodic cleaning of enclosure internal and external surfaces, filter integrity testing, filter replacement, change, periodic leak testing, and any required preventive maintenance for supportive equipment.

OVERALL QUALIFICATION/VALIDATION PERSPECTIVE

Despite what may appear to be a near-impossible and never-ending task, the qualification/validation of advanced aseptic processing technologies is not particularly difficult. Where realistic (the only kind which should be defined) requirements are established for the systems performance these systems can be readied for use rather simply. The classical qualification/validation methods used for other process equipment/facility systems are wholly adequate to bring these systems through validation. Experience with sterilization, process, and cleaning validation as well as some familiarity with ordinary clean rooms is certainly helpful.

REFERENCES

1. FDA. Guideline on General Principles of Process Validation Guideline, May 1987.
2. Agalloco J. Validation—Yesterday, Today and Tomorrow. Proceedings of Parenteral Drug Association International Symposium, Basel, Switzerland, Parenteral Drug Association, 1993.
3. ASTM 2500-07. Standard Guide for Specification, Design, and Verification of Pharmaceutical and Biopharmaceutical Manufacturing Systems and Equipment, 2007.
4. PMA. Validation Concepts for Computer Systems used in the Manufacture of Drug Products. Proceedings: Concepts and Principles for the Validation of Computer Systems in the Manufacture and Control of Drug Products, 1986.
5. ISPE, GAMP 5. A Risk-Based Approach to Compliant GxP Computerized Systems, 2008.
6. Pharmaceutical cGMPs for the 21st Century—A Risk-Based Approach, 2004.
7. ICH Q9. Quality Risk Management, 2006.
8. Agalloco J. Compliance risk management: using a top down validation approach. Pharm Technol 2008; 32(7):70–78.
9. Agalloco J, Carleton F, eds. Validation of Pharmaceutical Processes. 3rd ed. New York: Informa, 2007.
10. PDA TR#1, revised. Validation of Moist Heat Sterilization Processes: Cycle Design, Development, Qualification and Ongoing Control, major revision of PDA Technical Monograph. Volume 61, Supplement S-1, 2007.
11. PDA. Points to Consider for Cleaning Validation. PDA Technical Report #29, PDA. J Pharm Sci Technol 53(suppl 1) 1999.
12. DeVecchi F. Validation of environmental control systems used in parenteral facilities. In: Agalloco J. Carleton F, eds. Validation of Pharmaceutical Processes. 3rd ed. New York: Informa, 2007.
13. FDA. Guideline on Sterile Drug Products Produced by Aseptic Processing, 2004.
14. EMEA, Annex 1. Sterile Medicinal Products, 2008.
15. PDA. Process Simulation Testing for Aseptically Filled Products. PDA Technical Report #22. PDA J Pharm Sci Technol 1996; 50(suppl 6).
16. Akers J, Agalloco J. Isolators—validation and sound scientific judgement. PDA J Pharma Sci Technol 2000; 54(2):110–111.
17. Akers J, Agalloco J, et al. Design and validation of isolator systems for the manufacturing and testing of health care products. PDA Technical Report #34, PDA. J Pharma Sci Technol 2001; 55(suppl 5).

22 Isolator integrity leak inspection

Scott Pool

The purpose of this chapter is to guide users through the development process of an isolator integrity test program. Details of several leak detection methods are discussed to aid in the selection process. This chapter also offers practical isolator design considerations that will facilitate implementation of any integrity test program.

Why should an isolator be integrity tested? There are two straightforward answers to this question. Reason number one, and usually foremost, is to prevent what is inside the isolator from exiting, thus contaminating its surroundings. At first glance, this point may not seem important. Especially if the products processed inside the isolator are nontoxic. Although this is true, most users will want to sanitize the isolator interior with some type of gaseous sanitizing agent. The function of these agents is to kill microorganisms, which likewise makes them harmful to personnel. Therefore, containment of these agents is necessary for operator safety.

The second reason to integrity test an isolator is to prevent contamination from the surrounding environment from entering the isolator. If the isolator does not "isolate" the process from its surroundings, then it is not doing its job. Most users will internally pressurize their isolators during operation to minimize this possibility. Positive internal pressurization will continuously force air out through all open isolator leak paths. This constant flow of air will inhibit external contamination from entering the isolator. Routine integrity testing will identify leaks for repair to further reduce this concern.

In some cases, the products processed inside an isolator are toxic. In these situations, operator safety concerns usually require the isolator to be maintained at a negative internal pressure relative to its surroundings. This prevents the process materials from exiting the isolator in the same manner that positive pressurization prevents contamination from entering an isolator. The difference here, of course, is that airflow is from outside the isolator to inside.

Nothing is "leak free" and isolators are no exception. Typical isolator systems have numerous gasketed connection points, air-handling valves, floor drains, access doors, etc., which are all prone to leak. The first challenge, therefore, is to determine how much leakage is acceptable for the application. A leakage requirement of "none" or "zero" is unrealistic and impractical. In fact, every integrity test method available has some finite leak detection limit below which the leak rate is unknown. Once an acceptable leak rate is established, a process to reliably detect such an occurrence can be developed.

ACCEPTANCE CRITERIA

There are several issues to consider when determining appropriate acceptance criteria for an isolator integrity test plan. Most users will want to limit the release of isolator sanitizing agents into the surrounding clean room. A mathematical model to estimate acceptable sterilent leakage rates is given below. Some users may require a nitrogen-purged environment for processing oxygen-sensitive products in their isolators. Note that leakage of nitrogen, though nontoxic, can starve the surrounding environment of oxygen and thus put operators at risk. Therefore, an acceptable nitrogen loss rate must likewise be determined.

It is also important to consider the air makeup capacities of both the isolator air-handling system and that of the sanitizing equipment. An isolator system may not have a safety issue with a relatively large leak; however, the air makeup capacities of one of these systems may be exceeded resulting in poor isolator pressure control. Recall from the discussion earlier that precise pressure control is key for maintaining an isolator's environment.

After listing all of the relevant leakage concerns and determining their associated maximum safe leak rates, the limiting leak rate may be surmised. The limiting leak rate is the most stringent requirement of the group such that if the isolator passes this level of leak integrity, then all of the other considerations are likewise met and only one test needs to be performed.

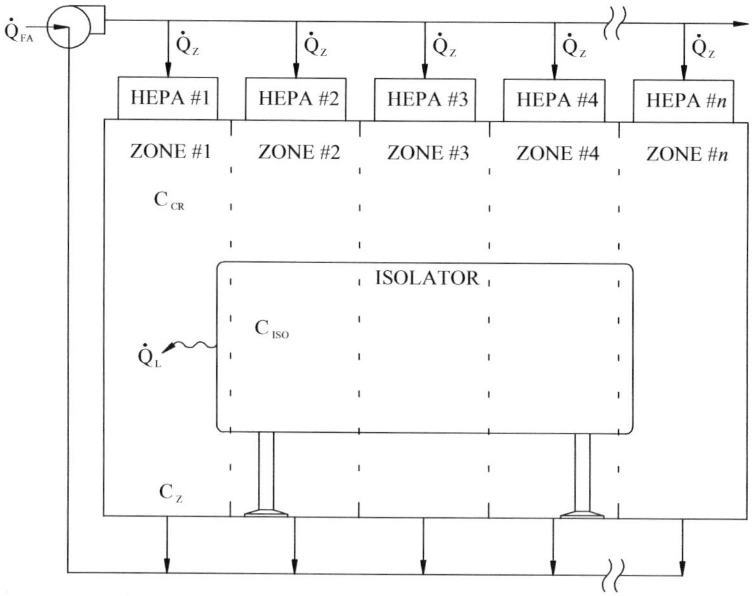

Figure 1 Schematic of a typical isolator installation in a clean room.

Make certain that your isolator vendor agrees to meet your requirements and has the necessary equipment to test it to the levels that you specify.

The following mathematical model describes how to calculate the sterilent gas concentration buildup in the clean room space surrounding a leaking isolator. Clean room design is beyond the scope of this chapter; however, certain assumptions must be made for these calculations. Figure 1 schematically depicts a typical isolator installation in a clean room. Note that the clean room has been sectioned into numbered zones by dashed lines. Each zone is serviced by one clean room HEPA filter (room inlet) and a paired clean room air return duct opening.

Where $\dot{Q}_L$ is the leakage air flow rate out of the isolator and into the clean room (L/min); C_{ISO} is the sterilant concentration inside the isolator (mg/L); $\dot{Q}_{FA}$ is the clean room fresh air makeup flow rate (L/min); $C_{CR}(t)$ is the clean room sterilant concentration (mg/L); $m(t)$ is the total mass of sterilant accumulated in the clean room (mg); V_{CR} is the air volume of the clean room (L) including the clean room air handling duct work volume.

The following assumptions must also be observed when using this analysis:

1. The sterilant mixes well and distributes evenly throughout the room.
2. The initial clean room sterilent concentration is zero.
3. The sterilant is stable over the course of the analysis.
4. The isolator leak rate and isolator sterilant concentrations are constants.

The sterilant gas concentration in the clean room is defined by the total mass of sterilent present in the clean room divided by the total clean room volume:

$$C_{CR}(t) = \frac{m(t)}{V_{CR}} \tag{1}$$

Conservation of the sterilant mass requires that the accumulated sterilant in the clean room must equal the sterilant entering the clean room minus the sterilant leaving of the clean room, which can be written as

$$\text{mass(accumulated)} = \text{mass(in)} - \text{mass(out)}$$

or

$$m(t) = \int C_{ISO}\dot{Q}_L \, dt - \int C_{CR}(t)(\dot{Q}_L + \dot{Q}_{FA})dt \tag{2}$$

Substituting Equation 1 for $m(t)$ in Equation 2:

$$V_{CR}C_{CR}(t) = \int C_{ISO}\dot{Q}_L \, dt - \int C_{CR}(t)(\dot{Q}_L + \dot{Q}_{FA})dt \quad (3)$$

Differentiate both sides of Equation 3 with respect to time.

$$V_{CR}\frac{dC_{CR}(t)}{dt} = C_{ISO}\dot{Q}_L - C_{CR}(t)(\dot{Q}_L + \dot{Q}_{FA}) \quad (4)$$

The solution to this first-order differential equation is

$$C_{CR}(t) = \frac{C_{ISO}\dot{Q}_L}{\dot{Q}_L + \dot{Q}_{FA}}\left[1 - e^{-\frac{t}{\tau}}\right] \quad (5)$$

where the time constant:

$$\tau = \frac{V_{CR}}{\dot{Q}_L + \dot{Q}_{FA}} \quad (6)$$

Equation 5 can be used to calculate the overall clean room sterilant concentration as a function of time due to a leak in an isolator. The time constant, τ, for this equation is the inverse of the number of fresh air changes per unit time for the clean room. It is important to note that these are fresh outside air changes and they do not include any air re-circulation component. Typical clean rooms have 10 to 20 fresh air changes per hour, which yields time constants of 3 to 6 minutes. After 5 or so time constants (18–30 minutes) the room sterilant concentration will plateau and the dynamic portion of this equation may be ignored. Because most isolator sanitization cycles are on the order of several hours, Equation 5 may be further reduced to the following:

$$C_{CR}\text{ (plateau)} = \frac{C_{ISO}\dot{Q}_L}{\dot{Q}_L + \dot{Q}_{FA}} \quad (7)$$

If the maximum allowable sterilant concentration is known, then the maximum isolator leak rate may be calculated by solving the Equation 7 for $\dot{Q}_L$. The maximum allowable sterilent gas concentration can usually be determined from the sterilant material safety data sheets or from other health and safety organizations.

$$\dot{Q}_L = \frac{C_{CR}\dot{Q}_{FA}}{C_{ISO} - C_{CR}} \quad (8)$$

Example

An isolator has a normal plateau gas concentration (C_{CR}) of 1.1 mg/L during its sanitization cycle. The isolator clean room has a fresh air make flow rate ($\dot{Q}_L$) of 70,000 L/min and the maximum safe sterilant concentration level for the clean room is determined to be 0.005 mg/L. Then the maximum total isolator leak rate as calculated from Equation 8 must never exceed

$$\dot{Q}_L = \frac{(0.005\text{ mg/L})\cdot(70{,}000\text{ L/min})}{1.10\text{ mg/L} - 0.005\text{ mg/L}} = 320\text{ L/min (11.3 SCFM)}$$

Typically, an isolator will have many small leaks instead of one large leak. This means that the leaking sterilant will distribute evenly throughout the clean room. If we assume a worst-case situation, where the entire leak is concentrated in one spot, then the clean room zone containing the concentrated leak would have a greater sterilant concentration than the rest of the clean room. The increased sterilant concentration can be calculated for a particular clean room zone for such a worst-case condition.

This is a simple case of two gas streams mixing. Gas stream number 1 is the air leaking from the isolator and stream number 2 is the air flow entering that clean room zone. Note that the air stream entering the zone will have some sterilant gas concentration due to build up in the clean room per Equation 8.

Two new terms must be introduced:

C_Z: the sterilant gas concentration for the zone (mg/L)
$\dot{Q}_Z$: the air flow rate entering the zone (L/min). Note that this is the total air flow through this zone.

Once again conservation of the sterilant mass gives the following equation:

$$C_{ISO}\dot{Q}_L + C_{CR}\dot{Q}_Z = C_Z(\dot{Q}_L + \dot{Q}_Z) \tag{9}$$

Substituting C_{CR} from Equation 7 into 9 and solving for the isolator leak rate eventually yields the following quadratic equation:

$$a \times \dot{Q}_L^2 + b \times \dot{Q}_L + c = 0 \tag{10}$$

Where the quadratic constants are given by

$$a = C_Z - C_{ISO} \tag{11}$$
$$b = (C_Z - C_{ISO})(\dot{Q}_Z + \dot{Q}_F) \tag{12}$$
$$c = C_Z\dot{Q}_Z\dot{Q}_F \tag{13}$$

Because only positive leak rates are of interest, the maximum allowable concentrated leak rate in a single clean room zone may be calculated using the quadratic equation:

$$\dot{Q}_L = \frac{-b - \sqrt{b^2 - 4ac}}{2a} \tag{14}$$

If we continue the example given above and further state that the air flow rate entering each clean room zone is 14,000 L/min then

$a = 0.005\ \text{mg/L} - 1.1\ \text{mg/L} = -1.095\ \text{mg/L}$
$b = (0.005\ \text{mg/L} - 1.1\ \text{mg/L})(14{,}000\ \text{L/min} + 70{,}000\ \text{L/min}) = -91{,}980\ \text{mg/min}$
$c = (0.005\ \text{mg/L})(70{,}000\ \text{L/min})(14{,}000\ \text{L/min}) = 49{,}00{,}000\ \text{mg L/min}^2$

$$\dot{Q}_L = \frac{91{,}980 - \sqrt{91{,}980^2 - 4(-1.095)(49{,}00{,}000)}}{2(-1.095)} = 53\ \text{L/min}\ (1.9\ \text{SCFM})$$

The worst case calculation for an isolator leak concentrated in a single clean room zone only allows a 53 L/min leak rate, whereas the overall clean room leak rate as calculated by Equation 9 allows 320 L/min (six times greater). The worst-case calculation is certainly more conservative. Users should exercise caution when selecting a calculation method to evaluate their isolator. Also note that the sterilant gas concentration will naturally increase closer to a leak origin. Operators should, therefore, limit their contact with an isolator that is being sanitized.

ISOLATOR INTEGRITY LEAK TEST METHODS

Once the maximum allowable leak rate has been determined, an integrity test method can be developed. There are several isolator integrity leak test methods available. They may be separated into two basic categories, leak locating and leak measuring. Leak-locating methods, as the name implies, pinpoint the location of a leak; however, these tests usually take a long time to perform and rely on an operator's skill and judgment. The results are also usually qualitative, not quantitative, which make it difficult to establish pass/fail criteria. Leak measuring tests, on the other hand, measure the overall performance of the entire isolator system at once. Generally speaking, the leak-measuring type test methods are faster and give a quantitative measurement of the entire isolator system performance. However, if the isolator performs poorly, they do not indicate the location of the problem and a leak-locating test must be performed. Most users will, therefore, need the ability to perform both a leak-locating and a leak-measuring type test. The leak-measuring method is typically used routinely just before isolator sanitization, and the leak-locating method is used only to find leaks if the leak-measuring test is unsuccessful.

INTEGRITY TEST METHODS

This section describes several common methods used for testing the integrity of an isolator. The basic procedure is outlined for each method, and the pros and cons for each are discussed.

Ammonia

This process is a leak-locating method that uses escaping ammonia vapor to pinpoint isolator leaks. Rags and bottles of liquid ammonia are first placed inside the isolator. After sealing the isolator, use the isolator's gloves, open the ammonia and soak the rags. Open pans of ammonia will also work well. The object is to saturate the air inside the isolator with as much ammonia vapor as possible. All of the isolator's air stirring fans and blowers should be turned on to assure that the ammonia vapor is distributed everywhere within the isolator. It is also a good idea to place a few strips of ammonia sensitive cloth inside the isolator (before generating any ammonia vapor) to verify that the ammonia concentration is sufficient.

Once the ammonia vapor concentration has completely turned the cloths inside the isolator blue, positively pressurize the isolator to its working pressure. This produces a pressure gradient to help drive the ammonia vapor out through any leaks. Large leaks can be detected with the human nose. An ammonia sensitive cloth can be used to detect smaller leaks. The cloth changes color from yellow to blue in the presence of ammonia. The cloth is blotted around all joints and seams then observed for a color change. Large leaks turn the cloth immediately whereas small leaks may require more hold time. Typical leaks of any consequence require hold times on the order of 5 seconds. Any ductwork on the low-pressure side of an air re-circulation blower should not be tested with the blower running. If a leak was present and the blower was running, air may be drawn into the isolator through the leak and thus avoid detection. Upon completion of this test the ammonia vapors must be aerated safely away from personnel.

The advantages of this method are that it will pinpoint the location of fairly small leaks. It is relatively fast to perform because many operators can work simultaneously. Also, ammonia is readily available and is relatively safe to use.

The disadvantages to this method are that the results are only as good as the operator(s) skill level. Operators can easily overlook a leak if they are not meticulous. Also, dealing with the leftover ammonia soaked rags can be a nuisance. Zip-lock bags introduced with the ammonia before the test will facilitate clean up.

Helium

This method is also a leak-locating method. It uses helium as the tracer gas to find leaks. A helium mass spectrometer is used to detect any escaping helium. This type of equipment is robust and is readily available from many commercial sources.

First the isolator must be filled with helium. Typically, large plastic bags are inflated with helium inside the isolator. Start with the bag collapsed to ensure that only helium is inside the bag. An opening for the air to escape from the isolator during the bag inflation must be provided. Once the bag is inflated, the isolator is sealed closed. The bag of helium can then be cut to release the helium into the isolator. This procedure minimizes wasted helium over a continuous helium flushing method.

A small wand or "sniffer" is then slowly passed over all of the joints and surfaces of interest. If a leak is detected, the helium mass spectrometer shows an increase in helium concentration which can give an estimate of the size of the leak.

The main advantage for the helium method is its sensitivity. Leak rates of 10^{-6} cc/sec are detectable with this method. Helium is also safe to handle; however, large leaks can starve the room of oxygen thus creating a hazard for operators. For safety, the background helium level can be measured by occasionally holding the sniffer probe away from the isolator.

The disadvantage to the helium method is that the equipment is expensive. The cost usually means that only one helium detection unit may be purchased and therefore only one operator can work at a time. This makes the test very time consuming. Because helium is a manual method, it too relies on the operator skill. Also, an inventory of helium must be maintained. Furthermore, small leaks requiring helium detection are usually of little consequence to a positively pressurized isolator.

Pressure Decay

This method is a leak-measuring type. The sealed isolator is internally pressurized from an external compressed gas supply. The air supply source is removed and the pressure is monitored for decay. If the pressure decays, it is assumed that air is leaking out of the isolator. This test method is often built into the sterilent gas generator equipment.

The advantages of this test are that it can be automated and it, therefore, does not rely on an operator's judgment or expertise. It also tests all isolator joints simultaneously and it does not require any special tracer gas. Best of all, it can be used to measure the isolator's leak rate which can be compared to the limits determined in the section above.

Boyle's Law may be used to calculate an average leak rate from the pressure decay data. The isolator's volume is assumed to be constant. Initially, the isolator begins with a known quantity of air molecules and ends with a known quantity of air molecules:

$$n_{\mathrm{i}} = \frac{P_{\mathrm{i}}V}{RT_{\mathrm{i}}} \text{ and } n_{\mathrm{f}} = \frac{P_{\mathrm{f}}V}{RT_{\mathrm{f}}} \tag{15}$$

where n_{i} and n_{f} are the initial and final number of air molecules (mol); P_{i} and P_{f} are the initial and final isolator internal absolute pressures. Note that the absolute pressure (Pa) is the gage pressure Pa + 101,325 Pa; T_{i} and T_{f} are the initial and final isolator absolute temperatures. Note the absolute temperature (K) is the temperature °C + 273; V is the isolators internal volume (L); R is the universal gas constant (8314 L Pa/K/mol).

The change in the number of air molecules or rather the loss of air molecules is given by

$$n_{\mathrm{LOSS}} = \frac{P_{\mathrm{atm}}V_{\mathrm{LOSS}}}{RT_{\mathrm{f}}} = n_{\mathrm{i}} - n_{\mathrm{f}} \tag{16}$$

where P_{atm} is atmospheric pressure (of the clean room); V_{LOSS} is the resulting volume of the air leaked into the atmosphere.

$$\frac{P_{\mathrm{atm}}V_{\mathrm{LOSS}}}{RT_{\mathrm{f}}} = \frac{P_{\mathrm{i}}V}{RT_{\mathrm{i}}} - \frac{P_{\mathrm{f}}V}{RT_{\mathrm{f}}} \tag{17}$$

The volumetric air loss (leakage) rate can be determined from the following equation where t is the time in hours between the initial and final pressure and temperature measurements:

$$\dot{V}_{\mathrm{LOSS}} = \frac{VT_{\mathrm{f}}}{t \times P_{\mathrm{atm}}}\left[\frac{P_{\mathrm{i}}}{T_{\mathrm{i}}} - \frac{P_{\mathrm{f}}}{T_{\mathrm{f}}}\right] \tag{18}$$

P_{atm} can be assumed equal to P_{f}. This further reduces the equation to

$$\dot{V}_{\mathrm{LOSS}} = \frac{V}{t}\left[\frac{T_{\mathrm{f}}P_{\mathrm{i}}}{T_{\mathrm{i}}P_{\mathrm{f}}} - 1\right] \tag{19}$$

This value can be compared to the maximum allowable leak rate to determine the acceptability of the isolator.

This loss rate is sometimes expressed as a percentage of the isolator's overall volume.

$$\mathrm{LOSS\%} = \frac{\dot{V}_{\mathrm{LOSS}}}{V}100 = \frac{100}{t}\left[\frac{T_{\mathrm{f}}P_{\mathrm{i}}}{T_{\mathrm{i}}P_{\mathrm{f}}} - 1\right](\%/\mathrm{hr}) \tag{20}$$

The disadvantage of the pressure decay leak test method is that it is extremely temperature sensitive. Small temperature changes can cause significant changes to the isolator's pressure. Isolators that cool down during the test will cause the air inside to contract, thus decreasing (decaying) the pressure even though the isolator may not be leaking. It can be frustrating searching for a leak that does not exist. Conversely, isolators that heat up during the test cause the air inside to expand, which can mask a leak. This could give the user a false sense of security. It is, therefore, necessary to turn off all heat-generating equipment that may cause a temperature fluctuation. It is also necessary to accurately monitor the air temperature inside the isolator during the test. The following analysis highlights the importance of temperature control during a pressure decay leak test.

Assume an isolator with a fixed internal volume V that is leak free. The initial pressure P_i and temperature T_i of the isolator are known and at some time later the final temperature T_f is measured. Boyle's Law may be used to calculate the final pressure P_f of the isolator.

$$PV = nRT \tag{21}$$

where V is the isolator volume; R is the universal gas constant; n is number of moles of air inside the isolator.

$$\frac{P}{T} = \frac{nR}{V} = \text{constant} \tag{22}$$

$$\frac{P_i}{T_i} = \frac{P_f}{T_f} \tag{23}$$

$$P_f = \frac{P_i \times T_f}{T_i} \tag{24}$$

$$T_f = T_i + \Delta T \tag{25}$$

$$P_f = \frac{P_i(T_i + \Delta T)}{T_i} = P_i + \frac{P_i \times \Delta T}{T_i} \tag{26}$$

The change in isolator pressure due to a change in temperature is given by

$$\Delta P = P_f - P_i = \frac{P_i \times \Delta T}{T_i} \tag{27}$$

Remember that the pressures and temperatures must be in absolute units when using these equations. A plot of ΔP verses ΔT is given in Figure 2. Notice that a change in temperature of

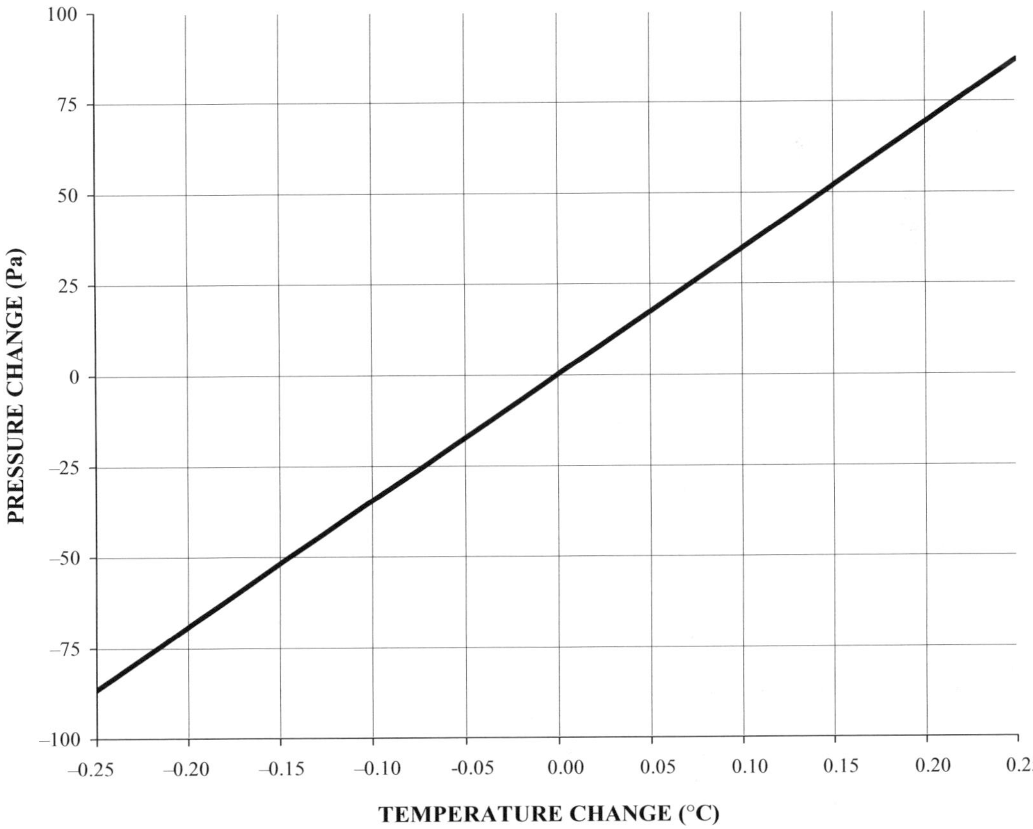

Figure 2 Temperature's effect on pressure for a fixed volume.

only 0.1°C (0.18°F) changes the internal isolator pressure by 35 Pa (0.14 inches of water column) regardless of the isolator's internal volume.

Another disadvantage to this method is that it is sensitive to pressure changes in the surrounding clean room. An isolator's pressure is usually measured relative to the clean room in which it resides. If the clean room's pressure is not stable, then the pressure decay results may be inaccurate. Personnel entering and leaving the room easily affect a clean room's pressure. It is a good idea to limit access during a pressure decay leak test.

Pressure Maintenance

Pressure maintenance is also a leak-measuring method. As the name implies, air is metered into a sealed isolator at a measured flow rate until the isolator's internal pressure is maintained at a constant level. The flow rate is modulated either automatically or manually to regulate the isolator's internal pressure at the working pressure. If the isolator temperature remains constant, the air flow rate into the isolator must equal the air flow rate out of the isolator (leakage). This method, therefore, measures the overall leakage rate of an isolator at its working pressure.

The advantages of this method are that it measures the isolator leak rate directly. Therefore, no calculations are necessary to determine the leak rate. It also does not require any special tracer gas.

The disadvantages to this method are the same as those for pressure decay. It is very temperature sensitive and the results are also affected by the stability of the clean room's pressure control. This method is better suited to large isolators that are more difficult to seal. Smaller relatively leak free isolators would require a very sensitive mass flow meter.

Isolator Design Considerations

The following points detail some isolator design considerations that can facilitate implementation of an integrity test program.

- Specify all instrumentation and controls to perform both a leak measuring and leak locating type test before purchasing an isolator. This will minimize costly retrofits and schedule delays.
- Consider all areas serviced by the clean room air handling equipment that surround the isolator. Contamination will be disseminated into these areas in the event of a mishap.
- Provide easy access to the upstream side of the isolator's air inlet valve and the downstream side of the air exit valve. This access can be a removable panel or duct section. If one of these valves fail, and thereby causes the isolator to fail the leak test, a means to confirm their integrity with a leak-locating method must be provided.
- Do not insulate air duct junctions or joints. The insulation can obstruct or mask a leak making them difficult to locate. If temperature control of the duct is an issue, consider controlling the room's environmental conditions around the duct work.
- Provide sensors to monitor the clean room for unsafe sanitizing agent concentrations. This provides a second layer of operator safety in case of a mishap.
- Most isolators will include some planned openings like product entry and exit mouse-holes. Closures for these openings must be provided during leak testing. Often these openings incorporate long tunnels to prevent particulate ingress. Simply capping this opening off may produce a dead leg for sanitization. Usually, a hose attached to the cap directed into an air return duct can create sufficient flow to sanitize the tunnel.
- Punctures in gloves are generally too small to be detected by the methods outlined in this chapter. Users should consider a separate integrity program for gloves.

CONCLUSION

A well-planned integrity test program is key for proper and consistent isolator operation. Operator safety and the maintenance of an isolator's environment are directly affected by an isolator's integrity. This chapter provides a method to achieve a practical integrity test program. It addresses how to develop acceptance criteria. It also discusses how to perform several different integrity test methods and offers practical suggestions to consider when isolation technology is employed.

23 Environmental monitoring of advanced aseptic processing technology

James Akers and James Agalloco

Advanced aseptic processing technologies (AAPT) began to appear in the manufacture of drugs and biologics in the late 1980s. The first of these systems were simple (comparatively speaking) adaptations of the flexible (polyvinyl chloride) wall isolators, which had been introduced for sterility testing only a few years before. From the beginning what attracted forward-thinking individuals to aseptic processing inside isolators was the potential of reduced contamination through the separation of human operators from the manufacturing environment. It did not take long in the implementation process for those same technologists to realize that reduced contamination was a reality of isolator technology rather than mere potential.

In the early 1990s, Dr. Richard Wood of Pfizer reported that he and his associates had performed over 6000 active air sampling exercises in an early flexible wall isolator without the recovery of a single-colony forming unit (cfu). Such performance was at that time unattainable in human-scale manned clean rooms and is still unreachable nearly 20 years later. In addition, the elimination of airlocks through the use of rapid transfer ports (RTPs or DPTEs) along with decontamination using chemicals such as peracetic acid followed by vapor phase hydrogen peroxide (VPHP) eliminated the second most prominent source of microbial contamination in clean rooms, namely the transfer of microorganisms along with materials, tools, components, and other supplies required for processing or testing into the isolator.

There were many twists and turns in the adoption of isolators and other advanced technologies, particularly in the United States where obstacles seemed to appear at nearly every turn. However, through this entire period of time the promise of dramatically improved environmental control performance in both isolators and other AAPT has been consistently realized. This chapter examines what this new reality of reduced contamination in AAPT is revealing and how it should alter the monitoring of these far lower contamination risk environments.

THE EVOLUTION OF ENVIRONMENTAL MONITORING

Interestingly, during the same time period as the introduction of isolators, first for sterility testing and later for manufacturing, the pharmaceutical industry witnessed a dramatic upswing in emphasis on environmental monitoring (EM) as well. Beginning in the early 1980s prominent regulator inspectors changed the direction of EM and set into motion an evolution toward ever-increasing sampling intensity that continues today (1–3). Two key components in what became the favored model for EM were the establishment of alert and action levels and an emphasis on trend analysis. Accompanying, the alert and action level emphasis and trend analysis was a parallel attempt to employ various forms of statistics to support EM limit definition (4). That notion was accompanied by the idea that perhaps statistics could ultimately be used to confirm appropriate process control or even "sterility assurance levels." Initially, there were significant differences in alert and action levels, but as is typical with compliance driven specifications in aseptic processing a continuous tightening of expectations occurred such that by the middle of the decade beginning in 2000 action levels in the ISO 5 environment were often 0 CFU, and the action level 1 CFU. John Sharp a former UK medicines inspector termed this phenomenon the "regulatory spiral" (5). It now appears that the introduction of advanced technologies only served to quicken the rotation of the spiral and drive continuous reduction in the radii at each turn.

In retrospect, it now seems evident that from the onset of advanced aseptic process those systems should have been subject to EM requirements that varied considerably from clean room practice.[1] However, the enthusiasm for the benefits that seemed arise from the ongoing and

[1] It seems equally clear that the evolving clean room EM practice although beneficial in the early days ultimately reached a point of diminishing returns by the late 1980s.

ever upward spiraling intensity of EM waned, when clean room EM concepts were applied to isolators; and later to other advanced technologies without any real modification from standard clean room practice. In fact, some regulatory inspectors even suggested that because isolators were less prone to contamination than clean rooms, that EM programs for these devices should be even more intense than those used for EM in clean rooms. This makes no scientific or risk analysis sense at all, and appears to be nothing more than the belief that if you do not find a needle in the haystack at first, then the only logical recourse is to look even harder rather then give up the futile quest.

HONEY I SHRUNK THE CLEAN ROOM

There are those that to this day continue to see isolators, or closed restricted access barrier systems (RABS) as really nothing more than small clean rooms. To people inclined to consider separative technologies in that way it has always seemed logical to treat these shrunken "clean rooms" in exactly the same manner in design and process control as a true human-scale clean room. Hence, in spite of the much smaller enclosed volumes of isolators and to some extent closed RABS, the design parameters for air velocity in these advanced designs has paralleled those used for human-scale clean rooms. Similar emphasis on air stream visualization has been applied to isolator or closed RABS designs in spite of their unmanned operating condition. In addition, it seemed intuitively obvious to too many isolator project and compliance audit teams that the same EM practices should apply as well.

It is now known beyond a doubt that these philosophies are wrong, the "honey I shrunk the clean room" description of separative technologies is at best incomplete and at worst just plain incorrect. The unmanned environment of modern AAPT has only one thing in common with the manned clean room and that is that the air enters the workspace through HEPA or better quality filters. The manned clean room and the isolator or AAPT system could not be more different in terms of contamination control capability and their ability to reduce microbial risk in aseptic processing. As system designers continue to reduce the impact of personnel sourced contamination through the reduction and ultimately the complete elimination of human interventions altogether, the differences in performance have become even more profound.

The rationale for the differences in design and performance are shown clearly by the Akers–Agalloco risk analysis model in aseptic processing and by the studies done by Katayama et al. on various types of "real-world" aseptic processing technologies (6–8). What has emerged is an understanding that the further system designs move toward the elimination of personnel the greater the reduction in contamination risk potential will be observed.

Given the evolution of EM over the last two decades and the emphasis it receives in quality audits, it is improbable that the authors could have written anything more controversial than the last sentence of the previous paragraph. In many cases, the review of EM data is the most time-consuming aspect of a typical aseptic processing audit or inspection. However, what is there to audit if the user reports that in the last 2 years they have had only three EM isolates on their fill line, or even more strikingly that they have had no recoveries of EM isolates or media fill test positives at all.[2] In these two cases, the review of EM data and investigations would take either dramatically less time than that for a conventional clean room, or no time whatsoever. Because if the answer is that no contamination was observed there is really nothing to review. One could discuss the choice of sampling locations and volumes but it is expected that a wise auditor would quickly grasp that where no contamination is observed the system is operating below the analytical limit of detection making these details are of no consequence at all.

A NEW QUESTION EMERGES

The performance of AAPT in terms of contamination control makes it logical to ask a question regarding EM and diminished returns on investment and effort that have never been asked (although perhaps should have been asked) in the context of conventional manned clean rooms.

[2] Suggestions that the detection of such a level of contamination should result in rejection of the material without further consideration should be immediately discounted. Aseptic areas have never been "sterile." The presence of detectable microorganisms in them should neither be surprising, nor indicative of process failure.

That question is simply this, in the wake of irrefutable evidence that what contamination remains in an AAPT is consistently or even completely below the limit of detection of the EM methods employed what possible sense does it make to continue testing with these same methods? It is appropriate to remember the well-known "bon mot" attributed to Einstein and others, "one definition of insanity is to continue to do the same thing again and again while expecting a different outcome." Typically of course, this quote is offered up in aseptic processing as a criticism of those making the same risk increasing mistake over and over again. However, it seems equally applicable to the continued use of a method that provides no quantifiable effect in the measurement of, or if you prefer analysis of, risk. It is tempting to simply stop this chapter now and assert that the preponderance of evidence appears to indicate that the value associated with traditional microbiological EM in AAPT is so low that there is no justification for continuing the practice.

However, that assertion is disquieting in the extreme to both those who have practiced traditional EM for years and still believe in (or haven't yet grasp the limitations) of the exercise, and those compliance focused individuals who believe that should they stop doing microbiological EM they would put themselves and their firm in a position of extreme vulnerability. These points of view are understandable, scientifically invalid though they may be. Readers of this text would be equally dissatisfied if this chapter said did not answer the question, "What can replace microbiological EM in the process control of AAPT?" Therefore, this chapter explores what monitoring/control alternatives are available as industry moves to a future in which all aseptic processes will be advanced and direct human interventions will be a thing of the past. However, before suggesting other means of addressing environmental integrity of AAPT systems it is appropriate to consider why EM has come to have expectations associated with its practice that are scientifically untenable.

PROVING STERILITY THROUGH ENVIRONMENTAL MONITORING—A CONCEPT OUT OF TOUCH WITH REALITY

Again the reader may feel upon first inspection that the authors have written another phrase with the intention of being argumentative or even provocative. After all because EM has been considered an essential part of an overall sterility assurance program, how can its perceived value be tossed aside by the suggestion that the use of EM as a means of assessing sterility is unrealistic? There are sounds reasons for so doing, but to understand these reasons clearly it is necessary to take a critical look at the most common belief structures in conventional aseptic processing and ask challenging questions about their validity.

From its origins into the early 1980s, EM was considered only a means to ensure that an aseptic processing facility was able to operate within a general state of control. Two decades or more ago it was fully accepted that low level contamination was likely perhaps even certain to be recovered during routine surface, active air, and personnel monitoring in manned aseptic processing environments. Gradually, as clean room design improvements, better gowning materials/practices, and equipment automation made it increasingly unlikely for positive samples to be observed the notion that clean rooms should be "sterile" became more prevalent. It seems possible, maybe even probable, that the recommendation of zero as an "alert level" arose from the fact that a typically low percentage of samples did in fact evidence any contamination. Perhaps it also seemed logical to suggest that as the products manufactured by aseptic processing are labeled "sterile," EM recoveries or in the current jargon "hits" are a priori evidence of a loss of sterility. Really, one should not expect to make a sterile product in a nonsterile (or perhaps more accurately a nonaseptic) environment and obviously any environment in which microbiological contamination can be recovered is inarguably nonsterile.

This logic runs head into an immutable scientific truth which is that unless the available methods used to conduct monitoring can in fact measure the attribute called "sterility," said methodology is unsuitable by definition as an indicator of "sterility." So, can microbiological monitoring measure or prove the existence of, even for a snap shot in time, the existence of a sterile environment? Regulations and guidance appear to have evolved based around the belief it is possible to at least "know" when sterility is absent, this is in fact not possible (9,10). Of course if that is true, and it is, surely must also be true it is not possible to "know" when sterility is present either.

Examining the challenge of provable sterility further it is reasonable at some point to ask what "sterility" in fact really is. It is possible to advance a number of definitions, but it is probably most logical to start with the definition that is most widely accepted in science, which is *the complete absence of microorganisms capable of reproduction.* One could, of course, use a definition that appears to be even more rigorous, which is the complete absence of any evidence of life, for example, active metabolism. However, it really does not matter as contemporary EM technologies are incapable of proving sterility by either definition.

Why can't a very large number of EM samples on surfaces, air, and personnel prove sterility? Actually, there are several reasons, but the first among them is that to prove the complete absence of something (microbial contamination) is to prove a negative absolute. Thus, periodic unitary samples even of very large size and incredible intensity would not be sufficient. Nor would continuous sampling at discreet critical locations done for the entire period of an aseptic processing operation be sufficient. No, to prove the absolute that is sterility it is necessary to sample every cubic millimeter of air that enters and exits the environment during the entire process. This of course makes a 4-hour exposure of the 100 mm settle plate a hopelessly futile exercise if the measurement of sterility is really the intent. This is continuous monitoring only because this relatively small plate samples only a tiny fraction of the air around the critical zone and is exposed for a long time, but time of exposure really isn't the issue here, the relative lack of sensitivity and coverage of the sampling method is.

So, the horns of a dilemma emerge very clearly as does the logic (or lack of logic) behind two decades of supposed EM evolution. Obviously, the way things have evolved in EM many in industry seem to think that to claim effective control over the aseptic environment the only approach must be to increase sample intensity. The problem is that a firm can never increase sampling intensity or sample volume enough to make a reasonable statistical approach to the measurement of sterility, even if recovery and growth methods were both universal in their ability to recover and perfect in terms of sensitivity; and quite obviously they are neither. Consider a clean room of 100 m^3 total volume and an air exchange rate of 200 air changes/hr 20,000 m^3 of air flows into and out of the room each hour. Sample sizes in aseptic processing for either total particulate (often wrongly called "nonviable" monitoring) or active microbial air sampling are typically around 1 m^3 and it can take several minutes or even a half an hour to take such a sample. If 100 such samples are taken under constant operation and it is assumed that it took at least 10 minutes to pull a 1 m^3 sample it can be quickly calculated that it is possible to evaluate only 600 m^3 in an hour. This sampling volume or intensity would be staggering in that it would require no less than 300 plates/hr to be incubated or approximately 2400 for a typical 8-hour shift. Yet, for all this considerable effort, expense and intrusion (which comes with their own set of risks to the process), 97% of the air entering this sample environment passes through without being evaluated. One can see very clearly that the higher sampling intensities that have evolved over the last two decades, although undoubtedly well meaning, have been quite futile measured against what would actually be required from a sampling point of view to prove sterility. It must be restated that sample volume is only one of the issues, sensitivity and universality of recovery are equally important and if anything even more problematic

For the sake of further evaluation make the assumption that it is possible to actually conduct the 60,000 samples/hr required to sample the entire air volume entering the room described in the previous paragraph. Wouldn't it be possible then to know that "sterility" had been achieved? Would it be possible to devise some super sampler that could sample all the air and return it to the environment uncontaminated (a very tall order as people would have to load and unload this mind-boggling number of samplers, it is certain that some adventitious contamination would occur calling the entire endeavor into question)? To measure sterility it would be necessary to meet yet another requirement. There would need be available an analytical method so sensitive, universal, accurate, and precise that it could be relied upon to recover any viable organism present in the room. Because sterility is the objective the sampling cannot be restricted to just the mold or bacteria present, it is essential to expand the expectation to include all obligate intracellular parasites such as virus as well. Of course, there are many pathogens to say nothing of saprophytic organisms that could never be recovered or grow under the generic culture conditions currently employed. This forces an important realization, which is quite simply that a 0 CFU result on an EM sample cannot mean *sterile* and but rather *nothing detected*.

These realities also point out other inconvenient truths, including the fact that media fills cannot prove sterility even if the media fill requirements were increased to 1,000,000 containers per test run.[3] It must also be recognized that the sterility test in spite of its euphemistic title can't prove "sterility" either, not just because of sample size limitations inherent in this destructive test method, but also because it too is limited in microbiological sensitivity. Or, to put it another way, all the microbiological methods used in "validation," product release testing and monitoring in aseptic processing have a limit of detection considerably higher than zero.

ABSOLUTE PROOF OF STERILITY ELUDES US

Quite often in discussions about the limitations of sterility testing, process simulation testing and EM nonmicrobiologists among the regulatory community, standard-setting organizations, and industry attack the inadequacy of microbiological analysis. The authors of this chapter have often been confronted with someone who suggests that the measurement systems should be able to measure "sterility" and the thing holding industry back must be the inadequacy of the methods themselves. More recently, there are individuals who have suggested that if industry would implement instrumental and more rapid microbiological analysis then it could surely measure "sterility."

Chemical analysis is far more precise and accurate than microbiological assays, including the latest rapid or instrumental methods. However, analytical chemistry can't measure the absolute absence of a material either. In terms of universal recovery of contaminants chemical assays fall short as well, as no single method can measure the absolute absence of everything. Everyone seems to understand when there are situations in cleaning validation where the limit of detection of an assay specific for a single contaminant is insufficiently sensitive and thus unable to measure the trace quantities that might put the process at risk. However, those same people somehow seem to believe that it should be possible to use microbiological assays to measure the absolute absence of all microbial contamination.

To state the obvious, the problem of measuring sterility is not one of inadequate methodology it is rather one of insufficient understanding of the real problem. Absolutist mentality seems to accompany the claim of "sterility" on a label, but this attitude is so completely wrong that it is surprising that it is not routinely discussed for what it is. What it is, is of course a mistake that manifests itself to one degree or another in many current EM standards and guidelines and which has plagued advanced aseptic processing as the first isolators came into use over 20 years ago. It is wrong-headed absolutism that led some in industry to think that there had to be a way to prove that isolators could be a suitable replacement for terminal sterilization and to thus embark on the completely futile path of trying to prove a 10^6 sterility assurance level (SAL) in these systems. Initially, some thought the failure to accomplish this goal was because the microbiological methods weren't good enough, actually though it was a failure in the human thought process not an analysis failure. The absurd suggestion that some inspectors made that isolators should be subject to more testing in the form of greater EM sampling and bigger process simulation tests results is busy work, may actually increase the contamination potential and is completely unnecessary because it will not enable us to make more confident claims regarding "sterility."

So, the authors offer this first law of aseptic processing process control:

It has neither been, nor will it ever be possible to measure the attribute of "sterility" by any current or anticipated microbiological assay.

It is appropriate to consider what realistically attainable goal might be established for aseptic processing. It's really quite simple, and one that industry has consistently achieved for many years—assurance of patient safety for sterile products manufactured aseptically. The

[3] Despite FDA's recent change to their current good manufacturing practices (cGMP) regulations, it is widely acknowledged that there are no accepted means to "validate" aseptic processing. Media fills regardless of their size cannot "validate" aseptic processing, they can be considered another form of environmental monitoring subject to the same limitations described herein.

absolute nature of "sterility" confounds our ability to attain it; however avoiding contamination in sterile products through the use of aseptic processing is accomplished on a daily basis. Considering the aseptic limitations inherent in subsequent activities associated with administration of sterile products to actual patients, the industrial preparation of those products is perhaps the most certain part of the entire process. Sterile products are certainly safe as delivered in their final package; once the container is opened, the activities of reconstitution, admixture, and administration are without a doubt less certain!

The objective in commercial-scale operations, therefore, must be to ensure patient safety rather than prove sterility.

MOVING FORWARD POSITIVELY

The objective of this chapter is not to treat EM negatively, but rather to carefully consider its true analytical capability and limitations so that it may be used wisely and effectively. It should be quite obvious that EM has reached a point of diminishing return and that as an industry modern aseptic processing facilities have already exceeded the point where EM is no longer a value-added exercise in the assurance of safety.[4] It seems counterproductive to continue to pretend these limitations don't exist and that absolutist thinking is anything other than pointless. However, the assertion of process control in an effort to ensure microbiological safety and the existence of a validated state of control when using AAPT is a necessary requirement.

It is essential to have means of assuring product/patient safety, it is just that the way in which industry has gone about it has been entirely wrong, and the idea that "sterility" can be proven in the absolute sense is really quite naïve. Rather than dwell further on the weaknesses of long-standing aseptic process control thinking and its general inapplicability to the vastly cleaner environments that are can be expected in the future; it is appropriate to consider new metrics that better utilize resources and provide the information needed in the most efficient means possible.

The first and most important positive step that must be taken is to disabuse ourselves of the notion that as sterility is the absence of microbiological contamination, microbiological means must be used to measure safety. Absolutist mentality has sent industry into a cul-de-sac, and the only positive way out is to make a U-turn.

This leads us to offer our second law of aseptic processing process control:

Microbiological analysis is not required to demonstrate product safety in advanced aseptic processing.

This is not as heretical as it may seem. In fact, EM is not routinely used in aseptic surgery and hasn't been for many years because it has been understood in that discipline that the microbiological data collected was not a reliable predictor of risk. The newest aseptic food processes are also devoid of EM for similar reasons. Also, the effort and cost required to collect the data were not found to be value added.

In conventional aseptic processing it is understood that it is encouraging to determine that the majority of the samples do not reveal microbial growth. This is reflected by the most recent proposed revisions of USP <1116>, which addresses itself to the microbial control of classified environments, and suggests that <1% contamination recovery rates should be routinely attained in ISO 5 environments. Of course, it should be understood that in microbiological sampling zero does not mean no organisms present ("sterile") but rather no contamination detected. So again, although it might be comforting to suppose that the overwhelming predominance of zeros in conventional clean room ISO 5 critical zones indicates that the environment is at least *mostly* sterile; however that is not what the data are really telling us.

In the case of isolators and other advanced aseptic processing in which humans are not conducting direct interventions the probability of recovering organisms is 100- to 1000-fold less than in manned environments. This, quite reasonably, argues for less "viable" monitoring not more.

[4] By this point in the chapter the reader should be willing to fully acknowledge that the measurement of sterility is impossible and hence attempting to do so is a less than zero sum game.

WHERE WOULD CONTAMINATION IN AN AAPT COME FROM?

Well, the likelihood of it being derived from people is exceeding low, which is the whole point of advanced aseptic processing. Nevertheless, this has not stopped speculation about other sources of contamination, which are the following:

1. Gloves—It is certainly true that in the early days of isolator based sterility testing and in isolator production systems installed as recently as the mid-1990s glove leaks and low-level glove contamination were observed. The glove in fact was identified as the principle weakness in these systems and the route by which contamination of human origin could still reach the critical zone within an isolator. The introduction of contamination through gloves is significantly less of an issue now than it was 12 to 15 years ago. First, gloves in the 1980s through 1990s were primarily of Neoprene construction and gloves made of this material become friable over time and after numerous exposures to VPHP. Today nearly all gloves are Hypalon a material that is both highly tear and puncture resistant and far more resistant to VPHP. Also, the wearing of an underglove is more common and elaborate glove integrity testing and management programs are now in place. Also, ergonomics have improved, automation has increased and in some isolators gloves are now used infrequently or even not at all. So, at this time gloves are no longer sources of significant contamination risk and the time is approaching when they will be far more rarely used or even eliminated altogether.[5]
2. Leaks—In the early stages of AAPT with the then available isolator technology there was concern that leaks in the enclosure could be significant risk modalities. It was hypothesized by some that small leaks combined with rapid air flow in the enclosure could result in the entrainment of contamination via the Bernoulli or venturi effect. This hypothesis has not been confirmed and there has been no report of contamination entering an isolator through such leaks. Of course, all mechanical things leak, but isolators for aseptic processing are maintained at a positive pressure relative to the surrounding room which means there is adequate air overspill to ensure that the enclosure remains free of contamination.[6]
3. RTPs—A real cause célèbre in the 1990s was the potential of the so-called "ring of uncertainty" as a source of contamination. It was noticed that the very apex of the lip seal where the two RTP flanges are sealed would not be treated with VPHP during the decontamination process. Even when the concern about this potential contamination source was greatest no contamination event was confirmed. Also, a number of countermeasures were put into place including false containers, which allowed the ring to be treated or at least half of it to be treated. Manual decontamination and heat sterilization have also been employed to mitigate this perceived risk. Where product contact parts are moved into the enclosure using RTPs the "ring of uncertainty" can be covered by a sterilized skirt or insert to ensure that there is no opportunity for these components to contact the "ring." Lastly, many critical transfers are now done through e-beam or VPHP tunnels, and VPHP passboxes that have come into wider use.
4. "Mouseholes"—So-called open isolators, which are systems that use "mouseholes" to allow materials to enter and exit the enclosure were once thought to be at risk from contamination entering from the external environment. One regulatory guidance document even suggested that insects could fly through an isolator opening and into the enclosure. Or course, isolators that use mouse holes are equipped with ample compensating air overspill and typically operate at a pressure of +30 to 50 Pa relative to the surrounding environment. Experience has confirmed that mouse holes are not a significant contamination source.
5. HEPA filters—This is the last and most recent hypothetical isolator problem and like the four listed before it, this one has also been thoroughly debunked. The argument put forth was the HEPA filters are not "microbially retentive filters" and are therefore not of sterilizing

[5] Gloveless isolators are increasing being utilized in aseptic food production, and are available for pharmaceutical application as well.

[6] The same air overspill concept is what protects the manned aseptic processing area from contamination from the surrounding lower pressure and less clean environments.

grade. It therefore, stands to reason that unless the air was sterilized by some other modality such as heat the air could not be sterile. Actually, at the flow rates they are designed to accommodate HEPA filters are extremely effective, typically 99.97% to 99.997% of all 0.3 μM particles are removed from the air stream. In many modern isolators and AAPT the make-up or fresh air is filtered through a HEPA prefilter at its way to the air plenum in the ventilation system. Because these systems typically re-circulate 80% to 90% of the air passing through the enclosure, the majority of the ventilation air passes through the HEPA filters many, many times per hour. Of course it is impossible to know if this air is truly sterile, because the residual level of microbial contamination is below the current level of detection. Continuous total particle counting in static isolators has shown zero contamination even after as many as 72 hours of sampling.

It was clear from the very beginning that the level of contamination in isolators was extremely low and there is now similar experience with results from other types of AAPT as well. As industry moves toward an era of more complete automation and gloveless separative technologies microbiological risk will be even less of a concern.

Thus, we offer our third law of aseptic processing process control:

As the need for human intervention is reduced or eliminated, the less valuable microbiologically focused EM becomes.

REASONABLE MICROBIOLOGICAL MONITORING

The authors are unconvinced that traditional viable monitoring is capable of providing useful information regarding contamination risk or patient safety. It is widely thought that EM might still have benefit in terms of providing some means of detecting a catastrophic failure. However, in the very unlikely event of such a breech occurring total particulate analysis using an electronic counter or changes in internal pressure would be a superior approach. These systems give immediate feedback and could provide data regarding changes in environmental control performance in something approaching real time.

This is somewhat different than what is typically called in this industry "nonviable particulate" monitoring. It would be more accurate to call this analysis "total particulate monitoring" as in the previous paragraph. These systems count all particles and do not selectively count only those that are "nonviable." In fact, systems are now emerging that use spectrophotometric methods to resolve putatively viable organisms from nonviable particulate. These systems can even recover the viable but not-culturable organisms that may make up as much as 40% to 50% of the total environmental population. Although experience with these systems is limited, they may provide a means of getting environmental control data quickly and efficiently.

Despite this treatise, the long association of microbiological EM with aseptic processing is likely to continue as the regulatory expectation is that viable EM will be done. However, as the idea that more monitoring is required in AAPT than in manned clean rooms has been thoroughly debunked. It is our position that only routine active air and surface monitoring should be performed:

1. Active air sampling should be done within the enclosure at not less than two locations. The settling plate is not sensitive enough to be of much value and should not be done although in some jurisdictions it remains an expectation. There is no value in doing air sampling more than once per day given that its sensitivity is not really sufficient for this analysis.
2. Glove and surface sampling should only be done at the end of a campaign. It is illogical to do in-process sampling as it is not desirable to leave media residues in a working AAPT. If gloves are physically leak tested after use, this has a higher level of sensitivity regarding contamination risk than microbiological monitoring. However even leaks detected on the gloves may not be definitive evidence of contamination (11). Therefore, only limited surface monitoring should be done and realistically the need for this sampling is technically questionable.
3. Continuous total particle counting can be done: the probe(s) should measure the air approaching the point of fill/seal or manufacture. This way the assessment of air quality would not be affected by process generated particulate.

SUMMARY

EM in AAPT should not blindly follow the existing flawed manned clean room paradigm. The risk levels are entirely different and the already limited sensitivity of traditional microbiological methods makes them even less valuable in these low contamination background environments than they are in manned environments. The authors recognize that this change in approach will require changes in industry and regulatory understanding of the utility of EM and ultimately revisions to existing cGMP and guideline documents. Realistically, a reassessment is already overdue even in the conventional manned clean room concept.

It should be recognized that these technologies have not merely shrunk the clean room they have essentially eliminated the major sources of contamination. Further refinement is already underway for the systematic elimination of even very minor contamination sources. Continuing with traditional approaches to in-process control is illogical and scientifically wrong in AAPT systems. New and more enlightened approaches based upon evidentiary science are required. One would not use a World War II era air-speed indicator that was able to measure only to 350 knots on a modern fighter capable of 1200 knots. Similarly, one should readily understand that 1950s technologies such as touch and settle plates cannot provide useful information in AAPT and this will become even truer as these technologies continue to evolve and improve. Already today, active air sampling has proven of almost no value in current AAPT designs and settle plates are even less useful.

It is senseless to cling to the past as industry moves into the future. We sincerely hope that process control in AAPT will be discussed from only a scientific and engineering perspective and that industry can move forward with a truly clean sheet of paper. Only then will approaches to process control be properly vetted. The era of risk- and science-based approaches to regulation and quality by design (QbD) should allow for the flexibility technological advancement of this magnitude necessitates.

REFERENCES

1. Tetzlaff R. Regulatory aspects of aseptic processing. Pharm Technol 1984; 8:39–44.
2. Avallone HL. Control aspects of aseptically produced products. J Parenteral Sci Technol 1985; 39:75–79.
3. Avallone HL. Clean room design, control and characterization. Pharm Eng 1982; 46:33–34.
4. Wilson JD. Aseptic process monitoring—a better strategy. J Parenteral Sci Technol 1997; 51:111–114.
5. Sharp J. Letter to the Editor. J Parenteral Sci Technol 1993; 47(1):2–3.
6. Agalloco J. Akers J. Risk analysis for aseptic processing: the Akers–Agalloco method. Pharm Technol 2005; 29(11):74–88.
7. Agalloco J. Akers J. Simplified risk analysis for aseptic processing: the Akers–Agalloco method. Pharm Technol 2006; 30(7):60–76.
8. Katayama H, Toda A, Tonkunaga Y, et al. Proposal for a new categorization of aseptic processing facilities based on risk assessment scores". PDA J Pharm Sci Technol 2008; 62(4):235–243.
9. EMEA. Annex 1, Sterile Medicinal Products, 2008.
10. FDA. Guideline on Sterile Drug Products Produced by Aseptic Processing. 2004.
11. Sigwarth V. Gessler A. Stark A. Relevance of Physical Glove Integrity Testing to Microbial Contamination of Isolator Systems. Presented at ISPE meeting. Prague, Czech Republic, 2005.

24 Decontamination of advanced aseptic processing environments

James Agalloco and James Akers

INTRODUCTION

The control of microbial contamination is a critical requirement for environments used in aseptic processing. The first inclination of many practitioners (and unfortunately many regulators) is to seek sterility for that environment as that would seemingly assure the greatest potential for success. Expectations for sterility (or near sterility) of the environment are implied by statements found in US Food and Drug Administration's (FDA's) latest aseptic processing guidance (1). That guidance document includes such statements as:

"Samples from Class 100 (ISO 5) environments should normally yield no microbiological contaminants."

"Air monitoring samples of critical areas should normally yield no microbiological contaminants."

"Modern aseptic processing operations should normally yield no media fill contamination."

In a traditional manned aseptic processing environment, it is simply not possible to achieve sterility, and although decontamination of those environments is an expectation there is a simple reality that prevents decontamination from achieving a stable microbial control level that approaches the ideal of "sterility." This is because in a manned environment, human operators function as mobile contamination generators and contribute levels of mostly transient contamination. The level of contamination operators contribute will vary primarily as a function of the strenuousness with which they are required to work. Also, the contamination produced by operators is primarily airborne; decontamination of surfaces although often a positive contamination control activity, it is largely ineffective against the airborne personnel-contributed contamination most likely to put product at risk. Given the analytical limitations of microbial analysis one cannot reasonably expect monitoring to prove "sterility" either. So, although necessary and useful, neither treatments to eliminate contamination nor attempts to measure contamination enable us to achieve the condition of "sterility" in manned aseptic processing operations.

Therefore, when personnel are introduced into an aseptic processing environment intimations of sterility are certainly excessive. Microbial contamination has been ever present in manned aseptic processing, yet operational success has steadily progressed. The Parenteral Drug Association's (PDA) periodic surveys on aseptic processing practices revealed a steadily improving performance capability (2). Nearly all of the improvements evidenced by industry's advances in aseptic processing were accomplished prior to the advent of the newer technologies such as isolators and restricted access barrier systems (RABS).

The treatments used for control of microbial populations in manned aseptic processing need not be perfect. That could be restated as they neither need sterilize, nor meet the requirements for of sterilization validation to be acceptable. In fact, given the toxic nature of decontamination agents, they cannot be used at times when the manned aseptic environment is at greatest risk, which is when human operators are present and product is at risk. Thus, in the manned aseptic clean rooms, the environment is essentially microbially compromised at all times during operation and comes closest to the desired germ-free condition only when sporicidally decontaminated and free of personnel.

Because the operators (including those that would perform the environmental decontamination and monitoring) are contributing microorganisms throughout the process, the heating, ventilation and air conditioning (HVAC) system and procedural controls serve to protect the exposed materials from contamination throughout the process. RABS and isolators provide better separation between the personnel and the exposed sterile materials, but the same limitations exist albeit to a lesser extent. The initial microbial state of the environment is important, but certainly not the only consideration with respect to assuring acceptable aseptic processing in these facilities.

Isolators are aseptic processing environments in which sterile materials are handled and in some cases assembled into finished sterile dosage forms. Their application for aseptic processing mirrors that of a manned clean room in which similar procedures have been conducted for many years. Isolators provide a near-absolute separation between personnel and products, and if sterilized (as opposed to decontaminated) the microbial control goals some regulations imply are possible. Should isolators be sterilized prior to the aseptic process, after all wouldn't that afford greater confidence in the aseptic operations to follow?

First, one must consider whether that expectation is a reasonable one. To explore this, recall the distinction between aseptic and sterile: aseptic means free of pathogenic organisms; whereas sterile means free of all life forms. Our industry has blurred the distinction between aseptically produced and terminally sterilized products. It is recognized that terminally sterilized products are inherently safer than those which are aseptically produced, although the level of risk associated with any product labeled sterile can vary considerably based on how a drug, biological, or device is admixed, administered, or used. Many sterile products must be produced aseptically because the product cannot withstand a terminal treatment in its final container. The use of an isolator for aseptic processing will not be improved by treatment of the internal environment to eliminate (sterilize) all microorganisms. Manned clean rooms have been successfully used for aseptic processing for over 40 years, and although these modern clean rooms control microbial contamination effectively they have never been nor will they ever be "sterile." That an isolator should be sterilized, just because it can, ignores the difficulties created by harsh chemical treatments on process materials and equipment. The soft parts of the isolator (gloves, half suits, and other plastic materials), biological substances, elastomeric materials, equipment parts, and electronic components can all be damaged or altered by the conditions required to attain sterility, at least as sterility assurance is defined in the validation of sterilization process in industry where extreme levels of overkill are commonly targeted. An effort to attain internal sterility at the present level of isolator design would result in potential loss of isolator integrity and likely substantial adverse impacts upon many of the other items necessary for aseptic processing.

The goal of the decontamination treatment is the establishment of an environment essentially free or in the case of manned clean rooms sufficiently free of microorganisms. This can be accomplished in the clean room by using manual sanitization of the internal surfaces by gowned personnel. In an isolator, it is realized by treating the internal volume with most commonly a sporicidal vapor and less frequently an atomized liquid or gas. The treatment provided to reach this state need not meet the higher standards for sterilization to be suitable for aseptic processing. The most prevalent definition of overkill sterilization states:

> Overkill sterilization is a process where the destruction of a high concentration of a resistant microorganism supports the elimination of bioburden that might be present in routine processing. That objective can be demonstrated by attaining any of the following: a defined minimum F0; a defined time-temperature condition or a defined log reduction of a biological indicator. (3)

Delivering an overkill process is the common objective in the sterilization of many items, especially where the materials being processed are intended for human use. The high margin of safety afforded provides an acceptable level of risk to the patient. It provides for a far lower than one chance in a million that an organism might survive the process. In fact, overkill sterilization may produce probability of nonsterility of tens of orders of magnitudes less. That far exceeds what is required to mitigate risk in an aseptic processing environment; the clean room or isolator is after all not going to be injected into a human. All that is required for aseptic processing is an environment sufficiently free of contamination such that patient risk is low and well controlled.

In clean rooms, this is routinely accomplished by manual disinfection of surfaces with a non-sporicidal agent,[1] although sporicides are generally also employed on a less frequent basis.

[1] Sporicidal treatment of classified environments is customarily performed on a periodic or as needed basis, as an adjunct to substantially more frequent decontamination with phenolic or quaternary ammonium compounds.

The use of a sporicide injected automatically by a validated process at a scientifically established dose with uniform distribution for the decontamination of an isolator providing multiple log reduction of a spore (substantially less than the 12 logs required for an overkill process) is far more effective in the elimination of microorganisms than what is accomplished manually by personnel in a clean room. The PDA has suggested the complete kill of a resistant spore with an initial population of 10^3 (effectively a 5–6 log reduction when multiple biological indicators (BIs) are used) is sufficient to render the isolator free of detectable microorganisms (4).

If a 12-log reduction (overkill sterilization treatment) is provided to an isolator there are several potential negative consequences:

- Longer dwell periods are required to achieve greater kill with extended exposure of the materials inside the isolator to the chemical agent.
- Longer exposure periods result in increased interaction between the agent and exposed materials/surfaces risking component failure and higher agent residuals.
- Longer exposure periods result in the potential for increased penetration into porous materials causing greater interaction as well as substantially longer aeration periods.
- Longer overall cycles reduce the operational availability of the isolator.
- The oxidizers used for vapor or gas decontamination may cause product damage at concentrations of 100 PPB or less, this means exposure levels and outgassing may be critical.

Sterilization is not a reasonable objective for isolator microbial control, particularly when the isolator is not the item that must be sterile. The isolator only provides the environment in which the aseptic process occurs. A common term for the antimicrobial treatment needed for isolator is decontamination. It differs from sterilization only by degree and level of documentation. In the pharmaceutical industry, we define sterilization as not more than one contaminated unit in a million, but this is an arbitrary risk analysis criterion. An isolator that is decontaminated to an appropriate level is considerably safer than a manually decontaminated clean room; in fact the absence of contamination generating personnel in separative technologies would make them safer even in the absence of decontamination.

Validated and automatically controlled decontamination treatments of isolators that provide a 5 to 6 log reduction (complete kill of a 10^3 challenge) of a resistant spore are more able to reduce microbial populations to lower levels relative to manual disinfection of a clean room by gowned personnel. It is important to note that the 10^3 spore challenge population is a minimal requirement and actually complete kill of a 10^6 spore challenge population in the validation of isolator decontamination is far more common. The manual disinfection of a clean room is subject to substantial variations in efficacy, after all the process is only as effective the operators' proficiency. Where sporicidal agents are used in clean room disinfection they are only used intermittently, with the bulk of the regimen provided by nonsporicidal agents. The personnel performing the manual disinfection are another significant shortcoming; the very personnel charged with applying the disinfecting materials are contributing microbial contamination in the clean room by their very presence and their physical exertion while conducting disinfection.

As the goal of the sporicidal treatment is elimination of microorganisms from an operating environment, rather than preparation for human injection, sterility as defined by at least a 12-log reduction in a resistant biological indicator is an unrealistic goal. If attaining a sterile state within the isolator were possible without risking material damage, increased aeration time, and decreased capacity, then perhaps it would be a reasonable requirement. As sterility in the classical sense cannot be accomplished without compromising other considerations, then less lethal decontamination is more appropriate.

DETERMINING APPROPRIATE PROCESS OBJECTIVES FOR ASEPTIC PROCESSING COMPONENTS

In the use of isolators or RABS for aseptic processing some parts of the system must be sterilized; for example, product contact parts, whereas others need only be decontaminated, for example enclosure internal surfaces. This is wholly consistent with the practices employed in manned clean rooms and should not be altered when the aseptic process is conducted in an isolator or RABS.

Sterilization of Product Contact Materials

The sterilization requirements for product contact parts or container/closure systems within advanced aseptic processing systems are identical to those established for conventional manned aseptic processes; a probability of a non-sterile unit (PNSU) of 10^{-6} or better. Direct or indirect connection of autoclaves, dry-heat ovens, or tunnels for these materials to the enclosures is relatively straightforward. On a smaller scale, the transfers can be accomplished using either transfer isolators or RTP containers. Aseptic connections of any type for liquid product or inerting gases must be made within the enclosure for maximal mitigation of risk. Sterilization-in-place (SIP) capable of being hard piped to a connection point within the enclosure is the lowest risk means of supply. Stopper bowls and component delivery systems are better treated in situ by the same vapor or gas process used for isolator decontamination. It is often impractical and generally more risky to attempt to sterilize these systems out of place and install them aseptically within the isolator. Also, sterilizing them and then installing them when the isolator is "open" achieves nothing in terms of added safety.

Gas Decontamination of the Isolator and Internal Equipment Surfaces

Decontamination is a more reasonable objective than sterilization for the nonproduct contact surfaces of isolators. A 5 to 6 log reduction of resistant BIs is certainly sufficient (the complete kill of indicators with a population of 10^3 spores). Isolators are unfriendly environments for microbial survival and colonization; the complete kill of a 10^3 population is far more effective than manual decontamination of a clean room by gowned personnel. There is a special category of RABS (cRABS) designed that are decontaminated in a room in a similar fashion and then operated as a RABS with air overspill to the background environment.

High Level Disinfection of the RABS and Internal Equipment Surfaces

High-level disinfection has been defined by the International Society for Pharmaceutical Engineering (ISPE) with respect to RABS as "... capable of destroying all organisms with the exception of high numbers of resistant spores" (5). That definition was adapted from an earlier definition originally developed by Block (6). The treatment of the internal surfaces of a RABS is accomplished by aseptically gowned personnel. The early stages of the treatment could be accomplished with the RABS open, whereas the last and more critical surfaces would be decontaminated using gloves installed on the RABS. A sporicidal agent would be used, but the manual nature of the application limits its overall effectiveness as does any treatment performed when the doors are open. Alternatively, RABS with or separate from the surrounding environment can be treated with vapor phase hydrogen peroxide (VPHP) achieving a level of spore log reduction compliant with the minimal recommendations for isolators.

Methods for Introduction of Wrapped Sterile Materials

Many aseptic processes require items that have been previously sterilized by radiation or other means be introduced into the aseptic environment after exposure to a less capable environment. With clean rooms, this is often accomplished by manual decontamination using a sporicidal agent often in conjunction with a double-door airlock or pass-through. Using an isolator or RABS, the wrapped parts or components can be introduced through a tunnel in which surface sanitization of the package is performed. The tunnel replaces the pass-through or airlock of the conventional clean room. These methods are intended to surface sanitize the exterior of the package only because the interior of the pack and the components are already sterile. The decontamination of the wrapping is intended only to preserve the conditions within the enclosure as materials are introduced. The use of multiple sterile layers is commonplace to provide a means for minimizing bioburden on materials as they are introduced.

Critical Aspects in Environmental Decontamination

There are a number of essential requirements for environment decontamination of enclosures or environments that must be addressed. These are applicable regardless of whether the objective is sterilization (as some firms have sought) or decontamination. Sterilization or decontamination using either vapors or gases has proven consistently efficacious. However, they impose different challenges and requirements regarding cycle development, process control, and validation.

Dosage of the Decontamination Agent

To assure consistent lethality in a sterilization/decontamination process, it is essential that a constant amount of the chemical agent be present. With gas sterilization this is usually accomplished by recirculation of the gas. Ethylene oxide (ETO) sterilizers will sometimes use large external blowers to help insure uniform gas concentration across the chamber. When isolators were first decontaminated with VPHP it was recognized that thorough mixing of the vapor to ensure uniformity of distribution provided clear advantages in decontamination effectiveness, this resulted in the placement of circulation fans to assist in achieving uniform lethality. With the introduction of large-scale filling isolators equipped for unidirectional air flow internally, it was sometimes found that in some cases this circulation alone was sufficient to assure uniform vapor distribution. As there are no reported adverse effects of placing internal fans within enclosures, their inclusion in the design is recommended. They certainly do no harm when in operation during the exposure to the agent or during the aeration of the isolator after the treatment. In room decontamination, internal circulating systems can help provide more uniform conditions than is possible solely from the room HVAC system.

Concentration measurement was at one point thought to correspond well to VPHP decontamination effect, but several studies have demonstrated that this correlation is not reliable. At the present time, this can only be accomplished at reasonable cost for chlorine dioxide (ClO_2). The instrumentation for measurement of H_2O_2 is prohibitively expensive for more than a single-point determination, whereas in-process concentration measurement of other agents (O_3 and peracetic acid) is not presently available. It is important to note though that the conditions for VPHP vaporization as well as the mass of solution vaporized can be consistently controlled to a very high level. This in combination with well-controlled vapor distribution results in uniform and consistent decontamination.

The presence of hydrogen peroxide can be confirmed by chemical indicators, and where they can be observed during the exposure phase they can provide some indication of concentration uniformity. If the distribution of the H_2O_2 is consistent, the chemical indicators should change color at similar times, although variability as high as 50% is possible. There are no chemical indicators available for use with the other decontamination agents.

Relative Humidity

Just as achieving a constant gas concentration is necessary for effective treatment; so is a constant and typically elevated level of humidity. Although agents used for gaseous decontamination agents are different, they all require the presence of humidity to achieve efficient sporicidal effect. It has been well understood for many years that humidified spores are more permeable to gaseous agents. In O_3 (which is not widely used in the decontamination of isolators or clean rooms) and ClO_2 processes, the humidity is introduced prior to the addition of the gas, whereas the vapor processes using H_2O_2 and peracetic acid add water in either the vapor or liquid state as part of introducing the decontamination agent.

The measures used for assuring uniform concentration of the decontaminating agent will also provide for even distribution of the humidity across the isolator. Its measurement at multiple locations is substantially easier than gas concentration however there have been relatively few reports of multipoint measurement having actually been used.

Temperature

The process temperature is an important factor in the lethality of any decontamination process. Temperature has been shown to increase lethality in chemical sterilization or decontamination processes. Of course, as liquid water is always in equilibrium with its gaseous equivalent, water vapor, the ability of an environment to sustain a concentration of water varies as a function of temperature, the higher the temperature the greater the concentration of water vapor an atmosphere can support in the gas phase. Thus, the requirement of water vapor introduction often in the form of steam means that gas processes will always have some vapor component. The temperature may be highest with some VPHP generator systems close to the inlet point and this can result in poor saturation levels and as a result lower lethality. Some vapor processes have the added complication of having a changing temperature during the process. The addition of a hot vapor to a room temperature chamber over an extended period of time results in a process that may not reach a steady-state condition. This has profound effects in the use of H_2O_2 and is described in greater detail in the appendix to this chapter. Both the higher temperature circumstance at the inlet and the rising temperature during injection are not significant issues in all VPHP generator systems.

Generally, modest temperature differences across enclosures appear to have little impact on the lethality. All of these agents are strong oxidizers and the rate of chemical reaction (and thus microbial inactivation) is relatively constant over a fairly wide temperature range. Rapid decontamination can be achieved at elevated temperature, but only when the injection rate is increased to achieve saturation or even condensing conditions throughout the target.

It is worth noting that ClO_2 is explosive at temperatures in excess of 40°C, so caution must be exercised when it is used especially around heat sterilizing equipment.

UNIFORMITY OF CONDITIONS

To achieve consistent results in a decontamination (or sterilization) process, uniformity of conditions is highly desirable. The greater the turbulence inside the enclosure the more uniform the process parameters are likely to be and the more consistent the results obtained. Some vendors have attempted to rely on unidirectional air flow (as provided in many filling isolators) to provide uniform conditions. This may be acceptable, however, the reasons unidirectional flow is desired for aseptic processing are exactly why it is nonoptimal for the decontamination process. It is strongly recommended that the enclosure be as well mixed as possible, and the use of additional internal fans to promote greater mixing is often advantageous.

BIOLOGICAL INDICATORS

Confirmation of process lethality for decontamination is established through the inactivation of resistant microorganisms. The most common choices for the agents used for isolators are *Geobacillus stearothermophilus* (for H_2O_2 and peracetic acid) and *Bacillus subtilis* (for ClO_2 and O_3), though the relative resistance of these organisms to any of these agents is not substantially different (7–9). What is certain is that these organisms are more resistant than the majority of expected bioburden organisms that might be encountered. The relative resistance for the indicator organisms relative to bioburden varies but is typically 1 to 2 logs greater.

A variety of biological indicator presentations have been used with these agents, ranging from paper strips, fiberglass discs to stainless steel coupons. Regardless of the indicator type selected, it is essential that the resistance of the indicator to the process be understood. The supplier of the indicator must play a major role in this process, and close coordination between the supplier and the end user is essential.

Much has been made of so-called "substrate effects" in which firms have exposed resistant indicators on a variety of materials to confirm the effectiveness of the process. This appears to be little more than a "make-work" exercise, as although the apparent resistance changes from material to material, once a "worst-case" substrate has been identified by one researcher; there is no evidence to support a different result obtained elsewhere. The substrate for the biological indicator is really of little relevance; it is the relative resistance of the spores on the indicator to the bioburden that plays a greater role in cycle effectiveness.

It is likely that what has been defined as substrate effect is at least in part a result of the high spore populations used in decontamination challenges. It has become commonplace to use populations of one million or more spores per carrier, which parallels the typical moist heat practice. However, the vapors and gases used for isolator or clean room decontamination do not penetrate spore clumps or envelopes with the efficiency of steam. One should choose a substrate that provides for consistent lethality over time, and once that has been identified use it for all studies. That is a practice that has been successful for sterilization validation for decades. That substrate effects exist should not come as a surprise to anyone; making too much of the minor differences between one substrate to another is unfortunate. The most logical substrate to employ is stainless steel as nearly all product contact material treated directly by gas or vapor during decontamination is manufactured from this material. Also, studies on various carrier material have consistently shown that stainless steel is quite representative. There is really no point in using alternate substrates, stainless steel has proven quite satisfactory in practice over a decade of studies.

All of these agents are surface sterilants that penetrate rather poorly, especially relative to steam or even ETO. Because their penetration is relatively weak relative to other sterilizing methods, the biological indicator packaging plays a vital role in the resistance. It has been shown that H_2O_2 biological indicators packaged in Tyvek are harder to kill than "naked" or un-enveloped BIs (10). Chlorine dioxide BIs packaged in glassine envelopes may exhibit resistance increases of twofold or more (11). Biological indicators on different matrixes have been shown to give very different results. Glass fiber filter paper as used for BIs in steam sterilization resulted in extremely variable results with H_2O_2, this variability depending to a significant degree upon the degree to which spores populations were free of organic and inorganic contaminants. As mentioned previously, glass fiber filter papers have been replaced in many cases by stainless steel carriers for excellent practical reasons (12).

There are some cautions with the use of biological indicators of which the reader should be aware. Proper preparation of the BI is all important, the preparation must be extremely clean; the presence of cellular debris or organic salts from media or buffer solutions can cause substantial variations in indicator performance. The *D* value for the challenge organism should not be spore population dependent; this is an indication problematic spore preparation or perhaps inoculation. The use of commercially prepared BIs is highly recommended as the vendors have substantially more experience with their preparation than most end users.

It is wise to test each lot of BIs to verify its resistance; counting the population of spores is not enough. The resistance of the spores can be determined for comparative purposes in a small isolator using a fraction-negative approach at the intended cycle parameters. The user should be aware that "*D* value" claims are not generally appropriate with BIs marketed for use with VPHP. There are at least three commercial VPHP processes and BIs will exhibit different resistance characteristics under different test conditions. Resistance determinations performed under different conditions that those used by the vendor in making their "*D* value" claim can result in markedly different results. Standardized conditions for "*D* value" determinations do not exist for VPHP and given the different process systems in use resistance claims made by BI vendors must be taken as broadly indicative only. These so-called "*D* values" do not have the reliability of those associated with BIs used for moist heat, dry heat, or even ETO applications.

DECONTAMINATION CYCLE DEVELOPMENT AND VALIDATION

The providers of the decontamination equipment all provide assistance with cycle development for their system. Regardless of the equipment or agent chosen, it is essential that the approach provide assurance that the routine conditions used for decontamination (or sterilization if that is the intent) are defended by appropriate challenges. A well-defined rationale for this is an essential part of the validation report for the treatment. There have been concerns raised regarding the use of fraction negative studies in the validation of decontamination processes in isolators. That perspective is unfortunate, because fraction negative studies are essential to properly defining the length of the treatment process. If total kill analysis is used, make certain to allow enough lethality to actually get there. The addition of some "cushion" in terms of resistance is recommended. The use of a "half-cycle" approach as is common with ETO sterilization is ill advised. It can result in very long process times in some systems and processes, and the security afforded by the "half-cycle" approach is unnecessary and often illusory.

One of the major considerations in cycle development is identifying locations for the placement of the biological indicators. Typical locations include those portions of the isolator that are most important for production use; those proximate to where the aseptic process will take place. If the intent is to sterilize anything in the isolator, those items should typically have BIs with a population of 10^6 exposed in or on them. Other locations typically evaluated are the corners of the isolator and other locations where achievement of suitable levels of saturation or condensation in vapor decontamination might be difficult. Even where gases are employed, water vapor is typically a critical consideration as relative humidity levels of 60% or more are required for most efficient lethality.

There are no defined rules for the number of BIs to be used. In large systems ($>4\ m^3$), 30 to 50 or more may be required. In smaller isolators ($<1\ m^3$), 10 to 15 BIs are generally adequate, whereas in moderate-sized installations, 25 to 30 BIs are typically enough. The decontamination of entire suites using these agents may require the use of many more BIs that are necessary for an enclosure.

One note of caution must be stated in this exercise, it is certainly possible to place BIs in locations where they will not be fully inactivated by the process. This would be particularly true of locations that can be found in many isolator systems where the BI would be obscured or even completely occluded. That these locations should exist may trouble some; however, the goal of the treatment is to ready the environment for use in aseptic processing, not to render it sterile. The essential concern is that the critical areas more likely to engender process risk are treated appropriately to fully eliminate microorganisms. This is not only a realistic goal; it is routinely attainable. In the nearly two decades of aseptic manufacturing in isolators or aseptic chambers as these devices are called in the aseptic beverage industry, there have been no reports of product risk arising from ineffectual decontamination. This fact taken alone seems sufficient to confirm that the processes employed for decontamination, though they may differ in processing design or philosophy have been more than adequately robust in terms of performance.

Decontamination Interval

The interval between decontamination cycles is often a part of the overall validation effort and may be tied to the use of the system on a campaign basis. This interval may be established by performing media fills at the beginning and end of the desired campaign duration, with environmental monitoring over the entire course of the time period. The PDA has developed guidance in this area that may be of assistance (13). Sterility test isolators are qualified in a similar manner with mock sterility testing or bacteriostasis/fungistasis testing conducted over the course of the decontamination interval. In filling enclosures, the current trend is for the interval to be limited to a number of consecutive batches of the same products. There is ample evidence that the microbiological tests industry has long relied upon in aseptic processing are of diminishing value in advanced aseptic processing. Isolators, for example, very infrequently result in microbial recovery and even less frequently have media fill positives been reported. This likely means that these traditional methods for environmental assessment in clean rooms are largely ineffectual at measuring any potential residual microbial contamination present in isolators. As such the use of media fills or environmental monitoring to define campaign length may be of less value than physical parameters such as maintenance of a consistent positive pressure and consistent total particulate levels where continuous monitoring with electronic particle counters is employed.

REVALIDATION FREQUENCY

Decontamination is considered to be such an important component of the sterility assurance for an aseptic processing system, that annual revalidation is considered appropriate. In this effort a single confirming study using biological indicators is used to reconfirm the continued effectiveness of the decontamination treatment. If a more resistant BI than originally employed is utilized for the revalidation, some unexpected positives may result. The decontamination process has not changed; however, a change in the resistance may suggest that it is not as effective. Before beginning the revalidation, the resistance of the BI to be used should be determined, and the expectations for its inactivation adjusted appropriately. Caution must be exercised to avoid defining the revalidation effort into failure unintentionally.

Residuals

The user will need to validate a safe level of sanitizing agent residual after the treatment. Outgassing measurements can be difficult and technique dependent. Residues on nonproduct contact surfaces may be noncritical to the process depending upon the characteristics of the products being manufactured in an enclosure. Where residues on product contact materials are a concern these must be measured directly. Items that are more susceptible to retaining residual sterilant are often those that are wrapped in Tyvek®, sealed in plastic, or themselves manufactured from polymeric materials. In considering whether a material will allow the passage of H_2O_2 and thus be a potential problem with residuals postaeration, the moisture transmission can be a reasonable predictor. Those materials that are permeable to moisture (an easily located piece of information) are often those that are permeable to hydrogen peroxide. Similarly, those materials that readily adsorb water will also tend to adsorb hydrogen peroxide.

MATERIALS ISSUES

The decontamination agents are all highly reactive chemicals. It is important to recognize that there is a trade-off between microbial kill and adverse material effects. In attaining a greater kill (as is often the objective when sterilization is the target), the dwell period where materials are in contact with the agent is extended. Longer exposure times are sometimes associated with negative effects on the materials in contact with the agent. The authors have experienced embrittlement of gloves, breakdown of polymers, corrosion of surfaces, and discoloration of materials after repeated exposure to lengthy cycles. Neoprene gloves that were once the norm in isolators and RABS systems have largely been replaced by Hypalon gloves which are not as subject to degradation in the presence of powerful oxidizers. To ensure long life of the equipment, the processing time should be minimized to what is sufficient to provide the required log reduction. The use of half-cycle approaches that arbitrarily double the exposure time beyond what is needed to attain the needed log reduction can chemically stress the materials exposed to the agent unnecessarily.

Aeration and Outgassing

A major element of the decontamination process is the establishment of the aeration period at the conclusion of the treatment. This step is important to process reliability as it assures that the materials exposed to the agent are not adversely affected by the treatment. It needs to be established as a part of the decontamination cycle development to define the required aeration period before activities can commence. The common (and sometimes necessary) answer to what residual level to aerate to is often the 8-hour time-weighted average (TWA) defined by OSHA for the agent used. This may be appropriate in some instances (e.g., sterility testing) where residual agent can impede microbial recovery; however, in many instances operations can commence while the level is still somewhat higher. It must be recognized that the limit is an average acceptable value over an 8-hour period, and that the residual level will continue to decrease over time. Thus a value of 5 ppm of H_2O_2 at the end of the aeration may be fully acceptable if the production activities to follow are not impacted at this level. The TWA limit for H_2O_2 is 1 ppm, whereas ClO_2 and O_3 both have a TWA of 0.1 ppm.

The materials present in the isolator chamber can be major contributors to H_2O_2 aeration difficulties. Items that are permeable to moisture are subject to penetration by H_2O_2 and if these materials are exposed in long decontamination periods, desorption, or outgassing of the H_2O_2 in or on these items back into the air can be rate limiting. One of the ways to overcome this is to limit exposure times (thus decontamination as a goal may be preferable due to its shorter exposure requirements and consequently lower time for adsorption of H_2O_2).

Aeration can be somewhat improved by increasing the number of air changes in the isolator; however, if adsorption and outgassing are significant factor with the materials being decontaminated, increasing the number of external air changes may have limited impact.

Process Safety

The chemical agents for use in decontamination are potent chemicals and personnel safety must be a consideration in their use. When rooms and enclosures are decontaminated by personnel, personal protective equipment may be required in the preparation of materials; application to surfaces and verification of adequate aeration posttreatment. The measures to be taken will vary with the materials being used; however, those agents that are most effective against microorganisms, especially spores, are also toxic to humans. Where the agents are introduced into these areas in a semiautomated or automated manner, the essential safety concerns are altered but not eliminated. The environments surrounding the treated area/enclosure may also experience unacceptably high levels during and after the process. If the environment is to be routinely decontaminated pressure tight doors, safety interlocks, emergency exits, and other measures may be necessary. Localized alarmed monitoring systems may be used if deemed appropriate.

Safety of the surrounding environment can be affected by leakage of gas or vapors from the decontamination process into the surrounding environment. The equipment used for the decontamination or the isolator itself may have an integrated leak test capability, which may be used as a prerequisite to each decontamination cycle. The typical precycle leak test uses pressure decay and its greatest benefit is in alerting the staff that the unit is not properly secured before the introduction of the agent. The leak detection acceptance criterion should not be set so sensitive that it will detect very small leaks as that will create more of a nuisance than any benefit. During the automatic decontamination of isolators, personnel should refrain from using gloves and half suits during the exposure cycle and through the early portion of the aeration period.

Other Points to Consider

Once the decontamination process is over, the environmental conditions inside the isolator are maintained by the ventilation system and "other" factors including separative technologies. It is not reasonable to think that every piece of equipment/item contained in an enclosure can or should be "sterilized." Decontamination is really all that should be demonstrated. After all, it is not as if the enclosure isolator will be injected into a patient, and thus attaining sterility for it is not a meaningful concern.

CONCLUSION

The decontamination (or sterilization if that is the intent of the treatment) of target enclosures, chambers and environments is readily attainable using any number of different materials that are lethal to microorganisms. The effectiveness of the treatment can be established using resistant biological indicators. Regardless what the goal of the process is, it is certain that at the end of it the enclosure will present a far lower product contamination risk than possible in any manned environment used for aseptic processing.

APPENDIX 1

DECONTAMINATION METHODS FOR ENVIRONMENTS AND ENCLOSURES

INTRODUCTION

The decontamination of environments and enclosures can use any number of different chemical agents—H_2O_2, ClO_2, O_3, or peracetic acid (CH_3COOOH). Hydrogen peroxide is by far the most commonly used isolator decontamination method and was first introduced in the early 1990s. Several manufacturers offer generators to deliver H_2O_2 for reproducible decontamination with substantial documentation (see chapters 25–28). Chlorine dioxide is an effective sporicide and may see greater usage in the future for decontamination. Peracetic acid was the first available agent for isolator decontamination and is still used in some sterility testing units (PVC) and a few production applications as well. Other agents are possible for these applications, but there limited use does not warrant further discussion.

An important distinction must be made with respect to the commonly used agents. Chlorine dioxide is a gas at the conditions of use, but requires the presence of water vapor for effective sporicidal effect. Thus, chlorine dioxide does depend upon the distribution of a vapor and its penetration into spores and packaging materials. Hydrogen peroxide and peracetic acid are liquids at room temperature. Peracetic acid is introduced as and remains a liquid until the aeration phase of its use. Hydrogen Peroxide is commonly introduced at elevated temperature (slightly greater than 100°C) into a room temperature environment. Its ability or need to remain as a vapor throughout the decontamination is a point of considerable discussion. That it may condense creates some difficulty in parameter measurement, nevertheless regardless of its state (gas, vapor or liquid) H_2O_2 is lethal to spores. There is however ample evidence that VPHP is maximally efficient as a sporicide when it condenses or is very near to the saturation point.

HYDROGEN PEROXIDE DECONTAMINATION

VPHP is the most widely used method for the decontamination of isolator enclosures and is increasingly used for the treatment of clean rooms and RABS and as such will be the only decontaminating agent covered in detail in this appendix. Hydrogen peroxide or H_2O_2 falls into a broad category of sporicidal antimicrobial agents that are classified as oxidants. Other widely used sporicides that fall into the same general category as hydrogen peroxide include ozone, peracetic acid (and other super oxides), halogens (including chlorine, chlorine dioxide, iodine, and sodium hypochlorite. The sporicidal properties of oxidants in general and H_2O_2 in particular have been recognized for decades. H_2O_2 has been widely used as a surface sterilant at liquid concentrations of >4% and as a skin disinfectant at concentrations of 3% or less for many years.

Given its common use in medicine as a sterilant and disinfectant the antimicrobial and the sporicidal properties of H_2O_2 have been widely studied. Abundant information is available regarding the sporicidal effectiveness of H_2O_2 at a variety of concentrations (14). It was determined many years ago that mixtures of H_2O_2 and peracetic acid have a more powerful sporicidal effect that either of these compounds does when used alone (15). However, the strong odor associated with peracetic acid and that agent's corrosiveness (it is an organic acid) makes it unappealing for use in the decontamination of complex manufacturing equipment that are composed of many different materials. Because H_2O_2 alone does not leave toxic residues and decomposes to water and oxygen it is a useful agent for the sterilization of materials/surfaces that may come into contact with sterile products. H_2O_2 is widely used for the sterilization of containers (particularly in aseptic beverage production), plastic films, medical devices, and in some rare cases process piping.

The earliest isolators used for sterility testing were decontaminated using H_2O_2 in combination with peracetic acid. Throughout the decade of the 1980s, this combination remained the method of choice for isolator decontamination. However, following the introduction of H_2O_2 generators in the early 1990s it has supplanted peracetic acid and become the predominant decontaminating agent in both sterility testing and production environments. According to recent surveys, nearly all isolator manufacturing systems installed and validated in recent years have used H_2O_2 as the decontaminating agent.

H_2O_2 was first introduced using a free-standing generator with a closed, single-loop configuration in the late 1980s. This system is still widely used today. The process consists of a H_2O_2 reservoir that contains 30% to 35% H_2O_2 in a mixture with water (and stabilizers). The target is dehumidified by the dry air stream to a user selectable target value between 10% and 30%. The liquid H_2O_2 is pumped from this reservoir at a rate that is controlled gravimetrically—the flow rate can be chosen by the user. The H_2O_2 is vaporized at temperatures of ~100°C into a dehumidified air stream and blown into the target system at a user selected air flow rate. The injection of vapor H_2O_2 continues for a user-defined time period and the injection rate is chosen to deliver a calculated concentration based on the volume of the target system and assumptions regarding the decomposition rate of the vapor H_2O_2.. In this closed-loop configuration the H_2O_2 in the exhaust "leg" of this loop flows through a mixed-bed catalyst decomposing the H_2O_2 into water and oxygen. This air stream is returned through the dehumidifier removing residual water and picks up freshly vaporized H_2O_2 on its way to the inlet point within the target system.

In the mid-1990s adaptations of the closed loop H_2O_2 generator began to appear that operated in an open-loop configuration. This obviated the limitations imposed by the restricted capacity of the desiccant drier system. Shortly thereafter modular generators designed to operate in an open-loop configuration where introduced as was a generator that employed a continuous duty refrigerant drier that did not require regeneration. Other commercial generators have been introduced that use dual-loop configurations in which the humidity control loop is separated from the H_2O_2 injection loop. There are also generators that are built into the isolator and vaporize H_2O_2 directly onto a hot plate located in the isolator air handler plenum. In recent years, studies have shown that dehumidification of the target many not be required and may even be counterproductive. Therefore, systems are now available that delete the dehumidification phase of the process.

At the present time, H_2O_2 generators are available from several vendors and some of these systems have unique operational philosophies and process control systems. Although different in many ways, all of these units vaporize hydrogen peroxide and have the ability to control the rate of injection (where continuous or intermittent dosing is used) or amount of material of injection (where a single dose is employed) and the total exposure time.

Outline of the H_2O_2 Decontamination Process

The H_2O_2 decontamination process can consist of up to four "phases" or steps. The equipment vendors may use different terms to describe these phases. These four phases are dehumidification, conditioning, decontamination, and aeration.

Dehumidification

The purpose of the dehumidification phase is to reduce the ambient moisture level within the isolator enclosure so that the concentration of H_2O_2 can be maximized. H_2O_2 is commonly vaporized from mixtures of H_2O_2 and water (the percentage of the mixture used varies with the vendor). Some equipment vendors describe the H_2O_2 process as a "dry" one. These vendors generally recommend that condensation during the H_2O_2 process be avoided. Reduction of ambient moisture within the enclosure allows a higher injection rate of H_2O_2/water mixture while avoiding condensate formation. The reduction of humidity prior to a gas or vapor antimicrobial process is atypical. Generally, gas sterilization processes require an increase in humidity (sometimes called preconditioning) for optimal kill effectiveness. Not surprisingly, this has become a point of controversy in H_2O_2 decontamination. Some scientists and vendors claim the H_2O_2 use is a wet process and that effective spore kill occurs only when microcondensation of the H_2O_2 occurs on the surface. Proponents of the microcondensation approach often set humidity targets that are higher than those advocated by those whose objective is a dry process. At least one vendor has eliminated dehumidification entirely because of its counter intuitiveness. From a practical perspective humidity targets of 5% to 70% have been successfully used, where success is defined is a reproducible spore log reduction. At the present time humidity targets below 20% are rare and some published studies have indicated that higher humidity levels should be used (15).

When large rooms or enclosures are to be decontaminated, some form of external dehumidification is often employed. External dehumidification can substantially shorten the time required to reach the humidity set point, and of course where modular generators are used that lack a separate dehumidification process an external drier is essential. Process monitoring during dehumidification consists of one or more humidity sensors that provide data to the control system.

Conditioning

The purpose of the conditioning phase is to inject H_2O_2 at a high rate that enables the calculated concentration to be reached as rapidly as possible. The operating parameters for the conditioning phase are generally not established until the target concentration is determined. During the conditioning phase an injection rate higher than sustainable throughout the process is utilized to increase the internal concentration of H_2O_2 to the desired steady-state condition more rapidly without condensation. The conditioning phase has been eliminated by vendors that focus on a condensation approach.

Decontamination

This comprises the dwell portion of the cycle where H_2O_2 is either circulated continuously (Steris, Bioquell), injected intermittently (Skan), or introduced all at once (Shibuya). The fundamental differences in these approaches focuses on the nature of the kill being performed: whether it is a gas or liquid phase process. Although the debate persists as to whether H_2O_2 is a dry or microcondensing process, it is accepted that spore-killing effectiveness is reduced if the concentration is well below the dew point. The narrower the temperature spread within the enclosure the better as this assures constant relative humidity and VPHP concentration relative to dew point. Unfortunately, temperature spreads of 5°C to 10°C are not uncommon in larger systems. Design features, such as auxiliary circulation fans to maximize turbulence during the process can narrow the temperature spread and also enhance agent/humidity distribution. It is important to note that vapor concentrations will be highest at the point of injection; therefore fans that will enhance mixing can improve concentration uniformity by moving hot H_2O_2 rapidly away from the injection point.

Aeration

There are two critical factors that must be considered in achieving aeration of H_2O_2. The first and most important factor is the air exchange rate. Studies have shown that higher the fresh air exchange rate, the more rapid the aeration phase. For the most rapid aeration fresh air exchange rates of 100 changes per hour or more should be considered. No other factor will have as great an effect on reducing aeration time. The second key factor is outgassing (desorption) of materials exposed to H_2O_2. Outgassing time can be reduced by selecting materials that are less likely to absorb and retain H_2O_2. Although the starting point for aeration time can be calculated using dilution rate equations, it is also possible to measure concentrations using sensors or test tubes that are relatively accurate to H_2O_2 at levels of <5 ppm. The only certain way to develop aeration processes is through empirical measurement.

Decontamination Using ClO_2

The use of halogens in the decontamination of manufacturing equipment and environments must be done with careful attention to concentration and exposure as these agents too can be highly corrosive even to stainless steels. Halogen-releasing compounds such as chlorine dioxide may prove to be a valuable alternative in the decontamination of isolators, rooms and in other pharmaceutical applications. However, the use of halogens will generally require careful consideration in the selection of materials and components for the construction of isolators. At a minimum initial passivation of stainless steel and regular repassivation will be essential if chlorine dioxide or other halogenated sporicides are to be used. Chlorine dioxide is discussed in detail in Chapter 28.

REFERENCES

1. FDA. Guideline on Sterile Drug Products Produced by Aseptic Processing, 2004.
2. Agalloco J, Akers J, Madsen R. Aseptic processing: a review of current industry practice. Pharm Technol 2004; 26(10):126–150.
3. Agalloco J. Understanding overkill sterilization: Putting an end to the confusion. Pharm Technol 2007; 30(5):S18–S25.
4. PDA. Design and validation of isolator systems for the manufacturing and testing of health care products, PDA Technical Report #34. PDA J Pharm Sci Technol 2001; 55(5 Suppl).
5. ISPE. Restricted Access Barrier Systems (RABS) for Aseptic Processing, ISPE Definition, August 2005.
6. Block S. Disinfection, Sterilization and Preservation, 2001; Philadelphia, PA: Lippincott Williams & Wilkins.
7. Rickloff JR, Orelski PA. Resistance of Various Microorganisms to Vaporized Hydrogen Peroxide in a Prototype Table Top Sterilizer. Proceedings of the 89th General Meeting of the American Society for Microbiology; Washington, DC: 1989.
8. Sigwarth V. Skan AG. Process Development of the Skan Integrated System, SIS 700, H2O2 Decontamination Method, Process Description and Qualification Guide, Basel, Switzerland, 2002.
9. Sintim-Damoa K. Other gaseous sterilization methods. In: Morrissey RF, Phillips GB, eds. Sterilization Technology. New York: Van Nostrand Reinhold, 1993:335–347.
10. Grignol G, Eddington D, Karle D. et al. Chemical and Biological Aspects of Hydrogen Peroxide Gas. Proceedings of the ISPE Barrier Isolation Technology Conference, Washington, DC: 2000.
11. Kowalski JB. Sterilization of medical devices, pharmaceutical components, and barrier isolator systems with gaseous chlorine dioxide. In: Morrissey RF, Kowalski JB, eds. Sterilization of Medical Products. Champlain, NY: Polyscience Publications, 1998:313–323.
12. Reference?
13. PDA. Process Simulation Testing for Aseptically Filled Products. PDA Technical Report #22 Revision, pending publication by PDA.
14. Block SS. Peroxygen compounds. In: Block SS, ed. Disinfection, Sterilization, and Preservation. 4th ed., 2001; Philadelphia, PA: Lippincott Williams & Wilkins.
15. Watling D, Cian R, Parks M, et al. Theoretical analysis of the condensation of hydrogen peroxide gas and water vapour as used in surface decontamination. Bioquell 2002.

25 Hydrogen peroxide gas decontamination

James R. Rickloff

The use of advanced aseptic processing equipment has gained wide acceptance over the past several years as an alternative to the conventional clean room for the testing and manufacture of sterile health care products. The availability of an automated, reproducible decontamination process significantly contributed to this technology shift. The Parenteral Drug Association (PDA) has defined an aseptic isolator as a sealed enclosure supplied with air through a microbially retentive filtration system (HEPA minimum) and is able to be reproducibly decontaminated prior to use (1).

There has been a great deal of debate on terminology applied to isolation technology due to its use in other industrial and healthcare settings. For example, isolator "sterilization" issues have been the focus of many industry sponsored conferences over the past two decades although the complexity of the equipment involved makes it very unlikely that isolators and their contents are truly being sterilized. The industry consensus at the present time is to eliminate detectible levels of microorganisms on nonproduct contact surfaces within the isolator environment. This should be accomplished by treating a precleaned and properly designed isolator with a sporicidal agent in a quantifiable and reproducible manner with contact points kept to a minimum during the decontamination cycle. Product contact equipment and piping must be sterilized prior to use and this is still generally accomplished using moist heat.

The most common germicide being used to decontaminate isolators is hydrogen peroxide (H_2O_2). The sporicidal properties of this chemical have been recognized for years in both its aqueous and gaseous forms; the latter being applied to most isolator applications over the past two decades (2,3). The purpose of this chapter was to provide the reader with an overview on the basics of H_2O_2 gas decontamination and to describe how the sterilant should be properly applied to isolator systems. The latest in validation techniques and sterilant monitoring requirements are discussed from a user and regulatory perspective.

TECHNOLOGY OVERVIEW

History

Although sterilization using gaseous agents has been practiced for over five decades, H_2O_2 gas did not begin to gain acceptance as a sterilant until the early 1990s. The sporicidal affects of the gas were actually discovered in 1979 (4,5). The first data on its efficacy suggested that concentrations as little as 0.5 mg/L (360 ppm) could render an item sterile whereas at a lower temperature when compared with ethylene oxide.

The American Sterilizer Company (AMSCO) in Erie, PA, licensed the technology from American Hospital Supply Corporation in 1980 to explore potential hospital applications, such as the replacement of ethylene oxide for the terminal sterilization of thermolabile medical instruments and supplies. The initial focus of AMSCO's development program was to obtain Environmental Protection Agency's (EPA) approval of the sterilant to verify that there were no outstanding health or safety issues involving the use of H_2O_2. The sterilant received its registration number in 1985 for use in a 2 ft^3 microsurgical instrument sterilizer. Additional research demonstrated that H_2O_2 gas was capable of inactivating a wide range of bacteria, bacterial spores, viruses, molds, and fungi. *Geobacillus stearothermophilus* spores have thus far been shown to possess the highest resistance to H_2O_2 gas (6–8). This may be due to the amount of manganese that is bound to the spore coat during the sporulation process, which would decompose H_2O_2 molecules during their transport through the spore coat. Unpublished data from AMSCO showed the presence of a "brown" precipitate when a column of a dilute *G. stearothermophilus* spore suspension was ozonated for a brief period of time. The same precipitate was not evident when other spore suspensions (*Bacillus atrophaeus* and *Clostridium sporogenes*) were treated in a similar manner.

Subsequently, the development program proceeded to determine the feasibility of "scaling" the technology up to larger volumes to pursue a variety of potential hospital and industrial applications. During that effort, it was shown that exposed surfaces could be sterilized by the vaporization of aqueous H_2O_2 into a flowing air stream and then delivering the mixture to sealed enclosures at ambient pressure and temperature. Flow-through equipment using the process became commercially available in 1990 with the introduction of the VHP® 1000 biodecontamination system. This new process was also reviewed and the sterilant approved by the EPA for applications involving the decontamination of sealed enclosures. It is a dry process resulting in no condensation of the active ingredient onto surfaces. This noncondensation feature provides an additional benefit of excellent material compatibility.

"VHP" is a registered trademark of STERIS Corporation and should only be used in conjunction with their equipment that has been designed specifically to vaporize aqueous H_2O_2 and controllably deliver the gaseous form of the oxidant to a sealed enclosure. The term "vapor" has been used over the years to describe the sterilant generated from that equipment. However, a vapor has been defined as (*i*) visible particles of moisture floating in the air as fog, mist, or steam or (*ii*) the gaseous form of any substance, which is usually a liquid or solid (9). To avoid further confusion, this chapter specifically describes the application of H_2O_2 gas (concentrations are maintained below the dew point at a specified temperature and humidity) to isolator-based systems.

Mechanism of Action

The literature still remains inconclusive as to the exact kill mechanism for either the liquid or gaseous phase of H_2O_2. The hypotheses for spore destruction that appear most frequently in the literature are DNA attack, enzyme destruction, and/or the disruption of the spore coat (10–13). The authors also mentioned that metallic salts, ultraviolet light, heat, and plasma have been shown to enhance the sporicidal action of H_2O_2. When used alone most of these treatments do not possess sporicidal properties, but their presence catalyzes the breakdown of the oxidant. One intermediate breakdown product of that catalysis is the highly reactive hydroxyl free radical whose half-life is in the thousandths of a second. This would suggest that H_2O_2 molecules must first penetrate into the cell before a synergistic radical formation process could affect the cell's active sites.

Factors Affecting Sterilant Efficacy

There are three major processing parameters that affect the inactivation of microorganisms by H_2O_2 gas. They are sterilant concentration, exposure time, and percent saturation, the latter being influenced by the temperature and/or humidity level in the enclosure. The presence (or absence) of air or other inert gases does not affect the ability of H_2O_2 gas to inactivate organisms; however, it can assist in, or obstruct, the delivery of the sterilant. In a flow through system, the air acts as a carrier to deliver the sterilant vapor to the sites to be decontaminated.

Selectively increasing the concentration of the sterilant has been shown to directly increase the microbial inactivation rate, as is the case with other sterilants. The maximum allowable (noncondensing) H_2O_2 gas concentration can be increased by raising the temperature of the enclosure and/or by using a more concentrated aqueous sterilant, as shown in Figure 1. The trade-off here, of course, is that it takes time to heat and then cool an enclosure prior to use and additional handling precautions are recommended as the aqueous H_2O_2 concentration is increased. Pharmacia (Kalamazoo, MI) was able to successfully use both features in a large filling isolator application where an automated clean-in-place (CIP) system and hot air drying provided consistent surface temperatures of around 35°C (6,14). H_2O_2 gas concentrations of 1.7 mg/L were obtained during the Pharmacia studies when 50 wt% H_2O_2 was flash vaporized into the infeed, filling, and outfeed sections of the isolator. An exposure time of less than 60 minutes was required to consistently sterilize numerous biological indicators under such conditions.

Flash vaporization differs from natural evaporation in that it produces a mixture of H_2O_2 and water vapor that has substantially the same weight percent composition as the multicomponent liquid (15). The validity of calculations for estimating the maximum allowable H_2O_2 gas concentration in air at a given temperature and humidity (Fig. 2) was questioned by Marcos-Martin et al. (16) who stated that "condensation is a phenomenon that cannot be avoided." Studies conducted by STERIS Corp. (formerly AMSCO) validated that flash vaporized H_2O_2

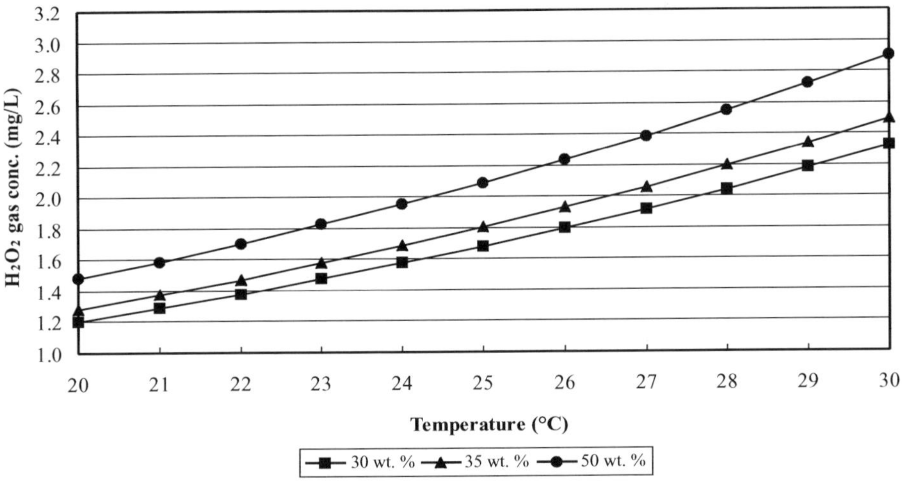

Figure 1 Dew point gas concentration for various temperatures upon the flash vaporization of different aqueous H_2O_2 solutions into a 10% RH air stream.

could exist in the gaseous state at high concentrations within an isolator and that the physical state (i.e., gas or condensate) at various surface temperatures were predictable (17).

An increase in exposure time will also result in a corresponding increase in microbial inactivation if all other process parameters remain constant. A linear regression analysis of *G. stearothermophilus* spore survivors at varying exposure times did not show an initial lag phase or tailing in kill rate that has been observed for aqueous H_2O_2 (18). Rather, the sporicidal activity of H_2O_2 gas against various lots of *G. stearothermophilus* spore suspensions when dried on stainless steel was found to follow first-order kinetics.

Increasing the temperature and/or decreasing the background humidity in an enclosure without increasing the H_2O_2 gas concentration tends to decrease the overall microbial inactivation rate by reducing the percent saturation of the gas. Percent saturation is the ratio of the actual concentration within an enclosure to the dew point concentration. A threefold variance in *D*-value can be seen in Figure 3 where 1.6 mg/L of H_2O_2 gas was tested in an isolator under varying degrees of water vapor content (19). The need for moisture in inactivating bacterial

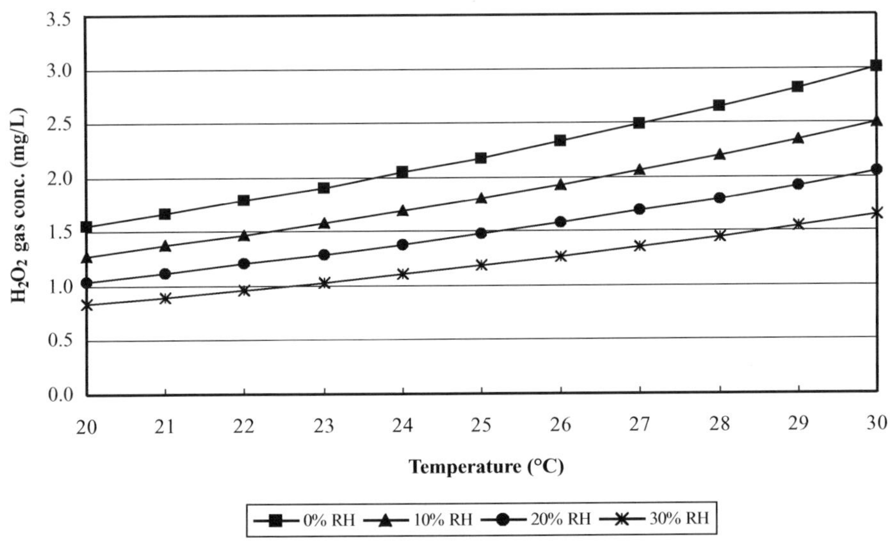

Figure 2 Effect of temperature and humidity on dew point gas concentration for flash Vaporized 35 wt. % H_2O_2 solution.

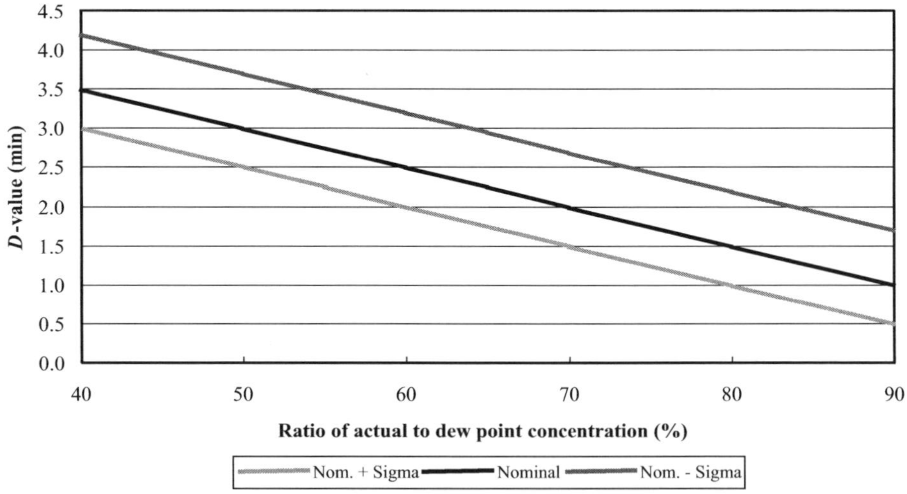

Figure 3 Effect of percent saturation on H_2O_2 gas *D*-value when tested at 1.6 mg/L (Best Fit Data Obtained from VHP1000 Cycle Development Guide).

spores is not unique to this technology as 10-fold and 120-fold variances in *D*-value have been documented for ethylene oxide and heat processes, respectively (20,21). This factor, although not necessarily controllable in a typical isolator, can be accounted for during the validation process, which is discussed later in the chapter.

The concentration of H_2O_2 gas within an isolator will be reduced by its reaction with various surfaces that the molecules come in contact with. Decomposition, absorption, and/or adsorption tend to keep the isolator concentration below the theoretical inlet concentration, although losses from the vaporization process (<5%) also contribute to the difference. In addition, exceeding the dew point will lead to condensation of the sterilant on cooler surfaces, which will lower the gas concentration in warmer areas of the isolator. With the exception of condensation, all of these factors remain constant from one decontamination cycle to another; therefore, they can also be accounted for during cycle development and validation.

STERILANT GENERATOR DESCRIPTIONS

A variety of decontamination equipment designed to safely deliver H_2O_2 gas and meet current good manufacturing practices specifications is currently available to the pharmaceutical and biotechnology industries. Several types of generators lead to the formation of condensate and those are discussed in other chapters. It has been reported that H_2O_2 gas generators have been integrated into nearly 90% of production isolator and sterility testing isolator applications (2,3). Decontamination cycles consist of multiple phases that are continuously monitored by internal sensors along with cycle parameters that are controlled within defined specifications. Typical cycle phases include dehumidification to a specified set point, conditioning to reach the desired sterilant concentration, exposure at the desired concentration, and subsequent aeration to remove residual H_2O_2 from the enclosure. The following descriptions provide a brief overview on the features and operating requirements for existing H_2O_2 gas generators in chronological order based on market entry:

Portable Closed-Loop Generators

AMSCO (Apex, NC) introduced the VHP1000 Biodecontamination System to the pharmaceutical industry in 1990 as the first portable, stand-alone H_2O_2 gas generator for the biological decontamination of clean, hard, dry surfaces within sealed enclosures (Fig. 4). The proprietary control system provided for the precise control of all critical cycle parameters already discussed, as well as the pressure or vacuum of the enclosure undergoing closed-loop decontamination. The unit also provided two outputs and three inputs for connection to external devices, which could be activated during the cycle.

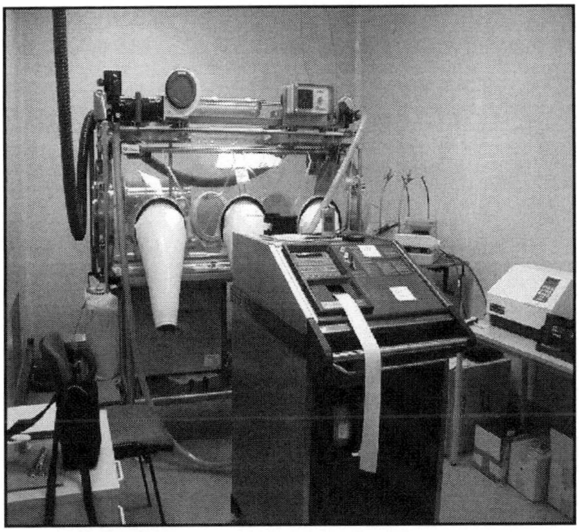

Figure 4 VHP1000 generator attached to a flexible wall transfer isolator.

The design incorporated several features that were requested by potential end users who, at that time, were primarily based in the laboratory. Some of these features (utility requirements, fully self-contained, cost, etc.) limited the scope of the system to enclosure volumes of less than 1000 ft^3 (28 m^3) internal volume. The desiccant-based drying system could only absorb so much moisture before requiring regeneration, a sterilant reservoir capacity of 1000 g, and a maximum airflow rate of approximately 20 ft^3/min (34 m^3/hr) limited the length of cycles and/or maximum gas concentrations that could be achieved in a larger enclosure.

Despite these limitations, there are currently over 700 validated systems in use around the world. Production isolator applications that have been installed over the past decade have overcome many of the generator's limitations by incorporating internal drying and external exhaust systems at much higher air exchange rates to improve upon cycle times. The installation of VHP1000 generators in series has also been used in an effort to increase gas concentrations in large isolator systems. There are several design issues that must be considered prior to going down this path, which are discussed later in the chapter.

STERIS Corporation (Mentor, OH) acquired AMSCO in 1996 and STERIS has continued to support the VHP® Sterilization Technology through continued research and development of enhanced decontamination systems for the pharmaceutical marketplace. The company released a second-generation "extended duty" H_2O_2 gas generator in 2001 that was designed to inject one cartridge worth of sterilant (1000 mL) before regeneration was required. The primary advantage of the VHP1000ED generator was that regenerate time could be reduced by nearly 80% when compared to the standard VHP1000. The manufacturer has offered a range of control options including Allen-Bradley, Siemens, and Mitsubishi PLCs, which streamlined the interfacing of the decontamination equipment to the isolator's control system. Several hundred of these units are now in service around the world.

Modular Open-Loop Generators

STERIS introduced the VHPM1000 modular generator in 2001 for large-scale isolator and room applications for volumes up to 5000 ft^3 (142 m^3). The system consists of three modules (generator, cartridge interface, and either an Allen-Bradley or Siemens operator interface), which are integrated into an isolator at locations where they would be most convenient to the operator (Fig. 5).

This generator operates in an open-loop configuration whereby dry air is passed through the generator a single time. The H_2O_2 gas-laden air stream is circulated throughout the enclosure prior to being exhausted to the outside of the building. In addition, the VHPM1000 does not have an internal desiccant system; instead it relies on connection to a dry air source for enclosure dehumidification. The dry air source needs to be controlled in terms of flow rate as most of it bypasses the generator module. The H_2O_2 gas-laden air from the generator is mixed with

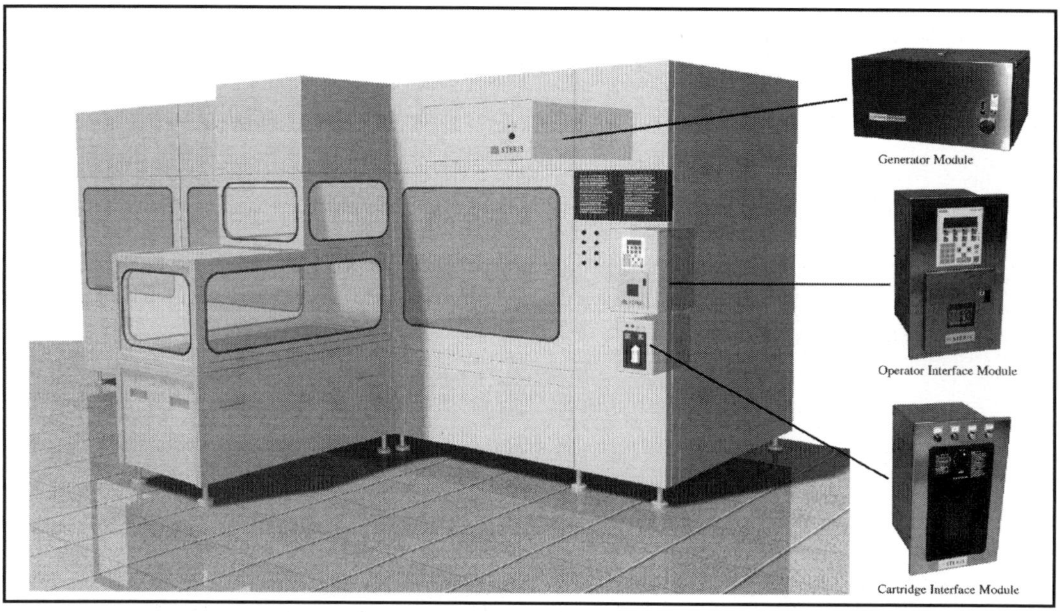

Figure 5 VHPM1000 integrated with HVAC and production isolator for continuous duty. *Source*: Photo courtesy of STERIS Corp.

the bypassed air for delivery to the isolator. Airflow rates in excess of 100 ft^3/min (170 m^3/hr) are used in combination with increased sterilant injection rates, which permits an increase in the allowable gas concentration inside the enclosure. This is possible because the higher air exchange rate through the enclosure reduces the impact of sterilant half-life on the gas concentration. Another advantage of the higher air exchange rate is a reduction in isolator aeration times.

The VHPM100 small-volume generator became available to the industry in 2007 for enclosures ranging in volume from a few cubic feet up to 500 ft^3. It was designed to be permanently mounted to the enclosure being decontaminated (space saver in small laboratories) and it can be configured to operate in either a closed-loop or open-loop arrangement. It can be operated independently as a stand-alone machine, but may also be operated through interface to external equipment. This interface provides many options, including data communication via the Allen-Bradley or Siemens PLC communication protocols, as well as discrete I/O interfacing. In most cases, this interface is used to start decontamination cycles, abort cycles, and monitor the system status.

DECONTAMINATION CHAMBER DESIGN ISSUES

Gas Distribution

The gas distribution characteristics of an isolator system is important to consider during the design phase of a project as areas that are minimally exposed to H_2O_2 gas will prevent decontamination in a reasonable time frame. There are means available to optimize gas distribution, but the user should not expect an isolator's air circulation system to accomplish this alone if numerous isolator sections are used and/or if complex equipment is housed within them. Positioning fans in certain areas within an isolator, such as shown in Figure 6, has worked well in eliminating zones of poor gas distribution.

Decontamination cycles for some system designs have been validated without the need for fans. The isolated filling line shown in Figure 7 provides unidirectional airflow around conveying and filling equipment within two separate isolator sections. The equipment was designed to minimize low air flow areas near and/or underneath their surfaces. H_2O_2 gas distribution between isolator sections was optimized by using two VHP1000s in series that were connected to a properly designed manifold system (see "Use of Sterilant Manifolds" section). The system also used sleeve holders that allowed the majority of the gloveport sleeve surface

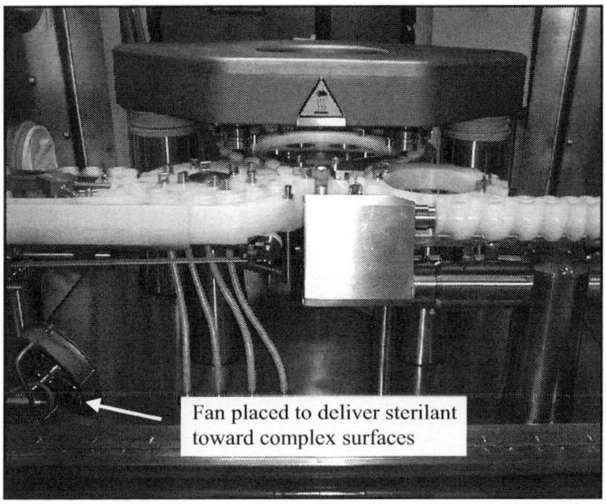

Figure 6 Optimizing H_2O_2 gas distribution through the use of circulating fans.

area to be placed outside of the unidirectional air flow pattern in an effort to minimize shadowing above critical surfaces (Fig. 8). The placement and sterilization of biological indicators verified that the sterilant could penetrate to the back portions of the sleeves. The isolator pressure when set at 0.20 inches of water column (50 Pa) during the decontamination cycle was sufficient to remove overlapping material within the sleeve areas.

Use of Sterilant Manifolds

There have been some rather complex isolator designs proposed over the years where sterilant generator inlet and return pipes were added on as an afterthought to make the system decontamination "capable." H_2O_2 gas concentration and distribution patterns were then found to be

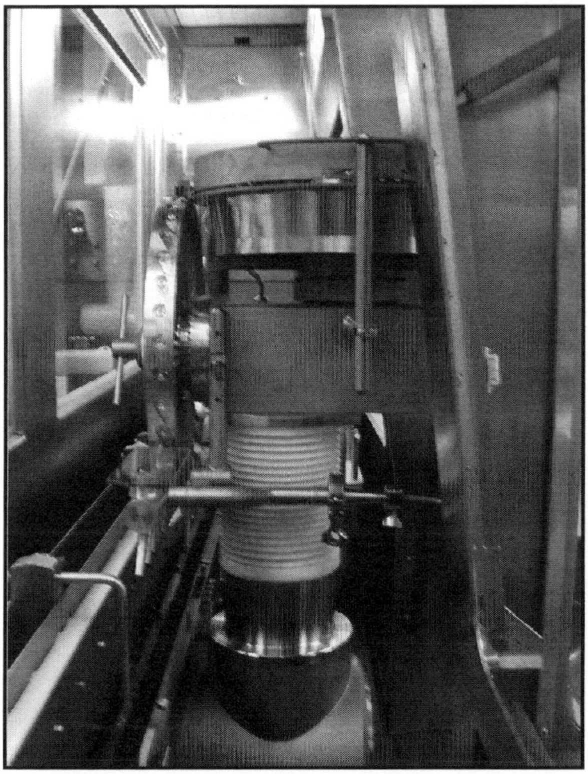

Figure 7 Optimized isolated filling line design (circulation fans not required).

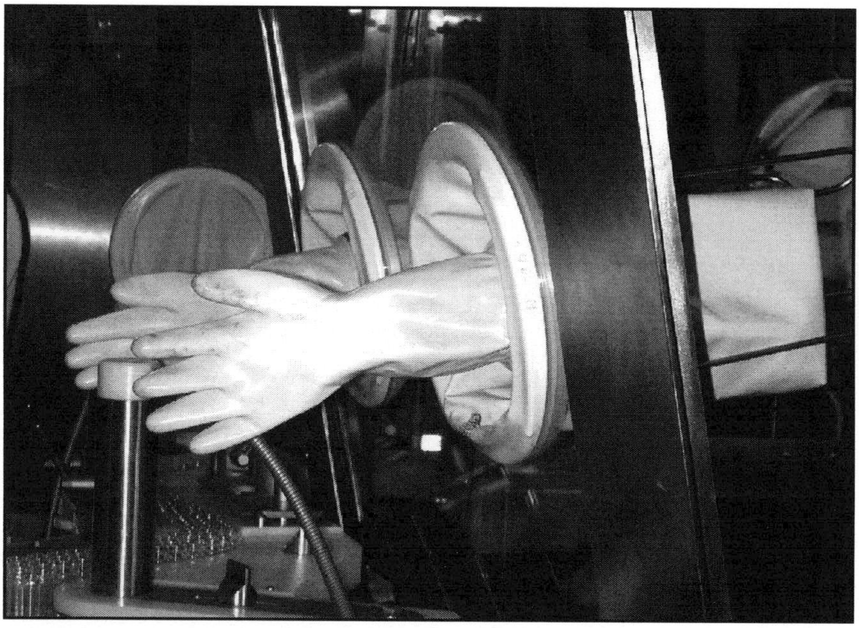

Figure 8 Use of sleeve extenders minimizes shadowing of critical surfaces undergoing decontamination.

less than ideal during cycle development, which forced some companies to lower the spore reduction requirement in specific areas of an isolator. There is no need to lower the spore challenge for the decontamination process if the sterilant chamber (isolator) is properly designed. Some isolator systems may need additional sterilant inlets and/or multiple (or larger capacity) generators to achieve a sufficient gas concentration throughout larger enclosures. Proper air flow balancing will need to be considered when splitting a generator's inlet air stream to various sections of an isolator with percentages typically based on the volume of that section.

The variable speed blowers that are installed within the stand-alone generators already discussed are subject to air flow restrictions when the outlet backpressure reaches certain levels. The isolator manufacturer should be able to provide air flow versus pressure drop curves to allow the maximum air flow for their particular system to be predicted. The pressure drop will increase as the length of pipe and the quantity of elbows and valves on the system increases. Smaller ID pipe will also have a greater pressure drop when compared with larger pipe sections. The pressure drop can be calculated for each individual system by estimating the equivalent length of straight pipe for the inlet and return piping (include bends and valves in the estimation) and then inserting that value into the following equation:

$$\Delta P = 1.73 \times L \times v^2/25{,}000 \times d$$

where ΔP is the pressure drop (inches of water column); L is the equivalent length of straight pipe (feet); v is the velocity at specific air flow rate (ft/sec); d is the pipe diameter (inches).

The effect on a generator's maximum air flow rate can then be estimated from the isolator manufacturer's flow curves.

Developing a manifold system that will minimize pressure drop is important because, as mentioned previously, the maximum H_2O_2 gas concentration will decrease at lower air exchange rates (sterilant half-life effect). Condensation must be avoided in the manifold piping, which will require the installation of heaters and insulation over the sterilant inlet pipe(s).

Manifold systems have also been designed and installed in facilities that require the remote location of the sterilant generator(s) due to space and/or safety requirements. Flow balancing, pressure drop, and the prevention of condensation need to be addressed in these applications, as well. Generators have been installed as far away as 100 feet from an isolator system without affecting the maximum airflow rate of the unit or the ability to decontaminate the enclosure. The time spent early on in the decontamination system design phase will pay dividends, especially when validation of the equipment becomes critical path on the overall project timeline.

Decontamination of Vacuum/Gas Lines

Due to the low vapor pressure of H_2O_2 gas and its tendency to decompose into water vapor and oxygen, various areas of an isolator may not experience sporicidal levels of the sterilant by diffusion alone. Pharmacia (Kalamazoo, MI) and Sanofi Pasteur (Swiftwater, PA) have discussed the use of facilitated flow or suction to deliver H_2O_2 gas through CIP piping, utility lines, environmental monitoring devices, and stopper wheels that were installed within their isolated filling lines (6,22). Figure 9 depicts the use of small vacuum pumps that are H_2O_2 compatible to deliver the sterilant through piping. The gas was returned to the system via the HVAC plenum or the generator's sterilant return line. Each of the piping sections was successfully challenged with biological indicators during the validation process. Ideally, the gas distribution requirements should be specified to the system supplier during the equipment design phase to avoid the sometimes difficult task of a field retrofit.

CYCLE DEVELOPMENT AND VALIDATION

All critical components on the commercially available generators, including pressure sensors, temperature sensors, blower controls, and mass measuring devices (electronic balance) need to be calibrated prior to validation activities to assure proper performance. Operational qualification testing should then performed to verify that critical cycle parameters remain within the manufacturer's specified tolerance limits as exceeding them can have a negative impact on the sporicidal efficacy of H_2O_2 gas. Ask the manufacturer of your sterilant generator for those tolerance limits. Each cycle phase should be tested to confirm the consistency of these critical parameters. The pressure control capabilities of the system should also be demonstrated by connecting the generator to each isolator. If included in the isolator design, redundant pressure monitors on independent ports should be tested to confirm that readings are consistent with the pressure control system on the sterilant generator. It is also recommended to test all alarms and aborts that are specifically related to efficacy and for operator protection.

Cycle development calculations use known (internal volume including the ductwork) and estimated (minimum surface temperature) isolator variables in determining sterilant injection and airflow rates, which should then be optimized experimentally. These studies can be placed in separate protocols to assist in generating acceptance criteria for the actual performance qualification (PQ) or included in a separate section of the PQ document if acceptance criteria

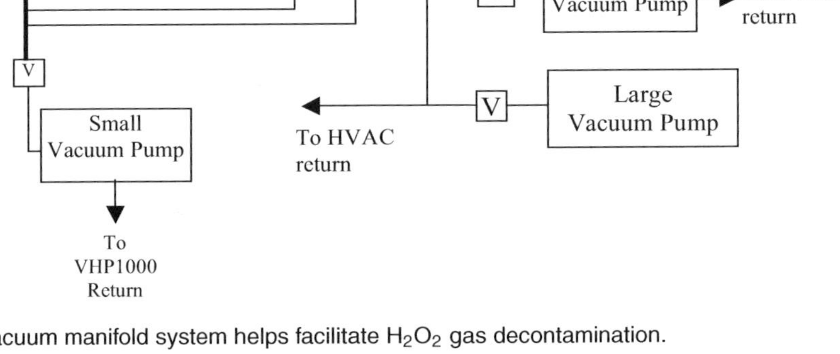

Figure 9 Vacuum manifold system helps facilitate H_2O_2 gas decontamination.

have already been defined. Thermocouples and chemical indicators should be used to determine the surface temperature and gas distribution characteristics of the isolator. The actual minimum surface temperature at the end of dehumidification replaces the estimated temperature used for base cycle calculations and parameters are then optimized, if necessary. The chemical indicator data is extremely useful in determining the need for additional fans and/or a change in the sterilant inlet manifold for multiple isolator systems prior to initiating the PQ.

D-Value Studies

Variable lot-to-lot resistance has been evident over the years for biological indicators used in the validation of H_2O_2 gas decontamination cycles (Fig. 10) (23). Because the United States Pharmacopeia (USP) has not yet established a resistance requirement for any biological indicators used within isolators, it is recommended that each lot be tested for resistance prior to the execution of a validation or requalification study (24). The resistance value of a biological indicator is characterized in terms of a *D* value, which is the exposure time required to cause a one logarithm, or 90%, reduction of a homogeneous population of bacterial spores under a specified set of conditions.

Many variables can affect the outcome of a *D* value test. It is imperative to provide a steady-state sterilant concentration, air temperature, and humidity during exposure of the biological indicators and then ensure that they can be maintained within a defined range during each replicate test and from study to study. *D* value tests are typically performed in triplicate under square-wave conditions, which means that the lag time associated with preexposure conditioning and postexposure aeration are eliminated.

The instrumentation used to evaluate the sterilization resistance of spore crops must be consistent with existing standards related to the performance evaluation of biological indicators (25). USP does recognize that approved BIER-type vessels are currently unavailable for isolator sterilants. However, the comparison of relative resistance among different lots of biological indicators in isolators is still possible if the factors mentioned earlier are taken into consideration.

One approach is to place the biological indicators in a sterilant impermeable container and seal it prior to placement into the isolator. The corners of prepackaged biological indicators can be fitted into springs to ensure their proper exposure to the sterilant and to prevent them from blowing around an isolator if fans are used for gas distribution. The sealed containers are added to the isolator along with a sufficient number of sterile buffer or recovery media tubes

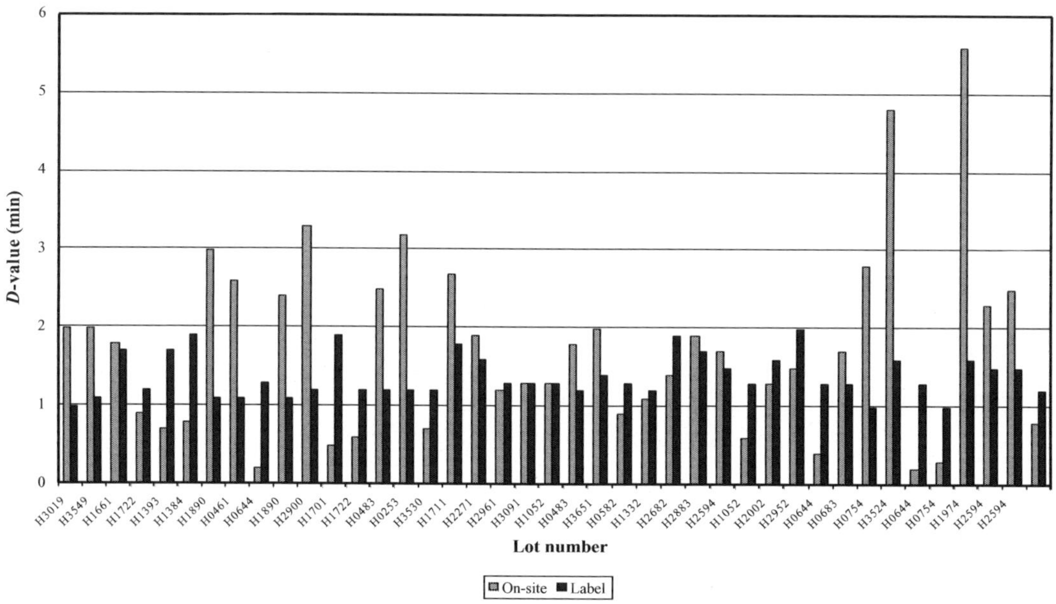

Figure 10 Apex Labs BI *D*-value comparison between manufacturer's label claim and data obtained on-site (1999 through 2005).

containing an appropriate neutralizer (catalase) and sterile forceps for carrier recovery. Once sterilizing conditions have been achieved in the isolator, the sealed container is opened and a timer is started. Replicate numbers of biological indicators are then aseptically transferred into individual recovery tubes after various exposure times. Following aeration, the recovery tubes can be removed for serial dilution plate counting (sterile buffer) or for immediate incubation (media).

An alternative method is to use a carrier holder and transfer system that permits the rapid entry of biological indicators into an isolator environment and their subsequent withdrawal upon completion of a particular exposure time (Fig. 11). For nonabsorptive carriers, this approach would eliminate the need for a neutralizer in the recovery buffer or media.

In using the Stumbo–Murphy–Cochran method of analysis, an estimated *D* value is calculated for each exposure time yielding fractional positive/negative data. The resulting *D* values are then averaged to obtain the final result for that test. Limitations associated with this method include the inability to always determine confidence intervals and a possible bias if the *D* value is based upon one dichotomous result (one data point). The procedure is easy to use in that it only requires the placement of exposed carriers into recovery media and determining the initial biological indicator population. The formula for estimating a *D* value is shown below:

$$D = U/\log_{10} N_o - \log_{10} N_u$$

where U is the exposure time (minutes); N_o is initial number of organisms per replicate; N_u is the ln (n/r): where n is the total number of replicates; r is the number of replicates negative for growth.

The *D* value data shown in Table 1 was obtained using *G. stearothermophilus* (ATCC #12980) spore suspensions that were dried on various surfaces and tested inside isolators of generally less than 60 ft^3 (1.7 m^3) in volume while connected to a VHP1000. The data suggest that the methodology employed was capable of achieving similar results between replicate tests, the spore suspensions (or biological indicators) tested back in the mid-1990s may have had a greater resistance to H_2O_2 gas, and current lots of suspension (or biological indicators) have had average *D* values ranging between 1.0 and 3.0 minutes when exposed to approximately 1.8 mg H_2O_2/L of air at 30°C. The gas concentration was estimated from the injection and air flow rate values and aqueous H_2O_2 concentrations shown in the table.

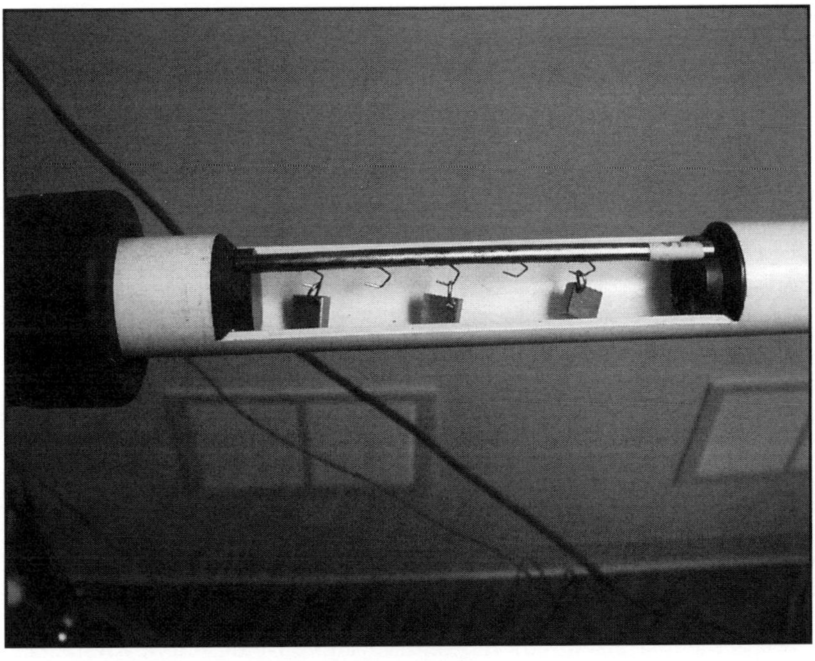

Figure 11 Test carriers placed in a *D*-value transfer apparatus.

Table 1 H_2O_2 Gas *D*-value Data Obtained Using *Geobacillus stearothermophilus* Spores (ATCC #12980) Under Defined Test Conditions Inside Various Isolators

				Study averages					
			H_2O_2	Inj. rate,	Airflow rate,	Air temp.	Replicate #		
Year	Facility	BI Description	(wt. %)	g/min	ft^3/min	(°C)	1	2	3
1995	A	Stainless, user prepared	30	1.7	10.7	28.0	7.0	6.6	4.8
1995	A	Filter in Tyvek®	30	1.7	10.7	28.0	10.2	10.1	8.4
1996	B	Stainless, user prepared	30	1.5	10.5	27.9	6.2	7.8	7.6
1996	B	Filter in Tyvek	30	1.5	10.5	27.9	7.0	7.4	7.1
1997	C	Stainless, user prepared	35	1.5	10.5	26.9	1.3	1.9	1.4
1997	D	Stainless, user prepared	35	2.5	15.9	28.5	2.1	1.9	1.1
1998	C	Stainless, user prepared	35	1.5	10.5	27.2	2.9	2.0	1.6
1998	E	Stainless, user prepared	35	1.2	10.7	35.5	15.0	13.7	17.7
1999	C	Stainless, user prepared	35	1.5	10.5	25.7	2.6	2.0	1.4
1999	F	Stainless in Tyvek	35	3.0	20.6	28.8	2.2	1.7	2.0
2000	C	Stainless, user prepared	35	1.5	10.3	27.1	2.0	2.6	0.5
2000	F	Stainless in Tyvek	35	3.0	20.6	29.5	1.8	1.8	2.3
2000	G	Stainless, user prepared	35	2.5	15.8	28.5	2.5	2.5	2.6
2000	H	Stainless in Tyvek	35	1.5	10.6	30.9	3.0	2.8	3.3
2001	C	Stainless, user prepared	35	1.5	10.5	27.5	4.3	4.9	3.1
2001	C	Stainless in Tyvek	35	1.5	10.5	30.7	1.6	1.6	1.9
2001	F	Stainless in Tyvek	35	3.0	20.7	29.0	1.6	1.9	2.0
2001	I	Stainless in Tyvek	35	2.2	18.6	32.7	2.9	2.7	2.5
2001	J	Stainless in Tyvek	35	1.5	10.5	28.7	2.0	2.2	1.6

Biological Indicators

USP defines a biological indicator as a characterized preparation of specific microorganisms resistant to a particular sterilization process (25). Biological indicators are used in isolator applications as the primary measurement requirement during the development and validation of decontamination cycles. The manufacturer must provide data on the stability of the spore population and its resistance throughout the labeled shelf life of the indicator. Data should be available to indicate that the chosen microorganism (usually a bacterial spore) is more resistant to the sterilant than the typical bioburden, including spore-forming organisms. Kokubo et al. (7) provided such information in 1998 for H_2O_2 gas where it was shown that the *D* value for the commercial strain of *G. stearothermophilus* (ATCC #12980) was 10-fold higher than the most resistant wild-type spore.

Test carriers (stainless steel or aluminum) inoculated with an appropriate spore suspension and dried prior to use has been the standard biological indicator for isolator decontamination applications over the past 15 years. Users have typically chosen to validate their isolator systems using the most resistant bacterial spores, although specific requirements have not been established. Commercially prepared test carriers come individually packaged in an overwrap material that does not adversely affect the performance of the indicator or the sterilant. A Tyvek® package has been successfully used for various H_2O_2 gas biological indicators as the gas will penetrate through it and there is little or no absorption into the fibers. The overwrap material will add resistance to the indicator, but the manufacturer can take this into account when deciding upon an acceptable level of resistance for the suspension and/or on its initial spore titer. It is still the manufacturer's responsibility to provide stability data for this type of biological indicator if labeled for use with a particular sterilant.

The debate continues on what spore challenge level should be used to validate an isolator decontamination process. PDA has suggested that the decontamination method should be able to provide a 3-log reduction of biological indicators known to be resistant to the agent employed (1). US Food and Drug Administration (FDA) has recommended a 4- to 6-log kill against an appropriate, highly resistant biological indicator, although the 4-log reduction was only recommended for controlled, very low bioburden materials such as items introduced into a transfer isolator including wrapped sterile supplies that are briefly exposed to the surrounding clean room environment (26). The recommended spore titer on the test carrier for demonstrating such a log reduction is also open for debate, because it depends on the choice of validation method (complete kill, fraction positive/negative, overkill, or bioburden). FDA is not a proponent of the fraction positive/negative data to estimate spore log reduction inside isolator systems. Finally, exposure times should be increased for actual (production) decontamination cycles to account for potential variables in the process; however, the doubling of the validated exposure time for nonproduct contact isolator surfaces seems unwarranted. The majority of users have added 20% to the validated exposure time to account for potential equipment variability.

This author's recommendation is to use a test carrier inoculated with at least 10^6 spores that possess a defined resistance to H_2O_2 gas and then verify that each carrier can be consistently sterilized during the validation of a "robust" decontamination cycle. This has been consistently achieved within properly designed decontamination chambers (isolators) during their validation and requalification over the past 15 years (27). The quantity of biological indicators used to challenge the decontamination process can range from a low of around 15 to a few hundred depending upon the internal volume and load within the isolator system, the intended use of the isolator and possibly because of the claims referenced in a validation master plan. The FDA's inspection arm is well aware of what the gas can and cannot do. The development of a robust decontamination cycle capable of achieving its intended purpose under a variety of conditions may help minimize 483 citations on decontamination processes, such as the ones described at ISPE's Barrier Isolation Technology Conference in 2001 (27).

Materials and Critical Surface Testing

The inactivation of spores that are dried on various materials of construction of an isolator is interesting data to gather for any new decontamination process. This information can provide the justification on the use of a particular material for biological indicators. The equipment vendor and/or other interested parties should generate the data and then share it with industry at conferences and in industry-sponsored journals. Performing this delicate work during the validation of every isolator is simply asking for trouble. There have been comments made over the past few years implying that *D* values vary with the materials on which spores were inoculated. In fact the most likely scenario is that a "tail" is occurring in the inactivation curve due to improper preparation and/or cleaning of the carriers. Data has been generated on the ability of H_2O_2 gas to decontaminate a variety of isolator materials in times similar to that of stainless steel suggesting that there were no significant differences in *D* value (6,23,28). Whichever carrier material is chosen, the substrate must be carefully assessed to assure that residual levels of H_2O_2 will not inhibit the germination of bacterial spores upon their placement into recovery media. Neutralizers such as catalase for H_2O_2 gas may be required in some instances.

The sterilization of biological indicators above or around a stopper hopper or bowl does not imply that those product contact surfaces are sterile and it should not be stated as such in a validation protocol or master plan. There may be several areas on complex pieces of equipment where sporicidal levels of the gas would have difficulty reaching in a consistent manner. The focus should rather be placed on the steps that would be taken to minimize bioburden on those surfaces prior to initiating the decontamination cycle. In addition, you may want to include some discussion on how those areas will be monitored for viable contamination after the completion of a filling campaign. The direct inoculation of spore suspension or placement of numerous test carriers on these product contact surfaces is once again increasing the risk of obtaining false positive test results.

Temperature Distribution

The maximum allowable H_2O_2 gas concentration within an isolator is based upon the background humidity level and the minimum surface temperature at the initiation of sterilant

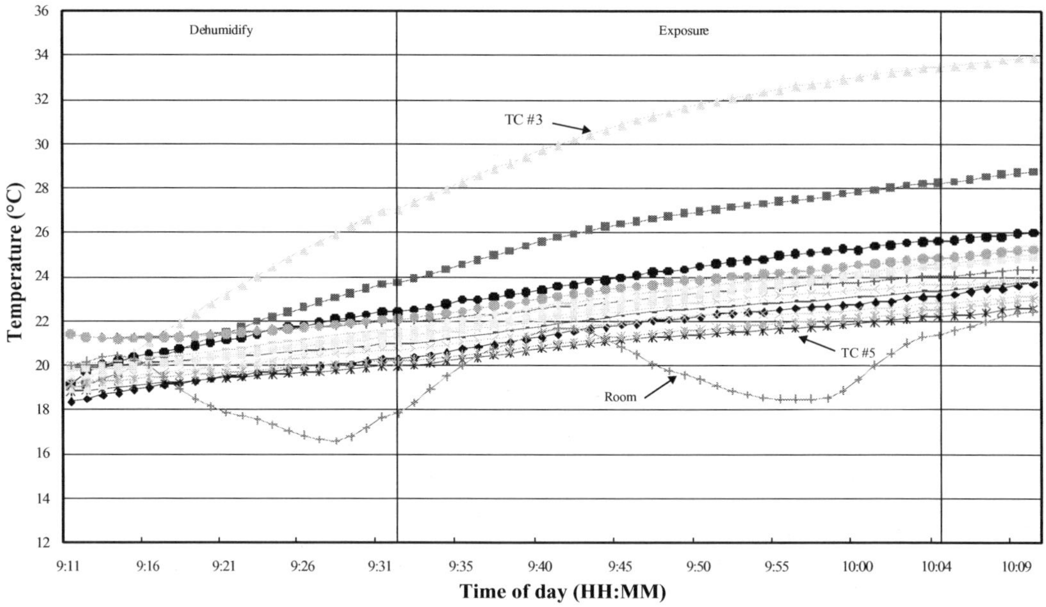

Figure 12 Isolator surface and room air temperatures during a VHP1000 decontamination cycle.

exposure. The coolest point in an isolator represents the location at which condensation would first occur when an excessive H_2O_2 gas concentration is used. Condensation will reduce the gas concentration in warmer areas of the enclosure; thereby complicating the development and validation of this type of decontamination cycle. Conversely, it was mentioned previously that temperature could indirectly affect sterilant efficacy in that an increase in temperature will lower the percent saturation and half-life of the gas. With these facts in mind, numerous thermocouple studies need to be performed during cycle development and the PQ to establish a temperature distribution pattern within the isolator and for the surrounding room (Fig. 12).

From a decontamination cycle perspective, it is important to demonstrate that day-to-day variability in room temperature stays within some acceptance window because the room can impact isolator surface temperatures. Areas that are designed to control the air temperature to within $\pm 2°C$ of the set point should not negatively impact H_2O_2 gas decontamination cycles. If day-to-day variability in room temperature is greater than that, there may be a need to establish the noncondensable gas concentration on the anticipated cool temperatures and then base the decontaminate phase time on sporicidal data obtained under warm room (worst case) temperature conditions.

The sterilant generator itself can also affect isolator temperature at least for enclosures that are less than a few hundred cubic feet in internal volume. Choose conservative dehumidify phase times in the event that a generator's desiccant system is warm or has little remaining capacity. The absolute humidity set point may not be reached within the allotted time and additional dehumidification may increase isolator temperatures to levels that may negatively affect sterilant efficacy.

It is equally important to demonstrate consistency in the range of isolator surface temperatures during at least the exposure phases of a decontamination cycle. Experience has shown that the average minimum and maximum surface temperature during exposure can fall within $\pm 5\%$ of their triplicate test averages (29). This information will provide further evidence that the decontamination cycle is being performed with an isolator and surrounding room that are in some state of control. It should be remembered to validate the time required to lower isolator temperatures back down to ambient temperature after continuous operation and/or if heat is employed to dry the equipment after cleaning.

Gas Distribution

The locations selected for the placement of chemical and biological indicators should be based on the physical configuration and anticipated air flow characteristics of the isolator. The focus during preliminary decontamination cycle development studies should be to verify or optimize the adequacy of the gas mixing capabilities of the system. Production isolators employ unidirectional airflow to control particulate counts during operation. They also house a great deal of equipment and these factors, when combined, typically lead to less than ideal sterilant distribution. The use of chemical indicators can quickly identify problem areas and engineering means are available to improve gas distribution within an isolator during decontamination (installation of fans, change in blower speed, etc.). It is not advisable to increase the gas concentration or the exposure time just to eliminate random positive biological indicators in occluded areas of the isolator. This may negatively impact sterilant performance and/or lead to material compatibility problems within the isolator due to condensation. Optimize the process first and then demonstrate that it is consistent and reproducible during the validation effort.

Sterilant Removal

According to OSHA, the permissible exposure level (PEL) for H_2O_2 gas is 1 ppm based on an 8-hour time-weighted average. This is an occupational exposure limit and has nothing to do with what an acceptable level would be within an isolator. The amount of aeration time needs to be validated in triplicate for each isolator application. The acceptable residue level will vary depending upon the intended use of the isolator and can range anywhere from below the detection limit to double-digit part-per-million levels. It is the responsibility of each user to demonstrate that the decontamination process does not negatively affect the product being manufactured or tested in the enclosure.

The amount of time involved in removing sterilant residues will vary due to absorption of the sterilant into materials and on the design of the isolator itself. If turnaround time is critical, design time should be spent reviewing the options on construction materials and/or exhaust methods. The introduction of fresh air at high exchange rates is customarily relied upon to rapidly remove the sterilant from isolators. Dilution has been the solution to many problems in the past and it will work here as well provided that it is done in a safe and consistent manner. Others have taken the approach to generate product stability data to known H_2O_2 concentrations and then aerating their isolators accordingly. Whichever way a company decides to go in terms of isolator design or stability testing, they should confirm that sterilant residue levels remain acceptable when the isolator is placed back in production mode in the event that the fresh air exchange rate is reduced at that time.

Generator Equivalency Testing

Sterilant generators should not be considered equivalent unless proven through validation studies (24). In reality, it may be easier to demonstrate that the validated decontamination cycle is conservative enough to account for any slight differences that may exist between generators. At a minimum, a single spore inactivation test and a single aerate test should be performed on an individual isolator to demonstrate that the decontamination cycle is not affected by a change in sterilant generator. If a difference in generator performance is demonstrated, another cycle may need to be validated for each isolator within the system.

There are now several applications around the world that use multiple H_2O_2 gas generators that operate in series to decontaminate numerous isolator sections at one time. This complicates the equivalency process especially if the end user wants to relocate generators to another system or if a spare generator is installed in one section due to service or calibration issues. For one such application, it was decided to use a near infrared H_2O_2 gas sensor to determine if critical cycle parameters from multiple gas generators could be maintained within defined tolerances (30). Baseline data were established on eight generators and the average gas concentrations were found to be within $\pm 10\%$ (± 3 standard deviations) of the overall mean. These values were within the critical control tolerances specified by the manufacturer. Conservative decontamination cycles were also developed, which provided greater confidence that the system would perform as intended if the need arose to swap generators. This monitoring procedure was also implemented for routine generator performance evaluations.

Residue Effects

The majority of sterile isolator applications have involved some sort of sterile material transport in and out of the enclosures during routine operations. In most cases, a decontamination step is used prior to isolator entry to remove bioburden on the external surfaces of containers or overwrap packaging. It may be necessary during validation studies to confirm that the decontamination process does not adversely affect the contents inside these items if the lack of microbial inhibition is a specific test requirement. For example, it is critical to demonstrate that the exposure of product or media containers to an isolator sterilant will not lead to a false-negative sterility or environmental monitoring test result, respectively. Typical sterilant ingress methods and one approach on how to include a variety of test supplies into a H_2O_2 gas residue effects study are discussed below.

A thorough review of all container/closure systems requiring decontamination needs to be performed and documented in terms of a description, volume, and materials of construction. The complete product matrix can be tested for sterilant penetration by using the validated decontamination cycle and a chemical assay. Although there are several quantitative assays available for the determination of low-level H_2O_2 concentrations, the use of a semiquantitative assay can quickly provide the necessary data to justify the bracketing of similar product or process containers (Fig. 13). This information can help keep the number of required microbiological test procedures to a minimum. Typically, the worst-case container/closure sample for various configurations will be the one that holds the smallest liquid volume as this would lead to a higher H_2O_2 concentration if penetration occurred at a similar rate.

Inoculate buffer-filled product containers with less than 100 viable microorganisms of some of the strains listed in USP's General Chapter on *Sterility Tests* <71> along with an environmental isolate or two, if desired (31).

The standard packaging for many gamma-irradiated settling or contact plates may be inadequate to prevent the ingress of H_2O_2 gas. It is essential to confirm that settling plates, Rodac® plates, and/or other media-containing sample devices can be decontaminated without affecting the growth promoting ability of the media. Test samples should be exposed to the validated decontamination cycle (back-to-back cycles have also been used) and then used per standard operating procedure (opened to the air or brought in contact with a decontaminated surface) prior to their removal from the isolator. The samples are then inoculated with less than 100 viable microorganisms of some of the strains listed in the USP General Chapter on *Sterility Tests* <71> along with an environmental isolate or two, if desired and incubated.

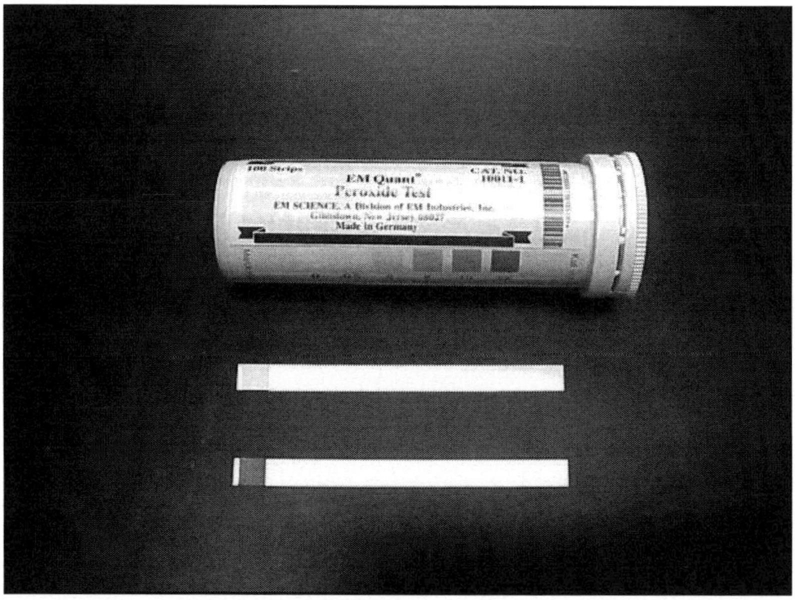

Figure 13 Semi-quantitative test strip used for the assay of aqueous H_2O_2.

There has also been an increase in vendor-supplied data on products claiming to be unaffected by their exposure to typical decontamination cycles. Bässler et al. (32) presented findings on the exposure of Sartorius gelatin membrane filters to H_2O_2 gas and found that there was no difference in the colony growth properties of the gassed filters in either single- or triple-wrapped packages. The data appear valid for *B. subtilis* spores; however, the vegetative forms of various other microorganisms were not tested during that study. Other studies have relied upon chemical indicators to demonstrate a lack of penetration through packaging; however, these devices will not change color to low levels of the sterilant, which could still inactivate some vegetative strains of microorganisms. BD Biosciences (Sparks, MD) has completed validation studies on BBL Isolator Pack™ prepared plated media, which used nine different microorganisms under defined test conditions. The results of their internal study were successful, but the company correctly stated that each isolator decontamination cycle must be validated independently as cycle parameters will vary from one site to another. Millipore has also evaluated a new line of agar plates for viable air monitoring in isolators that contain a neutralizer for H_2O_2, which likewise need to be validated for each application.

Residue effects tests are different from the sterilant ingress studies mentioned earlier in that all ingress variables are tested at once. The testing of sterility test supply materials (filter sets, media bottles, rinsing solution bottles, etc.) and at least one of each product container type from sterilant ingress testing are exposed to the validated decontamination cycle (back-to-back cycles have also been used). Following the validated aerate/exhaust time, recovery tests are performed to provide assurance that sterilant residues in or on the items or in the air, if present, will not lead to a "false-negative" sterility test. This is confirmed microbiologically using buffer-filled containers that are inoculated with the test microorganisms already discussed. The anticipated lowest operational air exchange rate through the isolator should be used during this study to verify conformance under worst-case sterilant residue conditions. All of the exposed samples and the positive controls should be positive for growth after their incubation.

STERILANT MONITORING

Process Related

There has been a great deal of debate over the last couple of years on the need to monitor the H_2O_2 gas concentration in production isolators. Some of the issues that have delayed their implementation include the lack of a recommended monitor, questions on calibration, location of the probe(s), and interpretation of the results. FDA is aware that there are still some unknowns to the technology, but would still like to see some measurement of sterilant concentration within large production systems instead of relying on indirect measurements from the generator (injection and airflow rates) (27).

A near-infrared guided wave H_2O_2 vapor monitor from Ocean Optics (Dunedin, FL) has been installed in several applications over the past few years. Most companies have only used the monitors during the development of decontamination cycles whereas some firms have kept them in the isolators to document the gas concentrations for use in approving equipment release for filling operations. The monitor provides a real-time value for both gaseous H_2O_2 and water concentrations (in mg/L) along a light path, as shown in Figure 14. Applying this technology to the control versus monitoring of H_2O_2 gas concentration becomes quite complex due to the changing background humidity levels (via sterilant decomposition) and surface temperatures in an isolator. The control systems for some of newer generators discussed earlier have been designed to receive such feedback, but the wide range of isolator temperatures may make it difficult to actually control the process by this method.

Personnel Related

Because isolators usually contain in excess of 1.0 mg/L (720 ppm) of H_2O_2 gas during a decontamination cycle, a real-time monitor should be available to detect an accidental release into the surrounding work environment. The toxic effects of H_2O_2 gas include irritation to the respiratory tract, eyes, and skin. Hand-held systems, such as the ones shown in Figure 15, have been available for years and studies have been undertaken to document their accuracy and interferences (33,34). Dräger peroxide detector tubes were unable to accurately measure the H_2O_2 gas

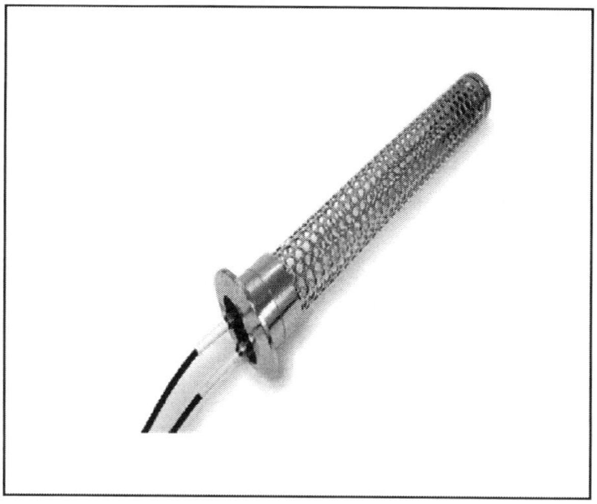

Figure 14 Guided Wave probe used for measuring H_2O_2 and water vapor in an isolator.

concentration when the relative humidity was below 20% whereas the Pac III electrochemical sensor was capable of providing accurate readings from 0.2 to 4.0 × PEL with no humidity effect.

Fixed-position electrochemical monitors are also available, which can provide a visual and audible alarm in the event of detecting H_2O_2 gas in the 1 to 2 ppm range (Fig. 16). An output is provided, which can provide a cycle abort signal when electrically interfaced to the sterilant generator. The sensing head should be mounted in an area where it is most likely to detect the gas while remembering to consider the physical and chemical properties of H_2O_2 when selecting a location.

SUMMARY

Validation data on the use of H_2O_2 gas for sophisticated isolator applications has been shared at conferences and in the literature over the past decade. In several cases, essential process variables have been overlooked and questions have been raised on the consistency of H_2O_2 gas generators and/or the devices used to qualify them (biological indicators). These issues may

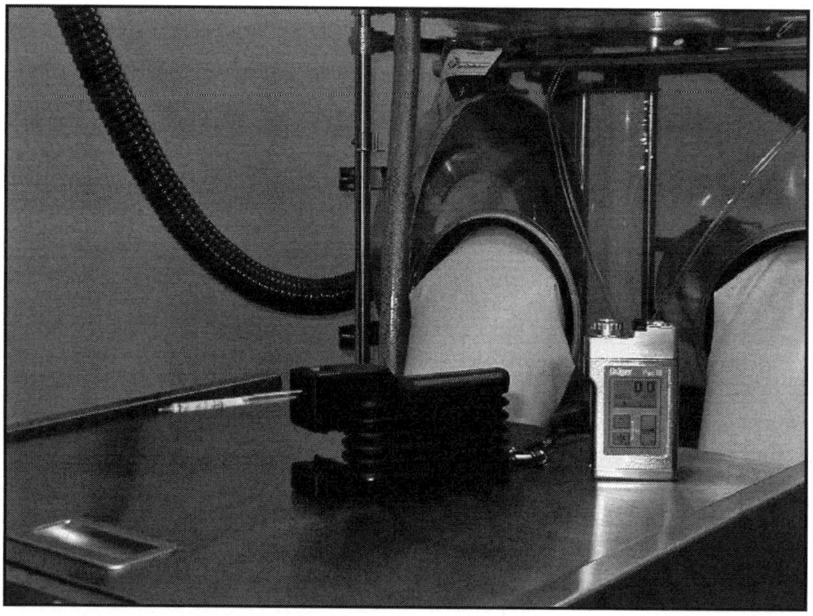

Figure 15 Common methods used for measuring low levels of H_2O_2 gas.

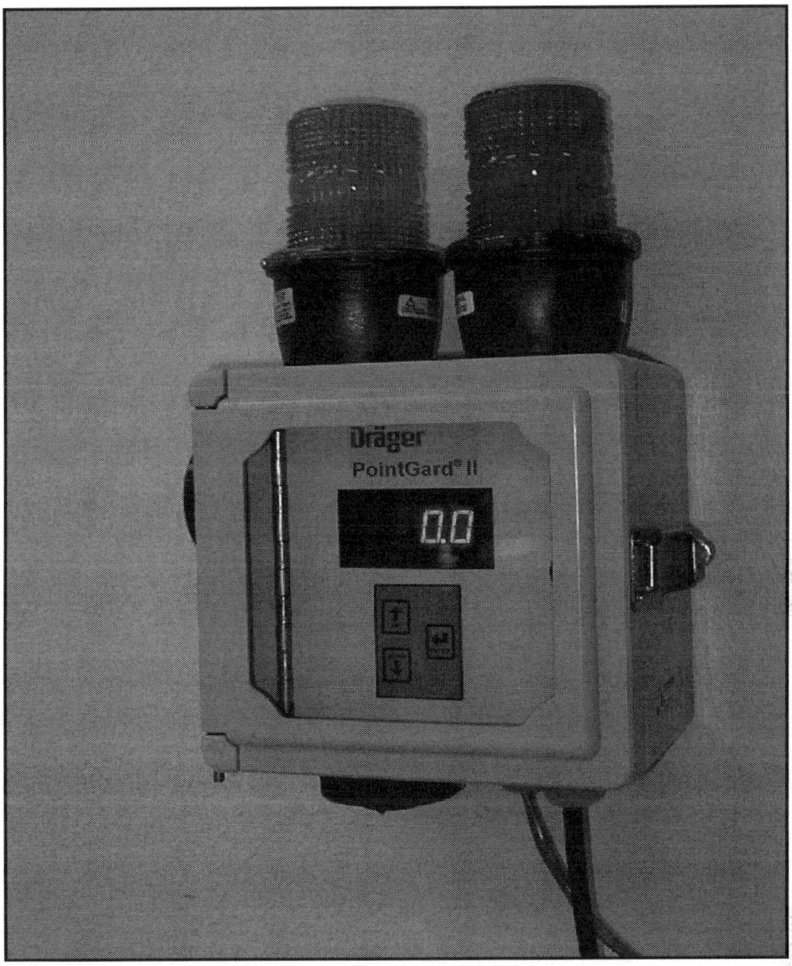

Figure 16 Fixed position H_2O_2 gas monitor with a two-level alarm.

in fact be due to a general lack of experience and/or guidelines on how to properly apply the sterilant to isolators. This chapter provides an overview on the technology, touches upon some of the key requirements for properly integrating sterilant generators into isolators, and it revisits the essential validation aspects of decontaminating isolators with H_2O_2 gas. Hopefully, this information has stressed to the reader that a properly designed decontamination chamber can lead to the development of a robust H_2O_2 gas decontamination cycle that will be reproducible under worst-case conditions.

REFERENCES

1. Kirsch J. Design and validation of isolator systems for the manufacturing and testing of health care products. PDA Technical Report No. 34. PDA J Pharm Sci Technol 2001; 55(5 Suppl TR34):1–24.
2. Lysfjord J. Porter ME. Barrier Isolation—History and Trends, 2008 Preliminary Data. Proceedings of the ISPE Conference on Engineering Regulatory Compliance; June 2–5, Arlington, VA.
3. Wagner CM, Raynor JH. Industry survey on sterility testing isolators—current status and trends. ISPE J Pharm Eng 2001 21(2):134–140.
4. Moore FC, Perkinson LR. Hydrogen Peroxide Vapor Sterilization Method. U.S Patent No. 4,169,123. September 25, 1979.
5. Forstrum RJ, Wardle MD. Cold Gas Sterilization Process. U.S. Patent No. 4,169,124. September 25, 1979.
6. Davenport SM. The Tip of the Iceberg—Designing and Implementing an Unsinkable VHP Cycle for Decontamination of an Isolator System. Proceedings of the ISPE Barrier Isolation Technology Conference; 1999, Arlington, VA.

7. Kokubo M, Inoue T, Akers J. Resistance of common environmental spores of the genus bacillus to vapor hydrogen peroxide. PDA J Pharm Sci Technol 1998;52(5):228–231.
8. Rickloff JR, Orelski PA. Resistance of Various Microorganisms to Vaporized Hydrogen Peroxide in a Prototype Table Top Sterilizer. Proceedings of the 89th General Meeting of the American Society for Microbiology; 1989, New Orleans, LA.
9. Neufeldt V, Guralnik DB, eds. Webster's New World College Dictionary. 3rd ed. New York: Simon & Schuster, Inc, 1997:1475–1476.
10. Pollard EC, Weber PK. Chain scission of ribonucleic acid and deoxyribonucleic acid by ionizing radiation and hydrogen peroxide in vitro and in *Escherichia coli* cells. Radiat Res 1967; 32:417–440.
11. Kawasaki, C, Nagano H, Ito T, et al. Mechanism of bactericidal action of hydrogen peroxide. J Food Hygiene Soc Jpn 1970; 11:155–160.
12. Bayliss CE, Waites WM. The combined effect of hydrogen peroxide and ultraviolet irradiation on bacterial spores. J Appl Bacteriol 1979;47:263–269.
13. Sintim-Damoa K. Other gaseous sterilization methods. In: Morrissey RF, Phillips GB, eds. Sterilization Technology. New York: Van Nostrand Reinhold, 1993:335–347.
14. McNassor GB. The Final Chapter—Biological and Process Validation of an Integrated High Speed Filling Isolator at Pharmacia & Upjohn. Proceedings of the ISPE Barrier Isolation Technology Conference; 1999, Arlington, VA.
15. Bier ME. Method of Vaporizing Multicomponent Liquids. U.S. Patent No. RE. 33,007. August 1, 1989.
16. Marcos-Martin M, Bardat A, Schmitthaeusler R, et al. Sterilization by vapour condensation. Pharm Technol Eur 1996; 8:24–32.
17. Grignol GD. Eddington DK, Rickloff J. Chemical and Biological Aspects of Hydrogen Peroxide Gas. Proceedings of the ISPE Barrier Isolation Technology Conference; 2000, Arlington, VA.
18. Lewis JS, Rickloff JR. Inactivation of Bacillus stearothermophilus Spores Using Hydrogen Peroxide Vapor. Proceedings of the 91st General Meeting of the American Society for Microbiology; 1991, Dallas, TX.
19. Rickloff JR. Hydrogen Peroxide Gas and its Use in Sterilizing Barrier Isolators. Proceedings of ISPE's 6th International Congress of Pharmaceutical Engineering; 1994, Philadelphia, PA.
20. Whitbourne JE, Reich RR. Ethylene oxide biological indicators: need for stricter qualification testing control. J Parenteral Drug Assoc 1979; 33:132–143.
21. Drummond DW, Pflug IJ. Dry heat destruction of *Bacillus subtilis* spores on surfaces: effect of humidity in an open system. Appl Microbiol 1970; 20:805–809.
22. Diehl MW, Edwards LM. Qualification and Regulatory Issues for a CBER Licensed Isolated Filling Line. Proceedings of the PDA Isolation Technology Conference; 2000, Irvine, CA.
23. Rickloff JR. Historical Perspective on the Decontamination of Isolators Using Hydrogen Peroxide Gas. Proceedings of the ISPE Barrier Isolation Technology Conference; 2005, Arlington, VA.
24. PIC/S Recommendation. Isolators Used for Aseptic Processing and Sterility Testing, September 2007.
25. Biological Indicators for Sterilization <1035>. In: USP 30 – NF 25. The Rockville, MD: United States Pharmacopeia, 2007:2099–2101.
26. Center for Drug Evaluation and Research (CDER) and Center for Biologics Evaluation and Research (CBER). Guidance for Industry, Sterile Drug Products, Produced by Aseptic Processing—Current Good Manufacturing Practice. Rockville, MD: U.S. Department of Health and Human Services, Food and Drug Administration, 2004.
27. Friedman RL. Aseptic Processing Isolators. Proceedings of the ISPE Barrier Isolation Technology Conference; 2001, Arlington, VA.
28. Miller MJ. A Comprehensive Strategy for the Use of Biological Challenges on Isolator Materials of Construction. Proceedings of the ISPE Barrier Isolation Technology Conference; 2007, Arlington, VA.
29. Rickloff JR. Key aspects of validating hydrogen peroxide gas cycles in isolator systems. J Validation Technol 1998; 5(1):61–71.
30. Rickloff JR. The Use of a Near Infrared Sensor to Determine the Range in H2O2 Gas Concentration for Multiple Sterilant Generator Applications. Proceedings of the PDA Spring Conference; 2000, Orlando, FL.
31. Sterility Testing <71>. In: USP 30 – NF 25. Rockville, MD: The United States Pharmacopeia, 2007:1878–1883.
32. Bässler H-J, Nieth KF, Herbig E. Tests on the colony growth properties of Sartorius gelatin membrane filters after exposure to vapour phase hydrogen peroxide. Eur J Parenteral Sci 1996;1(2):55–57.
33. Puskar MA, Plese MR. Evaluation of real-time techniques to measure hydrogen peroxide in air at the permissible exposure level. Am Ind Hygiene Assoc J 1996; 57:843–848.
34. Park J, Plese MR, Puskar MA. Evaluation of a New Personal Monitor Employing an Electrochemical Sensor for Measuring Hydrogen Peroxide in Air. Proceedings of the American Industrial Hygiene Association Conference; 2001, Orlando, FL.

26 Isolation technology: hydrogen peroxide decontamination

David Watling

INTRODUCTION

Much has been written and spoken about the processes involved in the decontamination of surfaces by using gaseous hydrogen peroxide, often without detailed reference to the equations governing the physical chemistry or reliable experimental data. It would seem logical that to achieve a proper understanding of the way in which the process works it is sensible to undertake a rigorous analysis, first of the physical chemistry, and then to establish how this will affect the application of the process to real situations. It may be expected that such an analysis would provide benefits both in terms of the reliability of the process and also the rate of kill that may be achieved.

Three important claims have been made about the process as used during the 1990s. These are that hydrogen peroxide vapor decomposes at room temperature according to a half-life rule, that the kill is achieved by the dry vapor, and that condensation must be avoided. Examination of the literature suggests that all of these assertions may be inaccurate and a detailed investigation is therefore required.

There are, of course, a number of parameters that must be controlled during hydrogen peroxide vapor phase decontamination and a proper understanding of the relationship between these would be expected to lead to consistent and reliable decontamination cycles. This chapter attempts to explain these relationships and points out how they may be controlled.

It should be remembered that hydrogen peroxide vapor decontamination is a nonpenetrative surface process and is only suitable for clean surfaces.

Physical Chemistry—Equilibrium Vapor Pressure

The purpose of studying the vapor pressure relationships of water and hydrogen peroxide is to establish at what point condensation will occur. If a liquid is placed in a closed vessel and maintained at a constant temperature the liquid and vapor phases will come to an equilibrium state. In this equilibrium state the number of molecules leaving and entering the liquid phase will be equal. Raising the temperature will cause an increase in the number of molecules leaving the liquid phase, thus raising the vapor pressure, until a higher equilibrium vapor pressure is reached.

For multicomponent solvent mixtures with constituent activities proportional to their respective mole fractions, that is, ideal solutions, the vapor pressure exerted by each component may be determined using Raoult's Law viz:

$$p_{\mathrm{A}} = x_{\mathrm{A}} p_{\mathrm{A}}^{0} \tag{1}$$

Where p_{A} is the vapor pressure exerted by component A, when the mole fraction is x_{A} and p_{A}^{0} is the vapor pressure that would be exerted by the pure substance at that temperature. The liquid mole fraction of substance A is defined as the number of moles of substance A divided by the total number of moles of all substances in the solution.

Equilibrium mixtures of hydrogen peroxide and water depart sufficiently from the ideal, as not to obey Raoult's Law and thus a modified form, taking into account the activity coefficients, must be used to determine the equilibrium vapor pressures viz:

$$p_{\mathrm{W}} = \gamma_{\mathrm{W}} x_{\mathrm{W}} p_{\mathrm{W}}^{0} \quad \text{and} \quad p_{\mathrm{H}} = \gamma_{\mathrm{H}} x_{\mathrm{H}} p_{\mathrm{H}}^{0} \tag{2}$$

The subscripts w and H refer to water and hydrogen peroxide.

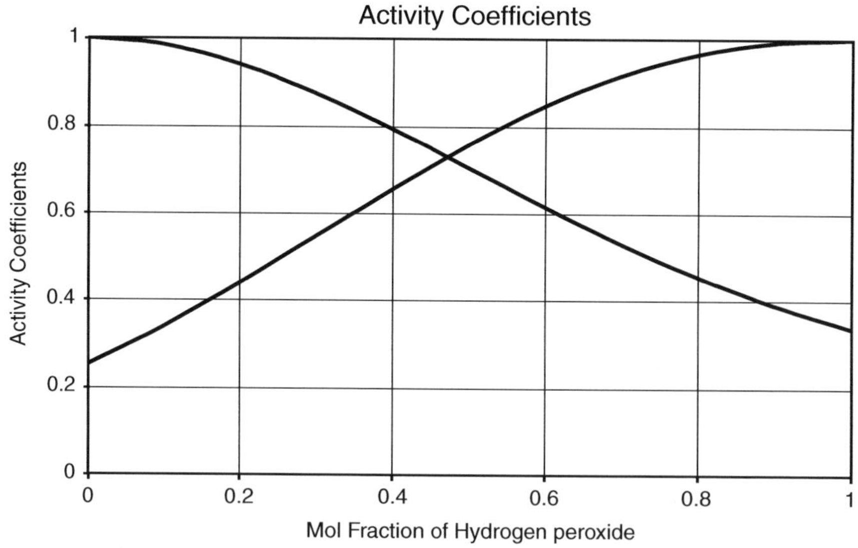

Figure 1 Graph of the activity coefficients of hydrogen peroxide and water against the Mol fraction of hydrogen peroxide.

The values of p_W^0 and p_H^0 may be found from the equations derived by Keyes (1) and Scatchard et al. (2), and are as follows:

$$\log p_W(T) = G + A/T + B \log T + CT + DT^2 + ET^3 + FT^4 \quad (3)$$

where $A = -2892.3693$, $B = -2.892736$, $C = -4.9369728 \times 10^{-3}$, $D = 5.606905 \times 10^{-6}$, $E = -4.645869 \times 10^{-9}$, $F = 3.7874 \times 10^{-12}$, $G = 19.3011421$, and T is the absolute temperature.

$$\log p_H(T) = D + A/T + B \log T + CT \quad (4)$$

where $A = -4025.3$, $B = -12.996$, $C = 46055 \times 10^{-3}$, $D = 44.5760$, and T is the absolute temperature.

Activity coefficients were calculated by Scatchard et al. (2) and reviewed by Schumb (3); equations for the activity coefficients are shown below and the values plotted in Figure 1, it will be noticed that they are always less than unity.

$$\gamma_W = \exp\left\{\frac{(1 - x_W)^2}{RT}[B_0 + B_1(1 - 4x_W) + B_2(1 - 2x_W)(1 - 6x_W)]\right\} \quad (5)$$

where R is the universal gas constant, B_0 is $-1017 + 0.97T$, $B_1 = 85$, $B_2 = 13$, and T the absolute temperature.

$$\gamma_H = \exp\left\{\frac{x_W^2}{RT}[B_0 + B_1(3 - 4x_W) + B_2(1 - 2x_W)(5 - 6x_W)]\right\} \quad (6)$$

By substituting Equations 4 and 6 in Equation 2, it is possible to calculate the equilibrium vapor pressure of hydrogen peroxide above any aqueous solution at any temperature from freezing to boiling. A similar calculation may be made using Equations 3 and 5 for the equilibrium vapor pressure of water.

The graphs shown in Figures 2 and 3 have been generated from these equations.

Physical Chemistry—Rapid Evaporation and First Bead of Condensation

Raoult's Law states that the equilibrium vapor pressure of each component of a solution will be directly proportional to the mole fraction of the component in the solution, and as the vapor pressure of pure hydrogen peroxide is much lower than that of water at the same temperature,

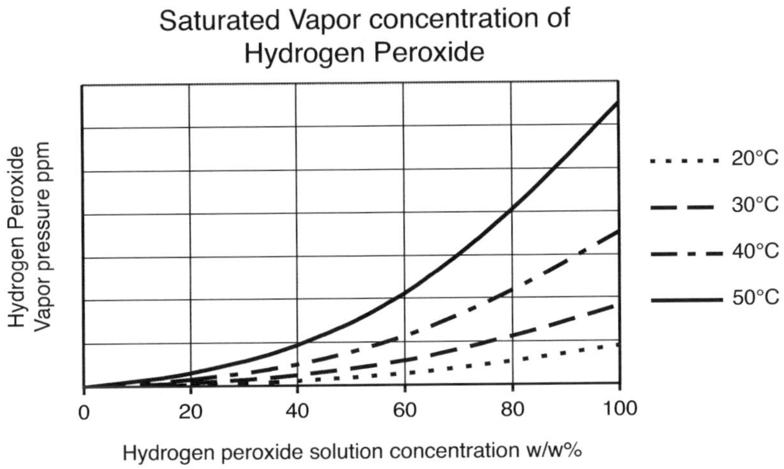

Figure 2 Graph of saturated hydrogen peroxide vapor concentration against hydrogen peroxide solution concentration.

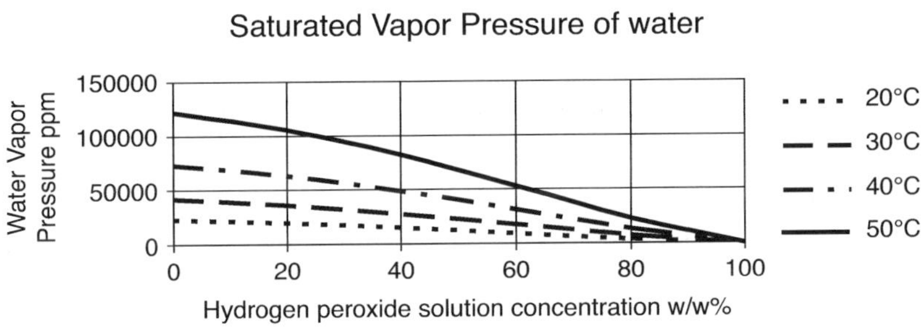

Figure 3 Graph of saturated water vapor concentration against hydrogen peroxide solution concentration.

it therefore follows that at any temperature the mole ratio of hydrogen peroxide to water in the vapor phase will always be lower than in the liquid phase when the system is in the equilibrium state. Figures 2 and 3 show that above a 50% w/w solution of aqueous hydrogen peroxide at 30°C, the vapor pressure of water is 23,117 ppm and that of hydrogen peroxide is only 771 ppm.

During hydrogen peroxide vapor decontamination cycles the hydrogen peroxide solution is "flash evaporated," a process that will cause all of the hydrogen peroxide and water to be turned into vapor. This generates a vapor mixture of the same proportions as the original solution giving a higher hydrogen peroxide vapor concentration than would be found under equilibrium conditions. We will use the term "rapid evaporation" in place of "flash evaporation" as dropping a solution of hydrogen peroxide on a heated plate to cause evaporation is not strictly "flash evaporation."

Normally such a "rapid evaporation" process is conducted so that the vapors are carried away in a stream of hot air. Should this stream of air contain any moisture then this will be added to the total water vapor in the system. If this stream of air carrying the rapid evaporated hydrogen peroxide solution is passed into a chamber then the vapor concentration may be raised to a level at which condensation will occur due to the lower temperatures encountered in the chamber.

If condensation is to occur, it must do so in equilibrium with the surrounding vapor at the moment that the condensation forms. As the rapid evaporation process generated vapor that was at a higher hydrogen peroxide concentration than is achieved in the equilibrium state, it follows that the condensation will be at a greater concentration than the original liquid providing the carrier gas is reasonably dry.

The concentration of the condensate will depend on the concentration of the evaporated liquid, the moisture content of the carrier air, and the temperature at which condensation forms. Any moisture in the carrier gas will reduce the concentration of the condensate. If for example the relative humidity (RH) in the chamber into which the vapor mixture is to be passed is 100% then as soon as any of the hydrogen peroxide and water vapor reaches the chamber, condensation would form but at a very weak concentration. A different situation arises if the carrier gas has a low water content and the humidity in the chamber is very low; this causes the initial condensate to form at a higher hydrogen peroxide concentration than the source solution.

As already stated, if hydrogen peroxide solution is rapid evaporated into a dry stream of air and passed to a chamber at a lower temperature there will come a point in time when the vapors become saturated and condensation forms. This condensate will be in equilibrium with the vapor and because the vapor was generated by rapid evaporation the condensate will be at a higher concentration than the original liquid. But if the process of rapid evaporation is continued the mass of condensate will increase until eventually all of the hydrogen peroxide solution will have been transferred to the chamber, at which time the vapor pressure of the hydrogen peroxide and water will be at the equilibrium pressures of the original solution at the temperature of the chamber, providing both the carrier gas and the chamber contained no water vapor, and the concentration of the condensate will also be reduced as the vapor and condensate will always try to stay in equilibrium.

This reduction in the concentration of the condensate and the hydrogen peroxide vapor concentration starts as soon as the first bead of condensation has formed. The system is never in a static equilibrium state because as more vapor is added and condenses, it changes the concentration of the condensate and hence the equilibrium point.

If this process is conducted when the chamber contains air that is not dry, but has some water content, then this will alter the vapor concentration at which condensation will occur and reduce the concentration of the first bead of condensation. At very high RH in the chamber, say at 70% and above, the concentration of the first bead of condensate will be lower than the original liquid and increase as more vapor is added to the chamber.

A complete mathematical analysis of the process of condensation from rapid evaporated liquid has been analyzed by Watling et al. (4) starting with the equations for the equilibrium vapor pressures of aqueous hydrogen peroxide solutions. The calculations to determine the moment at which the first bead of condensation is formed and the subsequent vapor concentrations following the onset of condensation can only be done using an iterative technique. To simplify these calculations a computer program was prepared on the basis of the equations derived by Watling et al., which is able to predict the vapor concentration during a decontamination cycle, an example of plots generated using these techniques is shown in Figure 4.

Three levels of humidity inside the chamber at the start of the cycle were chosen to demonstrate the effect on vapor concentration during a decontamination cycle. It is obvious from Figure 4 that with a low level of humidity in the chamber a higher hydrogen peroxide vapor concentration is reached, peaking at about 1100 ppm with a starting RH of 10%. The peak of the

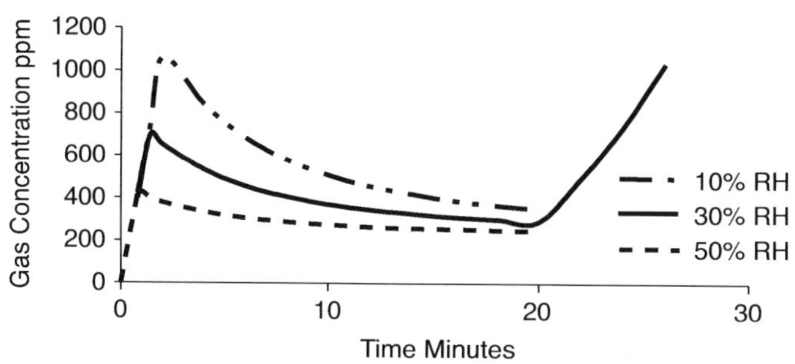

Figure 4 Gas concentration in a 1 m^3 chamber at various starting values of RH with a liquid injection rate of 2 grms/min @ 22°C.

hydrogen peroxide vapor concentration represents the point where the vapors have become saturated and the first beads of condensation form. As stated earlier at this point in the cycle the vapor concentration will start to fall as the vapors continue to condense. The very rapid rise in the hydrogen peroxide vapor concentration for the 30% RH plot arises after 20 minutes because of aeration. (Aeration is that part of the decontamination cycle where the hydrogen peroxide and water vapors are removed from the chamber.) For the purpose of the calculation it was assumed that aeration would start at 20 minutes and that fresh dry air is fed to the chamber to remove the hydrogen peroxide and water vapors. Displacing the vapors within the chamber with clean air changes the vapor pressure balance and because water has a much higher vapor pressure than hydrogen peroxide the water evaporates from the surface condensate more quickly. The preferential evaporation of the water from the condensed film increases the hydrogen peroxide concentration of the condensed film thus raising the equilibrium vapor pressure of the remaining condensate. This causes an increase in the hydrogen peroxide vapor concentration.

It should be noted that once condensation has formed the vapors and condensate are trying to reach equilibrium, but as this is a dynamic process this quasi-equilibrium state is always changing. It also follows that the concentration of the condensate will mirror the vapor concentration. Taking the example of the vapor profiles shown in Figure 4, the first bead of condensation will have higher hydrogen peroxide concentration than the evaporated solution. This concentration will fall as the mass of condensate increases and rise again during aeration.

Types of Hydrogen Peroxide Generators

There are two types of commercially available stand-alone hydrogen peroxide vapor generators. Although they both generate hydrogen peroxide vapor by the rapid evaporation process they are characteristically very different in the way in which the hydrogen peroxide and water vapor concentrations are managed.

Both designs circulate the air or air/vapor mixtures through the chamber to be decontaminated and return it to the generator. This has the advantage that the vapor is contained in a closed loop and may be decomposed within the loop thus avoiding the release of any toxic vapor to the environment.

The original design, first commercially produced in the late 1980s, is shown schematically in Figure 5 and may be described as the single-loop generator. In this design the air or air/vapor mixture from the chamber first passes through a catalyst inside the vapor generator. The catalyst decomposes any hydrogen peroxide present to water and oxygen. The vapor then passes through a dryer before further quantities of fresh hydrogen peroxide solution are rapid evaporated into the gas stream. After leaving the vapor generator the air or air/vapor mixture is

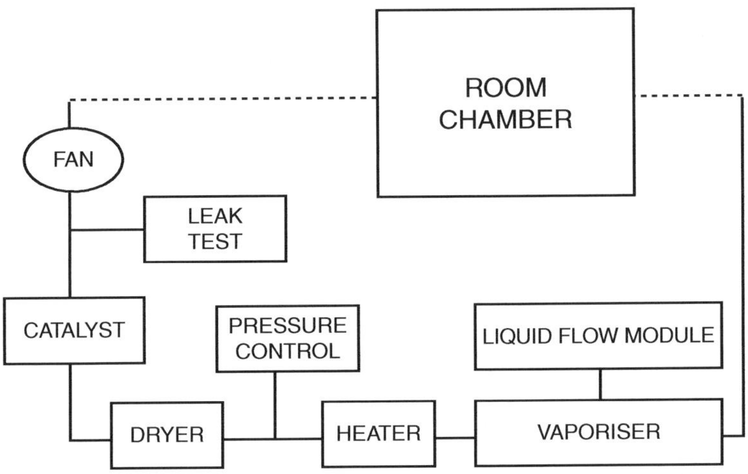

Figure 5 Schematic diagram of a single loop hydrogen peroxide vapor generator.

delivered to the chamber. A blower inside the generator circulates the air or air/vapor mixture round the closed loop.

The decontamination cycle is in three phases, the first is dehumidification, during the second phase hydrogen peroxide is evaporated and the final phase is aeration; the evaporation phase is often in two parts, a high evaporation rate to quickly raise the vapor concentration followed by a lower rate to maintain the required concentration.

During the first phase air is circulated round the closed loop and the dryer reduces the moisture content of the air. No hydrogen peroxide is evaporated during this phase of the cycle. Once the required level of humidity has been reached the rapid evaporation system is switched on and hydrogen peroxide solution is evaporated into the circulating gas stream.

If the evaporation phase is in two parts then during the first a high hydrogen peroxide evaporation rate will be used to quickly raise the vapor concentration. Once the desired concentration has been achieved, the evaporation rate is reduced to maintain the vapor concentration for a sufficient period of time to achieve kill on the target microorganisms.

In some hydrogen peroxide vapor decontamination cycles the evaporation phase is limited to a high single rate of evaporation, the same rate being maintained for sufficient time to cause decontamination.

The injection phase is followed by the third and final phase of the cycle, which is aeration. During this phase the rapid evaporation system is switched off and the air/vapor mixture is circulated through the system passing through the catalyst and dryer, which removes the hydrogen peroxide and water reducing the concentration in the chamber, by successive dilution.

Aeration is frequently the longest phase of a decontamination cycle. It may be considered to be in three stages, the first is to evaporate any condensation that has formed during the evaporation phase of the decontamination cycle; the second is to remove the vapors from the chamber by successive dilutions. The third and final stage is to continue circulation of clean air allowing any hydrogen peroxide that has been absorbed into the surfaces of the chamber and contents to desorb and be removed. It is the removal of the absorbed hydrogen peroxide that frequently makes the aeration phase the longest part of a decontamination cycle.

It is important to note that in the single-loop system all of the hydrogen peroxide returning to the generator is decomposed and practically all of the water is removed from the recirculating air/vapor stream. This is important because it means that the liquid is rapid evaporated into dry air, which contains no hydrogen peroxide or water. The reason for adopting this technique was that it was believed that hydrogen peroxide would decompose during the injection phase and hence it would not be possible to control the concentration of the vapor being returned to the chamber.

The more recent design known as the "dual loop" an example of this type of generator is shown in Figure 6 and a schematic of the dual-loop configuration is depicted in Figure 7.

In this design the circulating air or air/vapor passes either down the dehumidification/aeration branch or the gassing branch. The "dual-loop" system is best explained by reference to a decontaminating cycle, which uses the same three phases as the "single-loop" design. During the first phase, the circulating air passes through the catalyst and dryer to reduce the humidity to the required value. This is followed by the injection phase when the air passes through the preheater and rapid evaporator. The two parts of the injection phase are similar to those in the "single-loop" system. During the first part a high liquid evaporation rate is used to rapidly raise the vapor concentration. This is followed by the second part when the liquid injection rate is reduced to maintain the required conditions. Finally the air/vapor mixture is diverted back through the dehumidification/aeration branch to remove the hydrogen peroxide and water. Once again this is frequently the longest part of the cycle.

The significant difference is that in the dual-loop system no hydrogen peroxide or water is removed during the injection phase, thus allowing for a rapid build-up in the water and hydrogen peroxide vapor concentration. This process depends on the fact that no significant quantities of hydrogen peroxide are decomposed during the cycle.

Three isolator manufacturers, namely La Calhène, Bosch and Skan, have designed and built vapor generators into their isolators. This has the advantage that the control system is incorporated into the isolator controls, but the disadvantage that the generator may only be used for one isolator. Steris also provides a vapor generator that may be built into an isolator.

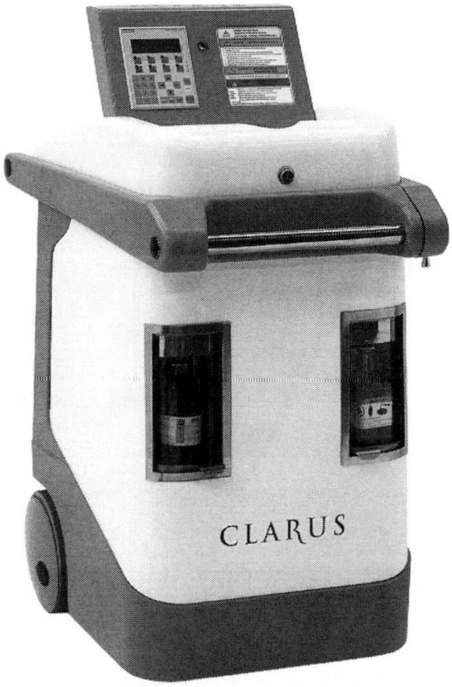

Figure 6 Clarus C hydrogen peroxide vapor generator by BIOQUELL.

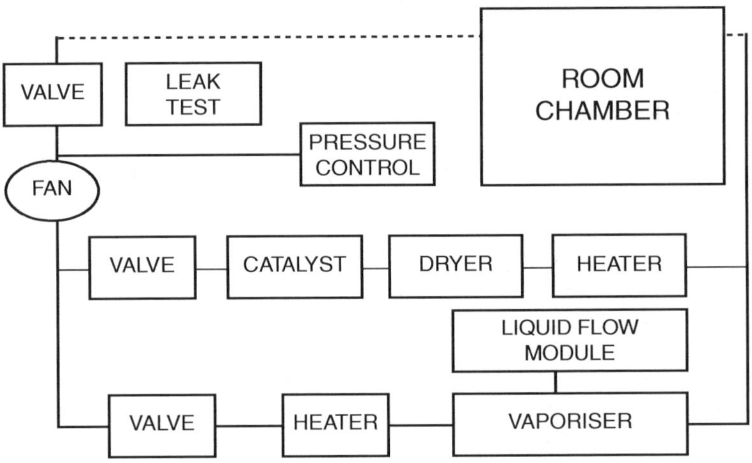

Figure 7 Schematic diagram of a dual loop hydrogen peroxide vapor generator.

All of these built in devices operated in the same way as either the single- or dual-loop generators and hence any analysis of their cycles may be undertaken using the principles already described.

BIOQUELL designed two vapor generators specifically for the decontamination of large chambers and rooms where the generator may be placed inside the room. This has the advantage that it is not necessary to run ducts into the room to carry the vapor in and out. One difficulty with large rooms is controlling the water content, or RH, of the room at the start of vapor generation. We have already seen that the water content of the chamber to be decontaminated has a significant effect on the maximum hydrogen peroxide vapor concentration and hence the concentration of the condensate. Once the first bead of condensation has formed the concentrate of the condensation tend toward that of the source liquid. By using an understanding

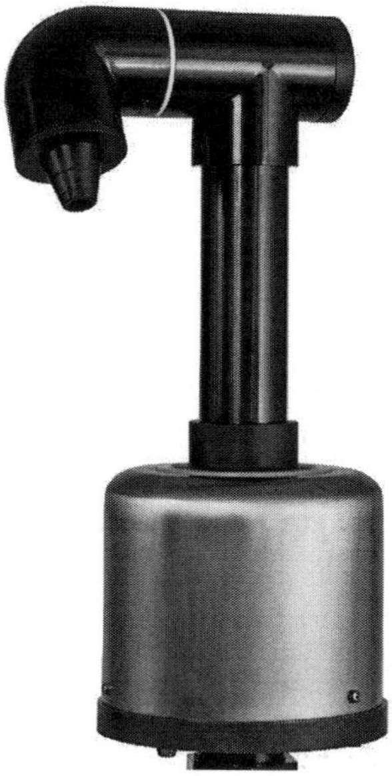

Figure 8 Dual rotating nozzle also seen in Figure 9 attached to the top of the hydrogen peroxide vapor generator.

of the physical chemistry and the starting conditions it is possible to adjust the cycle parameters to compensate for the initial RH within the room.

In large spaces, such as rooms, vapor distribution becomes very critical. This has sometimes been solved by the use of fans inside the room. A more elegant solution is shown in Figure 8. The dual rotating nozzle throws the vapor approximately 6 m with a velocity in the region of 20 m/sec. This type of nozzle is normally attached to a generator of the type shown in Figure 9. A further development of this technology is shown in Figure 10; in this generator the rotating nozzle has been replaced with a number of fixed nozzles pointing in different directions. Inside the generator is a bypass fan that produces a large air flow increasing both the velocity and volume of the air/vapor mixture delivered from the nozzles.

Biological Indicators and Kill Kinetics

The usual method of establishing if a kill has been achieved and hence the decontamination process has been successful is to use biological indicators (BIs).

The theory suggests that microcondensation is unavoidable in hydrogen peroxide decontaminations; it may also be advantageous. This section examines the evidence for the kill mechanism and reviews how this may impact on the use of BIs.

A BI is a number of microorganisms of known resistance to a specified sterilization or sporicidal process inoculated onto a carrier and contained within a primary pack.

There is considerable evidence that other gaseous decontamination processes are much more effective when the water content of the vapor is high. Porter et al. (5) reported the results of deactivation of *Bacillus subtilis* using peracetic acid (PAA). The tests were conducted by spraying a PAA solution containing 40% peracetic acid, 5% hydrogen peroxide, 39% acetic acid, 1% sulphuric acid, and 15% water into a chamber and allowing the vapor concentrations to stabilize. The test was conducted at various values of chamber RH.

The most important result that is drawn from this work is that optimal sporicidal activity apparently occurs at 80% RH. It would be expected from Raoult's Law that because the mole fraction of water in the sprayed liquid is 0.38 then condensation would start to occur at about 40% RH, the point at which Porter reported that kills start. This also accounts for the lower PAA vapor concentration reported at 60% and 80% RH as following the onset of condensation the vapor concentration would fall. One conclusion of Porter's paper is that PAA is more effective following the onset of condensation.

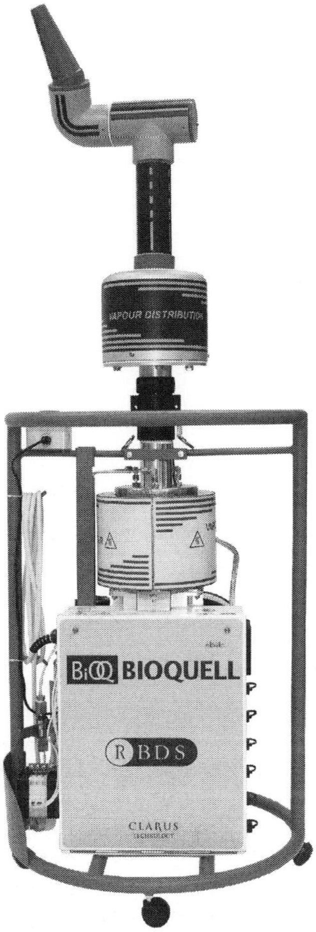

Figure 9 Clarus R. The first hydrogen peroxide vapor generator intended for room decontamination and designed to be placed inside the room.

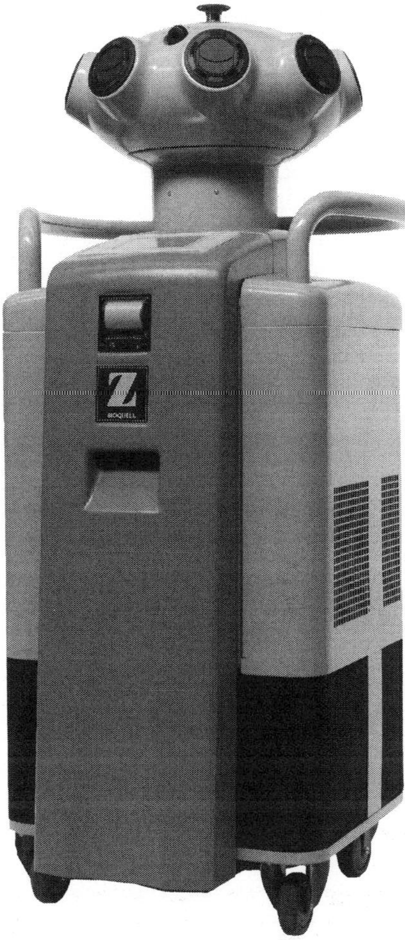

Figure 10 Clarus Z hydrogen peroxide vapor generator for room decontamination incorporating an aeration system.

The requirement for water is also highlighted in the European Standard (6) when advising on the mixture of formaldehyde solution and water that should be used to fumigate a microbiological safety cabinet. That document suggests that for each 1 m^3 of cabinet volume 60 mL of 36% w/w formaldehyde should be mixed with 60 mL of water and then boiled off inside the cabinet. Following this suggestion 98 g of water would be evaporated into each cubic meter of the chamber. As anyone who has conducted formaldehyde decontamination of a safety cabinet knows this is well in excess of the saturated vapor.

It is known that when both ozone and chlorine dioxide (both of which are gases at room temperatures) are used as gaseous decontamination agents that high levels of humidity are essential to achieve rapid and reliable cycles. All of this evidence suggests that gaseous decontamination is more effective when the level of humidity has reached saturation.

In a test conducted by the author an isolator was placed in an environmental chamber and connected through a utility port to a single-loop vapor generator. The vapor generator and isolator were arranged so that the vapor was delivered to the isolator and then exhausted to the outside, thus ensuring a flow of vapor through the isolator at known concentrations.

The temperature of the environmental chamber was set and the isolator was allowed to stabilize at the chamber temperature. *Geobacillus stearothermophilus* spore strips were placed on a wire hanger inside the isolator and removed at timed intervals. The results of the test at 40°C, 30°C, and 20°C are shown in Table 1.

Table 1 Results of a Test Showing Rapid Kill at 20°C Because of Condensation and No Kill at 40°C

At 20°C	At 30°C	At 40°C
Total kill at 15 minutes	Total kill at 40 minutes	Growth

The dew point of the supplied vapor mixture was approximately 30°C, and at temperatures above this value no kill was observed. At 30°C, the dew point temperature, kill took approximately 40 minutes, but at 20°C the time to kill was only 15 minutes. Thus in a dry gas, that is, at temperatures above the dew point, kill is either absent or very slow and where condensation is achieved fast kills are observed.

Unger-Bimczok et al. (7) reported in their paper a detailed study of the inactivation of *G. stearothermophilus* spores, using hydrogen peroxide and water vapor. In their conclusions they state

> *Based on the observations, it was suggested that the dominant kill factor is the overall deposition of water and hydrogen peroxide on the material surface to be decontaminated.*

They were also able to plot the kill kinetic curves at four different humidity levels at 400 and 600 ppm hydrogen peroxide vapor concentrations. It is interesting to note that some of these plots show significant amount of tailing.

It is clear that there is considerable evidence in the published literature that at room temperatures faster and more reliable kills are achieved after the onset of condensation.

There is much published literature about the choice of BIs for hydrogen peroxide surface decontamination that has led to the use of *G. stearothermophilus* as the standard organism (8) for this process. *G. stearothermophilus* not only appears to be amongst those microorganisms showing the greatest resistance to hydrogen peroxide vapor but also has the advantage that it is incubated at 58°C to 60°C and, hence reduces the risk of cross contamination during recovery and testing.

However, there are difficulties associated with any biological system; by their nature they are likely to be variable. This variability is usually compounded by the methods used in preparation, transport, storage, and recovery. Despite these problems with variability, BIs have become the "gold standard" used to evaluate a decontamination process. It was against this background that the PDA (Parenteral Drug Association) set up a task force to prepare some guidelines for the preparation and use of BIs for gaseous biodecontaminations. As part of their investigation the task force requested Bedfordshire University in the United Kingdom to photograph, using a scanning electron microscope, a number of commercially available BIs all inoculated with *G. stearothermophilus* onto stainless steel carriers. By kind permission of Dr. Graham Steele of the University of Bedfordshire four of these photographs are shown in Figure 11 and these clearly demonstrate the variability in the preparation of the indicators.

For a BI to give consistent results it is essential that it is prepared from a clean inoculum and that the spores are well separated on the surface of the carrier. With the degree of contamination shown in three of the photographs in Figures 11(b) to 11(d) and a process that is not fully understood it is not surprising that the results of some decontamination cycles are not always consistent.

There are further difficulties with the use of BI in vapor phase decontaminations. Two factors are usually considered to give reliable information about a BI; they are the number of spores on the carrier and the *D* value.

The *D* value poses some difficulty as it is defined as the time taken to achieve a decimal reduction in the number of viable spores when subjected to a known constant stress level. This difficulty arises because during a vapor phase decontamination the stress level is not constant and cannot be easily defined.

Consideration of the equilibrium vapor pressure during hydrogen peroxide decontamination quickly demonstrates the difficulty of having a constant and known stress level.

The theoretical plot in Figure 4 shows the predicted hydrogen peroxide vapor concentration during a decontamination cycle. During the first few minutes while the vapor concentration is rising there is very little stress on the microorganisms on the BI. At the peak vapor

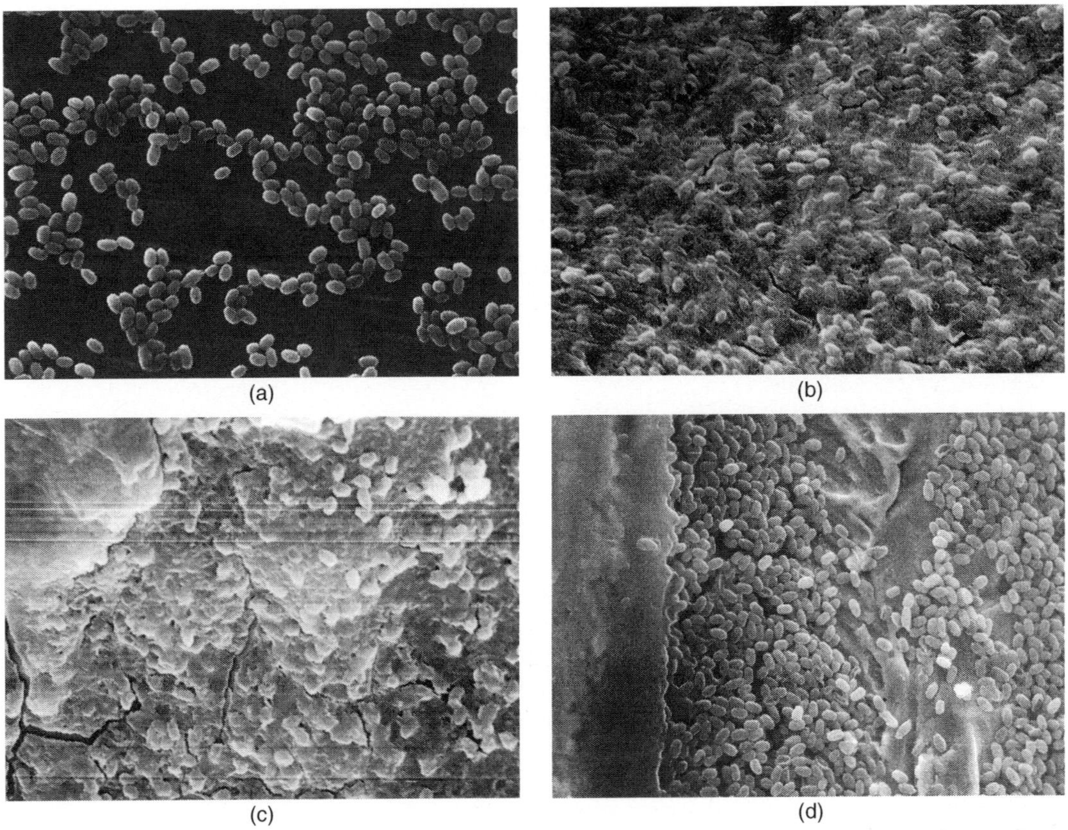

Figure 11 Scanning electron microscope photographs showing variability of the preparation of the biological indicators. 11(a) shows well-separated and clean spores whereas 11(b–d) show considerable debris and clumping.

concentration condensation will start to form in equilibrium with the vapor and hence these first few droplets will be at a high concentration. As the cycle proceeds to the vapor concentration falls and so will the concentration of the condensate, but this may be counteracted by the increasing thickness of the microcondensate layer. Thus, during the part of the cycle when condensation is forming both the concentration and thickness of the layer of microcondensation are changing with time; hence the stress level is also changing. Strictly speaking any *D* value calculated from a decontamination cycle where the stress levels are changing is not a true *D* value. It is also important to note that during the first part of aeration the microcondensate layer will be reducing but at increasing levels of hydrogen peroxide concentration. Any microorganism that has survived the vapor injection phase of the cycle may well not survive the aeration phase.

From the work of Unger-Bimezoz et al. (7) it is evident that there may be considerable tailing effects as the vapor and humidity concentrations are reduced. This leads to the question as to what tests should be applied to BIs to ensure consistent quality. The manufacturer will normally provided a certificate showing the enumeration and the *D* value, but the manufacturers' *D* value may not be relevant to the intended decontamination cycle.

What are required are tests that allow comparison between batch to batch and lot to lot of BIs. Assuming that the enumeration results are satisfactory then the problem rests on finding a solution to the death kinetics profile of the BI.

Manufacturers often quote *D* values of the order of 2 minutes with variations of perhaps half a minute. This variation may not seem very much but it represents a change in resistance of $\pm 25\%$. A more rigorous control over the quality of BIs used in validation work is essential to avoid the problems associated with revalidation, not because the vapor process has changed but because the resistance of the BI is not consistent.

The stress level during hydrogen peroxide vapor decontamination is not constant, but providing BIs are subjected to a consistent stress *pattern* then the results of different tests may be compared. A consistent stress pattern can be generated by always using the same vapor generator and chamber combination together with the same cycle parameters. The cycle parameters that must be controlled are the following:

- The temperature of the environment as this will change the wall temperature of the chamber.
- The starting temperature of the chamber.
- The starting RH within the chamber.
- The rate of evaporation of the hydrogen peroxide solution.
- The total mass of hydrogen peroxide evaporated.
- The concentration of the hydrogen peroxide solution.
- The temperature of the vapor mixture delivered to the chamber.
- The carrier gas flow rate.
- The location of the BIs within the chamber.
- The distribution of the vapor mixture within the chamber.
- The physical configuration of the chamber.

By placing the BIs into either growth media or buffer solution at timed intervals during the decontamination cycle it is possible to establish either the death kinetics by enumeration of those BIs placed in the buffer solution or the time at which the last BI showed no growth on incubation. Either technique will give a measure of the resistance of the BIs.

The decontamination cycle parameters should be adjusted so that the time interval between the removals of the sample BIs is much shorter that the expected kill time, as the sampling interval sets the sensitivity of the test.

Reaching saturation of the vapors is important as noted in Figure 12. This shows the relationship between the temperature of the vapors, the RH, and the hydrogen peroxide vapor concentration. It may be seen from Figure 12 that if the RH is 70% at a temperature of 32°C then the maximum hydrogen peroxide vapor concentration is 500 ppm. Above this point represents supersaturation and will lead to condensation.

Vapor Concentration for Dual- and Single-Loop System

In "Physical Chemistry—Rapid Evaporation and First Bead of Condensation" section, it was described how the vapor concentration changes during the decontamination cycle and also how the concentration of the condensate changes for a dual-loop generator. The calculation for the single-loop vapor generator is much more complex, because hydrogen peroxide and water vapor are removed from the circulating vapor mixture.

When using a single-loop generator the mass of water in the chamber at any time is the mass of at the start of the cycle plus the water content of the evaporated hydrogen peroxide solution less the water removed by the dehumidifier in the generator; this will depend on the efficiency of the dehumidification process. Likewise the hydrogen peroxide concentration depends on the mass of hydrogen peroxide evaporated less the mass removed from the circulating vapors.

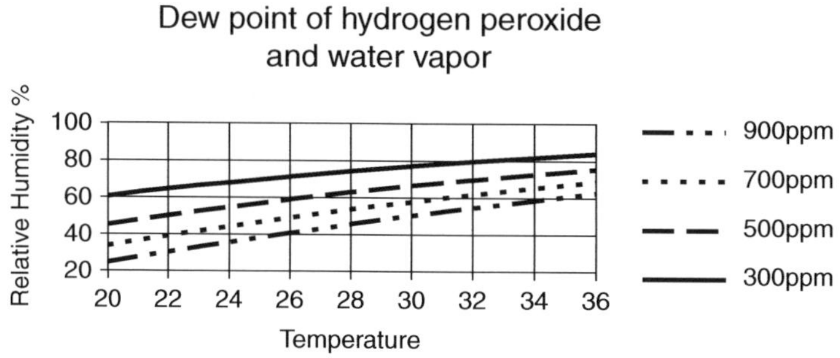

Figure 12 Graph showing the dew point of saturated water and hydrogen peroxide vapors over a range of temperatures.

The problem of knowing if the vapors are saturated is further complicated by the reduction of the evaporation rate of the hydrogen peroxide solution during the second part of the vaporization phase of the decontamination cycle. If the reduced evaporation rate is less than the removal rate of the hydrogen peroxide vapor from the circulating vapor then condensation within the chamber will evaporate leading to extended and unreliable cycles.

Such a problem does not exist with the dual-loop generator as no vapors are extracted during the critical part of the cycle and all of the hydrogen peroxide solution that is evaporated once the vapors become saturated is deposited as condensate.

Decomposition of Hydrogen Peroxide Vapor and Liquid

One of the major assumptions made during all of the calculations is that hydrogen peroxide vapor and liquid do not decompose by a significant amount during the decontamination process. Schumb (3) states that hydrogen peroxide vapor in a homogenous state is stable up to 425°C. This means that decomposition at room temperature would only happen if the vapor came into contact with a catalytic surface. Such decomposition could not be described as behaving according to a half-life rule. It is also stated by Schumb that liquid at 90% w/w and 50°C decomposes at a rate of only 0.001% per hour.

Some decomposition would be expected during a decontamination cycles as it is the action of the free radicals that are released during the decomposition process that deactivate microorganisms. However, the evidence from dual-loop cycles suggests that there is very little decomposition of the hydrogen peroxide either in the liquid or vapor phases. Any decomposition would result in an increase in the water content of the chamber and such an increase will lead to a reduction in the hydrogen peroxide vapor concentrations; which have not been observed.

Humidity

The term "RH" causes considerable difficulty when used to describe the moisture content of the vapor phase during hydrogen peroxide decontamination. Humidity is defined as the amount of water vapor in the air, and RH as the ratio of the water content of the air to the maximum possible water content in pure air, that is saturated water vapor, at that temperature expressed as a percentage. It must be remembered that in an atmosphere containing a mixture of hydrogen peroxide and water vapor that the vapors will become saturated, and hence cause condensation, before the RH reached 100%.

Consideration of Raoult's Law explains the problem that is encountered with a two component solution. Raoult's Law as stated in Equation 1 shows that the vapor pressure exerted by component A in a solution will depend on the liquid mole fraction of component A. Thus, if the mole fraction of water is 0.5 then the maximum water vapor content would be reduced by 50% assuming the system obeys Raoult's Law, and hence the maximum RH is reduced to 50%, as this represents saturated vapor.

Hydrogen peroxide decontaminations are frequently performed using 35% w/w solution, which is almost exactly 0.22 mol/mol. Thus according to Raoult's Law the maximum water vapor pressure in an equilibrium state would be 0.78 of the saturated vapor pressure at that temperature. It follows that if hydrogen peroxide obeys Raoult's law that it would be impossible to achieve a RH greater than 78%, because at this value the vapor would be saturated. In fact the real value will be lower than this because of the introduction of the activity coefficient that is always numerically less than unity, as shown in Figure 1.

Instrumentation

The previous sections discussed the equations that permit the vapor concentration, mass, and concentration of the condensate during a decontamination cycle to be calculated.

The two most important parameters are the vapor concentration and the mass of condensation. When the author started his investigation into hydrogen peroxide vapor decontaminations instrumentation was available to measure the vapor concentration, but not the mass or concentration of the condensate. However, there was some doubt over the accuracy of the vapor concentration measurements and work was commissioned at Southampton University in England to develop a calibration technique for the vapor concentration instrumentation; the technique was developed by Webb (9). It was based on the generation of a saturated vapor under known conditions and checking the vapor concentration using wet chemistry methods. Very good agreement was found between the theoretical value of the saturated vapor and wet chemistry, thus also confirming the equations of Scatchard (2). The saturated vapors were then used to calibrate an electrochemical cell that gave a linear output to within 1%. Other types of vapor sensors are available especially near infrared spectrophotometers, but these have not been calibrated to the same degree of accuracy. The electrochemical cell has the advantages of being relatively small and inexpensive, but suffers from slow response. Near-infrared instruments are much more expensive but have better response characteristics and are able to measure the water vapor concentration as well as the hydrogen peroxide.

Standard RH sensors suffer both from interference from, and incompatibility with, hydrogen peroxide. A solution to this difficulty was found by protecting a RH sensor with a sintered platinum filter. This decomposes any hydrogen peroxide to water and oxygen thus protecting the sensor but elevating the water content. The error, however, is small for at 20°C the equilibrium vapor pressure for 35% w/w hydrogen peroxide solution is 16,650 ppm for water and 183 ppm for hydrogen peroxide. The error, therefore, caused by decomposition of the hydrogen peroxide is only 1.1%.

A common method of measuring the hydrogen peroxide vapor concentration at the end of a cycle is with a Dräger tube, as they are relatively cheap to use and designed to give readings in the vapor concentration range of 0.5 to 10 ppm. The most commonly specified end point of a hydrogen peroxide gassing cycle is when the vapor concentration has fallen to 1 ppm, the occupational exposure limit. However care must be exercised as the Dräger specification sheet states that they should only be used when the water content is between 3 and 10 mg/L and the temperature range is 10°C to 25°C. Using these parameters it is possible to draw an operational envelope, shown in Figure 13. When used at too high a temperature the reading will be high, but the worst problems arise if they are used when the water content is below 3 mg/L. The chemical reaction in the tube is a water-based one and with very dry air at say 5% RH it is possible to get a reading of less than 1ppm when the vapor concentration may be as high as 80 to 100 ppm. This is particularly relevant when the aeration phase of the cycle is linked to a single-loop generator with a chemical dryer. Such systems produce air that is very dry, frequently much dryer than 5% RH.

No instruments were available to measure the rate of formation of condensation so a new instrument was devised based on the passage of light along the length of a glass window by total internal reflection. A schematic of the instrument is shown in Figure 14.

Light is focused into a parallel beam by a lens, and then passes through a reflecting prism and an optical pad into the window. The light is then transmitted along the length of

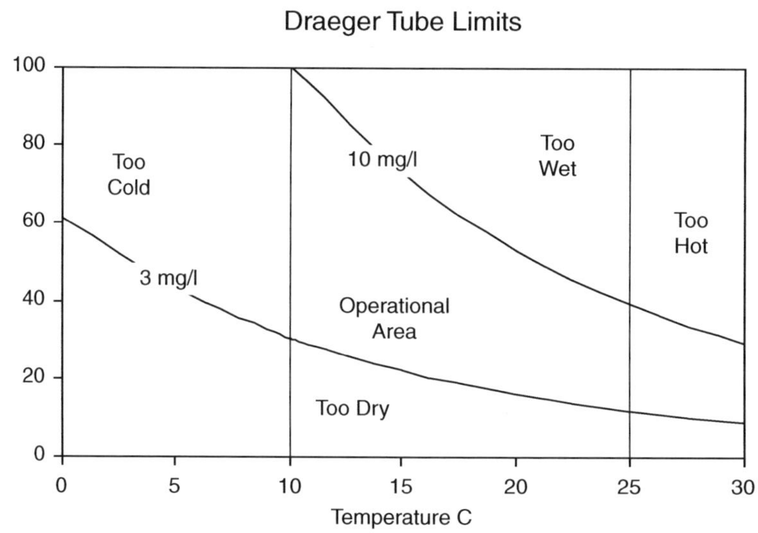

Figure 13 Operational envelope derived from Draeger specification sheets showing the operational limits of Draeger tubes.

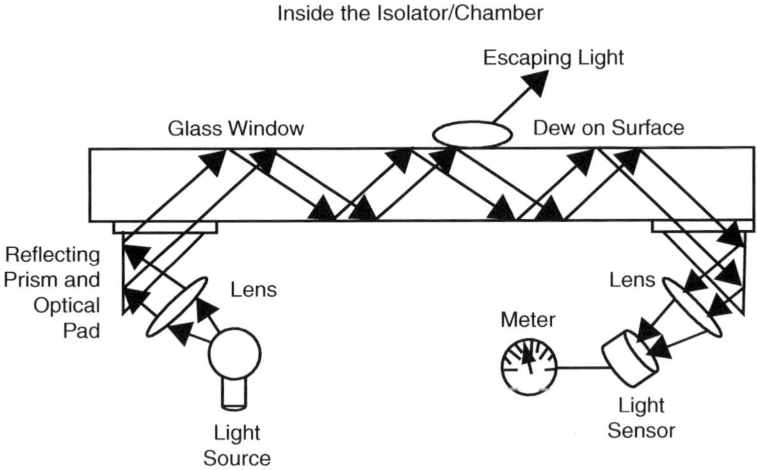

Figure 14 Schematic diagram of the optical condensation sensor.

the window until it reaches the second optical pad where it leaves the window and passes out through the second reflecting prism. It is then focused on the sensor by another lens. If a droplet of condensation forms on the surface of the glass it changes the refractive index allowing some light to escape and reducing the amount of light arriving at the sensor. The instrument was calibrated to read zero when the glass was clean and 100 when all of the light escaped from the surface. It should be noted that until the index rose to about 20 or 30 the surface condensation was invisible.

As soon as a droplet forms on the surface it creates a concentration gradient in the surrounding vapor. This gradient draws more vapors into the droplet causing it to grow until it touches an adjacent droplet and combines. This mechanism is important as it causes preferential condensation on the first droplets causing them to grow quickly.

No instrumentation has as yet been devised to measure the concentration of the condensate. The condensate film is often either invisible or only just visible and hence the instrumentation would prove very difficult. It is, however, possible to calculate the condensate concentration, as it must be in equilibrium with the surrounding vapor; thus if the temperature and vapor concentration are known it is possible to calculate the concentration of the condensate. A further calculation may be made to estimate the total mass of condensate.

At the present time research is being undertaken on new instrumentation to measure hydrogen peroxide vapor concentrations. These include spectroscopic methods, for example, tuned laser, Fourier transform infrared, ion mobility (calibration techniques) with some further work based on the formation and concentration of the condensate that can be used to estimate the hydrogen peroxide and water vapor concentrations.

Developing a Decontamination Cycle

For a decontamination cycle to be effective it is necessary that the vapor concentration is adequate, sustained for a sufficient period of time and that condensate has formed on all surfaces.

Having discussed the physical chemistry, hydrogen peroxide vapor generators, instrumentation, and the use of BIs it is now possible to use this information to develop a reliable hydrogen peroxide vapor decontamination cycle.

As may be expected, it is first necessary to make an estimate of the chamber volume to give an indication of the expected duration of the cycle and the mass of hydrogen peroxide solution required. This estimate may be made by calculation using the vapor pressure equations or equipment manufacturers may be able to help.

There are a number of techniques for the development of cycles but it is sensible to start with an investigation of the surface temperatures inside the chamber and the vapor distribution.

Surface temperatures should be mapped to find the hottest and coldest locations within the chamber. Providing the vapor distribution is even then these will be the last and first places to see condensation, the hottest location is likely to be the last place in the chamber where kill is achieved.

By placing chemical indicators, that change color when exposed to hydrogen peroxide, around the chamber and noting when they change color it is possible to find those areas within the chamber where the vapor distribution is poor and may cause difficulty.

Having found the most difficult locations in the chamber (i.e., the hottest and where vapor distribution is poor) it is then possible to decide the location of the BIs for the first development cycle. The number of BIs and their placement will depend on the size and configuration of the chamber, but as a minimum BIs should be placed at the most difficult locations, in each corner of the chamber and at the centre of each face. If possible BIs should also be placed so that they may be removed into either growth media or buffer solution at timed intervals so that the time to kill at that location may be established.

A cycle should then be run using the estimated parameters found from experience or the vapor equations. At the end of the cycle those BIs placed around the chamber must be collected using a sterile technique and placed in growth media and incubated to check for kill.

If all of the BIs from the locations inside the chamber show no growth then using the information from the timed BIs the cycle may be shortened until growth is found at one or more locations within the chamber. This will indicate the minimum cycle to achieve full kill and may be used to establish a satisfactory and reliable cycle.

However, if there are some survivors at locations within the chamber then a further longer cycle should be run until all the BIs within the chamber are killed, and this extended cycle may then be used to establish a satisfactory and reliable cycle.

A minimum of three development cycles should be run at a level that just ensures full kill and to this development cycle a safety margin should be added to ensure that all production cycles are reliable.

Care should be exercised in setting the safety margin and should always be based on sound scientific reasoning. Simply doubling the evaporation phase of the cycle may be a considerable overkill. The object of the safety margin is generally to double the killing time. If for example the BIs used for validation have a population of 10^6 microorganisms then the doubling of the cycle is intended to give a kill of 10^{12}, but the effective part of the cycle is not the whole part of the evaporation phase. It is only that part where the condensation has reached a level at which the kill commences and hence doubling this killing part of the cycle is all that is necessary to give log 12 kill.

Hydrogen peroxide biodecontamination is a surface condensation process and hence any change in the surface area to be biodecontaminated will necessitate a change to the gassing cycle parameters. Thus, a cycle developed for an empty isolator will almost always need to be altered for the same isolator when loaded with either product or equipment.

BIs by their very nature are variable and as such unexpected results may occur during cycle development. A useful technique to distinguish between a cycle failure and a rogue BI is the use of two BIs in each location. If the first gives an unexpected positive result the second BI is then available for analysis.

Equipment Considerations—Isolators

If the hydrogen peroxide and water vapor remained in the gaseous phase even when the temperature falls to ambient then the method of delivery of the gasses to the chamber would not be critical. The high concentrations of hydrogen peroxide and water vapor produced by the rapid evaporation process will condense at temperatures well above ambient. It is therefore important to make sure that the temperature of the vapor remains sufficiently high prior to entering the chamber to avoid condensation in the deliver systems.

The temperature of the gasses leaving the generator are generally in the region of 60°C to 100°C and condensation will normally appear if the temperature drops below about 55°C. To avoid condensation in the delivery hoses these should be trace heated and insulated. (For example with a circulating air flow of 60 m^3/hr at a RH of 40% and a hydrogen peroxide evaporation rate of 20g/min condensation will form in the ducts at 53°C.)

The vapors should be injected directly into the chamber to be decontaminated. If it is injected into a plenum chamber, for example, above the inlet HEPA filter, the vapor velocity will fall and because the plenum is at ambient temperature a substantial amount of condensation will occur before the vapors enter the chamber. The reason normally given for injecting the vapor into the supply plenum is to decontaminate the HEPA filters.

HEPA decontamination may be achieved by injecting the vapor directly into the chamber and then extracting above both the supply and exhaust filters. There may be an objection to this method on the grounds that the chamber is not protected by a HEPA filter in the vapor supply line. Placing a thermally insulated HEPA filter in the vapor supply at the interface with the chamber will overcome this objection.

On entering the chamber vapor should be distributed by either the use of nozzles that produce high velocity jets or the use of fans. Care must be exercised when using nozzles in small chambers to ensure that no hot spots are generated by focusing the jet onto either BIs or parts of the chamber surface or load. Particular attention should be placed on hot jets of gas/vapor mixture being focused on BIs as they have a small thermal mass, heat up very quickly, and hence become difficult to kill and unrepresentative of the surrounding surfaces.

As noted in "Types of Hydrogen Peroxide Generators" section, aeration is frequently the longest part of any decontamination cycle. This is because the catalyst in the vapor generator removes the hydrogen peroxide condensation and vapor. The flow through the catalyst is limited by the construction of the vapor generator, which in turn limits the rate of dilution of the hydrogen peroxide in the chamber. Additional aeration may be provided that bypasses the vapor generator or in some installations it is possible to use the isolator or room ventilation systems to vent the vapors to the outside, care being taken not to cause environmental damage.

Biodecontamination of Rooms

Three techniques have been used to decontaminate rooms. The earliest was simply to place a hydrogen peroxide vapor generator outside the room and pass the vapors through ducts into the room. It soon became obvious that this was not very efficient and a new generation of vapor generators were designed and manufactured that were placed inside the rooms. However, if a suit of room is to be decontaminated then this meant placing generators in each of the rooms so techniques were developed to use a dedicated system to distribute the vapors.

Having the vapor generator outside the room is similar to the techniques used in isolator decontamination. It is a useful technique if a vapor generator is available and the time taken to decontaminate is not critical. The main difference is that uniform vapor distribution is more difficult and will almost certainly require the use of fans inside the room. The location and type of fan will need to be recorded to ensure repeatability of the cycles. It will generally be necessary to trace heat the delivery and return ducts carrying the vapors to and from the room as this ensures that there will be no condensation in the ducts; which will evaporate during aeration thus prolonging the cycle.

The second technique of placing the vapor generator inside the room has the advantage that it is not necessary to make apertures into the room to run the ducts, and the problems of vapor distribution become simplified if the generator is equipped with nozzles that produce high-velocity jets. The example shown in Figure 9 does not have a catalyst or dehumidification system. Dehumidification of a large room is very time consuming and sometimes not possible so the process has to be run at whatever humidity is present at the start of the cycle. We have seen that condensation is the main factor in the kill mechanism and the concentration of the first bead of condensation will depend on the concentration of the source liquid, the temperature in the room, and the water content of the atmosphere. However, the concentration of the condensate will always tend toward that of the source liquid. It is therefore possible to decontaminate rooms, which have both very low and very high levels of humidity by simply adjusting the cycle parameters.

The vapor generator shown in Figure 10 has a built-in sensor that indicates when the vapors have become saturated and hence condensation has started. It is then only necessary to ensure that an adequate mass of hydrogen peroxide solution is evaporated following the onset of condensation to provide the necessary layer of microcondensation.

The third technique using a dedicated system to distribute the vapor is much more complex and requires the advice of an expert to design the system. A trace heated circulating duct has to be installed with outlets and returns in each room to be decontaminated. The hydrogen peroxide generator is connected to this circulating duct and the vapors injected into the circulating carrier gas. It is essential to keep this circulating mixture at a sufficiently high temperature to avoid condensation. One or more nozzles are provided in each room depending on the room size to ensure good vapor distribution. The pressure in the duct and the nozzles sizes are adjusted to ensure the correct proportion of vapor is distributed to each room. With large suites of rooms it is sometimes not necessary to decontaminate all of the rooms at the same time, by careful design of the nozzles and adjusting the duct pressure it is generally possible ensure the correct vapor distribution for a variety of room combinations.

Rapid Transfer Chamber

It has been noted especially in hospital pharmacies that there is an increasing requirement for multiple sterile transfers into dispensing isolators.

This challenge has been met by the design of a transfer port that is large enough to contain sufficient components to keep a hospital pharmacist busy for about 1 hour but have a complete load, biodecontaminated, and unload cycle time of less than 20 minutes. There are of course other applications of this technology, apart from hospital pharmacies, where such rapid sterile transfers are required.

To achieve such a short cycle time it is imperative to ensure that the vapor distribution inside the chamber is optimized and that the aeration rate is very high. The chamber shown in Figure 15 has an internal volume of 0.33 m^3 and may be connected at each side to an isolator,

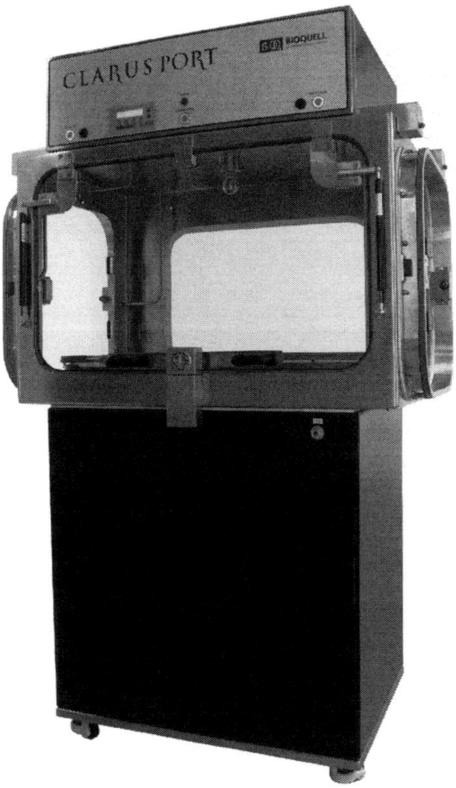

Figure 15 BIOQUELL rapid transfer chamber.

thus providing product to two isolators. The complete cycle time to achieve a log-6 reduction of *G. stearothermophilus* is about 20 minutes.

Efficacy

Hydrogen peroxide vapor is well established as a biodecontamination agent due to its "residue-free" nature (the only residues are oxygen and water) and its ability to be used at low temperatures. As with any other biodecontamination agents, hydrogen peroxide has been tested on many organisms and classes of organisms. However, because a great number of "common" microorganisms exist, efficacy testing remains an ongoing process.

There is in the literature a significant amount of information regarding the efficacy of hydrogen peroxide against a number of microorganisms, typically the paper by Heckert (10) about animal viruses and Kobubo (11) on the resistance of spores. This information can be used not only to look at specific organisms but also the efficacy of hydrogen peroxide vapor against types and groups of organisms.

It is important to understand that if a particular organism is not found in the literature, it does not mean there is no data available or that hydrogen peroxide is not effective against it.

CONCLUSIONS

From the analysis of the equations dealing with the physical chemistry of hydrogen peroxide and water it is now clear that the three original assumptions made about this process are all incorrect. Hydrogen peroxide either in the vapour phase or as an aqueous solution does not decompose according to a half-life rule. Although kill can be accomplished by dry vapor at ambient temperatures it is faster and more reliable once a layer of condensation has formed, and it is probable that in most biodecontamination cycles that are allegedly dry the process is in fact one of invisible condensation. Condensation is an important factor in achieving biodecontamination and is something that should be encouraged, not avoided.

Using the equations that describe the behaviour of vapour hydrogen peroxide and water has led to a better understanding of how this bio-decontamination process works. By a careful study of the behaviour of the vapours it has been possible to use this technology to biodecontaminate very large volumes while reducing the cycle times, thus further enhancing the value of this residue free biodecontamination process.

Hydrogen peroxide vapour phase biodecontamination has been in general use in the pharmaceutical industry since the early 1990s, but it is only now that as a proper understanding of the process is emerging that the true potential is being realised. It is clear from recent research that it may be used for very large spaces and also for the rapid biodecontamination of such items as transfer systems. There is at the present time no other process that has the same potential while being environmentally friendly having as breakdown products water and oxygen.

REFERENCES

1. Keyes FG. The thermodynamic properties of water substance 0° to 150°C. Part VI. Chem Phys 1947; 15:602.
2. Scatchard G, Kavanach M, Ticknor LB. Vapor—liquid equilibrium. VIII. hydrogen peroxide water mixtures J Am Chem Soc 1952; 74:3715.
3. Schumb WC, Sattersfield CM, Wentworth RL, eds. Hydrogen peroxide. Am Chem Soc Monograph.
4. Watling D, Ryle C, Parks M, et al. Theoretical analysis of the condensation of hydrogen peroxide gas and water vapor as used in surface decontamination. J Pharm Sci Technol 2002; 56(6):291–299.
5. Portner DM, Hoffman RK. Sporicidal effect of peracetic acid vapor. Appl Microbiol 1968; 16(11):1782–1785.
6. Biotechnology. Performance criteria for microbiological safety cabinets. EN12469:2000:41.
7. Unger-Bimezok B, Kottke K, Hertel C, et al. The influence of humidity, hydrogen peroxide concentratio, and condensation on the inactivation of *Geobacillus stearothermophilus* spores with hydrogen peroxide vapor. J Pharm Innov 2008; 3:123–133.

8. European Pharmacopoeia. Biological indicators for inspection of sterilization methods (Chapter 5.1.2). 3rd edn. Strasbourg, France: European Pharmacopoeia, 1980.
9. Webb B. A validated calibration method for hydrogen peroxide vapour sensors. PDA J 2001; 55(1):49–54.
10. Heckert RA, Best M, Jordan LT, et al. Efficacy of vaporized hydrogen peroxide against exotic animal viruses. Appl Environ Microbiol 1997; 63:3916–3918.
11. Kokubo M, Inoue T, Akers J. Resistance of common environmental spores of the genus *Bacillus* to vapor hydrogen peroxide. PDA J Pharm Sci Technol 1998; 52:228–231.

27 Single-injection vapor-phase hydrogen peroxide decontamination of isolators and clean rooms

Kunihiro Imai, Souma Watanabe, Yasusuke Oshima, Mamoru Kokubo, and James Akers

The decontamination of aseptic work environments has been practiced in the healthcare industry for decades. Prior to 1990, formaldehyde vapor was commonly used throughout the world for decontamination of clean rooms. The carcinogenicity associates with formaldehyde and its rather limited efficacy brought the use of formaldehyde to a halt. Formaldehyde, like nearly all gas or vapor decontamination methods, requires elevated humidity for maximum effectiveness, and unless clean rooms were designed specifically with formaldehyde "fogging" in mind, treatment was conducted at ambient humidity.

With the phasing out of formaldehyde "fogging" it became necessary to find alternative methods for clean room decontamination. Most firms moved to manual application of sporicides, often rotated with non-sporicidal germicides, to minimize residuals and corrosive effects of sporicides. These treatments are labor intensive and time consuming so unsurprisingly firms are exploring automated alternatives.

Research on sporicidal agents that could work effectively at temperatures close to those maintained in typical clean rooms has continued to be an area of active study. Some promising candidates have been advanced over the last 20-plus years. The combination of peracetic acid and hydrogen peroxide, which is known to be synergistic, has been used for the decontamination of aseptic enclosures such as isolators for both sterility testing applications and in some production applications including RABS. Chlorine dioxide, a well-known oxidizing gas has also been used for decontamination or sterilization at ambient temperatures. Also, ozone, which like chlorine dioxide and hydrogen peroxide is a powerful oxidant, has been advanced as a possible decontaminating agent for aseptic applications particularly in small enclosures such as pass-boxes or isolators (1,2).

The sporicidal efficacy of vapor-phase hydrogen peroxide (VPHP) was first reported in the late 1970s. This technology was licensed by American Sterilizer Corporation (AMSCO) in 1980 from American Hospital Supply Corporation and initial studies focused on the use of this technology in the sterilization of hospital equipment and supplies. However, by the mid-1980s isolators were introduced and initially used primarily in the conduct of the sterility test. As isolator technology came into wide spread use for production and research activities, VPHP rapidly became the method of chose for environmental decontamination.

Although the efficacy of VPHP against microorganisms was well established, the development of VPHP decontamination cycles and their subsequent validation proved to be a significant challenge. In the early years of isolator technology some proponents considered the isolator an "absolute barrier" or "sterile" enclosure, which was at least potentially capable of practical performance on par with terminal sterilization. This led to the notion that isolators must be sterilized, which resulted in the belief that validation of isolator "sterilization" with VPHP should require a validation and process control similar to that of the moist heat autoclave. After several years of vigorous discussion among industry, equipment suppliers and regulatory authorities it was finally generally accepted that *decontamination* was a more reasonable target that *sterilization*. Nevertheless, emphasis on validation of VPHP did not lessen and a demand for process monitoring, most specifically involving the accurate measurement of vapor concentration emerged.

The authors of this chapter have a collective experience of more than 60 years with both liquid and vapor hydrogen peroxide sterilization as well as decontamination methods (3,4). We have used several models of commercial VPHP generators and have undertaken applications research under a wide variety of temperature and humidity conditions in enclosures, and rooms of all practical sizes used in product testing and manufacturing. We describe in this chapter a method for VPHP decontamination developed and patented based on considerable research and development stemming from empirical experience in the design and validation of isolator systems. Subsequent studies found that this approach was eminently scalable and extremely efficacious in the treatment of even large clean rooms. The authors believe that this process model has not only efficiency advantages but also describes a process which is in concert with well-known microbiological principals regarding vapor and/or gaseous sterilization.

The experiments described in this paper were designed to evaluate key process control elements that had been thought to be required for optimal performance of VPHP systems. These concepts arose from the authors' hypothesis that there may be little or no value in the removal of moisture from a decontamination target prior to exposure to vaporized H_2O_2. In fact, it has been established with other forms of gaseous sterilization using oxidants such as ozone and chlorine dioxide that moisture levels above 65% were necessary for optimal kill effectiveness. It is also well known that elevated humidity enhances the efficacy of both ethylene oxide gas and formaldehyde vapor (1).

The authors also sought to experimentally evaluate the need for continuous replenishment of H_2O_2 vapor, as there have been indications that the half-life of H_2O_2 was sufficiently long that replenishment was unnecessary. Replenishment systems have been widely used since the introduction of VPHP (5,6). This is due in large measure to the fact that the commercial originators of VPHP designed their system around a replenishment model. Replenishment models were attractive not only because of the perceived need to replace rapidly decomposing H_2O_2, but because this concept was theorized to result in a quasi "square wave" cycle concentration model, which resembled in no small measure the typical BIER cycle used in *D* value determination of a moist-heat sterilization cycle (7). However, experience and laboratory research using near infrared (NIR) and electrochemical methods for H_2O_2 concentration measurement found that square wave cycles with stable target concentrations were somewhat to completely illusory depending upon the target and cycle conditions (4).

Thus, another factor that the authors of this work have extensively evaluated was the use of concentration monitors, specifically how well the measured concentration correlated with rate of spore inactivation. Information from the Steris cycle development guide appeared to indicate that vapor concentration measured in free air within the enclosure should correlate directly with the rate of spore inactivation. However, data published by Sigwarth and Stärk (8) indicated that relatively high rates of inactivation were possible with significantly lower concentrations of vapor. Also, the authors' previous experience indicated that a linear relationship between concentration in free air at a fixed temperature and rate of inactivation might not exist.

The authors' studies demonstrate that it is possible to eliminate the dehumidification phase of the process in nearly all clean room or isolator applications. These studies also indicate that it is not necessary to continuously inject vapor H_2O_2 throughout a cycle's exposure period. In addition, we have found that there is no need for an initial conditioning cycle phase in which H_2O_2 is injected at a higher rate measured in g/min than in the biodecontamination phase of the process.

EXPERIMENTAL METHODS AND CONDITIONS

The VPHP generator used to conduct the studies described in this chapter was developed and built by Shibuya Kogyo Company Limited (Kanazawa, Japan). The system operates at a fixed VPHP injection rate of 20 g/min. A process flow diagram of the generator as used in conjunction with an isolator target is shown in Figure 1.

Decontamination results for two very different targets are described in this chapter. A number of experiments were conducted in a 6.5 m^3 aseptic filling isolator. The isolator is a rigid wall unidirectional airflow design and encloses a vial-filling system capable of 300 units/min. The isolator and enclosed equipment are constructed primarily of 304 stainless steel and the isolator glazing is polycarbonate. Aeration was accomplished by direct venting at flow rates stipulated in the experimental data. The isolator and the filling equipment were manufactured by Shibuya Kogyo Co. Ltd., and the studies described herein were carried out at Shibuya's Morimoto factory in Kanazawa, Japan. A further study was conducted in a pharmaceutical clean room with an enclosed volume of 75 m^3 provided courtesy of Sankyo Pharmaceutical in Tokyo, Japan. VPHP was injected directly into the room environment using a Shibuya generator. Freestanding

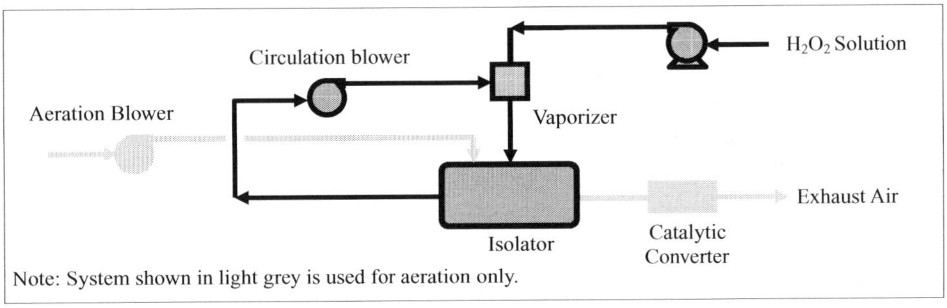

Figure 1 Process flow diagram.

circulation fans were employed to enhance the distribution of the vapor. A stand-alone aeration unit equipped with a catalytic converter accomplished the aeration of the clean room.

Biological indicators (BIs) were sourced from Apex Laboratories of Apex, NC, USA. The BIs consisted of *Geobacillus stearothermophilus* ATCC #12980 spores inoculated onto stainless steel substrates. The BIs were packaged in Tyvek envelopes. These BIs were chosen because they are representative of BIs most commonly used for cycle development and validation studies in VPHP applications. The nominal spore concentration per BI was approximately 2.0×10^6. The estimated population and nominal *D* value are given in each results table where relevant. It should be noted that the *D* values shown in the chart were provided by the vendor. The reader is reminded that *D* values are accurate only when conditions resulting in spore lethality can be accurately defined. In our experience vendors and some users may report *D* values as a function of vaporized H_2O_2 concentration. This however, can be misleading and may cause misunderstanding among users. As can be seen from the data presented in this chapter, a clear-cut correlation between concentration and lethality does not exist in the case of VPHP processes. There are many factors affecting VPHP "kill" effectiveness, including temperature, humidity, and dew point. We have often observed in fact an inverse correlation between airborne concentration and kill rate. This is due to the deposition of liquid H_2O_2 onto surfaces within the enclosure that we find correlates with superior kill effectiveness.

All BIs used in the studies reported in this chapter were cultured after each test in soybean casein digest agar and incubated at a temperature of 55°C for at least 7 days. Concentration of H_2O_2 vapor in all studies was done using a Draeger Polytron II. Low levels of H_2O_2 during and postaeration (1–3 ppm) were measured using Draeger test tubes.

RESULTS

Experiments were conducted to determine whether vaporized H_2O_2 of a volume sufficient to achieve decontamination could be delivered to an isolator target rapidly without the need for continuous replenishment throughout an exposure period.

In this experiment, no conditioning phase was used and H_2O_2 was vaporized and injected over a period of only a few minutes. After completion of the injection phase, dwell periods of various lengths were tested during which the recirculation blower of the isolator operated. In the study shown in Table 1 the isolator was initially dehumidified to 5% relative humidity (RH) and various injection quantities were tested. A rather sharp break point can be observed between 60 g of total injection in which 24 out of 30 BIs were positive for growth and 80 g,

Table 1 BI Inactivation as a Function of Injection Volume (Initial Humidity—5% RH)

Total VPHP injected	100 g	80 g	60 g	40 g	20 g
Initial isolator temperature[a]	32.0°C	32.5°C	33.0°C	31.0°C	32.2°C
Survivors/no. BIs tested	0/30	0/30	24/30	29/30	30/30

Positives/total BIs after 7-day incubation.
[a]Initial temperature is reported here only to confirm that it was consistent for each of the tested injection volumes.

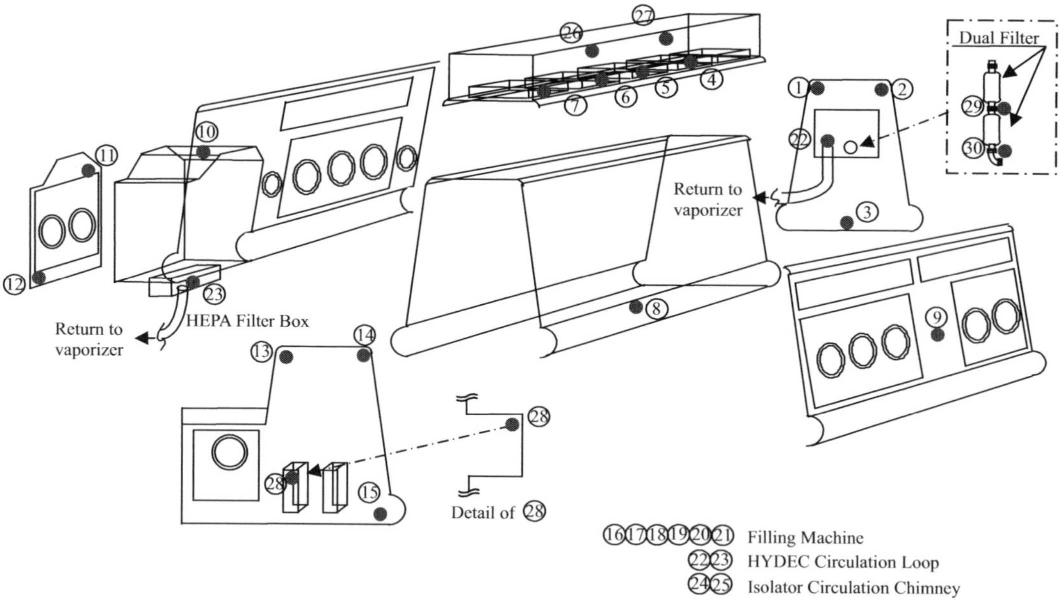

Figure 2 BIs placement diagram.

which resulted in no survivors. The injection rate of 20 g/min resulted in injection times in this study of 1 to 5 minutes. The results given in Table 1 were extremely reproducible and are representative of multiple experiments.

Figure 2 shows BIs placement for the isolator decontamination experiments.

Having established that effective VPHP decontamination could be achieved without continuous replenishment a series of experiments were conducted to evaluate the effects of initial relative humidity on lethality.[1] In these experiments the RH was varied between 5% and 70% and the 80 g total H_2O_2 injection quantity already demonstrated to be sufficient for complete inactivation of BIs at 5% RH was used in all test studies. The results given in Table 2 indicate that effective kill was achieved at relative humidities ranging from 5% to 70% RH. These data indicate that relative humidity is a less critical factor in VPHP decontamination than had been previously thought. These studies provided a strong indication that VPHP could be efficacious at any RH level used in isolators or clean room operations. Further studies to determine optimum RH for decontamination were required, and these tests provided further evidence that costly and often complex equipment and process control systems to control and monitor humidity in conjunction with VPHP decontamination could be effectively eliminated.

Experiments were designed to examine the influence of humidity on VPHP efficacy and to evaluate RH levels throughout test cycles. Comparative experiments were done at relatively high and low humidity values, the intention being to challenge the full range of humidity levels likely to be encountered under ambient conditions in a wide range of industrial environments. In this series of studies a Draeger Polytron II concentration monitoring system was used to determine the influence of humidity on the measured concentration of H_2O_2 vapor. A Vaisala humidity measuring system was used to assess humidity. The results are shown in Figure 3.

A constant injection quantity of 80 g was used in this experiment and no BI survivors were observed.

The results of this experiment demonstrated that there does not appear to be a correlation between measured H_2O_2 concentration and the absolute microbiological efficacy of the process. An identical 80 g total injection mass was used in each case and complete inactivation of

[1] The isolator diagram shows air return lines to the generator/vaporizer. However, this is for air movement only, there is no additional injection of vaporized H_2O_2 after the established injection mass target is reached.

Table 2 Injection Quantity Versus RH in Isolator Initial Study Temperature 20°C

Injection quantity	70% RH	60% RH	40% RH	20% RH	5% RH
100 g			0/30		
80 g	0/30	0/30	0/30	0/30	0/30
60 g	22/30	6/30	1/30	3/30	17/30
40 g	28/30	27/30	13/30	26/30	28/30

Positives/total BIs after 7-day incubation.

G. stearothermophilus spores on stainless steel coupons at a population of $>10^6$ were observed under all test conditions. Also, noteworthy from the results shown in Figure 3 is the interesting correlation between measured H_2O_2 concentration and humidity. Please note that the highest measured concentration was observed when humidity prior to injection was 5%. As the preinjection humidity was increased the measured concentration of H_2O_2 is corresponding lower.

An additional study regarding the effects of humidity was conducted and the results are shown in Table 3. The results of this study demonstrate that lower spore inactivation effectiveness is observed when relative humidity is low. It can be seen from these data that dehumidification prior to the start of injection is unnecessary and can be eliminated. Because dehumidification is not required the overall VPHP cycle or process time can be reduced, and dehumidification, which may contribute to an unwanted increase in enclosure temperature in isolators can be eliminated. Also, interesting is that regardless of the humidity a H_2O_2 injection can be found for any process that results in complete kill at a very broad range of humidities.

The authors observed an interesting phenomenon relating to inactivation efficacy, condensation and aeration, and RH. Data demonstrating this phenomenon is presented in Table 4. During these test cycles condensation was observed shortly after the start of the injection phase in each test shown in Table 4. In the case of relatively low initial humidity, condensate will disappear soon after the completion of injection. At higher initial humidity levels, condensation was observed until aeration began. However, once aeration started, all condensate disappeared completely and quickly. Also, at the start of aeration the vapor concentration increased rapidly as a direct result of evaporation of H_2O_2 from surfaces within the isolator enclosure. We observed no adverse effect to either process equipment or aeration time line in cycles where small levels of condensate were observed. Interestingly, it appears that for all the debate regarding visibly wet versus visibly dry VPHP processes, fully efficacious cycles can be developed around either approach. However, we have found that cycles in which condensation is observed are more robust in terms of antimicrobial effect.

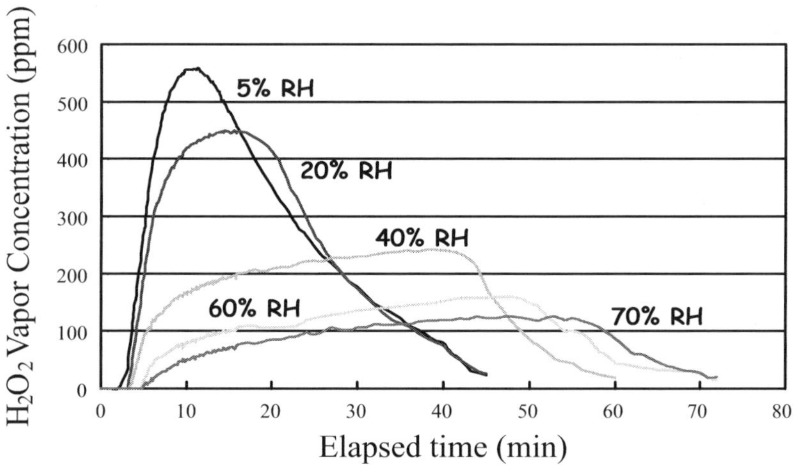

Figure 3 H_2O_2 vapor concentration versus RH at start of cycle.

Table 3 Relative Humidity at Process Start Versus Decontamination Efficacy

		RH (%)				
Injection quantity		**10**	**20**	**30**	**40**	**50**
40 g	#1		6/6	4/6	5/6	2/6
	#2		6/6	6/6	5/6	2/6
	#3		6/6	6/6	6/6	4/6
45 g	#1	6/6	4/6	0/6	0/6	0/6
	#2	6/6	5/6	1/6	0/6	0/6
	#3	6/6	6/6	1/6	1/6	0/6
49.5 g (45 × 1.1)	#1	6/6	2/6	0/6	1/6	0/6
	#2	6/6	6/6	0/6	0/6	0/6
	#3	6/6	4/6	2/6	0/6	1/6
54 g (45 × 1.2)	#1	5/6	2/6	0/6	0/6	0/6
	#2	6/6	0/6	0/6	0/6	0/6
	#3	6/6	1/6	2/6	0/6	0/6
58.5 g (45 × 1.3)	#1	0/6	0/6	0/6		
	#2	1/6	0/6	0/6		
	#3	1/6	0/6	0/6		
63.0 g (45 × 1.4)	#1	0/6	0/6			
	#2	0/6	0/6			
	#3	0/6	0/6			
67.5 g (45 × 1.5)	#1	0/6				
	#2	0/6				
	#3	0/6				

Note: The studies shown in Table 3 were conducted under the same operating conditions as those shown in Table 2. However, slight differences are observed with respect to efficacy. These differences are reflective of typical biological variability.

It is important to note that Table 2 includes results from BI locations that were "worst case" in terms of the difficulty to inactivate. On the other hand, Table 3 reflects data from BI locations chosen for relatively easy operator access.

Table 4 shows that the effective hold period for inactivation was established at 15 minutes after completion of injection regardless of initial humidity, in larger targets such as extremely large isolators or clean rooms we have found a 30-minute hold period to be most effective. The authors took particular note of this phenomenon in the refinement of this VPHP process. Table 4 suggests that spore inactivation is nearly complete at the end of the holding period in many cases. The authors also found that within the isolator the quantity of condensate is likely to increase during the hold period, probably due to slight decrease in ambient temperature. We also noted that condensation continued to be observed after the conclusion of the 15-minute hold period and in the absence of aeration; however, no further increase in condensate was

Table 4 Lethality at Critical Process Time

	Time		
RH (%)	**10 min later from start of holding time**	**At finish of holding time of 15 min**	**For 15 min after finish of holding time**
5	2/6	0/6	6/6
20	2/6	0/6	6/6
40	1/6	0/6	6/6
60	2/6	0/6	4/6

Isolator: 6.5 m^3 filling isolator; Positives/Total BIs after 7-day incubation; BIs: Apex Laboratories, *D* Value: 1.4 minutes.

Table 5 Lethality Data Starting Temperature Versus RH in Isolator

Temperature at start	70% RH	60% RH	40% RH	20% RH	5% RH
20°C	0/30	0/30	0/30	0/30	0/30
25°C	0/30	0/30	0/30	0/30	0/30

Total injection quantity: 80 g; Positives/total BIs after 7-day incubation.

witnessed. These results indicate that physical phase change from vapor to liquid H_2O_2 appears to correlate with highly efficient spore inactivation. However, when BIs were placed into the isolator at the end of what would have been the hold period, effective kill was not observed.

Experiments were conducted to evaluate the effect of temperatures on decontamination efficacy, and the results of this study are shown in Table 5. Generally, clean rooms housing isolators or used for aseptic processing are kept at temperatures in the range of 20°C to 24°C. Therefore, temperatures of 20°C and 25°C were chosen for the study. It is important to note that as the system described in this article injects H_2O_2 at a rather high rate and only during the initial minutes of the cycle there is comparatively little effect upon the ambient temperature of even a rather small enclosure compared to units that inject vaporous H_2O_2 in an approximately 100°C air stream throughout the process.

The data indicate that at a fixed total injection mass of 80 g over an initial RH range of 5% to 70% complete kill of 10^6 population *G. stearothermophilus* biological indicators was achieved at 20°C and 25°C in this particularly isolator enclosure. Therefore, no difference in efficacy could be seen between these two initial temperatures. Precise temperature control within a narrower range is not necessary and efficacy is assured at the normal temperature and humidity ranges one would expect to encounter in a typical clean room or isolator housed within a clean room. Studies were also done on the reproducibility of concentration as measured by the Draeger Polytron II. These data for three test cycles conducted at an initial RH of 40% and an 80-g injection mass are presented in Figure 4. The differences observed within the three test runs shown are small and appear to be within the normal variability one should expect within the system and the analytical method.

ROOM DECONTAMINATION

To evaluate the scalability of the process described in this communication a study was conducted in a pharmaceutical clean room with a total volume of 75 m^3. A total of 33 studies were done at total injection volumes of 100 to 480 g. It was determined that 200 g was sufficient to achieve a consistent and reproducible cycle with complete inactivation of 47 *G. stearothermophilus* BIs with a population of $>10^6$ on each coupon. The injection volume required for a target can be determined quickly and is a function of total volume and equipment/material surface area.

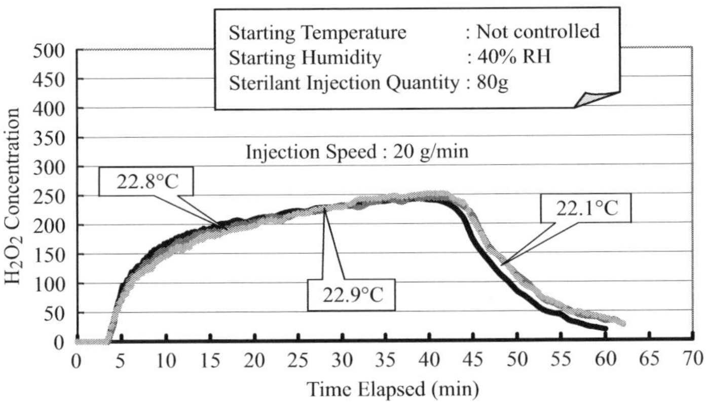

Figure 4 H_2O_2 vapor concentration reproducibility.

Table 6 75 m^3 Clean Room Decontamination Parameters/Results

Initial Temperature	20–24°C
Initial RH	50%
Total Injection Volume	200 g
Injection rate	25 g/min
BIs placed	47/test run
Total hold time	30 minutes
Total Process time including aeration	~5 hr
BIs positive	None
Residual at end of aeration	<1 ppm

Once this injection rate was found suitable, four additional test runs were done under identical conditions to confirm reproducibility. Distribution fans were placed within the room to ensure uniform vapor distribution and deposition. Cycle parameters and results are shown in Table 6. (Note that BI results and aeration outcome were the same for five consecutive tests conducted at the stated parameters.)

Single injection HYDEC® room decontamination systems have been installed in several aseptic processing facilities including those containing RABS. Complete kill of BIs with populations of 10^4 to 10^6 *G. stearothermophilus* sports have been inactivated on all surfaces including equipment, floors, ceilings, and walls in clean rooms as large as 200 m^3 total volume with cycle times of 8 to 10 hours. In all cases decontamination could be achieved overnight with aeration to <1 ppm H_2O_2 residual.

Studies have found that it is possible to decontaminate large parts hoppers, parts feeders used for large plastic bottles and drop dose tips in situ concurrently with room decontamination. This is significant since many of these parts feeders and hoppers are too large to sterilize out of place using an autoclave and aseptic assembly of these systems poses a far greater contamination risk owing to their size and complexity than decontaminating them in situ.

These studies indicate that is quite possible to achieve the same level of decontamination in clean rooms used to house RABS or fully automated processing equipment (defined as equipment that can be operated without human intervention) as can be routinely achieved in isolators. This capability creates the potential for advanced aseptic processing systems that marry different types of environmental control systems, and can result in advanced aseptic systems limited only by the imagination of the designers. In addition, given what has been learned about the efficacy of VPHP decontamination at a broad range of temperatures and ambient humidity levels, the engineer does not have to be concerned with extensive additional equipment to achieve humidity levels substantially lower than ambient.

Other Considerations in VPHP Decontamination

The authors do not want to leave the impression that VPHP is a panacea for all decontamination requirements. There are in our experience products that are quite sensitive to powerful oxidants such as VPHP. This is certainly true of biological macromolecules such as proteins, peptides, and nucleic acids. In depth studies are necessary to ensure that products do not have profound incompatibilities with VPHP. It is not uncommon for proteins and peptides to require residual levels in the range of 10 to 100 ppb.

It certainly is possible to achieve levels this low in VPHP processing, but in our experience special design of the isolator or RABS environment to be used is quite likely. Also, a careful balance must be drawn between decontamination requirements and low residuals. We have found that decontamination processes providing a four spore log reduction (which is different from complete kill of BIs with an initial population of 10^4) pose no microbiological risk to the aseptic process. The reader should consider that the regulatory standards allow for a 4-log reduction, and that sometimes it is best to avoid the validation practice of building "worst case" upon "worst case" (9,10).

Although it is generally possible to accommodate products that are exquisitely sensitive to VPHP, there may be circumstances where this is not possible. We do not believe, however, that this should serve to discourage firms that find product compatibility issues from using advanced aseptic processing technology. Rather manufacturers, regulatory authorities and validation engineers must understand that aseptic processing does not have to be all one way or another, flexibility is possible. Efficacy of the product must always take precedence, but in our experience an isolator that could not be decontaminated or a fully automated human free process even if VPHP decontamination (or the use of any other powerful oxidant for decontamination) is not possible. Our research indicates that such operations even without harsh sporicidal treatments are superior from a contamination control perspective to conventional aseptic processes.

Built-In or Free-Standing VPHP Systems?

We do not believe that there is a single correct answer to this question. Certainly, built-in VPHP generators have advantages particularly in smaller isolator systems or where portability is required. Built-in systems obviate the need to make tubing connections and therefore can provide a level of simplicity not possible with free-standing generators.

On the other hand, in large systems that might require multiple built-in vaporizers or generators another type of complexity arises. In this case the operation of multiple vaporizers or generators must be coordinated and supply of H_2O_2 to each of these systems must be accommodated. Also, should there be a mechanical or electrical problem with single built-in generator; the user will find that they may not have the ability to decontaminate the entire system. However, if a single high-vaporizer capacity free-standing unit is employed the user can employ a backup generator system should the need arise. We suggest that the user carefully consider their requirements/needs and determine which approach may be best for their production requirements. In our experience both built-in generators and freestanding generators have been used successfully on isolator systems for aseptic processing. There is no single right answer to the question of built-in or free-standing generators for isolator systems.

DISCUSSION

The authors are aware of the extensive prior debate on nearly all technical aspects of VPHP decontamination. The studies described in this chapter were not designed to address the issues that have been the subject of that debate, but rather to ask some fundamental questions relating to the practical aspects of Hydrogen peroxide decontamination in order to establish an effective generator. Specifically, it was our intention to determine if a simpler, quicker and more efficient method for VPHP could be developed. Our data show conclusively that it is possible to develop a system that is highly efficacious and broadly applicable to a wide range of targets including isolators, and clean rooms.

Our experiments found that VPHP is a robust process that is fully capable of decontamination at a wide variety of initial temperature and humidity conditions. We have also shown that continuous or even semicontinuous replenishment of hydrogen peroxide during the process is unnecessary. It is clear that VPHP decontamination is an effective process that effectively decontaminates over a wide range of operating conditions. This is logical when one considers that H_2O_2 is one of the most powerful oxidants known. H_2O_2 has a higher oxidation potential than either chlorine or chlorine dioxide and the hydroxyl radical which no doubt plays a vital role in H_2O_2 decontamination is exceeded in oxidation potential only by fluorine (11). Therefore, we believe that the real challenge in VPHP decontamination or sterilization is not antimicrobial efficacy, but rather developing a process that is efficient as well as effective.

Our studies have demonstrated that the key factors involved in the development of an efficacious process are total injection volume and the rapid injection of that total volume can be accomplished relatively rapidly and without any form of replenishment. Thus, cycle development can be simple because the hold time can be uniform. Hold times of 15 minutes are typical for isolator enclosures whereas 30-minute hold periods are typically used for large targets such as clean rooms.

The discovery that continuous or semicontinuous injection is unnecessary and that initial dehumidification is not required can both simplify and shorten the VPHP decontamination process time. The total H_2O_2 required by this process is typically substantially less than that required for replenishment processes. In any decontamination process, the user and process engineer must consider that antimicrobial processes always require a trade-off between kill effectiveness and damage to materials or product. Therefore, keeping the amount of H_2O_2 to the minimum required to achieve the targeted level of lethality or "kill" is advantageous in every respect.

Also, we believe that our finding that insertion of BIs into the enclosure at the end of the 15-minute hold period did not result in efficient inactivation appears to indicate that a chemical change had occurred, which resulted in greatly diminished oxidative capacity. Thus, it appears that the relationship of kill effectiveness to total injection volume most likely relates to providing sufficient VPHP to reach all surfaces within the enclosure or target. Longer hold periods and replenishment by further injection quantities do not enhance efficacy. Single injection nonreplenishment VPHP systems of the type described in this chapter have been installed and validated in more than 30 facilities for production and sterility testing in International Conference on Harmonization (ICH) zone countries.

REFERENCES

1. Joslyn LJ. Gaseous Chemical Sterilization. In: Block SS, ed. Disinfection, Sterilization and Preservation. New York, NY: Lippincott, Williams & Wilkins, 2001:337–359.
2. Block SS. Peroxygen compounts. In: Block SS, ed. Disinfection, Sterilization and Preservation. New York, NY: Lippincott, Williams & Wilkins, 2001:185–204.
3. Kokubo M, Inoue T, Akers J. Resistance of common environmental spores of the genus bacillus to vapor hydrogen peroxyde. PDA J Pharm Sci Technol 1998; 52(5):228–231.
4. Imai KS, Watanabe Y, Oshima M, et al. A new approach to vapor hydrogen peroxide decontamination of isolators and clean rooms. Pharm Eng 2006; 26(3):96–104.
5. Rickloff JR. Key aspects of validating hydrogen peroxide gas cycles in isolator systems. J Validation Technol 1998; 61–71.
6. Steris Co., Mentor, Ohio, Vapor Phase Hydrogen Peroxide Cycle Development Guide, 2001.
7. Pflug IJ. Variability in the data generated by laboratories measuring *D*-values of bacterial spores. PDA J Pharm Sci Technol 2005; 59(1):3–9.
8. Sigwarth V, Stärk A. Effect of carrier materials on the resistance of spores of *Bacillus stearothermophilus* to gaseous hydrogen peroxyde. PDA J Pharm Sci Technol 2003; 57(1):3–11.
9. Food and Drug Administration (FDA). Guidance for Industry: Sterile Drug Products Produced by Aseptic Processing—Current Good Manufacturing Practice (Appendix 1: Aseptic Processing Isolators). September 2004, 44–48.
10. Design and validation of isolator systems for the manufacturing and testing of health care products. PDA Technical Report No. 34. PDA J Pharm Sci Technol 2001; 55(5):1–23.
11. Kawasaki CH, Nagano T, Ito M, Kondo M. Mechanism of bactericidal action of hydrogen peroxide. J Food Hygiene Soc Jpn 1970; 11:155–160.

28 Chlorine dioxide decontamination/sterilization

Mark A. Czarneski

INTRODUCTION

Chlorine dioxide (CD) is a highly effective sterilizing agent that has many applications in the pharmaceutical industry including the decontamination of isolators and their contents and the decontamination of clean rooms. It has two primary features that make it extremely effective and well suited for use in isolators, clean rooms, and sterilization. It is a true gas at normal use temperatures and therefore is not susceptible to condensation issues and temperature gradients. It has a yellowish-green color, which allows its concentration to be precisely monitored and controlled by a UV–vis spectrophotometer. This gives the ability to provide tight process control from beginning to end.

CD is a single-electron-transfer oxidizing agent with a chlorine-like odor. This odor is the only similarity between CD and chlorine. Let us be clear, CD is *not* chlorine. CD can be generated in a variety of methods in liquid or gas. The following are some of the reactions that generate CD:

$$Cl_2 + 2NaClO_2 \rightarrow 2ClO_2 + 2NaCl$$

$$5NaClO_2 + 4HCl \rightarrow 4ClO_2 + 2H_2O + 5NaCl$$

$$2NaClO_2 + Na_2S_2O_8 \rightarrow 2ClO_2 + 2Na_2SO_4$$

$$2HClO_3 + H_2C_2O_4 \rightarrow 2ClO_2 + 2CO_2 + 2H_2O$$

$$2NaClO_3 + H_2SO_4 + SO_2 \rightarrow 2ClO_2 + 2NaHSO_4$$

CD chemical features and structure can be found in Table 1 and Figure 1.

CD's method of inactivation is different than chlorine (oxidation vs. chlorination), it is far gentler on materials, and provides a highly controllable and reproducible process. In addition, CD is compatible with many materials including stainless steel, aluminum, glass, and most plastics, which are found in isolator and clean room construction. The rapid sterilizing activity of CD is present at ambient temperatures and at relatively low gas concentrations of 1 (2) to 30 mg/L (3).

Sterilization with CD follows the same general processing steps as with other gaseous sterilants. As with ethylene oxide, moisture is required for optimal lethal rate and effective sterilization. With CD, moisture preconditioning is performed at 60% to 75% relative humidity (RH) prior to gas introduction (4). Gas is introduced to the desired concentration and held for a sufficient period of time to yield the required antimicrobial effect. Removing the CD by flushing with air or by evacuation terminates the process.

Use

CD is relatively new in its use as a gaseous sterilization agent. It has, however, a long history of use in other industries. CD is widely used as an antimicrobial and as an oxidizing agent in drinking water; poultry process water, and mouthwash preparations. It is used to sanitize fruit and vegetables as well as equipment for food and beverage processing. It is used to decontaminate animal facilities. It is also employed in the health care industries to decontaminate rooms, passthroughs, and isolators, and also as a sterilant for product and component sterilization. What's more, as an oxidizing agent, it is extensively used to bleach, deodorize, and detoxify a wide variety of materials, including cellulose, paper pulp, flour, leather, fats and oils, and textiles.

Worldwide, nearly 4.5 million pounds per day of CD are used in the production of pulp and paper make the industry the single largest user of CD (5). Many mills have now replaced chlorine gas completely with CD, thereby reducing their emissions of dioxin to "nondetectable" levels (6). Today, units producing up to 65 ton/day are operating in large softwood kraft pulp mills, though 5 ton/day units were typical in the 1950s.

Table 1 Chlorine Dioxide Properties

Chemical formula	ClO_2
Molecular weight	67.45 g/mol
Melting point (°C)	−59
Boiling point (°C)	+11
Density	2.4 times that of air

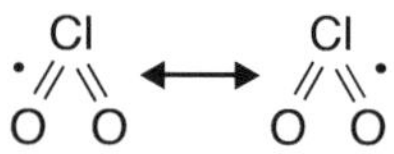

Figure 1 Chemical structure of chlorine dioxide (1).

About 5% of large water-treatment facilities (serving more than 100,000 people) in the United States use CD to treat drinking water. It is estimated that about 12 million people may be exposed in this way to CD. In communities that use CD to treat water for drinking uses, CD, is permitted to be present at low levels in the tap water (7).

It is also estimated that there were 743,015 pounds (337,026 kg) of CD released to the atmosphere from over 100 manufacturing, processing, and waste disposal facilities in 2000 (8).

History

CD was first prepared in 1802 by Chenevix. Humphrey Davy independently prepared CD in 1811, clarified its composition and proposed the name euchlorine. Over time CD has also been referred to as chlorine oxide, anthium dioxide, chlorine (IV) oxide, chlorine peroxide, chloroperoxyl, and chloryl radical. The CD prepared by Chenevix and Davy was prepared using a strong acid to liberate the gas from potassium and sodium chlorate. Davy found the molecule to be ClO_2, greenish-yellow gas with a molecular weight of 67.5 (9). It is highly soluble in water but does not dissociate and it has a chlorine-like odor. Despite numerous applications for CD in aqueous systems, many years passed from the time of CD's discovery until the utility of this powerful oxidizing agent in its gaseous form was recognized.

CD's special properties make it an ideal choice to meet the challenges of today's environmentally concerned world. Actually, CD is an environmentally preferred alternative to elemental chlorine. When chlorine reacts with organic matter, undesirable pollutants such as dioxins and bioaccumulative toxic substances are produced. Thus, the US Environmental Protection Agency (EPA) supports the substitution of CD for chlorine because it greatly reduces the production of these pollutants. It is a perfect replacement for chlorine, providing all of chlorine's benefits without any of its weaknesses and detriments. Most importantly, CD does not chlorinate organic material, resulting in significant decreases in trihalomethanes, haloacetic acids, and other chlorinated organic compounds. This is particularly important in the primary use for CD, which is water disinfection. Other properties of CD make it more effective than chlorine, enabling a lower dose and resulting in a lower environmental impact.

CD has been recognized since the beginning of the century for its disinfecting properties; these properties have led to the widespread use of CD in the treatment of drinking water. By 1996 CD was used in over 400 drinking water treatment plants in the United States (10). The Food and Drug Administration has allowed the use of aqueous CD in washing fruits and vegetables (11). Beyond this and numerous other aqueous applications, the sporicidal properties of *gaseous* CD were demonstrated in 1986. In other studies, it has been suggested that CD gas treatment was more effective in reducing bacterial population than was aqueous CD treatment (12). Subsequent to those studies, it has been shown that gaseous CD is a rapid and effective sterilant active against bacteria, yeasts, molds, and viruses.

CD was patented as a sterilant in 1985. The sporicidal activity of gaseous CD was demonstrated and, in 1988, it was accepted by the United States EPA for use as a sterilant. Sterilization studies with gaseous CD demonstrate its potential applicability for medical product sterilization.

Table 2 *D* Value Determinations Using the Stumbo–Murphy–Cochran Method (3 mg/L)

Gas conc (mg/L)	*U*	*n*	*r*	Nu	Log Nu	*D* value
3	21	10	0	N/D	N/D	N/D
3	24	10	1	2.30	0.362	3.92
3	27	10	1	2.30	0.362	4.41
3	30	10	2	1.61	0.207	4.78
3	33	10	6	0.51	−0.292	4.87
3	36	10	8	0.22	−0.651	5.05
3	39	10	9	0.11	−0.977	5.23
3	42	10	8	0.22	−0.651	5.89
3	45	10	10	N/D	N/D	N/D
					Average	4.88 min

Effectiveness

CD acts as an oxidizing agent and reacts with several cellular constituents, including the cell membrane of microbes. By "stealing" electrons from them (oxidation), it breaks their molecular bonds, resulting in the death of the organism by the break up of the cell. Because CD alters the proteins involved in the structure of microorganisms, the enzymatic function is broken, causing very rapid bacterial kills. The potency of CD is attributable to the simultaneous, oxidative attack on many proteins thereby preventing the cells from mutating to a resistant form. In addition, because of the lower reactivity of CD, its antimicrobial action is retained longer in the presence of organic matter.

A series of square wave studies was performed in a two glove 23 ft^3 flexible wall isolator *to* determine the effect of CD gas concentration on the inactivation rate of *Bacillus atrophaeus* spores. The *D* value (the time at a specified CD gas concentration required to reduce the microbial population by 1 log or 90%) of *B. atrophaeus* spores on unwrapped paper carriers, when exposed to CD gas concentrations of 3 and 5 mg/L, was determined using the Stumbo–Murphy–Cochran method.

Each biological indicator (BI) was stored at 75% ± 2% RH prior to entering the isolator and preconditioned in the isolator at 75% ± 2% RH for 30 ± 1 minute prior to CD gas exposure. The decline in %RH during the gas injection and exposure phases of the cycle was recorded for each of the *D* value runs.

Data calculations for the 3 and 5 mg/L exposure concentrations using the Stumbo–Murphy–Cochran are in Tables 2 and 3. The results can be seen in Table 4 (13).

Table 3 *D* Value Determinations Using the Stumbo–Murphy–Cochran Method (5 mg/L)

Gas conc (mg/L)	*U*	*N*	*r*	Nu	Log Nu	*D* value
5	18	10	1	2.30	0.362	2.94
5	21	10	2	1.61	0.207	3.35
5	24	10	7	0.36	−0.448	3.46
5	27	10	9	0.11	−0.977	3.62
5	30	10	10	N/D	N/D	N/D
5	33	10	9	0.11	0.977	4.43
5	36	10	10	N/D	N/D	N/D
5	39	10	10	N/D	N/D	N/D
5	42	10	10	N/D	N/D	N/D
					Average	3.56 min

Note: When the number of sterile replicates (*r*) is 0 or 10 the *D* value is not determined.
Stumbo–Murphy–Cochran formula:

D value = *U*/log No − log Nu

where *U* is the time in minutes, *n* is the number of replicates tested, *r* is the number of sterile replicates out of the number tested, Nu is the natural log of *n*/*r* [in (*n*/*r*)], No is the population of unexposed 81 (3.00 × 106 cfu/strip).
N/D, not determined.

Table 4 Results and Conclusion *D* Value Versus Chlorine Dioxide Concentration

Chlorine dioxide concentration (mg/L)	*D* value (min)
3	4.88
5	3.56
10	0.75
20	0.27
30	0.12

Cycle Description

The CD cycle is similar to the ethylene oxide cycle, in as humidity is required for process efficacy along with gas concentration. The process is the same for vacuum cycles to isolator cycles to clean rooms. The CD cycle can be carried out at pressures from negative pressures (2 kPa) to slightly above atmosphere. Figure 2 shows an example cycle of CD concentration.

The steps in the cycle are as follows:

- Precondition
- Conditioning
- Charge
- Exposure
- Aeration

Precondition

Precondition is the first step of the CD cycle where the chamber should be leak tested first. When using any sterilant it is good practice to perform a chamber leak test prior to each decontamination cycle to ensure chamber integrity. For an isolator or other atmospheric chamber, the pressure is raised to a pressure suitable to the target chamber, and then the chamber is held static for a period of time. The pressure difference from the beginning of the dwell time to the end is noted and if the pressure drop is not within acceptable parameters then the chamber must be properly sealed and retested before any sterilant in injected into the chamber.

Once the chamber has been leak tested, the chamber can be brought to the proper relative humidity set point (60–75%). Humidity can be generated in a variety of methods such as steam, fine particle size atomizers, hot plates, foggers, etc. Steam offers the quickest, cleanest, and most efficient way to raise humidity.

Conditioning

Once the humidity is at the proper level (60–75%), the cycle can advance to the next step, conditioning. During the entire conditioning time, typically 30 minutes for isolators and sterilizers and 10 minutes for clean rooms, the RH should be monitored. If the RH drops by any significant amount (5%) more moisture should be added to the chamber. Once the conditioning time is completed the next step starts.

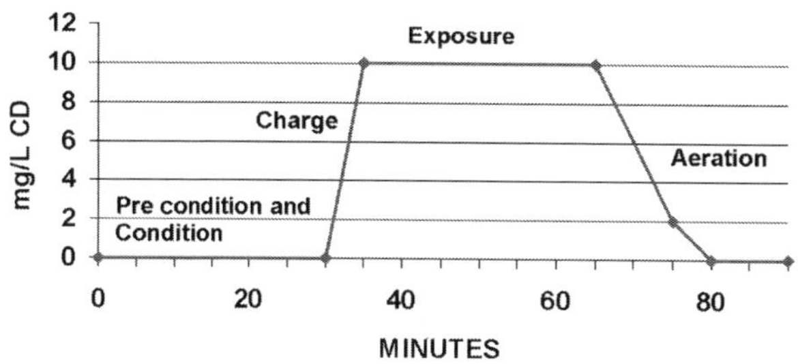

Figure 2 Cycle chart of CD concentration.

Charge

During Charge, CD gas is generated and introduced into the chamber to achieve a set concentration of gas. The target concentration is dependent on different factors: cycle time, consumable life, amount of reagent gas, ambient pressure cycle, vacuum chamber cycle, etc. If cycle time is extremely important a higher concentration is sometimes selected to achieve a faster kill. At higher concentrations the *D* values are much lower thereby shortening the overall cycle. If there are limited consumables or reagent gas on site then a lower concentration can be selected to preserve the consumables, but the exposure time must be extended accordingly. Under vacuum conditions the penetration of CD gas is quite remarkable. Usually a higher concentration is selected when using vacuum to ensure penetration into the smallest of places. CD is a surface sterilant and does not have the penetrating abilities of ethylene oxide. CD does not penetrate through plastic polymers such as (plastic tubing, bottle, bags, etc.) or through cardboard but it does reach tight areas (inside of syringes, bottles, tips, and caps). It does penetrate through breathable polymers such as Tyvek® and other porous materials used in filters and filter media. An additional benefit occurs as CD does not penetrate into the polymers, which can significantly reduce aeration time.

Concentrations range from 20 to 30 mg/L for sterilizers to 5 to 10 mg/L for isolators to 1 mg/L for rooms. Because CD is easily measurable in real time, the target concentration can straightforwardly be achieved each time and every time, thus giving the assurance of a repeatable and reproducible decontamination cycle. When gas concentration reaches the target concentration, the cycle proceeds to the exposure step.

Exposure

During exposure, the concentration of CD gas is monitored and maintained to keep the concentration at the target concentration for the entire exposure time (typically 20–30 minutes for isolators and sterilizers and 120 minutes for rooms). In addition, if gas concentration drops during the cycle, due to pressure relief or absorbance of CD into celluloid materials, the concentration is be made up to ensure gas concentration is constant during the entire decontamination exposure step.

Aeration

The aeration step starts once the exposure step is completed. In this step, the CD gas is removed from the chamber. For ambient chambers, this is accomplished by introducing air into the chamber and the removal of CD from the chamber to outside exhaust. Table 5 calculates the amount of CD used for a typical cycle in an isolator and clean room. Table 6 details the same cycle's aeration curve. As can be seen total aeration is achieved in 15 minutes for the isolator and 48 minutes for the clean room. These aeration times bring the chambers environment to the OSHA safe levels of 0.1 ppm.

Cycle Development

Moisture Conditioning

As already mentioned, the presence of moisture is critical to obtaining optimal lethal rate and effective sterilization with gaseous CD. Important points to consider with respect to moisture conditioning, when developing CD sterilization processes, are as follows:

Table 5 Quantity of CD for Given Chamber Size

Isolator volume (ft^3)	100 $\cong$ 28.32 m^3
Target concentration (mg/L)	5
Amount of CD in chamber	14.16 g
Clean room volume (ft^3)	10,000 $\cong$ 283.17 m^3
Target concentration (mg/L)	1
Amount of CD in chamber	283.16 g

Table 6A Aeration Rate for 100 ft^3 Isolator

Air exchanges	mg/L	ppm	Time (min)
1	2.5000	892.50	1
2	1.2500	446.25	2
3	0.6250	223.13	3
4	0.3125	111.56	4
5	0.1563	55.78	5
6	0.0781	27.89	6
7	0.0391	13.95	7
8	0.0195	6.97	8
9	0.0098	3.49	9
10	0.0049	1.74	10
11	0.0024	0.87	11
12	0.0012	0.44	12
13	0.0006	0.22	13
14	0.0003	0.11	14
15	0.0002	0.05	15

Note: Each air exchange 1/2 of CD is removed.
Exhaust rate (CFM) 100 ≅ 169.9 m^3/hr.

Table 6B Aeration Rate for 10,000 ft^3 Room

Air exchanges	mg/L	ppm	Time (min)
1	0.5000	181.00	4.00
2	0.2500	90.50	8.00
3	0.1250	45.25	12.00
4	0.0625	22.63	16.00
5	0.0313	11.31	20.00
6	0.0156	5.66	24.00
7	0.0078	2.83	28.00
8	0.0039	1.41	32.00
9	0.0020	0.71	36.00
10	0.0010	0.35	40.00
11	0.0005	0.18	44.00
12	0.0002	0.09	48.00

Note: Each air exchange 1/2 of CD is removed.
Exhaust rate (CFM) 2500 ≅ 283.17 m^3/hr.

For the sterilization of an isolator or similar sealed, enclosed space, is there control of the RH inside the chamber and what are the allowable minimum and maximum RH values? How do these values agree with the requirements for CD sterilization, 60% to 75% RH? If moisture is not controlled within the isolator or chamber, what are typical RH values in the chamber and the surrounding environment? Have seasonal effects been considered, such as lower RH in the winter?

For the sterilization of a load of material, within a chamber or a traditional sterilizer, what moisture condition has the load been exposed to/stored at prior to sterilization? Is there potential for seasonal RH variation that could affect the moisture condition of the load to be decontaminated? Does the load contain components or packaging materials that may become desiccated during storage in a dry environment prior to sterilization? This may affect the time required to fully moisturize the load. Could the density of the load or its physical geometry affect the penetration of moisture into least accessible areas?

Based on a large body of information, the following guidance can be given with respect to the moisture-conditioning step in the process.

In isolator-type applications, the use of a moisture conditioning step of 30 minutes at 60% to 75% RH prior to CD gas injection has been shown to be adequate in most situations.

The optimal RH is between 70% and 75%. At 55% RH, the lethal rate begins to be adversely affected and is seriously affected at RH values below 55%. Conditioning times of less than 15 minutes for sporicidal reduction is generally not recommended unless the RH of the chamber is constantly maintained within the range of 60% to 75% RH. Extended conditioning time (60 minutes) may be required in the case of dry environmental conditions inside a chamber or in the case of introduction of desiccated material(s) into a chamber.

The choice of a moisture conditioning time in a traditional sterilizer-based application is a function of the issues raised above as well as the approach used to perform the moisture conditioning. Passive moisture conditioning either in an external chamber or within the sterilization chamber itself can require protracted conditioning times especially with dense, desiccated loads. With passive moisture conditioning, appropriate validation studies are particularly important to assure moisture penetration into the least accessible areas.

In clean room applications moisture conditioning time can be performed during the charge phase. Because the chamber or room can be large, the charge can be as little as 15 minutes (for 1000 ft^3) or as much as 140 minutes (for 10,000 ft^3) room the conditioning occurs simultaneously during the charge step, thereby saving overall cycle time.

Exposure Time/Gas Concentration

Linear inactivation kinetics has been demonstrated with gaseous CD using the BI of choice for this sterilant, spores of *B. atrophaeus*. As with other gaseous sterilants, the lethal rate increases with increasing gas concentration. Early studies with a traditional sterilizer-based application used a gas concentration of 30 mg/L. This concentration was chosen in this particular situation due to the density and composition of the sterilization load. Work in isolator-type systems, which are generally not densely loaded and where much of the intent is surface sterilization, led to studies with lower gas concentrations, generally between 5 and 10 mg/L. Rapid inactivation of the BIs was observed with sterilization of 10^6 *B. atrophaeus* spores occurring in less than 15 minutes in almost all cases. In one application, testing was performed at a CD gas concentration of 3 mg/L with reproducible sterilization of 10^6 BIs. Concentrations for clean rooms and large volumes have used concentrations even lower. Concentrations have been as low as 1 mg/L. As would be expected, the required total gas exposure time is longer than that used at higher gas concentrations.

Based on studies using a number of test systems, the following guidance can be given with respect to choice of gas concentration and exposure time in process development studies:

In an isolator-type application, the recommended gas concentrations for process development studies are 5 or 10 mg/L. A very large number of sterilization exposures have been performed in isolators using a CD gas concentration of 10 mg/L. In almost all cases, complete kill of 10^6 BIs was observed with 15 minutes of gas exposure. At a CD concentration of 5 mg/L, complete kill of 10^6 BIs was observed with 30 minutes of exposure and positives started to occur at 20 minutes of exposure. In the event of a densely loaded isolator or a system with areas where gas penetration may be impeded, a longer gas exposure time may be required for similar sterilization efficacy. Also, the testing described here was performed in isolators with well-defined and effective circulation and/or recirculation systems; this ensured uniform gas distribution as measured by visual inspection, photometric monitoring and inactivation of BIs placed throughout the isolator and/or load. In process development studies with isolator-type systems, adequate circulation and uniformity of gas distribution must be carefully considered.

In a unique isolator-type application, a gas concentration of 3 mg/L has been successfully used. The enclosure being decontaminated was relatively large in volume (~5000 ft^3) and a rapid turn around time was not required, therefore a lower gas concentration could be employed. Due to the large volume, an extended time was required for the gas charge step to reach the 3 mg/L concentration. Because there is substantial biocidal activity during the extended gas charge step, the time required for the timed gas exposure step was found to be relatively short. If it is desired to use CD gas concentrations lower than 5 mg/L in an isolator-type application, it is recommended that careful consideration be given to the contribution of the gas charge, timed gas exposure, and aeration steps to the total biocidal activity. With the gas exposure time held constant, changes in the time required for either gas charge or aeration could significantly affect the total amount of biocidal activity. The potential for such effects should

Table 7 Example Chlorine Dioxide Cycles

Preconditioning		Chlorine dioxide exposure			
Min	% RH	mg/L	Min	# Nonsterile/ # Tested	Comments
30	75	10	5	10/10	Spores on unwrapped paper spore strips stored at 23% RH prior to use. Duplicate series of runs on different days.
30	75	10	10	5/10	
30	75	10	15	0/10	
30	75	10	5	8/10	
30	75	10	10	1/10	
30	75	10	15	0/10	
30	70	5	30	0/20	Spores on paper spore strips in Tyvek™ envelopes. Chlorine dioxide concentration of 5 mg/L.
30	75	10	15	0/10	Spores on paper strips, unwrapped
30	75	10	30	0/10	
30	75	10	15	10/10	Spores on paper strips in blue glassine envelopes
30	75	10	30	0/10	
30	75	10	15	0/10	Spores on paper strips in Tyvek™ envelopes
30	75	10	30	0/10	
30	75	10	15	0/10	Spores on glass fiber discs in Tyvek™ envelopes
30	75	10	30	0/10	

be taken into account in choosing and validating a gas exposure time. It is recommended that detailed process development and validation studies be performed to determine the appropriate gas exposure time and associated conditions. The reader is referred to ISO document 14937 for further guidance.

Examples of CD Process Development

Table 7 (14) presents examples of gaseous CD process development studies in isolator systems using 10^6 *B. atrophaeus* spores as the BI. This work evaluated different substrates, packages, and storage conditions.

Biological Indicators

Historical information has pointed to *B. atrophaeus* (ATCC 9372) spores as the appropriate BI for physical (dry heat) and chemical sterilants such as CD. To confirm this finding for gaseous CD, tests were done with *B. atrophaeus*, as well as other commonly used Bls.

Initially, four spore-forming organisms were selected; *Geobacillus stearothermophilus* (ATCC 7953), traditionally used in steam sterilization activities, *Bacillus pumilus* (ATCC 7953), most often used in irradiation studies, *G. stearothermophilus* (ATCC 12980), and *B. atrophaeus* (ATCC 9732). A study was developed to expose each type of BI to a standard CD cycle. In each of three runs, 15 Bls of each type were exposed to the CD standard cycle, removed from the chamber, and aseptically transferred to nutrient media. Microbial growth, as indicated by media turbidity, was recorded as a positive result. These exposures were performed in triplicate.

The results are shown in the Table 8. As can been seen in the Table, *B. atrophaeus* spores were consistently more resistant (highest number of Bls remaining nonsterile) than either the *G. stearothermophilus* strains or *B. pumilus*. Based on these data, the use of spores of *B. atrophaeus* as the BI for gaseous CD was affirmed.

Stability of Gas

CD is stable throughout even extended cycles but is not stable enough to be stored in pressurized gas cylinders. It is produced at the time and point of use. Throughout the cycle, it is stable and, unlike most of the H_2O_2 decontamination systems, it does not need to be continuously fed into and circulated through the chamber. Throughout the exposure step, the CD just sits in the chamber. Because CD is a true gas and does not condense, the stability of CD as the sterilizing agent is greatly enhanced over other methods. Because the CD concentration can be monitored

Table 8 Biological Indicator Resistance Study Results

Biological indicator	Run 1 # nonsterile/total tested	Run 2 # nonsterile/total tested	Run 3 # nonsterile/total tested	Total # nonsterile/total tested
B. atrophaeus (globigii) ATCC 9372	10/15	13/15	15/15	38/45
B. pumilus ATCC 27142	0/15	2/15	1/15	3/45
B. stearothermophilus ATCC 12980	1/15	2/15	2/15	5/45
B. stearothermophilus VHP	9/15	9/15	8/15	26/45

Cycle parameters: 30 mg/L gas concentration, 90% RH prehumidification, 6-minute exposure time.

and controlled, the concentration is precisely maintained throughout the cycle. Temperature variances within the chamber do not affect the concentration and this is significant in larger room decontamination applications where the temperature can vary across the facility. Equipment inside rooms also does not affect CD gas distribution as it affects H_2O_2 decontamination systems.

Measurement/Quantification

A spectrophotometer precisely monitors and controls the CD concentration from the charge step, through exposure, and throughout most of the aeration cycle until it gets to approximately 0.1 mg/L. This ability for real-time measurement addresses the FDA's call for concentration monitoring of sterilants. Because many things may affect a concentration (leaks, absorption, reaction, etc) monitoring is key to any process control. With this ability the variance from cycle to cycle does not exist with CD gas as it is monitored and maintained.

Because CD is a true gas and does not condense, aeration is very repeatable and can be validated to ensure that safe conditions are aerated to for repeat applications. There are also devices such as Draegar™ tubes and many different manufacturers that produce low-level sensors, which can be used to ensure that safe levels are attained once aeration is completed.

Safety/Toxicity

The OSHA 8-hour time-weighted average for CD is 0.1 ppm. The 15-minute short time exposure limit (STEL) is 0.3 ppm (15). CD is a respiratory/mucous membrane irritant. One of the great safety features of CD is that it has a 0.1 ppm odor threshold that makes it self-alerting (16). Most other sterilants need to be well over their STEL before they can be sensed or smelled. Because CD has such widespread usage in the water treatment and paper and pulp industries, there are is a wide selection of environmental monitors and personnel badges available. Also because of this widespread usage, there has been numerous safety studies conducted both for environmental effects, inhalation, as well as ingestion. Because it is also widely used in the food industry for sanitization and disinfection, there are allowable limits from the US government for ingestion. The EPA has set the maximum concentration of CD in drinking water at 0.8 mg/L (17).

Known Incompatibilities

CD reacts with carbohydrates, such as glucose, to oxidize the primary hydroxyl groups first to aldehydes and then to carboxyl acids (18). Ketones are also oxidized to carboxyl acids (19). Although CD has "chlorine" in its name, its chemistry is radically different from that of chlorine. When reacting with other substances, it is weaker and more selective. For example, it does not react with organic materials to form chlorinated species or with ammonia to form chloramine. CD oxygenates products rather than chlorinating them and thus trihalomethane formation does not occur (20). Therefore, unlike chlorine, CD does not produce environmentally undesirable organic compounds containing chlorine. CD, as with other oxidizers, causes oxidation to uncoated ferrous materials as well as other materials subject to oxidation. Control of moisture during the decontamination process mitigates the oxidation potential.

In-Process Controls

Process control is one of the greatest strengths of the CD technology and one that puts it worlds above other methods of decontamination. Because CD has a yellowish-green color, it can be precisely monitored with a UV-VIS spectrophotometer. This technological advantage allows the CD concentration to be precisely monitored and controlled from the Charge step, through exposure, and throughout most of the aeration cycle until it gets down to approximately 0.1 mg/L. CD is a true gas that distributes rapidly and evenly throughout the chamber. Because it is a true gas, issues with temperature gradients, cold spots, drafts from the heating, ventilation, and air conditioning (HVAC) system, outside humidity levels, heat sinks due to materials of construction, and other issues that can affect the condensation of vapor-decontaminating agents, do not affect the decontamination effectiveness of CD. Chamber mapping can also be performed with the built-in spectrophotometer to facilitate the validation effort. An RH/temperature probe monitors the RH and temperature conditions inside the chamber. Two differential pressure transmitters (the second for redundancy) monitor the chamber pressure. The tight process control and accurate concentration monitoring, along with a detailed run record, can lead to parametric release when used for product sterilization as well as expedite validation efforts for all applications.

Delivery Systems

The ClorDiSys^{TM} Solutions, Inc. Cloridox-GMP^{TM} Sterilization System (Fig. 3) is a CD gas generator system designed for use in any pharmaceutical, manufacturing, laboratory, or research setting. It provides a rapid and highly effective method to decontaminate a target chamber. The target can be any chamber such as an isolator (sterility test, filling line, containment), passthrough, processing tank or vessel, clean room, lyophilizer, etc. In addition, the system can be attached to most vacuum chambers to provide a method for component or product sterilization. The Cloridox–GMP^{TM} Sterilization System is portable in design and is comprised of a gas generation section and a sensing/electronic section. The system features a sophisticated sterilant concentration monitoring system to assure a tightly controlled decontamination process. All instrumentation, including the photometer for concentration monitoring, is easily calibrated

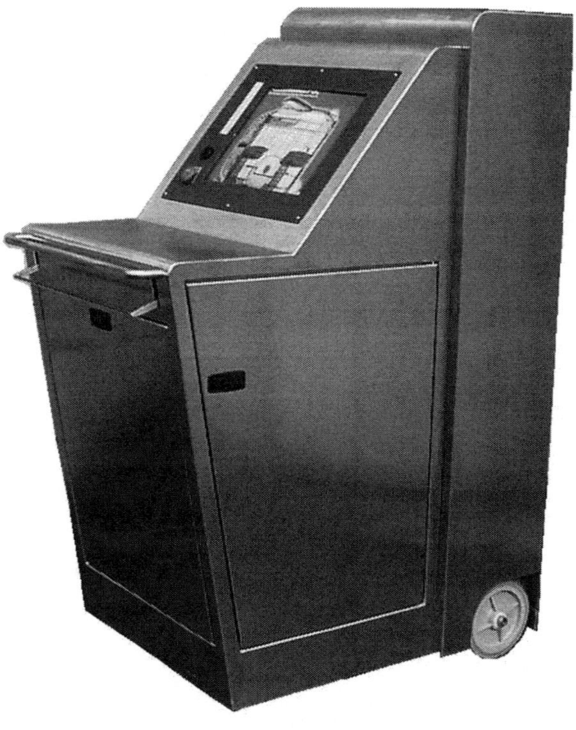

Figure 3 Cloridox-GMP CD gas generator system.

to traceable standards. The process is easy to validate due to the repeatable cycle, tight process control, and highly accurate sterilant monitoring system. A run record is produced that contains the date, cycle time, cycle steps, as well as relative humidity, temperature, pressure, and CD concentration. The human–machine interface system features a password protected, recipe management system with historical and real-time trending.

REFERENCES

1. Battisti DL. Development of a Chlorine Dioxide Sterilization System. PhD dissertation. Pittsburgh, PA: University of Pittsburgh, 2000.
2. Leo F, Poisson P, Sinclair CS, et al. Design, development and qualification of a microbiological challenge facility to assess the effectiveness of BFS aseptic processing. PDA J Pharm Sci Technol 2005; 59(1):33–48.
3. Jeng DK, Woodworth AG. Chlorine dioxide gas sterilization under square-wave conditions. Appl Environ Microbiol 1990; 56:514–519.
4. Czarneski MA, Lorcheim P. Isolator decontamination using chlorine dioxide gas. Pharm Technol 2005; 29(4):124–133.
5. The ClO_2 Fact Sheet. Available at http://www.lenntech.com/faqclo2.htm. Accessed May 12, 2010.
6. Stichfield AE, Woods MG. Reducing chlorinated organic compounds from bleached kraft mills through first stage substitution of chlorine dioxide for chlorine. Tappi J 1995; 78(6):117–125.
7. Agency for Toxic Substances and Disease Registry (ATSDR). Toxicological Profile for Chlorine Dioxide and Chlorite—Draft for Public Comment. Atlanta, GA: U.S. Department of Health and Human Services, Public Health Service, 2002.
8. U.S. Department of Health and Human Service. Draft Toxicological Profile for Chlorine Dioxide and Chlorine. Atlanta, GA: Agency for Toxic Substances and Disease Registry, 2002:103.
9. Davy H. On a combination of oxymuriatic gas and oxygen gas. Phil. Trans 1811; 101:155.
10. Richardsen SD, Thruston AD, Collette TW, et al. Future Use of Chlorine, Chlorine Dioxide, and other Chlorine Alternatives. New Orleans, LA: IFT Annual Meeting: Book of Abstracts, 1996:140.
11. Food and Drug Administration. U.S. Department of Health and Human Services. Secondary direct food additives permitted in food for human consumption. 21 C.F.R. Part 173–300 (chlorine dioxide). 1998.
12. Han Y. Linton RH. Nielsen SS, et al. Reduction of listeria monocytogenes on green peppers (*Capsicum annuum* l.) by gaseous and aqueous chlorine dioxide and water washing and its growth at 7°C. J Food Protect 2001; 64(11):1730–1738.
13. Czarneski MA, Lorcheim P. Validation of chlorine dioxide sterilization. In: Agalloco J, Carleton F. eds. Validation of Pharmaceutical Processes. 3rd ed. New York: Informa Healthcare, Inc, 2008:281–287.
14. ClorDiSys Solutions, Inc. Cloridox-GMP Sterilization System. System Operations Guide Appendix B. Microbiocidal Activity of Gaseous Chlorine Dioxide 2008. Accessed May 12, 2010.
15. Occupational Safety and Health Guideline for Chlorine Dioxide. http://www.osha.gov/SLTC/healthguidelines/chlorinedioxide/recognition.html.
16. American Conference of Governmental Industrial Hygienists (ACGIH) Threshold Limit Values (TLVs®) for Chlorine Dioxide.
17. Draft of Toxicological Profile for Chlorine Dioxide and Chlorite—for Public Comment. U.S. Department of Health and Human Services, Public Health Service Agency for Toxic Substances and Disease Registry (ATSDR), 2002.
18. Masschelein WJ, Rice RG. eds. Chlorine Dioxide Chemistry and Environmental Impact of Oxychlorine Compounds. Ann Arbor, MI: Ann Arbor Science Publishers, Inc, 1979:98, 111–145.
19. Kaczur JJ, Cawifield DW. Chlorine oxygen acids and salts. In: Arza Seidel, ed. Kirk-Othmer Encyclopedia of Chemical Technology. Vol 5. 4th ed. New York: Wiley, 1992.
20. Stevens AA. Reaction products of chlorine dioxide. Environ Health Perspect 1982; 46:101–110.

29 Current expectations for aseptic processing: a regulatory perspective

Richard L. Friedman

INTRODUCTION

In 2002, the Food and Drug Administration announced its current Good Manufacturing Practices (cGMPs) for the 21st century initiative (1). A critical objective of the initiative was to promote industry modernization. In accord with this objective, the Food and Drug Administration (FDA) has been encouraging pharmaceutical firms to adopt truly modern, robust aseptic processing technologies that will afford tangible safety benefits to sterile products.

Three elements are vital to a modernized approach to aseptic processing:

1. *Separation* of the aseptic processing line from the surrounding room environment, including the direct contamination risks posed by people.
2. Use of *automation* and integration to replace manual operations (interventions and other activities conducted by human operators) and transfers that still exist in legacy operations and are well-known sources of contamination risk.
3. Robust *advanced testing and monitoring* approaches to increase the amount of information on the state of process control.

This chapter will focus primarily on the first two elements, but will also consider the promise of the third.

IMPORTANCE OF A ROBUST ASEPTIC PROCESS DESIGN

There is no area of pharmaceutical manufacturing where strict adherence to cGMPs is more critical than aseptic processing. Aseptic processing is a true test of cGMP conformance, requiring daily vigilance in attending to the many critical details that establish and maintain an ongoing state of control (2). The objective is at once technically challenging and fundamental: to assure that each commercially distributed unit is safe for administration to patients. cGMP adherence starts with meticulous attention to many exacting needs that provide the foundation for a robust process, and operations that failed to meet this high standard have resulted in grave public health hazards (3,4). The FDA's 2004 guidance on *Sterile Drug Products Produced by Aseptic Processing* underscores the unacceptable risk to a patient from a contaminated drug.

> Sterile drug manufacturers should have a keen awareness of the public health implications of distributing a nonsterile product. Poor cGMP conditions at a manufacturing facility can ultimately pose a life-threatening health risk to a patient.

Consequently, establishing the capability to operate in a continuous state of control is essential. This capability is founded in a robust facility, equipment, and process design. Additionally, to ensure ongoing process control, a program for daily batch monitoring and periodic performance evaluation is critical to rapidly identify any potential risks to product sterility. As noted in ICH Q9 and Q10 (5,6), quality risk management and knowledge management provide the foundation for developing such design and control approaches, and sustaining any cGMP-compliant manufacturing operation.

Sterility testing methods, while useful for detecting major contamination in a batch, are analytically and statistically limited in their ability to detect very low-level batch contamination. As a result, the QC test used for batch release only provides a small part of the information needed to evaluate if a batch is sterile. Other data and information used to evaluate whether each dose in a given batch is produced safely are also similarly imperfect. Yet, in the absence of more extensive and sensitive measures of drug sterility, a number of major elements are integral to evaluate the ongoing capability of an aseptic process. Various measurements associated with each of these "macro" elements necessarily take on great prominence in assessing whether an

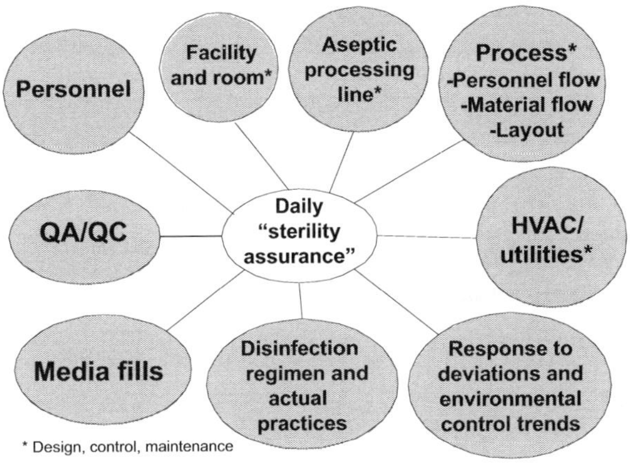

Figure 1 Macro model of daily sterility assurance: This illustrates the "macro" elements that help gauge state of control of a process. Data and information are obtained for each macro element from various personnel, facility, equipment, utility, and process monitoring systems, as well as from quality control tests.

aseptically processed batch (or a series of batches) is sufficiently low in contamination risk to merit being labeled as sterile (Fig. 1).

Many, if not all, of the risks associated with each of the macro elements in Figure 1 can be mitigated by modern design approaches. If assurance of sterility is not built into the manufacturing facility and process design by reducing or "designing out" identified risks, evaluation of daily operations will be too dependent upon monitoring and analytical uncertainty.[1]

Thus, at the core of the sensitive nature of aseptic processing is the *difficult detectability of episodic batch events that cause nonsterility*. The responsibility of a manufacturer to *detect and correct process events that may introduce invisible microbial contaminants*[2] into a product is a challenging one. Understanding the magnitude of this challenge to detect these risks in daily aseptic processing makes it clear why a firm must ensure that it has a robust design from the outset.[3]

A MAJOR STRIDE FORWARD

Since the 1980s, there have been steady and systematic improvements in aseptic manufacturing technology and process capability. The FDA's 2004 aseptic processing guidance, published under the cGMPs for the 21st century initiative, reflects FDA's risk-based and scientific approach by stating some important *design principles* (7,8). It is noteworthy that these principles are very much in accord with guidance produced in Japan and Europe in recent years (9,10):

1. The single greatest source of risk in aseptic processing is personnel-related contamination, and today's processing lines address this risk by incorporating the following into the aseptic line design:
    - *Automation* and integration of aseptic line operations to eliminate manual interventions wherever possible. As automation increases, the cumulative risk of production operators as vectors of contamination in the aseptic process will diminish.
    - *Separation* of the external clean room environment from the aseptic processing line. Use of isolators or a fully secured ("closed") restricted access barrier systems (RABS) is very common to accomplish this separation.
2. Design of personnel and material flow (e.g., material transfers) should be optimized to prevent unnecessary activities that could increase the potential for introducing contaminants to exposed product, containers, closures, or the surrounding environment.

At the time of the writing of FDA's 2004 guidance, significant industry progress to systematically improve aseptic processing was already under way. The introduction in the early 1990s

[1] Also note that most of this important data is not available in real time.

[2] It is also important to minimize the introduction of foreign particles into products, especially parenterals and ophthalmics. Visible particles should be strictly prevented by proper design, maintenance, and control.

[3] 21 CFR 211.42 and 211.113 of the CGMPs establish the requirement for a firm to design and build quality into the entire aseptic processing operation.

of isolators and restricted access barriers (i.e., this term refers to continuously secured lines that have special design provisions, and are properly operated and controlled during operations to maintain separation) led to major changes in aseptic manufacturing. The industry has continued to increase the usage of these separative technologies to ensure reduced contamination risk, greater process predictability, and improved consistency, thereby assuring cGMP compliance. There was a realization within industry that operations lacking these approaches were founded in a insufficient understanding of the many contamination vectors present in older operations that had resulted in too many well-documented failures. A more sophisticated understanding has resulted in the relatively widespread use of sound risk management approaches to develop new and modified process designs that better protect the exposed sterile product.

The industry and process equipment vendors deserve credit for their application of technological innovation that resulted in an important paradigm shift. This transition has been further facilitated by the FDA's 21st century initiative, and the 21 CFR 211 cGMP regulations, which do not specify which technologies to use, and instead promote continual improvement under a robust quality system that supports implementation of prompt adaptations in response to observed process deviations, weaknesses, or flaws. While they do not prescribe or prohibit specific technologies, FDA's cGMP regulations do require a drug company's management to assure that operations are properly designed, validated, and closely monitored to establish and maintain lifecycle robustness.

Yet it is important to note that the paradigm shift toward safer aseptic processing is not yet complete. Some aseptic operations that are unnecessarily vulnerable to contamination hazards remain in the industry. Antiquated design concepts continue to be perilously open to the adverse influence of external variables. These will always require a more cautious ongoing approach to validation and monitoring to determine if the process is dependable and capable of meeting its requirements.

These older, open aseptic processing systems will continue to receive extra regulatory attention because so many variables must be properly controlled to ensure consistent contamination prevention. FDA inspections have found noncompliant facilities that allow a major and persistent risk of sporadic contamination. These systems lacked the inherent process capability needed to substantially and robustly protect exposed sterile materials from external risks. Ultimately these firms realized the need for very extensive corrective actions to eliminate fundamental design flaws.

In summary, when assessing daily operational risks to the exposed sterile product, human performance is particularly unpredictable and difficult to measure, and at times serious risks to product sterility may be essentially imperceptible. Delicate heating, ventilation, and air conditioning (HVAC) balance issues, process flow (i.e., people, materials), equipment, transfers, and disinfection are also areas that loom large in assurance of sterility. The FDA guidance and an International Society for Pharmaceutical Engineering (ISPE) Baseline Guide (11) nicely articulate this holistic principle of the profound influence of external variables, particularly on traditional open systems, stating:

> Due to the interdependence of the various rooms that make up an aseptic processing facility, it is essential to carefully define and control the dynamic interactions permitted between cleanrooms (7)
>
> [An aseptic process requires] a strict design regime, not only on the process area, but on the interactions with surrounding areas and the movement of people, materials and equipment so as not to compromise the aseptic conditions (11)

Some Questions to Consider

Questions a manufacturer evaluating its aseptic processing operations might need to address include:

- Are your operations founded in 1950 to 1980s design knowledge that includes controlling the complex interactions of zoned clean rooms and heavy reliance on direct human interventions as features of the production process?

- Is a multidisciplinary process used to conceive design of your new or modified facility? Does this include a formal risk assessment program to assist in identifying and abating risk, particularly with respect to human contamination?
- Are process development scientists (e.g., microbiologists, engineers) aware of modern separation, automation, and testing approaches that can be used to improve process reliability, efficiency, and safety?
- Have modern transfer concepts been considered for your new operation?
- Have you evaluated equipment operation to determine the risk of corrective interventions and determined how they might be eliminated?
- Are your isolators and RABS designed with careful attention to ergonomics so that interventions, where unavoidable, can be managed with minimal risk?
- While using a RABS concept, are you able to operate the RABS in a truly continuously closed manner?

SEPARATION, AUTOMATION, AND TESTING

The implementation of advanced aseptic processing technologies invariably brings up many specific questions regarding terminology and design choices. With this in mind, this chapter will now address three specific focus areas—separation, automation, and testing—with a bit more specificity.[4]

Separation: Moving from Open to Closed Systems

The movement toward closed systems for aseptic processing has been an important advance to secure patient safety. For the purposes of this chapter, a closed system is defined as one that either has no openings to the external environment or is sealed by air over seal or pressure differential during operations.

When an *isolator* is used, the impact of surrounding areas while not eliminated is greatly reduced. Another popular separative design is use of a *closed RABS*. This design approach, while not as protective as isolators for various reasons, is also an advanced approach if access doors or hatches are only opened prior to operations for cleaning, sporicidal disinfection, and aseptic setup where needed. The key factor that is essential in achieving true separation for an isolator or closed RABS is that direct operator intervention is obviated at all times during production. All interventions must be performed using only the gloves built into the walls of the isolator or closed RABS.

Material transfer is a key element of all separative technologies. For isolators, it is important to prevent the breaching of isolation, and for closed RABS, it is similarly critical. For an *open* RABS, direct operator interventions by definition may occur. This means that the contamination control advantage, which accrues from the elimination of direct intervention, is not attained. Some of the operational concept and control procedures used by firms operating open RABS have not significantly increased confidence over older operations because direct interventions in open RABS are inherently riskier than isolator or closed RABS interventions that maintain system integrity using separative technology. It is not clear whether open systems can be considered a significant advance over many traditional operations already operating for many years with such a hybrid concept (line has extensive barriers; doors frequently opened) (12).

Additionally, RABS operations require fully gowned production staff. For open RABS, which allow direct operator intervention, intervention risks from these operators would continue unless stringent operational procedures that exclude any direct interventions are strictly followed with exceedingly rare documented exception. This means that gowning rooms and clean room zoning essentially follow the typical human clean room design model in scale and

[4] The reader is encouraged to work with cGMP compliance staff in the centers and district offices, and with review staff, during the conceptual design of a new facility, manufacturing line, or product to obtain initial input. After that initial feedback on a novel design, the manufacturer is ultimately responsible for demonstrating and justifying a sound design and control concept and adequate ongoing procedures to the FDA inspection team during cGMP inspections.

approach. The open RABS would be located in an ISO 7 (operational) clean room as a minimum, often with at least an immediately surrounding curtained area with ISO 5 HEPA filtered air, or even "wall-to-wall" HEPA filter ISO 5 operations. Thus, when considering new design options, it is important to be mindful that the lower level of separation in an open RABS design means that the surrounding room is more of a factor in contamination control than in isolators. And, a closed RABS provides a more robust separative concept that falls somewhere in between an isolator and an open RABS.

With this understanding of risk gradation, it becomes clear why the advantages of truly closed systems are so substantial. When a process is isolated, most of the focus can be on what happens within the confines of the "contained" environment of the processing line. The surrounding room environment for an isolator, while still requiring sound design and careful control, is far less critical to the prevention of risk than the manned clean room environment immediately surrounding a traditional (or open RABS) line. The newer separative technology systems compress the legacy clean room into a smaller facility footprint and provide major efficiencies through use of a more focused control approach.[5] Thus, a design decision to substantially "close off" the exposed sterile drug from external factors through separation technologies contrasts sharply with the old paradigm that is vulnerable to the impact of numerous complex clean room control variables in immediate and ancillary clean rooms.

Automation: Moving into the 21st Century

The 2004 FDA guidance notes the benefits of automation and integration. The following are three key excerpts:

> Any intervention or stoppage during an aseptic process can increase the risk of contamination. The design of equipment used in aseptic processing should limit the number and complexity of aseptic interventions by personnel. For example, personnel intervention can be reduced by integrating an on-line weight check device, thus eliminating a repeated manual activity within the critical area.
>
> Rather than performing an aseptic connection, sterilizing the preassembled connection using sterilize-in-place (SIP) technology also can eliminate a significant aseptic manipulation. Automation of other process steps, including the use of technologies such as robotics, can further reduce risk to the product.
>
> Use of a double-door or integrated sterilizer helps ensure direct product flow, often from a lower to a higher classified area. Airlocks and interlocking doors will facilitate better control of air balance throughout the aseptic processing facility. Airlocks should be installed between the aseptic manufacturing area entrance and the adjoining unclassified area. Other interfaces such as personnel transitions or material staging areas are appropriate locations for air locks.

There is widespread industry recognition of the significant benefit of many of these process improvements. It is standard design practice today for a processing line design to eliminate the risky open human manipulation of manually connecting a sterile holding vessel to the aseptic filling machine through integrating an SIP (sterilization-in-place)/CIP (cleaning-in-place) capable line. Similarly, firms are now routinely automating component charging or weight checking, resulting in significantly reduced risk of a previously repetitive and risky human intervention.

However, there remains a lot of room for progress in the area of automation. Automation has progressed more slowly than might have been anticipated in aseptic processing, although the technology is readily available. Many aseptic operations still require extensive manual activities and transfers. Unfortunately, jams, misfeeds, or other process malfunctions that lead to unplanned interventions continue to be well known and fundamental root causes of contamination, especially on lines that do not use a closed separative concept.

The concepts of separation (as discussed in subsection "Separation: Moving from Open to Closed Systems") and automation are not exclusive concepts, and are in fact very related.

[5] The shift to a more isolated environment requires a change in personnel skillset needs. Fewer operators to perform operations, and more automation experts, engineers, information systems specialists, and microbiologists are generally needed to address ongoing controls of these complex systems (including daily production floor issues such as maintenance and assessing SCADA system data).

Automation intertwines with separative part of design because the concepts of "restricted access" and "separation" are meant to preclude substantial involvement of people. When one observes a system that has a de facto operating approach (if not also SOP provisions) that permits opening of doors to RABS units for manual interventions, this would seem to reveal a process weakness in the separative design concept and also the lack of robust automation.

Some examples of automation found in many of today's aseptic designs include:

Automation and Integration—Some Examples

- SIP replacing manual aseptic connection
- Integrated transfers
  - Rapid transfer port
  - Decontaminating transfer port, for example, using hydrogen peroxide, chlorine dioxide, peracetic acid.
- Automated transfers
  - Lyophilizer loading was completely manual in the past, but over the last 20 years automated loading has become the standard for lyophilizer design. Firms now design the process flow to eliminate or dramatically reduce personnel involvement and instead use automated conveyance and loading or slot-type lyophilizer doors, which greatly reduce human borne contamination and also protect the lyophilizer environment.
  - Integrated dry heat tunnels are now used to ensure direct product flow without need for transport of batched sterilized (and depyrogenated) vials by gowned operator.
- Robotics
  - Firms are beginning to use robotic arms in place of humans (13). Robots that are amenable to high-level disinfection are commercially available and these units are also capable of operating in an ISO 5 or better clean environment, because particle levels are well controlled.
- Remote environmental monitoring devices
  - Total particulate counting systems operate remotely, and there are now monitoring systems that use spectrometry to get real-time information regarding airborne microbial contamination. These systems show promise in detecting viable but nonculturable bacteria as well. Systems for remote and fully automatic loading of active air sampling devices have also been developed. Such innovations can lead to a reduced likelihood for false positive results.

Testing

Many modern testing and monitoring approaches are available to manufacturers. There are promising new techniques for more rapid and comprehensive detection of environmental contaminants. Microbial identification technology has progressed tremendously in the last 10 years. More compact and capable nonviable particle monitoring systems can provide real-time process control data for use as an informative adjunct to traditional environmental monitoring methods.[6] Enhanced microbial identification methods (genotyping) help to correctly diagnose the source of sterility problems, reducing uncertainty and assumptions based on more tenuous data from the traditional identification technologies. This assists with investigations of certain environmental monitoring issues, along with sterility or media fill failure investigations.

In addition, better environmental data interpretations are now more common due not only to enhanced analytical capability, but also due to greatly improved trending systems. Many new analytical tools allow a firm to more reliably detect problems and measure process performance with respect to contamination prevention. These enhanced trending practices have been facilitated by software that has made collation and review of large quantities of data much more efficient and effective than in the past.

[6] This is particularly helpful in advanced aseptic processing at critical locations such as at an isolator egress port (e.g., "mousehole").

These advances are resulting in better and more comprehensive quality systems approaches to ensure the state of control of the aseptic process. The FDA has stated its interest in beneficial analytical advancements. The 2004 aseptic processing guidance recognizes the potential of such advances in this often-cited passage:

> Other suitable microbiological test methods (e.g., rapid test methods) can be considered for environmental monitoring, in-process control testing, and finished product release testing after it is demonstrated that the methods are equivalent or better than traditional methods (e.g., USP).

In addition, other FDA publications cite FDA's interest in beneficial analytical technologies. The FDA's final report on cGMPs for the 21st century (14) includes a section that highlights its new "science-based policies and procedures to facilitate innovation within the existing regulatory framework." Both the FDA aseptic processing guidance and the landmark guidance entitled "Process Analytical Technology (PAT)—*A Framework for Innovative Pharmaceutical Manufacturing and Quality Assurance*" are cited as providing encouragement for modern manufacturing approaches (15). PAT provides for timely process analysis to ensure feedback on ongoing manufacturing performance. This feedback then will promptly "feed forward" to ensure timely process corrections and ongoing maintenance of manufacturing control.

At the end of the day, improved tests, and better monitoring and trending systems, provide firms with important information to help identify root causes and control processes. With proper problem identification, a firm can then confidently direct resources toward effective resolution of the true root cause(s). As firms begin to more rapidly and accurately detect contamination risks and diagnose root causes, major sterility problems will be far less common.

CONSIDERATIONS FOR TECHNOLOGY SELECTION

There is considerable convergence between cGMP goals and good business practices for advanced aseptic processing, based on general industry trends with a variety of approved installations. Some of the distinctions that can be drawn between the technological choices are outlined in Table 1.

CLOSED SYSTEMS: MORE LATITUDE

FDA recently published a Q&A on the topic of closed systems, which reinforces incentives for isolated systems and FDA's risk-based approach to regulation (16). This Q&A provides an expectation for process simulation that recognizes the risk mitigation provided by a closed system.

> 10. What is the acceptable media fill frequency in relation to the number of shifts? Normally, media fills should be repeated twice per shift per line per year. Is the same frequency expected of a process conducted in an isolator?
>
> A firm's justification for the frequency of media fills in relation to shifts should be risk-based, depending on the type of operations and the media fill study design. For *closed*, highly automated systems run on multiple shifts, a firm with a rigorous media fill design may be justified to conduct a lower number of total media fill runs. Such a program can be appropriate provided that it still assures performance of media fills for each aseptic processing line at least semi-annually. The 2004 guidance for industry on *Sterile Drug Products Produced by Aseptic Processing* states that "[A]ctivities and interventions representative of each shift, and shift changeover, should be incorporated into the design of the semi-annual qualification program." In addition, the *EU Annex 1, Manufacture of Sterile Medicinal Products,* states that "Normally, process simulation tests should be repeated twice a year per shift and process."
>
> Certain modern manufacturing designs (isolators and "closed vial" filling) afford isolation of the aseptic process from microbiological contamination risks (e.g., operators and surrounding room environment) throughout processing. For such *closed* systems[7], if the

[7] The following footnote is appended to this FDA Q&A: "This does not apply to RABS (Restricted Access Barrier Systems)."

Table 1 Comparison of Traditional Versus Closed RABS Versus Isolator Aseptic Processing

Traditional (including open RABS)	Closed RABS[a]	Isolator
Significant costs of gowns	Significant costs of gowns	Significantly lower garbing requirements and substantially lower costs
Gowning/degowning time	Gowning/degowning time	Simple garb minimizes gowning time
Surface and air sampling daily	Surface and air sampling daily	Less frequent surface sampling
Lower automation, more interventions	Higher automation and integration, less personnel impact	Higher automation and substantial level of integration. Significantly less personnel impact.
Many manual activities	Less personnel intensive (SIP is widely used, CIP common, but manual aseptic equipment setup and sporicidal decontamination are still critical sources of variability)	Significantly less personnel intensive (SIP, CIP common, automated sporicidal decontamination cycle)
Daily dismantling, assembly of sterilized equipment	Potential for multiple consecutive days without disassembly, sterilization, and aseptic reassembly	Consecutive days without disassembly, sterilization, and aseptic reassembly
Environmental deviation investigations more frequent	Environmental deviation investigations typically less frequent than traditional lines	Environmental deviation investigations very infrequent
Focus on ISO 5 area, immediately surrounding clean room, and ancillary clean rooms	Focus on both ISO 5 and immediate surrounding area, with less focus on ancillary areas	Enclosed ISO 5 area is separated from room environment, and is the focus
Disinfection or decontamination procedures for processing lines and surrounding area are intensive, intricate, nearly always manual, dependent on thoroughness of operators, and of uneven efficacy	Disinfection or decontamination procedures for processing lines and surrounding area are intensive, intricate, often manual, dependent on thoroughness of operators, and of uneven efficacy	Decontamination procedures for processing lines and surrounding area are automated and consistently produce a microbe-free environment
Sterility failures still occur and require comprehensive, extremely time-intensive investigations into origin of problem and major losses of personnel time, operational time, and materials that went into the operation	Sterility failures less frequent	Sterility failures are rare
Media fill failures still occur; investigations of origin and scope of potential hazard are significant costs/investments	Media fill failures less frequent than traditional lines	Media fill failures very infrequent
Class 100 area is vulnerable. Numerous parts of operation potentially pose risks. Intricate everyday control	Simplifies operation in terms of process and material flow during operations	Simplifies operation in terms of process and material flow
Several rooms required for various process stages	Several rooms required for various process stages	Small facility footprint; generally fewer rooms to maintain
Elaborate multiroom pressure cascade needed	Elaborate multiroom pressure cascade needed	Simplified overall pressure cascade
Transfer to and from line provides some, or at times significant, risk	Transfer steps, if performed using robust transfer ports, are designed to prevent transmission of any contamination into the closed RABS during operations	Transfer steps, if performed using robust transfer ports, are designed to prevent transmission of any contamination into isolator
Material charging often performed by personnel	Charging performed through transfer ports. Mitigates risk	Charging performed through transfer ports. Mitigates risk
Intervention is generally performed by person operating in Class 10,000 environment	Intervention performed by person that has wall separating them from product	Intervention performed by person that is isolated from product

[a]Closed RABS refers to a system controlled so that it remains secure throughout aseptic manufacturing operations. For example, procedures ensure that doors are not opened at any time once manufacturing commences. When a door is opened, the aseptic manufacturing operation concludes and a new cycle of cleaning and decontamination precedes the next operation.

design of the processing equipment is robust and the extent of manual manipulation in the manufacturing process is minimized, a firm can consider this information in determining its media fill validation approach. For example, it is expected that a conventional aseptic processing line that operates on two shifts be evaluated twice per year per shift, and culminate in four media fills. However, for aseptic filling conducted in an isolator over two shifts, it may be justified to perform fewer than four media fill runs per year, while still evaluating the line semi-annually to assure a continued state of aseptic process control. This lower total number of media fill runs would be based on sound risk rationale and would be subject to re-evaluation if contamination issues (e.g., product nonsterility, media fill failure, any problematic environmental trends) occur.

CONCLUSION

Continued innovation and progress in aseptic processing is vital in our continued efforts to produce the safest possible medicines using currently available and proven technologies. The importance of exploiting current technological capabilities has been well demonstrated by significant industry and regulatory experience. Separative technologies such as closed RABS and isolators, and use of automation and enhanced control approaches, have been demonstrated to greatly reduce contamination risk and have enhanced patient safety. In contrast, significant sterility issues have occurred in operations that relied on insufficient understanding of contamination prevention and antiquated facilities. Based on the advancements of the last 20 years, and a receptive regulatory environment for innovation, one can be hopeful about what upcoming years hold in store for further technological advancement in aseptic processing. Many more innovative ideas to improve on the current processing paradigms will likely be offered for industrial adoption, and will further enhance assurance of consumer safety. The FDA, industry, and, most important of all, the consumers of aseptically produced health care products, will surely benefit from continued industrial modernization.

DISCLAIMER

This chapter was written by Mr. Friedman in his private capacity. This chapter reflects the personal views of the author and should not be construed to represent FDA's views or policies. No official support or endorsement by the Food and Drug Administration is intended or should be inferred.

REFERENCES

1. FDA. Pharmaceutical cGMPs for the 21st Century: A Risk-Based Approach. Washington, DC: US Food and Drug Administration, 2002.
2. Avis K. Personnel training—An academic approach. Bull Parenter Drug Assoc 1971; 25(5):235–238.
3. Friedman R. Aseptic processing contamination case studies and the pharmaceutical quality system. PDA J Pharm Sci Technol 2005; 59(2):118–126.
4. Blossom D, Noble-Wang J, Su J, et al. Multistate outbreak of Serratia marscesens bloodstream infections by contamination of prefilled heparin and isotonic sodium chloride solution syringes. Arch Intern Med 2009; 169(18):1705–1711.
5. ICH Q9. Quality risk management. Fed Regis 2006; 71(106):32105–32106.
6. ICH Q10. Pharmaceutical quality system. Fed Regis 2009; 74(66):15990–15991.
7. FDA. Guideline on Sterile Drug Products Produced by Aseptic Processing. Washington, DC: US Food and Drug Administration, 2004.
8. FDA Issues Final Report on 21st Century CGMPs. http://www.pharmamanufacturing.com/industrynews/2004/93.html. Published September 30, 2004.
9. Task Force on Sterile Drug Products Produced by Aseptic Processing. Guidance for Industry—Sterile Drug Products Produced by Aseptic Processing (with support from the Japanese Ministry of Health, Labor, and Welfare). 2005.
10. EMEA. European GMP, Annex 1—Sterile Medicinal Products. 2008.
11. ISPE Sterile Facilities Baseline Guide, International Society for Pharmaceutical Engineering. Tampa, FL, 1999.
12. Morris W. Health Authority Special Report: RABS Risks and Rewards—A Discussion with FDA's Rick Friedman and Brenda Uratani. Bethesda, MD: PDA, 2008:30.

13. DeSantis F, Amsberry K, Folks JL, et al. Aseptic formulation and filling using isolator technology. Pharm Technol Outsourcing 2003; 32–42.
14. FDA. Final Report on cGMPs for the 21st century. FDA, 2004.
15. FDA. PAT—A Framework for Innovative Pharmaceutical Development, Manufacturing, and Quality Assurance. 2004.
16. FDA. Questions and Answers on Current Good Manufacturing Practices, Good Guidance Practices, Level 2 Guidance Production and Process Controls. www.fda.gov/Drugs/GuidanceComplianceRegulatoryInformation/Guidances/ucm1. November 2009.

30 The evolution of advanced aseptic processing for pharmaceutical manufacturing: perspectives of a regulatory scientist[1]

David Hussong

This chapter will focus on a microbiology reviewer's observationson the evolution of the barrier system for aseptic processing of pharmaceuticals and the development of standards for their use. Some related information will be provided in this chapter that considers isolation systems for laboratory use, and isolators for sterility testing. Discussion of barrier systems will include restricted access barrier systems (RABS) and isolator systems (isolators). Some observations are offered on microbiological measurement of environments used for pharmaceutical manufacturing. The scientific review philosophy and the regulatory experience form the basis of this perspective.

The premarketing functions of FDA's review staff in the Center for Drug Evaluation and Research (CDER), the Center for Biologics Evaluation and Research (CBER), and the Center for Veterinary Medicine (CVM) include the scientific–technical evaluation of sterilization processes and their validation. Inspections are sometimes included as part of the premarket evaluation to ensure, for example, that the firm can maintain a consistent capability for meeting the commitments stated in the application. The postmarketing functions of FDA's field investigators include the assurance that the overall state of control is maintained and, where failures in products or control have occurred, appropriate corrective action is/was taken. Carrying out the premarketing and postmarketing functions in FDA consists of cooperative efforts between the review staff, compliance staff, and field investigators, with some variations in the implementation of those functions, depending upon the Center involved. The scientific review philosophy, statutory obligations, and the FDA experience have molded the way the pre- and postmarket functions are coordinated in the Agency.

ASEPTIC PROCESSING OF PHARMACEUTICAL PRODUCTS

Aseptic processing has been considered the most demanding of sterile manufacturing processes because of the need for existing environmental and procedural controls required to get the task done without contaminating the product units. Simple microbiological tasks such as culture transfer have made this point particularly clear to many technicians. For example, any tissue culture experiment includes scrupulous controls to prevent contamination and maintain culture purity.

"Aseptic processing," for the manufacture of sterile drugs, is a jargon derived from basic microbiological laboratory terminology. The expression, "aseptic process" suggests that it is not a sterile process, and is the result of medical microbiology terminology for handling laboratory cultures without infecting the technician or contaminating the culture. Unfortunately, many individuals have tried to equate this jargon with sterile manufacturing, and several have even written papers comparing the terms (1). These pursuits of equating jargon (aseptic processing) with a philosophical and absolute concept (sterile) seem like futile exercises since they ultimately demonstrate that the terms are not the same.

In contrast, terminal sterilization processes permit mathematical extrapolations that allow prediction to a point where survival becomes an improbable event. Louis Pasteur was the first to describe heat "sterilization" in his work that disproved spontaneous generation (2). The food industry advanced the science of heat sterilization with thermal measures and mathematical relations to microbial inactivation (3). These studies demonstrated that different foods (by pH

[1] These comments are those of the author only and do not necessarily represent the positions or policies of the FDA.

and carbohydrate content) influenced the requirement for heat of process (F_0) to achieve "sterility." In their examples, F_0 values ranging from 0.5 to 8.0 minutes were needed to achieve "sterility" (3). For pharmaceutical processes, terminal sterilization imparts the greatest confidence that the finished product has been rendered free of living microorganisms. However, the need for aseptic processes remains as more complex molecular materials heading toward the pharmaceutical market. Other parenteral products will require aseptic processing due to the need for medicines and container-closure systems that will not withstand terminal sterilization.

However, it is clear that sterility (an absolute concept) cannot be determined with absolute certainty. Microbiological death kinetics is expressed in logarithms, and so the population is always 10^n and will never reach zero, that is, sterility. Pflug and Smith (4) used mathematical extrapolation from thermal killing of spores, based on challenges with 1×10^4 spores added to each of 20 samples. In this example, a process imparting an equivalent heating time (U) of 12 minutes reduced the surviving spore population from 10^4 to 10^{-2} on each biological indicator, when the D_{121} value was two minutes. There are three points to emphasize here. First, this estimates probability of survival, not sterility. Second, this estimate is based on reliable assumptions about the resistance of the biological indicator relative to the expected bioburden. Third, survival endpoints can be projected to a fraction (10^{-n}) that represents improbable survival, based on a rigorous process. These assumptions and calculations cannot be applied to aseptic processing.

In the 1980s, a subtle change in the pharmaceutical manufacturing industry came about as a result of generic drugs. A great number of new manufacturers began to produce drugs, and many companies with experience in small-scale operations such as pharmacy, entered the manufacturing industry. Among the small-volume parenteral and ophthalmic drug manufacturers, many of the new companies chose technologies capable of making all of their products with the fewest filling lines to reduce the investment costs. Rather than constructing manufacturing facilities with aseptic processing and terminal sterilization capacities, these firms prepared all their products by aseptic processing. A great number of products came to market having been aseptically produced, although the products themselves were capable of being sterilized by terminal heat processes that offer measurable sterility assurance and simpler controls to assure sterility.

Regulatory agencies recognized that many aseptically manufactured products could be sterilized by terminal processes. In 1991, the U.S. Food and Drug Administration proposed a regulation that required terminal sterilization in an attempt to improve the safety of these drugs (5). Comments and discussion concerning this rule revealed concerns over the lack of measurable sterility assurance in products made by aseptic processing. To minimize these concerns, engineers pursued the integration of technologies developed for space exploration, electronics manufacture, and sterilization sciences. In 1990, a symposium on sterile product manufacturing described the future of aseptic processes as incorporation of robotics and systems that would remove personnel and other sources of contamination from the processing area (6). These proposals added measurable controls to aseptic processing, but they did not improve the measurable probability of nonsterility. However, they did generate a "warm feeling" about the direction of new processes, and that extended a general confidence in aseptically processed products as supported by media fill data that showed a limited freedom from microbial contamination.

EARLY BARRIER SYSTEMS

Other uses for barrier systems had already been accepted for various laboratory and production uses. The "glove box" concept from research laboratories had been adapted to the sterility test laboratory. Sterility test isolators were in use in a number of facilities. The review philosophy was that these offered a benefit to enhance confidence in sterility test data for release of the product by reducing false positives (false indications of contamination). Toward this end, it was to the benefit of the manufacturer to assure a clean and decontaminated isolator and less regulatory oversight was needed. "False–positive" results may have economic impacts and are unfortunate technical artifacts, but do not result in unsafe products going to market. Any public health consequence of false–positive results was due to reduced availability of product. It seemed a great irony that the inquiries concerning the laboratory practices relative to disinfecting these environments often focused on "what the regulators required" for adequate demonstration of disinfection. From the perspective of risk management, less regulation seemed the better choice. For reviewers, a false–negative result (a technically more likely event due to the methods used in sterility testing) was of greater public health concern.

Other isolators in use in 1990 included systems designed to put a physical barrier between operators and toxic or other dangerous drug ingredients. These systems are unique and use different air pressure and airflow characteristics. Their design is to keep the hazardous pharmaceutical materials from leaving the isolator, so airflow may be inward. This requires that the environments surrounding the systems should be suitable for aseptic processing, since the environmental air may enter the isolator.

TECHNICAL PROGRESS AND PROCESS MEASURES

The pharmaceutical industry has come a long way with aseptic processing in the past decade, but there remain weak links in the processing of sterile components to make sterile pharmaceutical products. The key to understanding this philosophy is found in the example that filters cannot provide the same certainty of yielding a sterile output as would a heat or radiation process. This applies to filters used for the product solution, as well as the filters used for the environmental air surrounding the manufacturing process. Additionally, equipment items that are constructed with tortuous pathways are prone to obstructions that reduce the contact and effectiveness of sterilants, and impair the testing of the sterilization validation. Such "difficult to treat" items would require processing that imparts a greater safety margin since process lethality is more difficult to measure, control, and predict. These practical concerns demonstrate the underlying fragility of a complex manufacturing system regardless of their technologically advanced nature.

In basic microbiology practices, cultures are transferred at a laboratory bench under minimum environmental controls and, with reasonable technical precaution, the technician and the culture remain uncompromised. In more stringent and complex processes, such as tissue culture, environmental control and enhanced personnel practices are necessary to protect the cell culture. Similarly, when more infectious biological agents are manipulated, biosafety cabinets and gloveboxes are used to contain the contagion. The oldest design of a barrier system is observed in nature, where skin provides the primary barrier to microorganisms. When the skin is injured, that protective barrier is compromised and infection is often the result. Extending this infectious disease concept to industrial technology, the utility of barrier/isolator systems becomes intuitive: separate the operator (a common source of contamination) from the processing environment and product quality will improve.

The technologies developed to control the environment for aseptic processes grew out of biomedical and space engineering. NASA's attempts to comply with the United Nations' "Treaty on principles governing the activities of states in the exploration of and use of outer space, including the Moon and other celestial bodies," resulted in a policy that the probability of contamination of a spacecraft should be less than 10^{-3} (7). Manufacturing controls and containment for these spacecraft were developed, including standards for clean rooms and workstations. An interesting concept that was developed from this program was that spacecraft would be manufactured with controls to limit its microbial contamination to less than 10^{8}, and the subsequent sterilization process should reduce this population by "12 decades" to a net 10^{-4} (thus achieving a 10-fold "overkill"). To this author's knowledge, this may be the first description of a 12-D cycle. NASA drove the sterile processing technology to great improvements. During this era, there were developments in environmental containment, such as glove boxes and biosafety cabinets. These relied on some barrier (either airflow or a physical wall) to prevent contamination from entering the area near aseptic processes. The growth of these technologies paralleled simple advances, such as high efficiency particulate air (HEPA) showers and curtained work areas in conventional aseptic manufacturing facilities.

In the 1970s, the World Health Organization described the production of small batches of biological products (usually made by operator-intensive processes) yielding 1000 or so product units, and the recommended maximum contamination rate for simulated procedures was 0.3% (8). By the time the 1987 FDA's Compliance Guidance on Aseptic Processing (9) was published, a generally accepted maximum contamination rate for process simulations was 0.1%. While an improvement, an alternative point of view concerning these criteria is that any acceptance of contamination events is a de facto demonstration of nonsterility in the process stream, and this was a logical concern.

THE BIRTH OF ISOLATORS FOR MANUFACTURING

Manufacturing sterile drug and biological products advanced through many "breakthroughs," which seems to be the nature of technology. For example, as mechanical filling replaced hand-held pipettes, there was improvement in process control and the ability to move the operator away from close contact with the process. As engineering improved, mechanical filling equipment was constructed that was suitable for use in smaller environments. However, that improvement only took product quality to a certain point and was limited by environmental control and sterile component manipulations. As each of these other limiting factors was addressed in technological improvements, the overall process control and product quality were enhanced. As the improved engineering of controlled microenvironments approached practicality, improvements in transfer ports (10) and filling equipment (11) came together in an uneasy marriage that created the prototypes of barriers in pharmaceutical applications. Complete isolation systems were the initial goal. However, the technology was evolving.

In addition to the isolator, another early barrier system prototype was the "Restricted Access Barrier System" (12), or RABS. This technology represented a compromise, possibly because the isolator system was perceived as too hard to validate. The stated goal of RABS was to improve the control of the process steps from filtered bulk solution to the sealing of the vials. These critical elements were correctly identified as points where improved control would result in greater confidence that the process will yield a sterile product. Points of concern were operator intervention, aseptic connections, storage, handling and transfer of components and equipment, and equipment setup. This system limited the area of potential incursion of contamination by constructing a rigid wall from the overhead HEPA filters to below the work surface. A combination of hydrogen peroxide and peracetic acid produced a *"High-Level Disinfection"* of the surfaces within the barriers, using a system of sprays and wiping. Packages entering the RABS were decontaminated under ultraviolet lamps, and the environment was continuously flushed with air from the HEPA filters.

The target for success of the RABS system was to do better than 0.01% contamination in the media fill demonstrations and to show greatly improved data from environmental microbiology surveys. Data from media fill experiments produced no positives from 218,000 "simulated fill" containers, and no colony forming units (CFU) from 440 cubic meters of environmental air, no CFU from 45 settle plates, no CFU for 167 glove samples, and no CFU for barrier and equipment surface samples. These data were far "cleaner" than industry standards for maximum acceptable values. What was not presented for control tests were data for conventional aseptic filling. This means that although the system presented is much better than the minimum standards for conventional aseptic filling in a clean room, it was not possible to state that the system was universally better than a well-operated clean room. After all, each system appears capable of producing sterile products. Problems arise when the system is not operated properly, and under those circumstances, the capability of the system is not achieved.

Very few experiments were designed to assess the limitations of controls used in aseptic processing. There are general or overall validation experiments that culminate in a media fill to simulate the combined processes for aseptic filling. However, the controlled variation of discrete variables for the purpose of determining their effect on contamination of manufactured product is rarely attempted. When these have been attempted, the results have suggested that environmental contamination is secondary to procedural deviations that introduce the environmental flora (13). By analogy, Jones et al. (14) showed very little impact of surrounding environments to media fill results for blow-fill-seal processes. The clear implication is that the operator and the environment pose less risk when they are separated from the critical filling areas. Barrier systems (isolators and RABS) provide a suitable barrier so that contaminants in the surrounding air have a minimum effect on the filling system. For filling traditional product containers such as glass vials, the advantages of barrier systems are obvious.

LESSONS FROM PROTOTYPES

The barrier users group (BUGS) struggled with an impossible philosophical task brought on by the imprecise jargon of the industry and regulators. In their symposium in 1995, BUGS described a prototype barrier/isolator constructed by the LUMs group (Lilly, Upjohn, Merck).

The system included an environment for critical process steps (handling sterilized components) that eliminated operator intervention during filling and closing operations when they may be exposed to the processing environment. The group used a hydrogen peroxide vapor with low levels of peracetic acid to inactivate *Bacillus subtilis* var *niger* spores used as biological challenges placed in the chamber's stainless steel surfaces. In other experiments, ultraviolet lamps were used for decontamination. Both prototypes were challenged with media fill studies that evaluated the "sterility confidence level" (or SCL), and while these systems provided excellent results they were not quickly embraced.

In the desire for technological advancement, isolator systems were also developed to provide complete separation of the critical operations. One prototype used a system that "localized" the production environment with a perceived advantage that hydrogen peroxide vapor in steam could be used to kill environmental microorganisms. They described the process as sterilization. However, sterility is an absolute term and had been equated with sterilization validation linked to a practical concept of demonstrating the massive kill of $\geq$1 million ($\geq 10^6$) resistant spores. This one-in-a-million concept from the realm of terminal sterilization would become an unfortunate stumbling block for many of the procedures and criteria used in subsequent attempts to bring barrier systems into production facilities.

However, the inactivation of microbes on an isolator wall is less critical to product sterility than the sterilization of product-contact filling equipment (13). Equipment such as sterile solution transfer hoses and filling needles are typically sterilized in place using steam, regardless of whether the filling process is in a conventional clean room or an isolator. Although product solution-contact items may release entrapped microbes directly into the drug solution, the barrier walls and noncontact surfaces rarely shed microorganisms and do not support their survival. This means the concept of eliminating microbes from occluded locations in filling pumps or transfer hoses appropriately demands a rigorous sterilization, but noncritical surfaces and equipment do not need antimicrobial processing any greater than decontamination. This is especially true when the system is adequately cleaned and dried (processing that can reduce microbial counts to negligible amounts), as would be expected of traditional clean rooms. In the traditional clean room, treatments are applied to control microbial contamination of surfaces. The Association for Professionals in Infection Control and Epidemiology defined sterilization, high-level disinfection, low-level disinfection, and cleaning (15). Spaulding (16) classified *semi-critical* items for hospitals as those items that come into contact with mucous membranes or broken skin and determined these items should be treated by *high-level disinfection*. This type of clinical use imposes far greater patient exposure than do environments surrounding a filling operation. Based on the rationale provided by Spaulding, the regulatory review staff considered the high-level disinfection process of manufacturing isolators to be adequate treatment for most isolator surfaces that provided an appropriate margin for safety. The level of contamination in the isolator is not expected to be great since the cleaning processes controls will include basic hygienic practices during, for example, installation of stopper bowls and vial feed equipment. The recommendation for *high-level disinfection* of these surfaces seems appropriate for the isolator since the number and resistance of organisms entering during setup and cleaning are adequately controlled by the decontamination process challenged with spores. By comparison, the traditional clean room would be maintained under environmental controls that would reduce those incidental contamination events.

As defined by APIC (15), high-level disinfection will destroy all microorganisms with the exception of great numbers of spores. If one compares the preparation processes used for traditional aseptic processing, those equipment pieces that convey drug solutions (e.g., piping or fill needles) are usually sterilized with a great margin for safety. This is generally performed by steam heat processes, and there is little concern for process time or deterioration of the materials because these are understood and controlled. Until the 1980s, many additional large equipment items such as stopper bowls were cleaned and sanitized before use, but not steam sterilized. During the 1980s, there was a transition to sterilizing these items in larger autoclave chambers, but sterilization of these was validated by microbial challenges of approximately 1000 spores, based on their very small bioburden population. Regulatory creep in the 1990s increased the biological challenge for these equipment items based on speculation that it was necessary, and to be consistent with practices in the food industry where the microbial load is greater. Considering the amount of handling this equipment encounters after sterilization, the value of the increased spore challenge (10^3 to 10^6) is less important.

Although the early prototype barrier and isolator systems yielded spectacular results, there were failures. This happens with any complex and evolving technology whether it is space flight or personal computers. However, failures that were observed in the BUGS prototypes arose from equipment (a stopper positioning device operating with vacuum) that was perceived to have little risk of imparting contamination. This experience was of great value, and demonstrates that the collective knowledge of the process development scientists is the most valuable asset in designing and establishing appropriate manufacturing systems. A trend in current regulatory thinking is that "risk assessment" can manage hazards. However, the example provided shows that risk analysis might fail to identify the point of risk. The failures in this event were in equipment that would have equally failed in any filling systems.

As of 1999, barrier systems were slow to be accepted by the industry in North America (17). It was reported that regulatory speculations had discouraged manufacturers into withholding investments in this technology (18). The reluctance was reportedly due, in part, to inappropriately applied design and sterilization paradigms to the barrier system. These include decontamination of environments demonstrated by biological indicator (BI) challenges that show "6-log kills," and even greater challenges in certain instances. Additionally, when validation engineers attempted to show the effectiveness of their overall process by evaluating the effect of the decontaminating agent on the BIs as a whole, the use of fraction negative calculation was sometimes rejected for this use. In the strict application of fraction negative analysis of heat processes, multiple BIs should be immediately next to the thermocouple. While it is true such analysis may not be strictly applied to sterilization assessments in isolators, these objections are inappropriate for decontamination of an entire chamber. Additionally, the use of conventional spore carriers bearing 10^6 spores is a very robust challenge for an agent that works by a surface-contact action. With hydrogen peroxide vapor agents applied for decontamination, the uniformity of a process cannot be assured without distributing BIs and the overall process effect can only be measured by combining the results of the BIs used in the overall process. In this way, the BI challenge assessment reflects the process effect on the isolator as a whole. However, BI data are not without pitfalls. It should also be emphasized that uniform biological indicators for hydrogen peroxide processes were not available when many processes were designed, so resistance (D-value) has not been carefully considered in the development of many decontamination processes. Several claims about hydrogen peroxide's disinfection capability are not relevant because of the concentration of the agent. There are limits to the concentration of disinfectant that may be used and this might affect the lethality of the disinfection process. Also, a small shift in resistance of a BI can have great impact on the apparent death kinetics. In addition, layers of spores are not natural events in either a clean room or a barrier system that is properly cleaned. The normal procedures for cleaning any aseptic processing environment, including isolators, should result in a very low environmental bioburden, possibly less than 10 CFU per 25 cm^2, and not 1,000,000 spores on 1 cm^2. To make this perspective meaningful, the role of cleaning to decontamination is important since appropriate cleaning is necessary if the disinfection is to be effective.

Other concerns that impeded isolator acceptance include glove integrity tests, material handling systems (transfer ports and mouse holes), and classification of surrounding environments. For manufacturing purposes, the control of these systems requires that the probability of product contamination from the environment be minimized, although data from recent studies of sterility testing isolators show this is not a source of contamination when other good techniques are practiced (19). Additionally, the chamber walls and other nonproduct-contact surfaces are unlikely sources of microbial contamination when routine aseptic procedures are followed. Emphasis on microbiologically prudent practices relating to component handling and critical equipment handling should be the area of emphasis, just as they would be in aseptic filling conducted in a conventional clean room. In fact, most recent product recalls (due to lack of sterility assurance) in the United States have been due to failure to perform the proper and routine practices associated with current good manufacturing practices (CGMPs), such as failure to adjust sealing equipment, failure to separate processed and unprocessed components, and failures to document subprocesses or process deviations.

ESTABLISHMENT OF REGULATORY STANDARDS

A driving factor for the industry's acceptance of isolator technology has been whether it is economically feasible. In their original proposals, the BUGS group wanted to install isolators into uncontrolled environments based on data showing the chamber could be rendered free of contamination and could maintain that. Regulatory apprehension was based on the lack of experience with the systems as well as the awareness that only a controlled environment would assure the opened isolator did not become extensively contaminated. In a meeting between BUGS and FDA in 1992, the conservative recommendation was offered by FDA regulators that isolators should be housed within a Class 100,000 (ISO Class 8) or cleaner environment. While this raised the costs of using an isolator system, it also offered the opportunity to minimize the preparation between campaigns or interventions. Compared to a clean room, the smaller isolators can economically maintain temperature and humidity with more frequent air changes. To assure the environment is protected from airborne particles, a greater air flow may be used in isolators. Due to more turbulent airflow in isolators, a greater airflow rate is used as well, especially when mouse holes are needed for continuous product discharge. The increase of airflow poses some risk because the HEPA filters are not sterilizing filters.

Historically, data from operation of these systems indicated that they maintain exquisite environmental control when all systems were operating appropriately. Ironically, anecdotal reports indicate that data were not enough, and the conventional clean room paradigm continued to creep in, often requiring interventions such as equipment replacement or environmental monitoring that intrude on the system and defeat the protections from intrusion that the isolator was designed to provide. In the case of environmental monitoring, there was lively debate about its risks and benefits for barrier systems. Since the isolators might be operated for weeks, microbial medium may need to be brought in and out of the system. This is not without risk. However, the failure to monitor the system during use means there would be inadequate documentation of maintained control. A compromise position proposed that microbiological monitoring could be performed during validation experiments, and physical monitoring would be sufficient during pharmaceutical manufacture, but that compromise was not universally embraced. The failure to reach an appropriate compromise was based on interpretation of regulations that require a system for monitoring environmental conditions for aseptic processing areas.

However, environmental monitoring methods for microbiology remain largely unchanged since 1881, when Fanny Hesse introduced the use of agar for bacteriological medium (20), replacing potatoes and gelatin as the solid surface for cultivating microorganisms. Cultivation on agar media is the foundation of the colony count, and most quantitative monitoring standards are based on "colony forming units." The problem is that these standards require cultivation methods that may not detect some or all the flora present. As shown by Carson et al. (21), microorganisms cultivate less easily after exposure to the environment. So a readily culturable laboratory strain of *Burkholderia cepacia* may not be recovered after acclimation to growth in distilled water. Similarly, when microbiological counts in clean rooms were performed using comparative methods that included conventional medium (Soybean Casein Digest Agar: SCDA) and low nutrient "oligophilic" Raven Medium, the results showed that SCDM underestimated the viable count by 10- to 100-fold (22). Again, the actual populations are not reliably evaluated by test methods that are based on conventional procedures developed out of clinical laboratory practices. Certainly, the detection of microorganisms in these environments is meaningful. However, results that are free of detected colonies have less meaning for evaluating a barrier system's environmental control.

New technologies have been demonstrated that may be able to detect viable cells by means other than colony formation or turbidity. For detecting microorganisms in finished product, alternate methods have been accepted for testing approved products prior to their release to the market. Among these methods are tests that assess adenosine triphosphate production or gases from physiologic activities related to growth. For testing airborne microorganisms, fluorescence from essential enzymes or cofactors has been used with detection levels greater than colony counts. This has been reported anecdotally on the outlet of HEPA filters, suggesting that they do not retain microorganisms absolutely. Further research studies are needed to understand the significance of these reports. It seems probable that regulatory standards may need to evolve from "colonies" or "turbidity" when dealing with environmental microbes. However, it is clear that measurement of the resident flora is not reliably done through conventional methods and the use of a well-characterized biological challenge for decontamination studies is essential for establishing a starting point for microbiological standards for cleanliness of isolators.

The Office of Pharmaceutical Science in the CDER is the operational unit where review of manufacturing processes for sterile human drugs is performed. Within the meaning of the FD&C Act (505(b)(4)(g)), "the reviewing division is the division responsible for the review of an application for approval of a drug under this subsection or section 351 of the Public Health Service Act (including all scientific and medical matters, chemistry, manufacturing, and controls)."

The CDER review staff believes that the barrier system user should establish appropriate controls and procedures for these systems' preparation and operations. This has included operation times, speeds, material transfer, physical environment (temperature, pressure, air flow, humidity), and challenges to decontamination. Intuitively, we have retained precedents for filter use, based on the similar use of filters for conventional aseptic filling and component preparation. The review staff considers environmental control in a barrier system to be superior to the control in a clean room, and is willing to accept that microbiological monitoring may be reduced. These opinions are based on media fill data showing the risk of contamination is much less. It is also accepted that barrier systems can operate for longer periods without detectable contamination. Once the isolator is clean, it will normally remain microbiologically clean until an intervention or failure occurs. Change out of equipment may be required in isolators, and the ideal situation would allow this without opening the walls. Within a RABS, should an intervention require opening the system, validation should be available to show what interventions are acceptable without cleaning and decontamination. This does not mean the system can run indefinitely or without periodic adjustment, disassembly, and cleaning. However, these periods may be defined by qualification studies based on the needs for manufacture of specific products. Changeover strategies will differ for large versus small isolators, and batchwise versus campaign manufacturing, and these strategies should be qualified as well. In the larger context, accepting these strengths and knowing the limitations will encourage the implementation of isolator systems. In the paradigm of "Quality by Design" this process knowledge is highly desirable.

Many unusual events have been reported and policies are developed often in reaction to rare events. Regulators often find themselves struggling with decisions that address a single event although the response has unintended impacts on many other systems. Reactionary policies that pose unnecessary demands on isolator users discourage manufacturers from considering isolator systems. There is a delicate balance to be struck because discouraging the use of isolators is a losing proposition for all of health care.

VALIDATING THE ASEPTIC PROCESS

The validation of an isolator's operations may be progressively done using the standard Installation Qualification, Operational Qualification and Performance Qualification to start its operations, and current regulatory review thinking advocates accepting concurrent validation as a means of implementing changes to extend an operational system's use period. As these systems mature, the risk-based policies will need to be revisited because many of these were developed from the paradigm of clean rooms for manufacturing. The isolator system used for manufacturing is a highly controlled clean room in miniature that requires fresh thinking. Environmental standards for these isolators typically call for maintenance of ISO Class 5 (Class 100) conditions, or better, even though those standards dramatically understate the environmental control found in isolator systems. The same general concepts for cleaning and disinfection should apply to filling environments whether in a clean room, RABS, or an isolator. The difference is that the RABS or isolator system will maintain environmental control longer.

One must carefully assess the strengths as well as the weaknesses of these systems. This is the foundation of the science and risk-based philosophy proposed by the FDA (23). To dwell inappropriately on speculative arguments about whether one thousand or one million spores need to be killed by the disinfectant used for the preparation of the isolator environment demonstrates misguided thinking about the utility of the process and misunderstanding of decontamination processes. Too often we suspect that regulatory approaches are risk averse and not science based. The barrier system was intended to provide better-controlled environments that protect the production process from intervention and particle shedding by operators (the most likely source of microbial contamination). Evidence of these systems' success is seen in the results of media fills. In the absence of these sources of contamination (personnel), simple cleaning and decontamination will reduce the microbial load to undetectable levels, and proper operation of the system will maintain the environment far cleaner than a conventional clean room. This may not achieve the regulatory paradigm associated with overkill sterilization, but that should not be the point. The isolator is not the product that needs to be sterile. The drug or device is the product that needs to be manufactured sterile. From a practical perspective, maintaining isolator environments with or undetected microbial levels yield freedom from contamination, and that means "sterile" products will come from the process.

REFERENCES

1. Sharp J. Sterile products manufacture—Sense and non-sense. Eur J Parenteral Pharm Sci 2003; 8(1):21–26.
2. Pasteur L. 1861. Ann. Sci. Nat., Ser. 4, 16:5. In Brock, TD. Milestones in Microbiology. Washington, DC: ASM, 1975.
3. Alstrand DV, Ecklund OF. The mechanics and interpretation of heat penetration tests in canned foods. Food Technol 1952; 6(5):185–189.
4. Pflug I, Smith G. The use of biological indicators for monitoring wet heat sterilization processes. In: Pflug I. ed. Selected Papers on the Microbiology and Engineering of Sterilization Processes. 5th ed. Minneapolis, MN: Environmental Sterilization Laboratory, 1977:207–216.
5. FDA. Proposed rule: Use of aseptic processing and terminal sterilization in the preparation of sterile pharmaceuticals for human and veterinary use. Fed Regist 1991; 56(198):51354–51358.
6. Archer JR. Robotics application in cell culture technology. In: Sterilization in the 1990s - Proceedings of the PDA/PMA Sterilization Conference - Sterilization in the 1990s; August 1990; Washington, DC.
7. NASA. Biological Handbook for Engineers. NASA CR-61237. Huntsville, AL: Marshall Space Flight Center, 1968.
8. World Health Organization. WHO Expert Committee on Biological Standards—Twenty-fifth Report. Geneva: WHO, 1973.
9. FDA. *Guidance for Industry: Sterile Drug Products Produced by Aseptic Processing—Current Good Manufacturing Practice*, 2004. Available at http://www.fda.gov/downloads/Drugs/GuidanceCompliance RegulatoryInformation/Guidances/ucm070342.pdf. Accessed June 7, 2010.
10. Marohl R, Jennrich C, Adams R. Sterilizable Transfer Port (STP)—Update. In: ISPE/PDA Joint Conference; January 1995; Atlanta, GA.
11. Sweeney MD. Validation issues for a production Barrier/Isolator sterile liquid filling system in a controlled environment. In: ISPE/PDA Joint Conference; January 1995; Atlanta, GA.
12. Davenport SM. Meeting the goals of increased sterility confidence for advanced aseptic processing—Implementation of a restricted access barrier system. In: Barrier Users Group Symposium; May 31, 1995; Bethesda, MD.
13. Lindsay J. Media fill challenges—PDA Training and Research Institute. In: PDA/FDA Joint Conference; September 2002; Washington, DC.
14. Jones DJ, Topping P, Sharp J. Environmental microbial challenges to an aseptic blow-fill-seal process—A practical study. PDA J Pharm Sci Technol 1995; 49(5):226–234.
15. Rutala WA. APIC guidelines for selection and use of disinfectants. Am J Infect Control 1996; 24(4):313–342.
16. Spaulding EH. Chemical disinfection of medical and surgical materials. In: Lawrence CA, Block SS. eds. Disinfection, Sterilization and Preservation. Philadelphia: Lea & Feabiger, 1968:517–531.
17. Lysford J, Porter M. Barrier isolation history and trends, a millenium update. Pharm Eng 2001; 21(2): 1–4.
18. Akers J, Agalloco J. Isolators—Validation and sound scientific judgement. PDA J Pharm Sci Technol 2000; 54(2):110–111.
19. Sandle T. The use of risk assessment in the pharmaceutical industry—The application of FMEA to a sterility test isolator: A case study. Eur J Parenteral Pharm Sci 2003; 8(2):43–49.
20. Groschel D. 100 Years of agar use in Microbiology. ASM News 1981; 47(9):391–392.
21. Carson LA, Favero M.S, Bond WW, et al. Morphological, biochemical, and growth characteristics of Pseudomonas cepacia from distilled water. Appl Microbiol 1973; 25(3):476–483.
22. Nagarkar PP, Ravetkar SD, Watve MG. Oligotrophic bacteria as tools to monitor aseptic pharmaceutical production units. Appl Environ Microbiol 2001; 67(3):1371–1374.
23. FDA. Pharmaceutical cGMPs for the 21st Century: A Risk-Based Approach. Final Report - Fall 2004. Available at: http://www.fda.gov/Drugs/DevelopmentApprovalProcess/Manufacturing/Questions andAnswersonCurrentGoodManufacturingPracticescGMPforDrugs/ucm137175.htm. Accessed June 7, 2010.

31 A perspective on European regulations for advanced aseptic processing[1]

James Agalloco and James Akers

INTRODUCTION

What is an Isolator from the Inspector's Point of View?

A section on Isolator technology forms part of the European Union Guide to Good Manufacturing Practice (EU-GMP), Annex 1 (see the text extract that follows) (1). However, no definition of an isolator is provided there or in the Glossary to EU-GMP. Annex 1 addresses the manufacturing of sterile medicinal products, which is of course an important point of emphasis for inspectors. The section detailing isolator applications is not expansive, and provides limited discussion regarding the various types or uses of the technology. This is relevant since another application of the use of isolators is in sterility testing. The EU-GMP has no reference to isolators from this perspective since the process for the undertaking of sterility testing is specified and described in the European Pharmacopoeia (The Harmonized Test for Sterility in Ph.Eur. 2.6.1 contains a very general statement about the testing environment and does not explicitly refer to isolator technology) (2). The different types of isolators are, however, described in other regulatory (or close-to-regulatory) documents such as the FDA Aseptic Processing guidance and the PIC/S Isolation Technology document, where the use of open and closed isolators is described (3,4).

The word "isolator" implies a piece of equipment that provides isolation from the surrounding environment—or more importantly, isolation from the personnel who operate within that surrounding environment since human beings are commonly acknowledged to be the greatest microbial threat to the integrity of the inside of an isolator. The term "barrier" is sometimes used generically, but it is not appropriate to refer to isolators using this term since "barrier" is used in other applications as will be evident shortly. An isolator provides a clean environment where microorganisms should be absent following appropriate sanitization. An isolator that is sufficiently closed to provide an enclosed area may be placed in a Grade D or Grade C environment for aseptic preparation.

Inspectors will endeavor to make a distinction and differentiation between an isolator and an open device that would be classified as an EU-GMP Grade A environment, such as a unidirectional air flow (UAF) cabinet. The results of this determination have a significant impact on the requirements for the surrounding environment. A Grade A unidirectional airflow workstation for aseptic work should be located within a Grade B environment. A restricted access barrier system (RABS) should be regarded as a segregated Grade A environment that has more in common with traditional clean rooms than with isolators and is also therefore accessed from a Grade B environment. In reality, RABS classification is developing into a complex system that depends on the completeness of segregation of the RABS from the external environment. While a specific RABS may be placed on a continuum somewhere between a traditional aseptic area and an isolator system, its exact position on a continuum is defined by the completeness of segregation between the internal and external environments.[2] They are still, however, regarded as not totally segregated and are expected to operate within a Grade B background.

[1] This chapter was adapted from an earlier work originally developed by Lennart Ernerot Ph.D. and Lilian Hamilton M.Sci. Additional input was provided by Dr. Martyn Becker, Dr. Nigel Halls, and Dr. Klaus Haberer. Without their considerable efforts this chapter would not have been possible.

[2] A continuum applicable to aseptic processing has been developed by PDA in TR #34, while an industry nonspecific continuum that can be adapted is provided in ISO 14644-7—Separative Devices.

Some examples on how to interpret and differentiate an isolator from a UAF-Grade A environment are as follows:

- A UAF workstation with horizontal flow outward under positive pressure that normally has one side completely open. The recommended surrounding for such a device is Grade B. If the air device is rotated 90° so that the filter opening faces the floor, it will become a vertical UAF cabinet. Product flows through the device as in a filling line within an open UAF, so that it should also be surrounded by Grade B for aseptic filling. Access to the system by aseptically garbed operator is accomplished with minimal control.
- The same basic device with surrounding walls that are closed and product transferred into and out from the device through restricted and controlled openings might be defined as a RABS that is protected from external contamination by continuous air overspill into the surrounding environment below the critical area. RABS may closely resemble isolators except that typically they are not "gassed"—internal sanitization is by wiping with disinfectants. A well-designed RABS can, while in operation, provide all the benefits of physical protection of the contents of the isolator, but cannot provide the same high degree of assurance of freedom of microorganisms from its internal surfaces as is provided by a validated decontaminated or "gassed" isolator. Personnel access is through fixed gloves installed in the wall of the system.[3]
- To be regarded as an isolator, the enclosure should be positively pressurized, the product pathway should be steam sterilized in situ if possible, and sterilized vials should be delivered directly from a depyrogenation/sterilizing tunnel directly attached to the device. The product exit from the system should be designed in a similar way in order to avoid entrance of air from the surroundings. Any interference from the immediate surroundings would necessitate better than the Grade D background environment for the isolator as specified in EU-GMP. The requirement for the background environment surrounding an isolator for continuous, aseptic filling may need to be higher than for an isolator where all materials are entered before the device is decontaminated. Isolators may range from small scale totally closed systems resembling glove boxes—having introduced all the items needed for a particular set of manipulations the isolator is closed and its internal surfaces and contents are decontaminated—to "open isolators" allowing (after decontamination) for continuous or semicontinuous in-feed of sterilized components and out-feed of sterile finished products. Between these two extremes are isolators that are apparently "closed" but into which items can be moved in and out after decontamination via specially designed doors (RTPs—rapid transit ports) that have been designed to allow such movement without compromising the microbiological quality within the protected area.

Regulators acknowledge the superior possibilities that isolator technology may provide and they also understand that the technology is still undergoing very rapid development (4). As a consequence not all inspectors are familiar or have even seen the most recent installations, so that it is important for firms to describe and justify their rationales and decisions for the installations made. When technology changes are extensive the inspection process would benefit from early involvement of the competent authority. In any case, the general requirement for extensive qualification and validation of the equipment and the process would not be substantially different from any other specialized technology.

REGULATORY DEFINITION OF ISOLATORS

GMP Requirements

The EU-GMP regulates manufacture of sterile medicinal products in Annex 1 (1). Paragraphs 21 to 25 cover isolator technology (see extract in the following text). Paragraph 21 recognizes the use of isolator technology as a means to potentially decrease the risk of microbial contamination for aseptically manufactured products. Much however depends on the construction of the isolator

[3] RABS designs where 'open door' interventions are an integral part of operation are actually clean room systems and not RABS.

as well as the choice of methods for transfer of materials into and out of the isolator, to determine whether this is properly achieved or not. The background environment should be controlled and for aseptic processing it should be at least Grade D. Some firms design the external environment to achieve Grade C to further mitigate contamination risk, even if Grade D performance is claimed. Since many companies must also comply with FDA requirements, Grade C (ISO Class 8) will be the norm since this is also the FDA requirement from the 2004 aseptic processing guidance (3). Production in isolators should be commenced only after appropriate validation and monitoring are carried out.

Other requirements for aseptically manufactured products in Annex 1 are also applicable when applying isolator technology. A few such examples are monitoring during operation, handling of components and starting materials, training of personnel, and high standard of personal hygiene and cleanliness.

There is no current guidance in EU-GMP for RABS and the expectations for these systems are necessarily "ad hoc" and are derived predominantly from the practices for conventional manned aseptic processing. A technical monograph is being derived by Pharmaceutical and Healthcare Sciences Society in the United Kingdom that defines the different types and uses of RABS. The most relevant section of the isolator technology paragraphs that appear in the following text is paragraph 22, which speaks about the material transfers that in many RABS designs resemble that used for isolation technology.

> Isolator Technology (From EU Annex 1)
>
> 21. The utilisation of isolator technology to minimize human interventions in processing areas may result in a significant decrease in the risk of microbiological contamination of aseptically manufactured products from the environment. There are many possible designs of isolators and transfer devices. The isolator and the background environment should be designed so that the required air quality for the respective zones can be realised. Isolators are constructed of various materials more or less prone to puncture and leakage. Transfer devices may vary from a single door to double door designs to fully sealed systems incorporating sterilization mechanisms.
>
> 22. The transfer of materials into and out of the unit is one of the greatest potential sources of contamination. In general the area inside the isolator is the local zone for high risk manipulations, although it is recognised that laminar air flow may not exist in the working zone of all such devices.
>
> 23. The air classification required for the background environment depends on the design of the isolator and its application. It should be controlled and for aseptic processing it should be at least grade D.
>
> 24. Isolators should be introduced only after appropriate validation. Validation should take into account all critical factors of isolator technology, for example the quality of the air inside and outside (background) the isolator, sanitisation of the isolator, the transfer process and isolator integrity.
>
> 25. Monitoring should be carried out routinely and should include frequent leak testing of the isolator and glove sleeve system.

PHARMACEUTICAL INSPECTION COOPERATION SCHEME

The PIC/S has issued an extensive perspective on isolation technology that outlines inspectional expectations for the industry (4). The PIC/S document is largely aligned with industry approaches with a single major exception. The document speaks about gas sterilization, whereas routine industry use of vaporized H_2O_2 now leans toward acceptance of sporicidal treatment as being accomplished by condensed liquid on the surface of the isolator interior.[4] This has significant implications with respect to the utility of physical measurements taken to demonstrate and document effective process parameters. Within its limitations, the efficacy of the typical

[4] See chapters 24 to 27 for expanded discussions of hydrogen peroxide decontamination.

vapor phase H_2O_2 decontaminating processes is excellent; however, correlation to physical measurements is still considered problematic.[5]

The PIC/S document is generally favorably disposed to isolation technology and frequently makes the point that environment performance expectations in isolator-based aseptic processing should be higher than that attainable in ordinary manned clean rooms. No specific mention is made in the document of RABS, although there are descriptions included of systems that resemble RABS. The absence of a clearly defined perspective is likely due to the smaller number of RABS installations upon which to base a regulatory stance.[6]

USE OF ISOLATORS

Typical Use

Since one of the main goals for inspectors is to ensure the protection of public health by the assessment of manufacturing operations and judging their compliance with appropriate standards of Good Manufacturing Practice, they typically focus on processes that assure product safety and in the supporting rationale and justification for the use of isolators.

Isolator technology can be utilized for many different reasons; they may be used in order to improve protection from microbial contamination in aseptic production or as a means to prevent cross-contamination (contamination of a starting material or of a product with another material or product). Another rationale for using an isolator could also of course be operator protection, as with the manufacture of radiopharmaceuticals or cytotoxic products. Isolators can also be used for handling of toxic starting materials; for example, in early development of new products when sufficient safety/toxicity data may not be available. A variation of this isolator rationale may be seen when working with nonsterile products containing highly toxic substances, and in installations where only containment is the goal, the designs and working practices may be markedly different.

Operator Protection

Operator protection is ordinarily not a concern for pharmaceutical inspectors. However, if the main purpose for using an isolator is operator protection, the inspection might focus on the design of the isolator to make sure that steps taken for operator protection will not compromise the quality of the product. Areas of interest would include pressure differentials and cleaning/sanitization; for example, with negative-pressure isolators or those with radiation protection using lead shields. The question an inspector will ask is—could the design increase the risk of microbial contamination of the product or could the lead shields be a problem when cleaning the isolator?

Aseptic Production

Product protection from microbial contamination during manufacture of sterile products is usually the main driver for the use of isolator technology. Aseptic processing is a difficult operation and is heavily regulated in order to maximize patient safety. An isolator-based aseptic process can be evaluated using a process simulation or media fill test. The acceptance criterion for process simulations should be zero growth; however, since it is not possible to prove a negative and as humans have to be involved in the processes, then it is logical to expect that there may be an occasional positive. EU-GMP is now harmonized with FDA requirements in that zero growth is the target (1,3). The presence of a single contaminant may not indicate a problem with the batch regardless of batch size. This is a significant improvement over the logical fallacy operated previously, where $<0.1\%$ contamination rate at 95% confidence was the stated acceptance criterion. This allows the unacceptable situation of four contaminants per

[5] FDA makes similar statements regarding concentration measurement in its 2004 Guideline on Sterile Drug Products Produced by Aseptic Processing. However, stating this as an expectation belies the inability of current analytical technologies to support it.

[6] The same situation prevails in the US, where FDA has not issued a document explicitly stating its expectations with respect to the use of RABS technology.

batch of 5000 units; nine per batch of 10,000 units, and so on being acceptable—even if those failures could be detected!

In the quest for better aseptic processing and safer products, the isolator will likely be one of the several possible answers to the problem. RABS endeavor to deliver comparable performance by enhanced separation of aseptically gowned personnel using isolator like design concepts albeit possibly without a constant pressure differential between the fill zone and that where the operator is located (normally Grade B). As the majority of RABS are manually decontaminated, it is unlikely that their decontamination process matches the certainty of that performed on an isolator system.

The use of isolators within an aseptic processing manufacturing environment is essentially of two kinds; large-scale, rapid operation within open systems that deliver the product through a "mousehole" into the external environment, and small-scale operations within a closed isolator. In small-scale production limited to the amount of material that can be introduced and manufactured between two decontamination cycles, it is easier to justify the isolator over other approaches since as long as sterile starting materials can be brought in and finished product removed without compromising the internal environment of the isolator the process can continue. The introduction and removal processes, however, pose some challenges to isolator integrity and these would be examined closely at inspection. Newer open systems allowing continuous production with integration of sterile (depyrogenated where necessary) components ingress, and the egress of closed seal containers requires added controls to assure their successful operation.

Sterility Testing

Sterility testing for products distributed in Europe should be performed in accordance with the European Pharmacopoeia. The method has a section "Precautions against microbial contamination," which allows sterility testing in an isolator though isolators are not explicitly mentioned. A PIC/S guidance document on sterility testing serves as an indication of what inspectorate thinking might be on this topic (5). Inspectors will focus on the number of false positive sterility tests and the rationale for declaring a test invalid. As isolators are often utilized for sterility testing to minimize the number of false positives, the user must consider the controls necessary to maintain aseptic conditions within the isolator.

ENVIRONMENTAL REQUIREMENTS

European Regulatory Requirements

The requirement for the background environment depends on the design of the isolator and its application. The EU-GMP requires the background environment to be controlled and at least Grade D for aseptic processing (1). Annex 1 also provides recommended limits for airborne contamination (particulate matter and microorganisms). There are also requirements on gowning, changing rooms, and airlocks for that level of environment. Environmental requirements for RABS are identical to the long established limits constituted for manned clean rooms, although experience has confirmed that the actual performance is typically significantly better than these requirements.

Justification for Choice of Aseptic Technology

The means for selecting an appropriate processing technology is not defined in regulation. Firms can select their desired approach to produce sterile products by aseptic processing free of artificial constraints imposed from the regulatory community. EMEA participants (as well as those from other regulatory bodies) have contributed to the industry documents that have helped shape the current technology choices (6,7). The choices made by the industry considering all of the relevant factors have been identified by Lysfjord and Porter (8,9).

Regardless of the specific choice made by a firm, the transfer of sterile materials and equipment into the processing environment is one of the most critical process steps and often justifies the use of an appropriate controlled background environment. The potential introduction of external contamination will raise expectations for additional protection of the environment such as better air filters, personnel and materials locks, frequent cleaning, and testing of environmental conditions.

Flow of Materials

The flow of material outside the critical aseptic environment isolator is often given less consideration since attention is usually focused on the process inside the critical zone. From a regulatory point of view the task is quite simple. Material brought into the critical areas should be in a condition that will not jeopardize the integrity of the isolator interior.

In marked contrast, the material introduction practices are of critical importance in RABS where the surrounding environment is Grade B and open door interventions may be required during the setup and operation of the system. The materials introduced into the surrounding environment in a RABS must not compromise the expected microbial conditions in that area, nor contribute to contamination ingress within the RABS.

Transfer of materials into and out of isolators is generally considered critical, as the material introduced into an operating isolator may be a vector for the potential introduction of microbial contamination. The transfer must therefore allow materials to enter/leave without any contamination risk for the isolator interior. As these materials are commonly automatically decontaminated or sterilized as part of entry into the isolator environment, the risk of contamination ingress is largely mitigated. The surrounding environment should be a sufficient barrier to reduce any contamination risks during transfer of goods.

A common mode for the transfer of materials is to connect different pieces of equipment to form a chain of simultaneously operating devices, where the transfer device and its contents have been decontaminated by, for example, the use of vaporized hydrogen peroxide. The filling isolator or RABS is therefore just one piece in the overall chain. The complete chain, however, must be properly designed from the point where cleaning or decontamination takes place until the finished sterile product safely leaves the last piece of equipment. Validation must verify that flow of air in different devices is operating without disturbing the specification in another device. Worst case conditions as well as emergency situations should be covered in order to demonstrate performance when the integrity of the isolator/RABS is at greatest risk.

Isolators should be operated without opening throughout the entire aseptic process, and an effective RABS should be operated in the same manner. This is rarely a major consideration for isolation technology, as these units are specifically designed to be operated in this manner. RABS designs are less standardized, and some RABS installations have been seen to require "open door" interventions to allow continued operation. The notion that a "restricted access barrier system" can be accessed in an unrestricted manner suggests that it is badly misnamed and is not a RABS at all, but merely an expensive and overly complicated manned clean room. An "unrestricted restricted access barrier system" is of course an oxymoron of the highest magnitude and should not be a part of any design for an aseptic processing system.

When isolator technology is used for labor or environmental protection from contaminants there are often other regulations to follow besides pharmaceutical GMP. Other regulatory precautions must not override the GMP aspects. The operational system should be designed such that all requirements are met. No regulator will accept compromises to GMP or patient safety in order to satisfy purely environmental or safety considerations.

PERSONNEL

Training of Personnel

Training should cover the setup and maintenance of the aseptic processing system and its surroundings as well as the immediate operations within the critical zone. The main benefit of using advanced aseptic systems and practices is the ability to create a *safe* barrier between product and people in order to protect them from each other.

Training of personnel should be conducted with the aim of keeping this barrier as effective as possible.

Training should also include all technical aspects of transfer of materials in and out, the work with gloves or half-suit as well as immediate maintenance and testing procedures. As for all GMP training, there should be a plan and records showing that operators, maintenance personnel, and anyone else whose duties take them into an aseptic processing environment have received sufficient initial as well as ongoing training.

Requirements on Protective Clothing

The EU-GMP requires personnel to use protective clothing appropriate for the process and the grade of the working area. Gowning requirements for all clean areas are specified within Annex 1.

However, inspectors will be interested in the rationale used for the choice of protective clothing and measures taken to protect the product (and the critical processing environment) from contamination. It is not uncommon that companies will apply higher demands on cleanliness using these advanced technologies due to the proximity of the protective system components to the critical process zone. Isolators may be placed in Grade D or cleaner and the personnel dressed accordingly. The intention, which appears appropriate, is to protect the isolator from contamination during preparation and cleaning before and after the production. It is usually open during only the cleaning portion of this process. RABS commonly require the same gowning requirements utilized for manned aseptic filling, as the background environment is typically no less than Grade B.

Gloves

At this stage in their evolutions, almost no pharmaceutical isolators or RABS will work automatically, so there must be devices to permit the handling of materials inside the enclosure. This may range from occasional corrections of automatic processes to extensive manual work. Glove ports or half-suits will be the normal way of achieving this. Open door activities, necessary for support of badly designed RABS operations, must be considered with skepticism. Access of that type is contradictory to the core goals of advanced aseptic processing.

Gloves should be sufficiently flexible to accommodate the intended work but they must also be resistant enough to allow for this work without tearing. They should also resist decontamination cycles utilized on the interior of the enclosure. The systems for fitting gloves and especially exchange of them are critical. If glove change is permitted without a subsequent decontamination cycle there should be proof available to verify that the changing of a glove will not pose a contamination hazard to the product.

Usually the operator will be expected to use additional gloves on their hands for hygienic reasons as to avoid direct contact with gloves attached to the enclosure when they are used by different people within the operational environment. A pinhole or tear in an enclosure glove may raise concerns for the contamination risk for the inside environment. Testing for the absence of pinholes and leaks in gloves and half-suits is considered critical from a regulatory perspective; however, there is growing evidence that the importance of this is overstated (10,11).

CLEANING AND DECONTAMINATION

Methods

Isolators and RABS as well all other equipment need to be maintained in a clean condition. After cleaning they should be visibly clean from potential contaminants. Inspectors will be interested in finding out if operators can reach all areas for cleaning and the extent to which the internal equipment has to be disassembled. If the isolator is used for different products, cleaning validation must verify that the cleaning method is efficient. Cleaning validation should include studies to show that the residual levels of cleaning agents are appropriate to manufacturing conditions. Cleaning agents must of course be compatible with the materials for the enclosure construction. If clean-in-place systems are used they must also be validated.

According to the European GMP, there is no requirement for a sterile environment during aseptic production, since this is not actually possible. EU-GMP uses the term "sanitization" (Annex 1 paragraphs 61–63 although it incorrectly refers to it as "sanitation") without specifying the level of microbial control to be achieved (1). The term "sterile" is normally reserved for finished products where the probability of detection of a nonsterile unit can be demonstrated to be less than 1 in 10^6.

The enclosure interiors should be classified as Grade A and should be monitored, with microbiological requirements being less than 1 CFU/m^3 (air sampling), less than 1 CFU per four hours on settle plates (diameter 90 mm) and less than 1 CFU on contact plates (diameter 55 mm). In order to achieve this during production the company needs to use efficient methods for decontamination, with the sporicidal effects of materials such as peracetic acid or hydrogen peroxide being appropriate in this context. The firm should provide a rationale for the choice of decontamination system used.

Specifications

Sterile manufacturers must be able to explain to the inspector why a specific method for cleaning or decontamination was chosen. Inspectors will wish to know if the method is repeatable and reliable and if results achieved are appropriate.

Specifications must be set and should include:

- Conditions for the cycle used such as temperature, time of exposure, humidity, concentration of agent[7] (where possible)
- The system configuration or load (empty or with equipment)
- Biological indicators (type of organism, resistance to agent, location).

Decontamination should not impact the products to be manufactured so that postdecontamination process ventilation must be addressed to demonstrate that there is no residual agent that could affect the product. The inspector will be interested in the precautions taken to prevent recontamination of surfaces during setup and operation.

VALIDATION

Validation Requirements

Isolation technology is part of an integrated process that includes equipment and devices for pretreatment, transfer, and handling of products. Most of the operations in a modern system take place in an automated manner but any aseptic processing system will also need a supply of sterile product, other materials, components, and environmental monitoring media. EU-GMP Annex 15: Qualification and Validation can be readily applied to isolator and RABS installations (12). As with all annexes, Annex 15 is not a stand-alone document but is predicated on the main chapters of EU-GMP and other relevant annexes such as Annex 1 for sterile medicinal products. An inspection will inevitably focus on all aspects of validation and the results documented.

Annex 1 to the EU-GMP in paragraphs 66–71 describes that the validation of aseptic processes should include the use of media fills. These paragraphs provide guidance regarding the number of filled units, which as already noted is harmonized with FDA requirements. In actuality the performance of advanced aseptic processing systems should be much better than this expectation, which also applies to the less capable manned clean room.

Maintenance

It is not enough to have a validated advanced aseptic processing system if it is not maintained properly. Maintenance consists of unplanned breakdown maintenance and planned preventive maintenance. Change control procedures must be adhered to.

During validation of the system, the end user is expected to identify and prepare relevant instructions including those necessary for maintenance. Such instructions could refer to a manual issued by the manufacturer of the isolator or RABS.

Preventive maintenance should include but not be limited to calibrations, changing of gloves, half- or whole suits, when, where, and what to lubricate, monitoring and changing of filters, checks to be done on fans, and other checks to be done on relevant parts of the overall

[7] Decontamination agent concentration measurement is a common regulatory expectation; however, there are significant limitations to its utility especially for vapor phase system, as two phases may be present throughout the decontamination process (see chap. 24).

installation. The inspector will look for a program for preventive maintenance and evidence for adherence to it.

Regarding repairs; there should be an authorized list of spare parts and a detailed engineering drawing. The inspector will look for operational and maintenance logbooks (or equivalent) to check what kinds of problems have occurred and how they have been solved, as well as for evidence of changes and therefore adherence to change control procedures. The inspector will also look for evidence to see that the isolator is cleaned and sanitized as planned.

REFERENCES

1. European Communities. EudraLex, The Rules Governing Medicinal Products in the European Union, Volume 4, Pharmaceutical Legislation, Medicinal Products for Human and Veterinary Use, Good Manufacturing Practices, Annex 1, Sterile Medicinal Products. European Commission, Brussels, 2008.
2. European Directorate for the Quality of Medicines. European Pharmacopoeia. 6th ed. Strasbourg, France: Council of Europe, 2007.
3. FDA. Guideline on Sterile Drug Products Produced by Aseptic Processing, September 2004.
4. PIC/S.Recommendations on Isolators Used for Aseptic Processing and Sterility Testing, PI 014–3, 25 September 2007.
5. PIC/S.Recommendations on Sterility Testing, PI 012–2, July 2004.
6. PDA.TR #34 Design and Validation of Isolator Systems for the Manufacturing and Testing of Health Care Products. PDA J Pharm Sci Technol 2001; 55 (5 suppl).
7. ISPE. Restricted Access Barrier Systems (RABS) for Aseptic Processing, ISPE Definition, August 2005.
8. Lysfjord JP, Porter M. Barrier isolator history and trends—2008 final data. Pharm Eng 2009; 50–55.
9. Lysfjord JP, Porter M. Restricted Access Barrier System (RABS)—2007 Final Data. Pharm Eng 2009; 56–59.
10. Sigwarth V, Gessler A, Stark A. Relevance of physical glove integrity testing to microbial contamination of isolator systems. Paper presented at: ISPE Meeting; September 20–21, 2005; Prague, Czech Republic.
11. Miller M, Walsh M. Case studies in the use of the BioVigilant IMD-A for real-time environmental monitoring during aseptic filling, intervention assessments and glove integrity testing in manufacturing isolators. Paper presented at: PDA Annual Meeting; April 20–24, 2009; Las Vegas, NV.
12. EMEA.EUDRALEX, Volume 4—Medicinal Products for Human and Veterinary Use: Good Manufacturing Practice, Annex 15 Qualification and Validation. European Commission, Brussels, 2001.

32 Advanced aseptic processing technologies in Japan

Tsuguo Sasaki and Morihiko Takeda

From history books on Japan, we learn that the society has actively imported, adopted, and promoted new and advanced cultures, political systems, scientific technologies, and other knowledge and inventions from the most esteemed foreign countries at the time. Over the 200-year period from 630 A.D., Japan achieved epoch-making growth during a time at which Chinese culture and Buddhism were introduced from the Tang dynasty, one of the most sophisticated civilizations at the time. The Meiji era, starting in 1868, brought about the end of Samurai history and opened the doors for the New Government to start modernizing Japan. The adaptation was broad and diverse, transfiguring Japan into a modern country, the first Western-style nation in Asia. The ensuing years after World War II was a time of recovery from devastation and of advancement to a country capable of manufacturing world-class industrial products based on science and technology. The Japanese people have long adored, respected, and studied the civilizations, cultures, and scientific achievements of advanced countries. Japan, through sending out its own human resources to other countries and inviting highly skilled specialists from abroad, has effectively utilized the knowledge acquired toward the growth of the nation. The country has long been accused of being skillful at imitating foreign ideas; however, the Japanese have demonstrated a high sense of ingenuity and curiosity, and great enthusiasm to take on new civilizations and cultures, and adapt them in their own way. They also have shown the necessary motivation and talent to further advance imported ideas to make them fit their own styles.

The drastic changes made in manufacturing technologies in the Japanese pharmaceutical industry over the past 30 years have been remarkable. Although the fundamentals of good manufacturing practice (GMP) and validation were imported from Western nations, current manufacturing systems are in no way inferior to those of the West. With the entry of foreign pharmaceutical companies into the Japanese market together with mergers with Japanese pharmaceutical companies, aseptic manufacturing processing has been enhanced to a level comparable to that in the West. This chapter briefly covers aseptic processing technologies currently available in Japan.

CHANGES IN STERILITY ASSURANCE LEVEL OF ASEPTICALLY MANUFACTURED PRODUCTS

The global view of pharmaceutical product manufacturing seems to indicate that aseptic manufacturing methods starting with the production of vaccines and antitoxins have made great advancements, with the production of antibiotics as a turning point. Penicillin G reported in 1942 not only provided immense benefits to both physicians and patients from the viewpoint of infection treatment but also has contributed to the development of the modern pharmaceutical industry. The discovery of streptomycin, tetracycline, and erythromycin following penicillin led to the development of a new drug manufacturing process. The introduction of sterile filtration, freeze-drying, and other new technologies appears to have set the foundation for aseptic manufacturing methods. The improvements in sterility assurance level (SAL) for sterile products over time can be seen with results of the sterility test for biological products carried out as a national control test to date (Fig. 1). When high efficiency particulate air (HEPA) and/or membrane filters were not available after World War II, the sterility of products was dependent on the effect of antiseptic agents formulated but eventually many lots of products were rejected by the sterility test. The rejection rate was as high as 10% despite very low detection sensitivity level (SAL approximately 10^{-1}), permitting speculation that almost all products were contaminated. The recent permissible contamination limit in the medial fill test has approached zero despite the increased number of units used in the test, a stark contrast from the 0.3% in 1973 (Table 1), evidencing drastic improvement in aseptic manufacturing technologies.

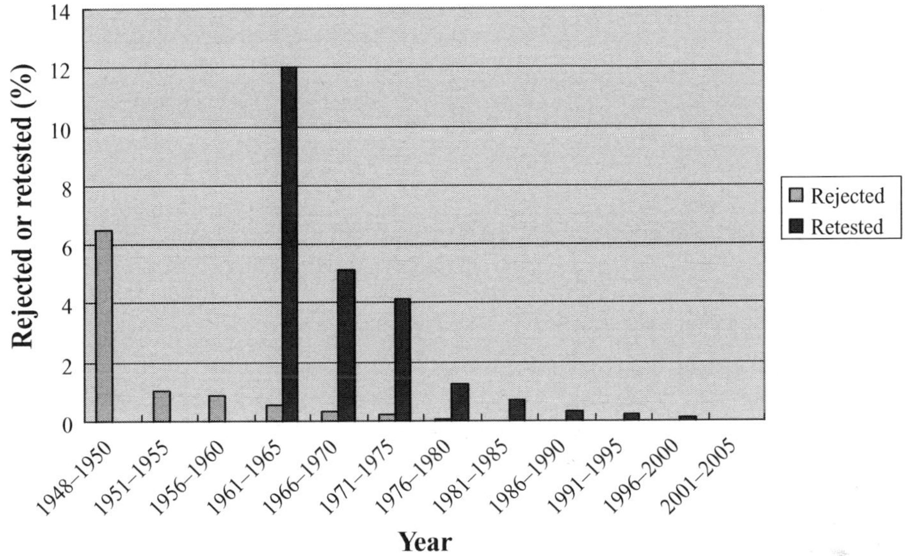

Figure 1 Summary of sterility test for biological products carried out as a national control assay in Japan (1948–2005).

PREREQUISITES FOR ACHIEVING HIGH STERILITY ASSURANCE LEVEL IN ASEPTIC MANUFACTURING

Sterile drug products are manufactured by aseptically handling sterilized parts of the products (e.g., containers, stoppers) using sterilized manufacturing equipment. Attempts for aseptic processing are challenged by various factors of contamination such as operators and manufacturing environment. In addition, manufacturing processing creates the possibility for microbial contamination, and the major source of contamination is humans. Sterilization itself is a technically

Table 1 Changes in Acceptance Levels of Media Fill Run

Requirement	Minimum units	Acceptance level
WHO (1973). General requirements for the sterility of biological substances. WHO Technical Report Series, No. 872	1000	0.3%
FDA (1987). Industry Guideline on Sterile Drug Products Produced by Aseptic Processing	3000	1 in 1000 with a 95% confidence level
Japanese Pharmacopoeia (1996). Media Fill Test	A large number of (media filled) units to detect 0.1% contamination rate	0.05% with a 95% confidence level
ISO 13408 (1998). Aseptic processing of health care products—Generals	3000	0.1% with a 95% confidence level
FDA (2004). Industry Guidance on Sterile Drug Products Produced by Aseptic Processing, EU-GMP Annex 1 (2008), ISO 13408–1 (2008): Aseptic processing of health care products—Generals	• <5000, no contaminated units should be detected. One contaminated unit is considered cause for revalidation, following an investigation • 5000–10,000, one contaminated unit should result in an investigation, including consideration of a repeat media fill. Two contaminated units are considered cause for revalidation, following investigation • >10,000, one contaminated unit should result in an investigation. Two contaminated units are considered cause for revalidation, following investigation	

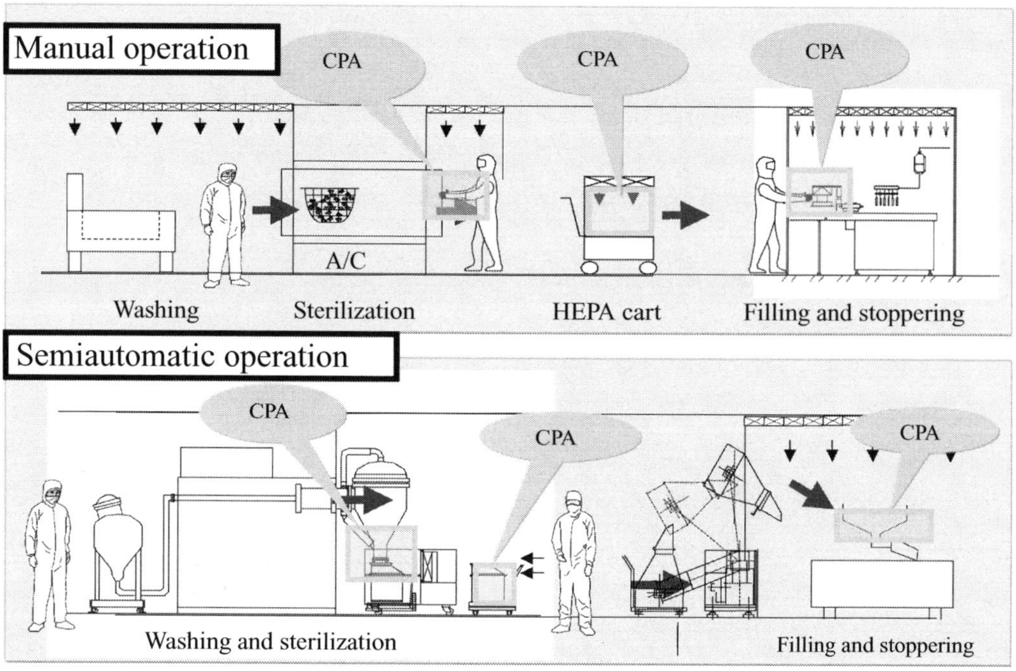

Figure 2 Example of critical processing area (CPA) showing human intervention. This figure illustrates washing, sterilization, and transferring of rubber stoppers to the filling machine.
Abbreviation: HEPA, high efficiency particulate air.

well-established process. Practical approaches to contamination containment may be focused on the aseptic filling of pharmaceutical solution into containers and maintenance of aseptic conditions throughout processing. These process operations pose the question, "which areas of manufacturing facility are critical in maintaining the sterility of drug products." Example of critical areas for contamination prevention may be transfer ports of an autoclave, interior of a HEPA cart during product transfer, and chambers for carrying sterile stoppers into a stoppering machine (Fig. 2), since these areas require the intervention of human operators or exposing products/materials to the environment. The assurance of sterility during aseptic processing can be implemented by a hardware and/or software approach. The software approach is heavily dependent on human operators; however, it is not possible to control the entire movement of humans by software applications. One of the basic approaches is to minimize the involvement of operators in controlled aseptic manufacturing to increase the SAL.

STERILE MANUFACTURING EQUIPMENT

The innovation of technologies for realizing manufacturing with a good balance of stable quality and high product output as best illustrated by Toyota's just-in-time system is the heart of the Japanese industry. Aseptic manufacture of drug products is also supported by this traditional concept of well-balanced quality and performance. The elimination of the major contamination source, humans, from an aseptic manufacturing process has been tried by developing closed processing systems and process automation system. Technologies thus developed are briefly summarized later.

Isolator Technologies

A high level of sterility assurance for drug products manufactured in an aseptic process essentially requires the minimization of human intervention in the process. One of the current best fits for this purpose is the isolator. One to three new isolators are introduced for drug production annually in Japan (Fig. 3). The grade of the environment surrounding the isolator is C in most cases, followed by B (Fig. 4).

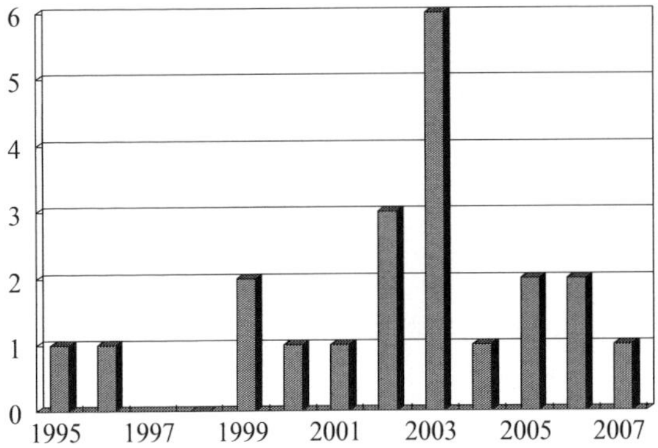

Figure 3 Annual numbers of isolators introduced in the production of sterile pharmaceutical products in Japan (from ISPE report).

Integrated Closed System for Sterile Bulk Products

Conventional aseptic manufacturing of bulk drug substance often uses freeze-drying technology. Until recently, a bulk material sterilized was typically processed by the following procedures: transfer to a tray, vacuum freeze-drying using a freeze-dryer, recovery of dried powder from the tray, crushing of the dried powder, and dispensation of the powder into a sterile container. A series of these procedures were undertaken by handling sterilized drug solution and dry powder in open air, requiring manual operations and ultimately increasing risk of contamination due to the exposure of drug solution or dry powder to the environment and humans. Today, these sequential operations can be performed in a closed system by using a freeze-dryer (developed by Kyowa Vacuum Engineering Co., Ltd.) (Fig. 5). The basic concept of the closed manufacturing system is the ice-lining technology—a method of forming an ice-lining layer between a heat transmitting medium (heat transfer surface) and drug solution to recover freeze-dried drug substance avoiding adherence of drug substance to the heat transfer surface (Figs. 6 and 7).

This closed-system technology has enabled technicians to freeze-dry, crush, and recover drug substances in a closed system without requiring the use of trays and other containers as the sources of contamination. The closed system is also capable of clean-in-place (CIP) and sterilization-in-place (SIP) to minimize the risk of contamination of bulk drug substance from the environment and/or humans. Furthermore, running costs of production can be greatly reduced since the system does not require the installation or use of a sterile filling facility, filling machine, and trays, which are essential in the conventional freeze-drying process.

Automatic Ampoule-Loading/Unloading Technology in Freeze-Drying Chamber

Automatic loading to and unloading from a freeze-drying chamber of freeze-dried drug products in ampoule requires highly automated technology. It has long been considered to be difficult to collect ampoules into trays following a rapid filling process (400 ampoule/min 1 mL); however, such an automated production line system is already in operation in Japan.

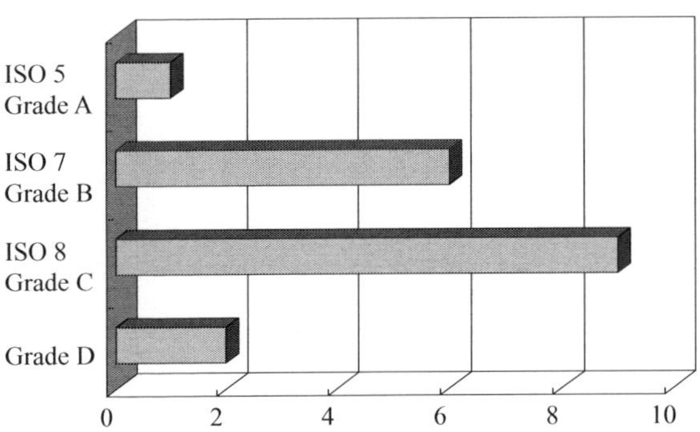

Figure 4 The environment surrounding isolators (from ISPE report).

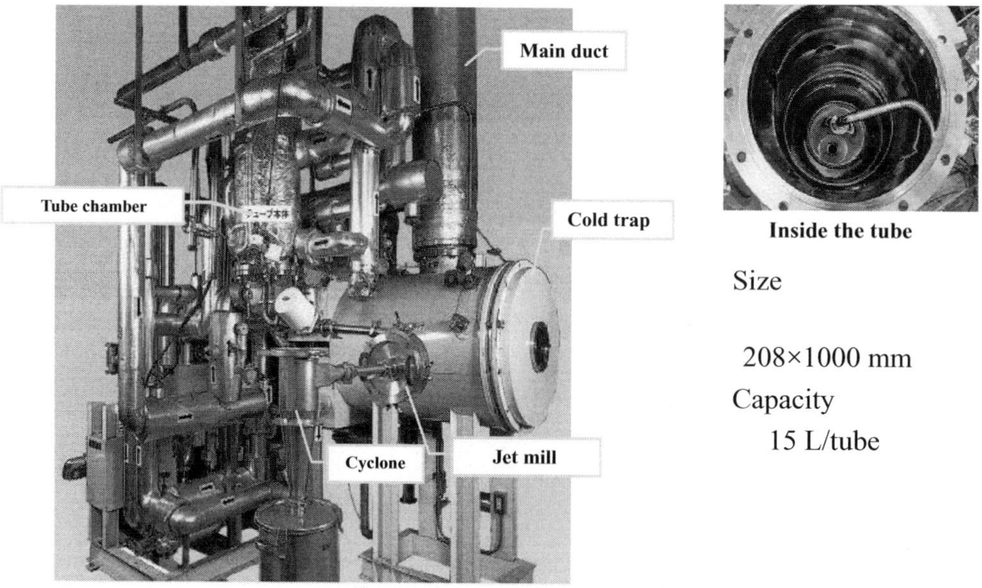

Figure 5 Outline of integrated closed system (ICS).

Arrangement of ampoules unloaded from the filling machine in trays requires the flow of ampoules to be changed from continuous to intermittent, since the action of arrangement itself is an intermittent action. A transportation apparatus (conveyer) capable of changing the transportation distance has been developed, allowing automated stable ampoule-loading/unloading procedures with trays.

There is also a production line system equipped with apparatus capable of automatically loading and unloading ampoules and vials of different sizes after filling. Production efficiency is compromised if trays or containers need to be changed according to the size of ampoules or vials. As a counter action to decreasing efficiency, a new type of tray equipped with a partition plate with spring has been developed. The handling of this tray has been automated and a production line system handling multiple sizes of ampoules and vials is already in commercial use.

Revolution Drive-Free Aseptic Isolators

The automation of ampoule or vial collection into trays in an aseptic isolator requires a built-in mechanism that can invert trays within an isolator. A multiarticulated robot is one solution;

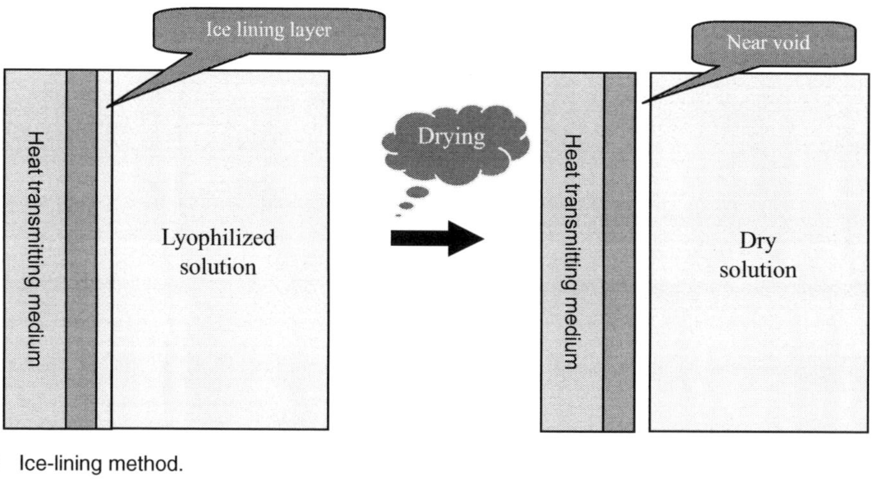

Figure 6 Ice-lining method.

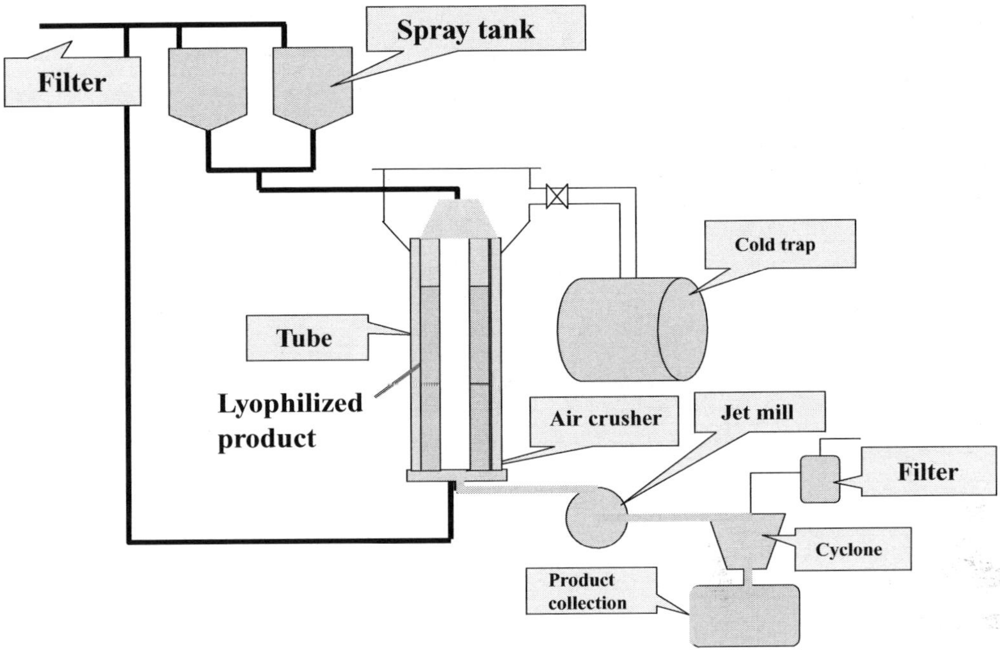

Figure 7 Flow of integrated closed system (ICS).

however, it creates waste space within the isolator. At present, a new apparatus that has a revolution drive not inside but outside the isolator to indirectly drive mechanical parts within the isolator is available for practical use (developed by IDK Co., Ltd.) (Fig. 8).

The above-mentioned technologies have been combined and a multiple production line system integrated with isolator-equipped ampoule filling, vial filling, ampoule sealing, and vial stoppering machines and, in addition, an automatic guided vehicle transporting ampoules and

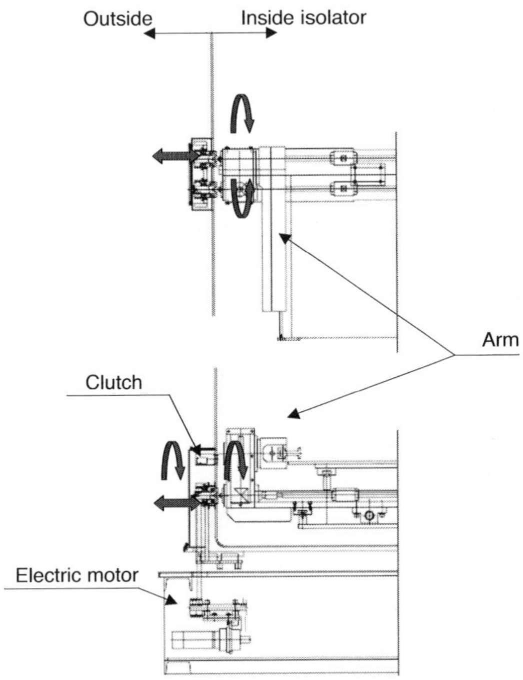

Figure 8 Principle of drive-free aseptic isolator.

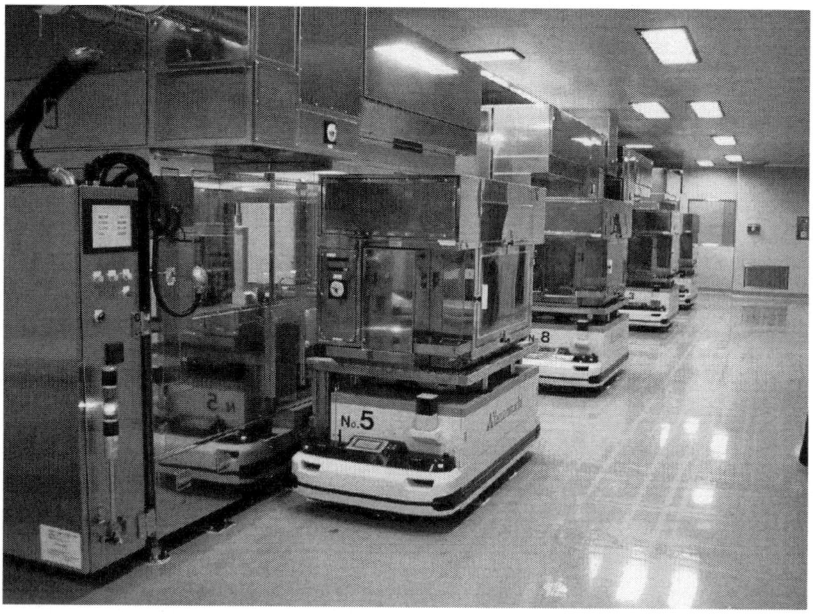

Figure 9 AGV station for lyophilizers in aseptic area.

vials collected in trays among these machines and as many as five freeze-drying chambers have been employed for aseptic product handling in controlled areas (Figs. 9–12).

FOREIGN SUBSTANCE INSPECTION APPARATUS

It may be a specific characteristic of the Japanese people, but consumers are keenly concerned about the contamination of foreign matters in pharmaceutical products. Pharmaceutical manufacturers are forced to invest an extensive amount of time and energy in preventing contamination during the manufacturing process. As an illustration of a company's measures, an automatic inspection apparatus developed by a Japanese pharmaceutical company Eisai Co., Ltd. is briefly described in the following section.

Development for Automatic Inspection Machine

Eisai Co., Ltd. started to develop a machine to inspect for insoluble foreign particles in order to improve the quality of their injectable pharmaceutical products. In 1970s, Eisai found the light

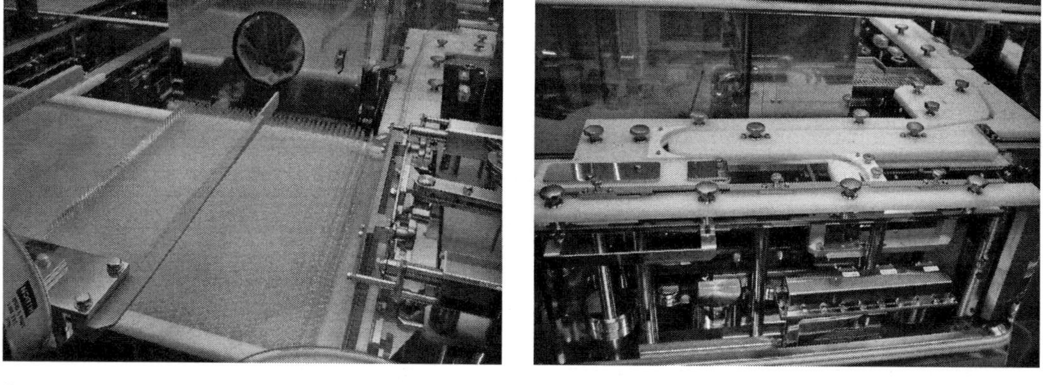

Figure 10 Ampoule collection and buffer conveyer in isolator (filling capacity: 400 ampoules/min for 1 mL and 2 mL).

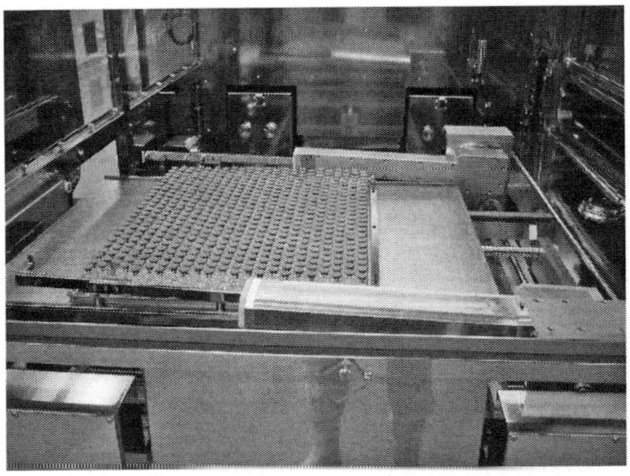
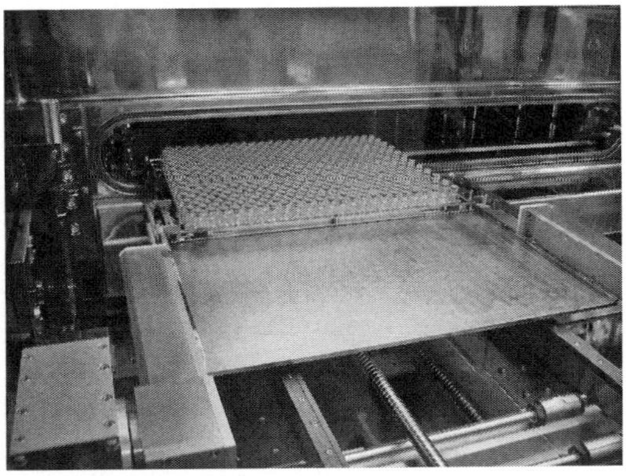

Figure 11 Vials/ampoules automatic loading for lyophilizer in closed RABS.

transmission SD (Static Division) System to be the most reliable and cost-effective method in order to detect foreign particles in products.

Based on the pharmaceutical manufacturers' requirement to inspect also the cosmetic defects such as crack or scratch on the container, Eisai Machinery added CCD camera and vision system for cosmetic inspection. Following the performance of the filling machine, Eisai Machinery also developed a high performance machine series Eisai Machinery Inspection System (EIS®), whose highest performance is 600 syringes/cartridges and 400 vials per minute (Figs. 13 and 14).

Layout of the Automatic Inspection Machine

The containers such as syringe or cartridges are supplied from upperstream machine through double infeed conveyors and transmitted to the oscillating star wheel on which serious cosmetic defects, such as missing cap and bend needle, are inspected by vision system and discharged, because such containers may damage the machine system and mechanism.

The containers are spun at high speed to remove most of bubbles, as bubble is sometimes a source of false detection of particles. If containers have no serious defect or bubble, they go

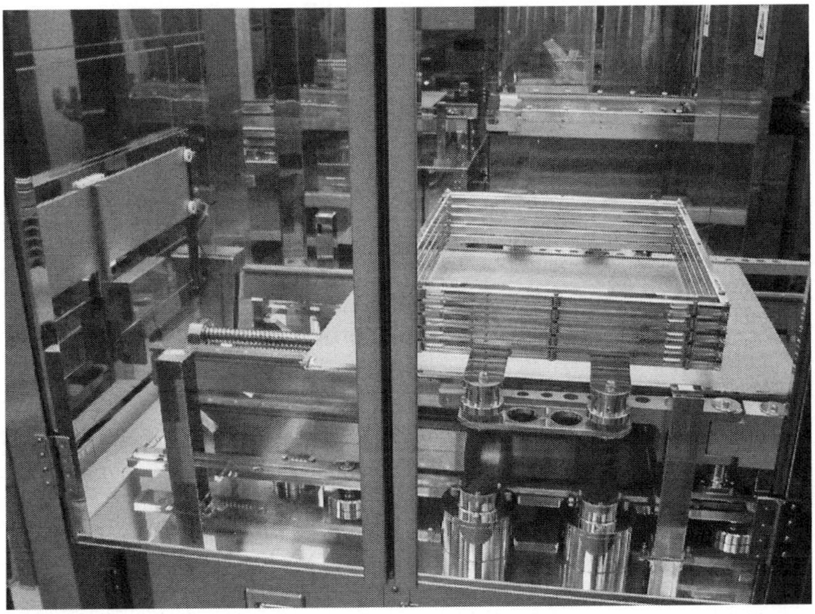

Figure 12 Tray stacking system in isolator.

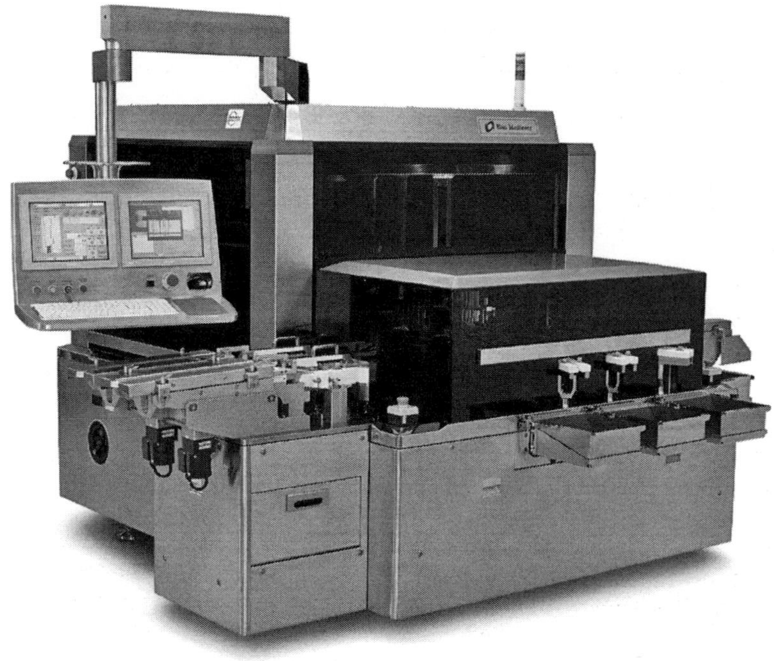

Figure 13 Outline of automatic inspection machine (EIS-A206 S).

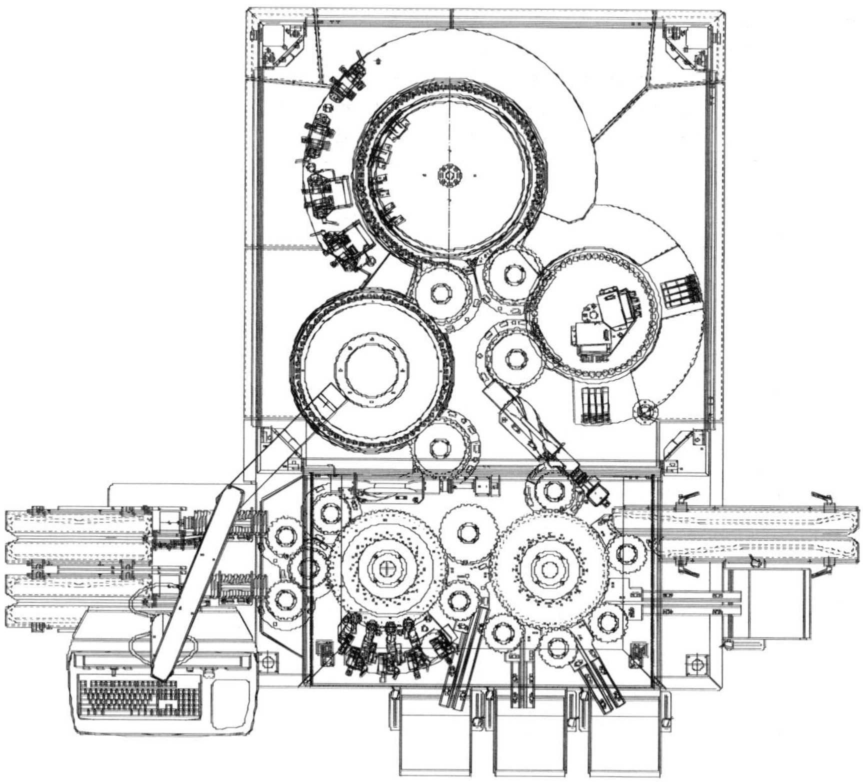

Figure 14 Drawing of machine layout (EIS-A206 S).

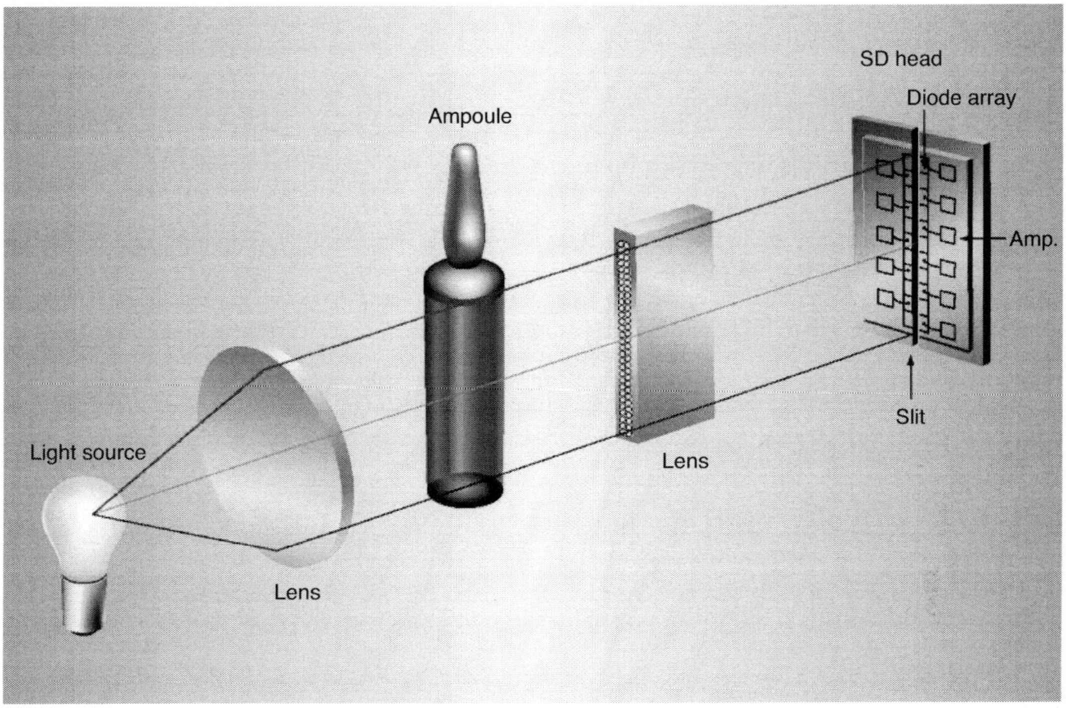

Figure 15 SD system.

to the camera table, where detailed cosmetic defects are inspected, for vials as example, such as body, neck and heel, fill level, cap/crimp/liquid color, and crimp.

Finally, the containers are inspected twice at SD table, on which particle contamination is strictly inspected. Accepted containers are selected mechanically and transferred into the outfeed conveyor, which is connected to the downstream machine. While rejected containers due to the inspections are brought to three separate reject trays (in this type three reject trays) based on customer's configurations.

Functions

SD System (Fig. 15)

SD system is a system where

- Light projector transmits the high intensity light beam perpendicular to the container.
- Stack of small sensors (light-receiving diodes) is located at the other side of the container.
- The container to be inspected rotates between 1000 and 5000 RPM before inspection and is suddenly stopped by a break just before inspection. At that time, container is stationary but the liquid inside it continues to rotate.
- Any particle in the solution blocks a portion of the transmitted light, casting a shadow that is detected by an array of small light-receiving diodes.
- The instantaneous change in the light intensity is measured, while printing on the container surface can be canceled.

By analyzing only the change in light intensity caused by moving particles, the signals can be distinguished from static light reduction caused by stationary object such as scratches, dirt, and printing on the container surface, significantly decreasing the rejection of qualified products (false rejects). Unlike camera-based systems that capture, process, and compare images, the SD system reads voltage fluctuation in real time.

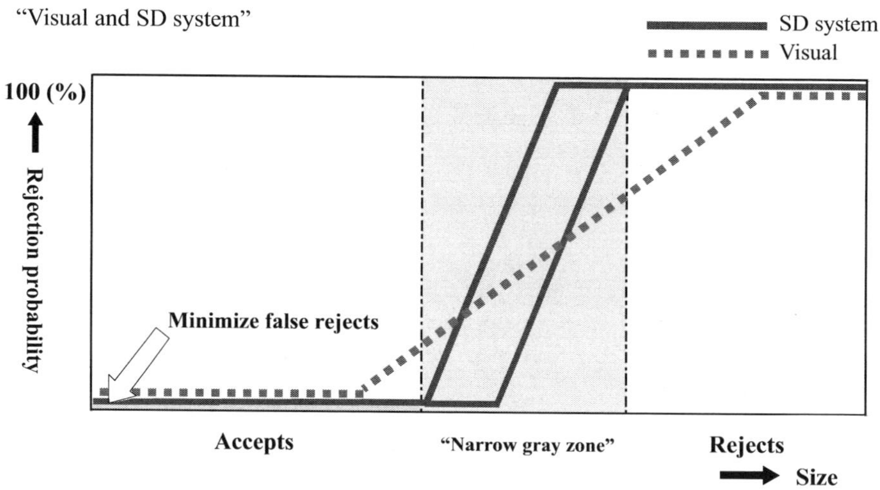

Figure 16 Foreign particle detection characteristic curve.

The key to detection, however, is not to reject good product. Because of narrow gray zone of SD system curve (Fig. 16), the system enables to minimize both the passing of bad products and rejecting good products.

Vision System

SD system recognized particles with the change of the shadow or light intensity, therefore cosmetic defects such as scratch, crack, aluminum crimp of vials and/or unmoving particles in the containers cannot be inspected by SD system. Such defects and particles can be rejected by the vision system inspection.

Cameras are set based on the inspection purpose, such as body crack and cap color. Up to 24 images can be captured with 360°C of the container at each inspection. Inspection results are determined at image processing circuit capturing images from spinning products.

Other Functions

In order to meet qualitative and productive requirement from global manufacturers, the latest machine (model EIS-A series) has following functions.

Retrieve system

EIS-A series store inspection data for each container. The data can be retrieved and used to fine-tune inspection parameters without running actual products through the machine. A graphical display provides visual verification of each inspection performed.

Spin control

For accurate particle inspection, new Controlled Spin System of EIS-A series keeps container at the proper spin speed by monitoring the feedback from rotating spindle cap.

Oscillating drive unit

In order to realize higher inspection speed without any loss of accuracy of detection and stability of the transportation, newly developed oscillating drive unit is used for EIS-A series (e.g., EIS-A206 S).

Furthermore, EIS-A series have preinspection oscillating drive mechanism that enables better inspection performance.

Transportation

EIS-A series have Automatic Reinspection function as optional. This function returns uninspected containers to the prespin table for a full reinspection (except containers on the

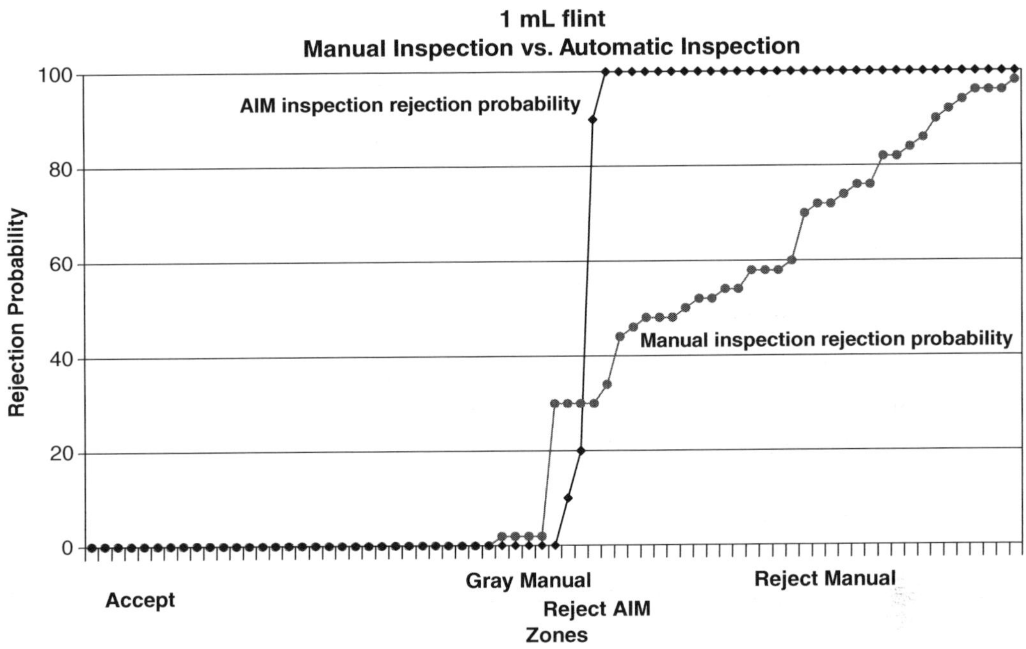

Figure 17 Rejection probability of manual inspection versus automatic inspection. *Abbreviation*: AIM, automatic inspection machine.

preinspection star wheel). Setting for such second pass inspection is user configurable through the human machine interface (HMI).

Additionally, EIS-A series has "Loop Validation" (optional), which allows product setup under actual production conditions by recycling test container set through the machine except preinspection area.

Advantage for Using Automatic Inspection Machine

Quality Improvement

Automated inspection systems are generally selected over manual and semiautomated visual subsystem in order to increase output and improve inspection accuracy. Figure 17 is plotted according to Knapp Study methodology comparing the rejection probability of samples using manual inspection versus automated inspection. An increased rejection capability of the automatic inspection in the reject zone shows improved security over that of the manual inspection.

Productivity Improvement

Michael de la Montaigne (Eisai Machinery U.S.A. Inc.) et al. performed a study from 2004 to 2005 to evaluate the economic efficiency of manual and automatic inspection method. Considering the fixed and variable costs including man power costs, the study indicated that automatic inspection's efficacy is more than double of the semiautomatic inspection machine and about 15 times of the manual system. The study also suggested that the initial high costs of the automatic system can be compensated by its higher efficiency within a couple of years.

ACKNOWLEDGMENTS

The authors gratefully acknowledge Eisai Co., Ltd., Astellas Pharma Inc., Kyowa Vacuum Engineering Co., Ltd., and IDK Co., Ltd. for providing their data and figures.

33 Pilot plants and isolation technology

James Agalloco

The development of many different pharmaceutical processes is facilitated by execution at an intermediate scale of operation in a facility that is often called a "pilot plant." Pilot plants in the global health care industry are used in support of bulk pharmaceutical chemicals, biotechnology processes, and dosage form manufacturing to define the process beyond what discovery scale efforts can. They often utilize small scale or lower throughput pieces of equipment requiring lesser quantities of material substantially reducing the consumption of what is often very expensive developmental material. Pilot plants are utilized for a variety of reasons including: preparation of materials for clinical or toxicology evaluation, optimization of process parameters, and evaluation of different lots of active raw materials.

The typical pilot plant uses equipment similar in design to that intended for commercial scale production albeit in smaller scale or capacity. Pilot plant equipment is customarily somewhat larger than laboratory apparatus, and though quite a bit smaller than commercial equipment. Pilot plants supporting parenteral formulation or biotechnology are often asked to provide environments in which asepsis or lesser degrees of microbial exclusion are provided. In many instances, containment and asepsis are required simultaneously, and the pilot plant must be capable of both worker and product protection.

Nearly all pilot plants are designed to be extremely flexible, able to match the capabilities of diverse production facilities, and able to provide the operating conditions for a variety of potential products and processes. Pilot plants may be subject to frequent alteration, to match either the evolving needs of an individual process that might require a subtle change, or the completely different processing requirements of a new product. The need for reconfiguration of the process equipment of a pilot plant can be almost constant. For most processes, whether for synthesis or formulation, liquid or solid, rearranging the equipment, or moving the material through the equipment in a different order is of little consequence. Aseptic processing is substantially different, sterile items must be protected from contamination, and any movement must consider the potential for environmental or operator-induced contamination. Aseptic facilities are designed for protection of sterile materials, and flexibility of arrangement is rarely a major consideration. The reconfiguration of an aseptic pilot plant would customarily entail physical rearrangement of the equipment, their background environments, and potentially the facility walls as well. This can create significant difficulties in capital cost, lost equipment time, and the attendant qualification/validation costs associated with the renovation. Isolation technology whether used for creating a microbially controlled processing environment, containment of potent compounds, or both at the same time may be an ideal solution for aseptic pilot plant applications, as the material protection is unaffected by repositioning of equipment, as the protection afforded by the use of isolation technology is unaltered by a change in the position of one isolator with respect to another.

Consider the process flow diagram shown in Figure 1, which depicts the actual process flows for a variety of closely related developmental products.

In this particular instance, the firm required asepsis, while also handling flammable solvents, and potent powder materials. Each of the blocks in the process flow diagram surrounded a single unit operation. Consider for a moment the difficulty in designing a pilot plant to accommodate these diverse requirements in which each piece of equipment was located in a separate aseptic environment. There is no single facility arrangement that could satisfy all of the required flow patterns without multiple points of crossover between personnel and material flows. Were all of the equipment to be located in a common classified area, flexibility of processing might be possible, however, at substantial compromise to worker protection and asepsis of the materials. Isolators afford a viable solution to the layout difficulties associated with the complex process flow a pilot plant must accommodate while simultaneously affording the necessary worker and product protection. In this example, the isolators intended for the various

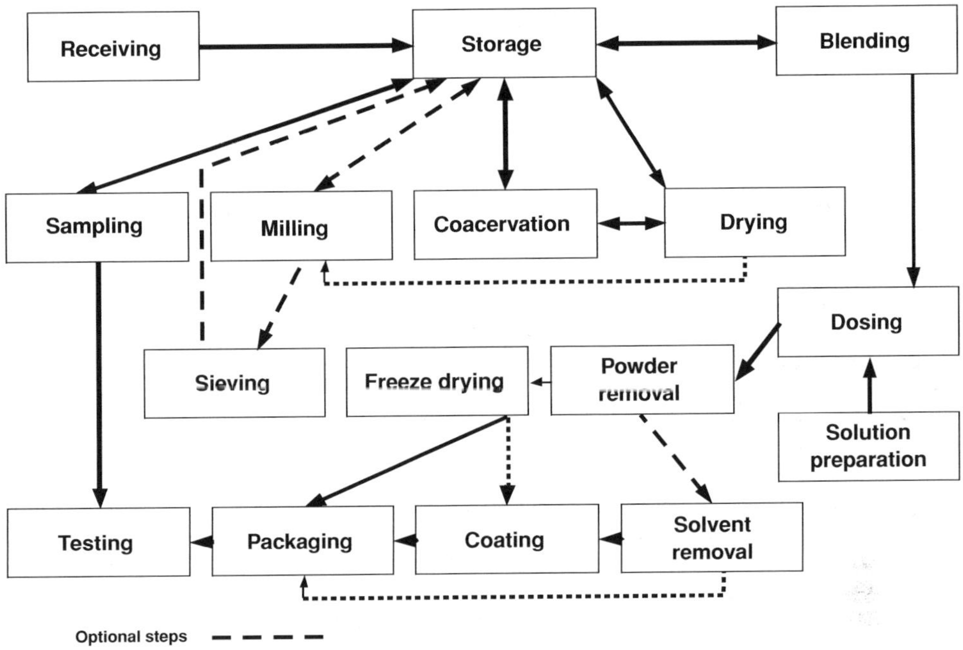

Figure 1 Process flow diagram for pilot plant.

unit operations were predominantly standard designs, while a limited number were custom designed to fit specific processing requirements. Each unit operation required for the process is performed within an isolator, with transfer isolators used to convey material between them. The relationship between the isolators can be compared with an archipelago (the unit operation isolators) served by a number of ferries (the transfer isolators). This approach to pilot plant design afforded total flexibility of operation, as the transfer isolators can be used to bring materials from any unit operation to any other while maintaining the required product protection and material containment required. As the project evolved, an analysis of the required attributes of the isolators for the various unit operations was performed. This revealed that the requirements varied according to the specific unit operations carried out within the various isolators (Table 1). In addition to the identification of the major design elements for the isolators, an equipment order sequence was developed that allowed for staged investment, as operational demands on the pilot plant increased. This design reflected some specific flows; however, it should be evident that the use of isolators allows for essentially total freedom of process sequence, any unit operation can follow or precede any other. For this project, other nuances were easily accommodated. Only those isolators that were potentially exposed to solvents would be explosion proof. Those isolators where neither solvents nor powders would be exposed could be flexible wall decreasing weight, and lead time. Provided the rapid transfer port (RTP) designs are compatible, the purchase could also be spread over multiple vendors to shorten the delivery schedule.

The use of isolation technology can provide advantages over a more conventional room-based pilot plant with less complex flow requirements:

- Where the process sequence might be altered or added to during the developmental effort, the use of isolation technology means that a new piece of process equipment can be introduced without an impact on the preceding or subsequent steps. Such a possibility would be more difficult were the equipment permanently installed in a room. A process step could just as easily be removed without impact.
- In the event, additional capacity is needed for a particular step in the process, a second piece of equipment can be brought online without interfering with operations in the existing equipment essentially doubling the output of that step without disturbing operations. Alternatively, a smaller capacity unit could be replaced with one of larger capacity.

Table 1 Isolator Design Overview

		#	Order group	Wall	Explosion proof
1	Dose forming	1	1	R	Y
2	Hopper	1	1	R	N
3	Kneeling transfer	1	1	R	Y
4	Milling/sieve	1	1	R	N
5	Autoclave interface	1	1–2	S	N
6	Coacervation	1	2	R	Y
7	Solution preparation	1	2	R	Y
8	Freeze-dry	1	2	R	Y
9	Dedusting	1	2	R	N
10	Transfer isolator	2	2	S	N
11	Package	1	3	S	N
12	Powder sample/repack	1	3	R	N
13	Oven interface	1	3	S	N
14	Transfer isolator	1	3	S	N
15	Blender/dryer service box	1	3	R	Y
17	Sterility test—$^1/_2$ suit	1	4	S	N
18	Sterility transfer	1	4	S	N

S, soft wall isolator; R, rigid wall isolator.

- Maintenance or modification of equipment can be carried out on any piece of equipment without fear that the service or maintenance personnel might disturb operations in other equipment or environments.

The use of isolators for individual unit operations in a pilot plant allows process changes to be accommodated without facility modification. The flexibility afforded by isolators allows the facility the ability to operate its equipment without the inherent limitations imposed by their physical arrangement within a more conventional facility dependent on classified rooms. Moreover, the use of isolation technology allows for changes in an individual unit operation without affecting the other unit operations. Process sequences can be altered as needed to suit changes in the process. A process that was originally executed in a sequence of A→B→C→D can be executed as B→D→C→A or C→A→D→B or any other desired sequence without any cost, or delay. Unit operation B could be replaced by unit operation E, doubled in throughput by the addition of a larger B, or perhaps a second B. Alternatively, a new unit operation F could be added at any point in the process sequence. Table 2 outlines the possible relationships among unit operations up to a total of four different activities. In classical pilot plants, equipment is sometimes rearranged to accommodate the specific needs of a particular process. With aseptic processing, where the protective environment surrounding the equipment is an essential part of the overall process, relocation of the equipment is far more complex. Lyophilizers, and filling machines, even for smaller scale production are difficult to relocate, and even if movable may require substantial requalification when relocated within a classified area. Thus, aseptic pilot facilities are only minimally flexible and substantial compromises may be necessary to accommodate the diverse needs of developmental activities. If any of the unit operations are performed more than once in the process (as might be possible with such unit operations as blending, milling, mixing, or sampling) the number of possible permutations is further increased.

Given that the number of unit operations in the typical pharmaceutical process is ordinarily substantially greater than four, the possible flow patterns (and room arrangements) for a pilot plant to accommodate can be extremely high. Isolation technology allows for total flexibility of arrangement something impossible with a fixed facility design, but an essential requirement in pilot plant operations. The rearrangement of classified rooms to accommodate the type of flexibility is impossible without interrupting operations, and results in substantial higher costs. A further benefit is that the background environment can be of a lower classification than that necessary for operational use, reducing both capital and operational costs over the life of the facility.

Table 2 Process Combination in 2, 3, and 4 Step Processes

Number of operations	Unit operations	Possible combinations	Number of possible combinations
2	A B	A→B, B→A	2
3	A B C	A→B, B→A, A→C, C→A, B→C, C→B, A→B→C, A→C→B, B→C→A, B→A→C, C→A→B, C→B→A	12
4	A B C D	A→B, A→C, A→D, B→A, B→C, B→D, C→A, C→B, C→D, D→A, D→B, D→C, A→B→C, A→C→B, A→B→D, A→D→B, A→C→D, A→D→C, B→C→A, B→A→C, B→C→D, B→D→C, B→A→D, B→D→A, C→A→B, C→B→A, C→A→D, C→D→A, C→B→D, C→D→B, D→A→B, D→B→A, D→A→C, D→C→A, D→B→C, D→C→B. A→B→C→D, A→C→B→D, A→B→D→C, A→D→B→C, A→C→D→B, A→D→C→B, B→C→A→D, B→A→C→D, B→C→D→A, B→D→C→A, B→A→D→C, B→D→A→C, C→A→B→D, C→B→A→D, C→A→D→B, C→D→A→B, C→B→D→A, C→D→B→A D→A→B→C, D→B→A→C, D→A→C→B, D→C→A→B, D→B→C→A, D→C→B→A	60

The use of isolators for parenteral pilot plants has been implemented in at least two projects where flexibility in operation was a determining factor. QLT Phototherapeutics constructed a pilot plant capable of filling syringes and vials incorporating freeze-drying, bulk processing, and terminal sterilization in 2004 to 2005 (Fig. 2) (1). The University of Kentucky utilized a similar concept on a somewhat large scale in the design of their Center for Pharmaceutical Science and Technology in 2005 to 2006, which had the capability of filling both potent and nontoxic sterile compounds (2). Each project began with the same basic goals of flexibility, expandability, and worker safety that were fully realizable only with isolation technology.

A closely related approach to that described in this chapter has been developed by Xcellerex of Marlborough, MA. They offer comparable flexibility for the processing of biological materials starting with cell culture and extending through to final purification. The various unit operations that comprise their FlexFactory^{TM} are performed in restricted access barrier systems (RABS) type enclosures that are intended for location in either ISO 7 or ISO 8 background environments (3). Aside from the differences in expected internal environmental conditions for early stages of production, the approach is essentially identical to that described for aseptic pilot plant operations and offers the same advantages.

There are firms that have recognized that efficacy testing in animals is simpler, easier, and substantially less expensive than safety/toxicity testing. These firms have placed new therapeutics into animals to establish their potential utility for a particular indication, before completing safety/toxicity testing. In order to produce the necessary clinical materials, worker

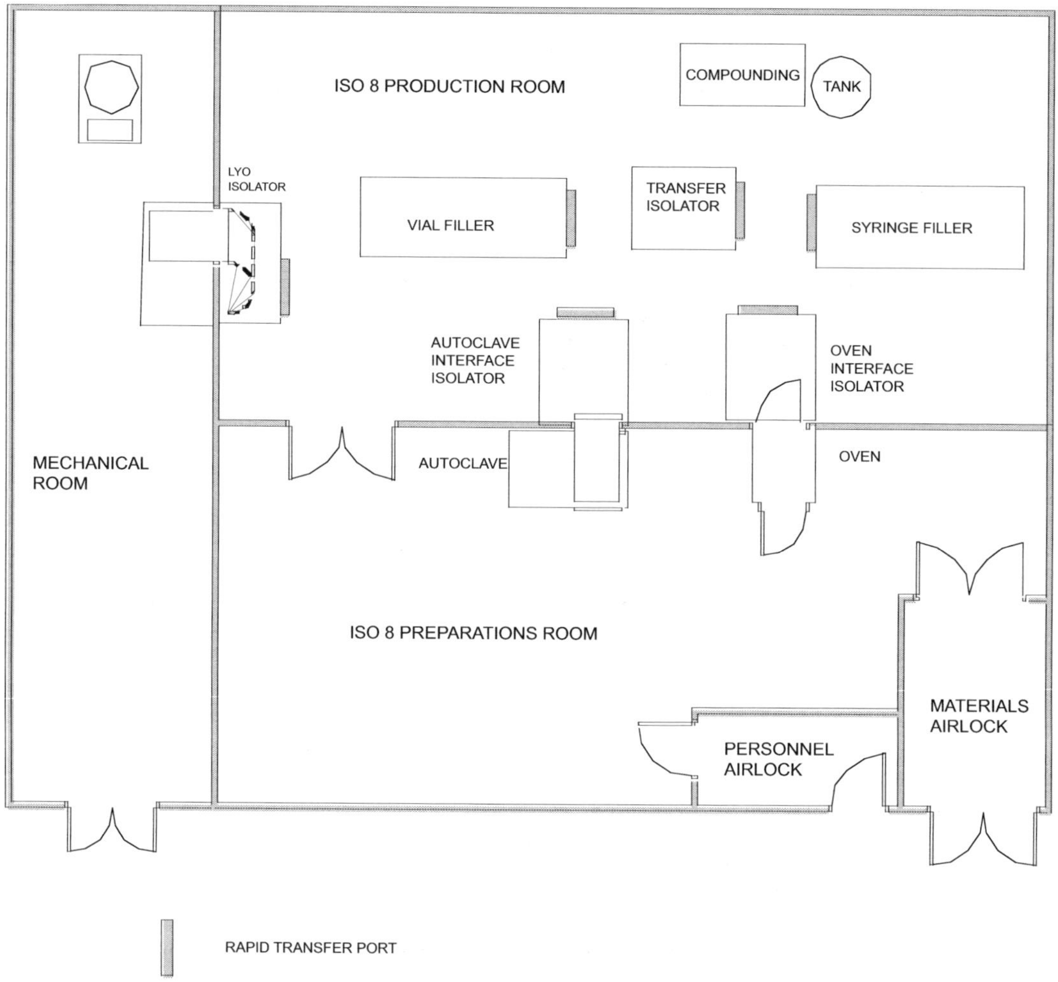

Figure 2 Conceptual drawing isolator based aseptic pilot plant.

protection is essential during every stage of the process as there is no available information relative to the materials potential effect on humans. Isolators that provide for enhanced worker safety can be employed in all aspects of the development/clinical manufacturing from API or biotech origin beginning at bench top scale of preparation. Given the changing nature of clinical production requirements, the aforementioned flexibility is an added benefit over the enhanced worker protection isolation technology inherently provides.

Isolation technology may be an ideal solution for pilot plant applications where either asepsis or containment is required. It can be expected that the future development of many health care products will increasingly rely on the use of isolators for aseptic and containment pilot plants to provide the necessary protection to both product and personnel.

REFERENCES

1. Procyshyn C. Case study: Clinical aseptic isolator manufacturing facility. In: Proceedings of ISPE Conference on Sterilization & Aseptic Processing for the 21st Century; June 7–8, 2006; Washington, DC.
2. Thomas P. Inside Kentucky's new aseptic thoroughbred. Pharm Manuf 2006; 5(7):18–21.
3. http://www.xcellerex.com/platform-flexfactory-biomanufacturing.htm. Accessed May 24, 2010.

34 Highly automated isolator-based vaccine filling—a case study

James Akers, Kazuhito Tanimoto, and Masahito Kawata

The global pharmaceutical industry has traditionally been considered a conservative industry slow to adopt technological advances such as computerized systems and automation. However, its conservative nature has not prevented a significant increase in the implementation of newer technologies for aseptic filling. Shibuya Kogyo Co., Ltd. introduced isolators for aseptic manufacturing into the Japanese market in 1994 and as of this writing has installed more than 175 isolators for aseptic processing, containment, and sterility testing in Japan, Asia, and the United States. Japan has become a significant center for the advancement of aseptic processing, and the variety of aseptic production applications for which isolators have been used is comprehensive and includes both large and small volume parenterals, lyophilized products, powder fills, combination products, as well as medical devices. In addition to advanced aseptic processing environments such as isolators, Japanese firms have been aggressive in their adoption of factory automation and robotics. Japanese pharmaceutical manufacturers hold themselves to very high standards regarding both overall product quality and economic performance as measured in yield and production uptime.

Japan has also been an active participant in the International Congress on Harmonization and has been progressive in the implementation of new standards reflecting the latest advancements in aseptic technology. In 2005, a document entitled *Guidance for Industry—Sterile Drug Products Produced by Aseptic Processing* (hereafter called the Guideline) was written by a joint task force comprised of industry, academic, government scientists, and regulatory experts. This comprehensive 99-page guidance document provides information on all aspects of aseptic processing including production facilities, utility systems, sterilization equipment, environmental management, process simulation, and ongoing process control. This guidance document provides useful information regarding the design and validation of advanced aseptic processing technologies such as separative technologies and blow/fill/seal.

According to the authors, readers unfamiliar with aseptic processing in Japan might believe upon reading the 2005 guidance document that Japanese performance standards regarding aseptic processing generally parallel those of Europe and the United States. The environmental monitoring recommendations, media fill procedures/acceptance criteria, and process validation expectations embodied within are fully compatible with those of the United States and the European Union. Since Japan as previously noted is one of the three constituent regions within the International Conference on Harmonization (ICH) as previously noted, this should not be surprising. However, aseptic technology specialists in Europe and the United States are relatively less familiar with Japan's practices. Comparatively speaking there has been little information available in Europe and North America regarding aseptic processing requirements and production facilities in Japan. The author's objective in preparing this chapter is to use this case study to make those outside Japan more familiar with that country's practice and their innovative approach to facility design and process control.

The authors believe that before describing the case study, the reader would benefit from a brief summary of Japan's aseptic processing guidance:

- Personnel—The guideline clearly states that human operators are the most significant source of contamination in aseptic processing and therefore stipulates a comprehensive set of objectives in personnel training. These include expertise in aseptic technique and a working knowledge of microbiology including specific knowledge "regarding species likely to be encountered" in routine monitoring. Additionally, personnel are to be thoroughly trained in the donning of gowns and comprehensively evaluated in their gowning capability and performance. Finally, workers are expected to have a working knowledge of the principles of cleaning and disinfection.

- Quality systems expectations are defined in the Guideline including documentation systems, general organizational structure, risk analysis, and qualification of equipment and process validation.
- Requirements for facility design and clean room classification are described in detail within the Guideline. Critical areas are required to meet Grade A expectations for both total particulate and microbiological contamination, and surrounding support areas are expected to comply with Grade B requirements. The conditions stipulated for the design, management, and control of aseptic processing environments are like those defined in the European Union Guide to Good Manufacturing Practices (EU-GMPs). Pressure differentials of 10 to 15 Pa are recommended between adjacent rooms of different classifications.
- Disinfectants and sanitizing agents much be demonstrably free of microbial contamination at the time of use, and disinfectant application methods must be verified/validated for effectiveness. Firms are also expected to ensure that residues of antimicrobial agents can be reduced to a predefined and safe level.
- Component preparation processes must be validated that demonstrate a 99.9% (3-log reduction) of bacterial endotoxin.
- Environmental monitoring in Grade A critical zones for airborne contamination must be conducted for each shift of operation. Personnel are also to be sampled for microbial contamination once/shift. Surface monitoring is to be performed at the end of each production operation, and total particulate monitoring is to be completed "throughout the entire aseptic procedure" in all Grade A environments.
- All product contact materials including container/closure systems and filters, for example, must be sterilized utilizing a validated sterilization process. The use of biological indicator challenge tests is required in the validation of sterilization processes. Specific guidance is provided on all sterilization methods used in industry, and a separate section is dedicated to directions for the use of sterilization-in-place systems.
- The Guideline recommends that where isolator systems are utilized in aseptic processing "the number of half suits, gloves, transfer ports, and connections ... to a minimum in order to reduce the chance of contamination." Isolators are also required to have a minimum positive pressure differential of 17.5 Pa relative to the surrounding environment, which is expected to meet Grade D requirements.
- Media fills must comprehensively challenge the entire process including all product contact equipment and must consist of at least 5000 units as a general recommendation. All shifts must participate in media fill tests and all production aseptic interventions must be included in each test. Media fills should cover the longest production time utilized in actual aseptic manufacturing.

The list above highlights Japanese Guideline recommendations on many of the most commonly discussed issues in aseptic processing. Space does not allow a full review of this very comprehensive document. However, the authors trust that the list clearly indicate to the reader that Japanese standards are well harmonized with those of Europe and the United States.

Japan, like the other constituents of the ICH, has its own very well-developed pharmaceutical manufacturing equipment industry. Japan is fully capable of supplying all the equipments and facility infrastructure required for a state-of-the-art aseptic processing facility.

The most modern Japanese aseptic processing installations utilize a great deal of automation, vision systems, and electronic process control. Japanese requirements for computer system validation have been pragmatic from a scientific and engineering perspective, and have not encumbered pharmaceutical manufacturers wishing to employ advanced process control technologies, robotics, and machine automation.

CASE STUDY—VACCINE ASEPTIC PROCESSING

This case study serves as an example of current Japanese thinking regarding aseptic processing. This aseptic processing manufacturing line is installed at the Handai-Biken facility in Kagawa, Japan, and is dedicated to the aseptic bottling of vaccines in vials. The facility was built and the equipment installed in 2004, it was fully commissioned, installed, and validated in 2005 after

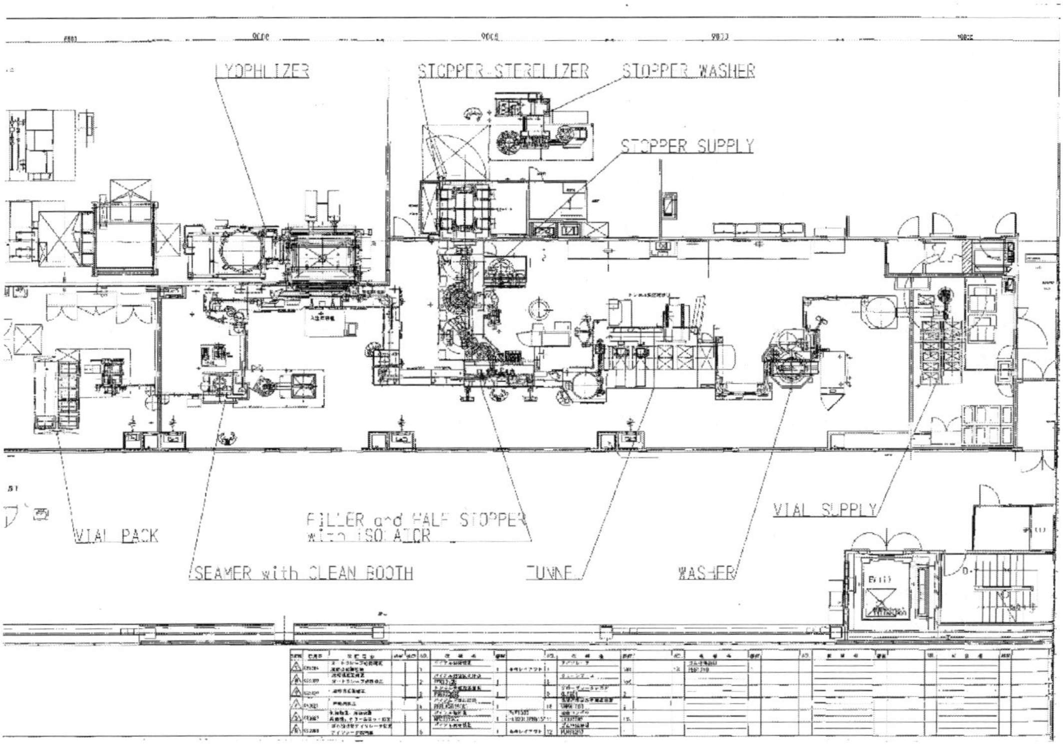

Figure 1 A top view of the installation layout.

which the commercial production of vaccines was initiated. The layout of the facility, which can produce both lyophilized and liquid-filled vials, is shown in Figure 1.

In this facility all product filling, lyophilization, and stoppering are conducted in vertical unidirectional airflow isolators, which are designed and operated to comply with IS0 14644 Class 5/Grade A requirements. The environment surrounding the isolators complies with ISO Class 7/Grade C requirements. Handai-Biken's carefully and thoroughly developed user requirement specifications for this project reflected the firm's focus regarding minimizing aseptic contamination risk and maximizing safety for the biological products to be manufactured using this production system. Given the focus upon risk mitigation, it is logical that two critical objectives for this production system were minimal particulate contamination and a diminished reliance upon human interventions. Additionally, productivity was considered a vital requirement. Therefore, a number of design features were implemented to ensure that the production line provides high production yields; which require minimal line stoppages, ease of changeover, and very high uptime.

ISOLATORS

The project consists of five isolator sections (described below) in order starting from the infeed side of the production line:

1. Interface/accumulator isolator between the tunnel and filler (3.9 m^3 total enclosed volume)
2. Filling/stoppering machine isolator (4.8 m^3 total enclosed volume)
3. Rubber stopper supply system isolator (16.9 m^3 total enclosed volume)
4. Lyophilizer conveyor isolator (3.9 m^3)
5. Automatic lyophilizer loading/unloading isolator (17.0 m^3).

The total enclosed isolator volume for these five sections is 47.4 m^3. For the purposes of vapor phase hydrogen peroxide decontamination, the isolators are divided into two sections.

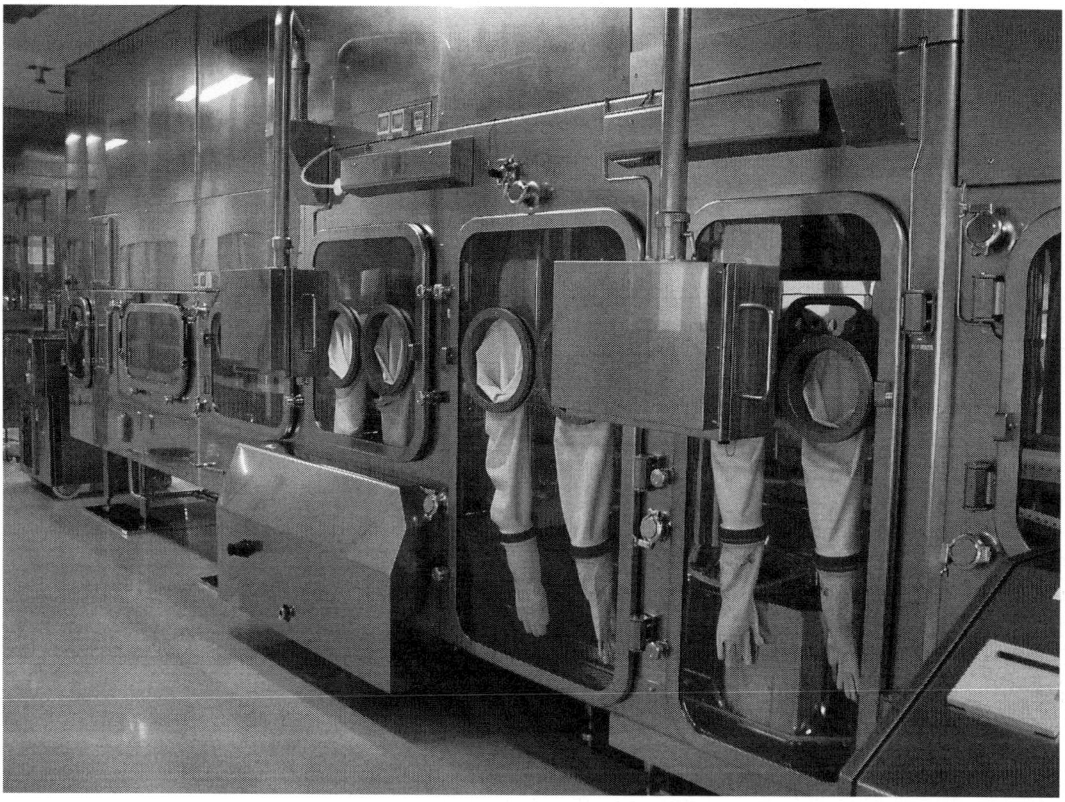

Figure 2 An external view of the isolator network within the ISO 7/Grade C surrounding environment.

Section one, which consists of isolators 1 to 4 above, has a total enclosed volume of 30.4 m^3, while the second decontamination group consists only of isolator 5. Decontamination is accomplished by VHPM1000S units sourced from Steris. The isolators are equipped with dehumidification units to reach the low humidity levels required by the Steris vapor phase hydrogen peroxide generators prior to the decontamination process (Fig. 2).

Decontamination of the isolators was validated using *Geobacillus stearothermophilus* biological indicators on stainless steel coupons with a population of 10^6 spores per indicator. The acceptance criterion for decontamination was complete kill of all biological indicators placed within the isolators.

PROCESS EQUIPMENT

Following are functional descriptions of each major piece of process equipment beginning with vial wash and ending with capping:

Vial Washer

The vial washer utilizes hot water for injection for vial washing. In typical washer designs, this results in the formation of water vapor under the top cover of the machine. Handai-Biken engineers were concerned about the negative air pressure that would develop within the top cover and in conjunction with Shibuya developed a double shell washer system in which positive HEPA filtered air is supplied between the outer and inner shells of the machine cover to eliminate the possibility of entrainment of particulate matter from the surrounding environment. This ensures that the vials are washed and handled in a high air quality environment and that risk from total particulate contamination is very low.

Dry Heat Tunnel and Interface Isolator

The dry heat tunnel is equipped with a fully dry heat sterilizable cooling zone. The tunnel's cooling zone can be sterilized by dry heat at 170°C for 20 minutes during changeover periods. This dry heat cooling zone sterilization process is fully validated. A vial counting system is used in front of the tunnel inlet to form a single row to ensure smooth feeding of glass with minimum pressure on the glass pack as it passes through the tunnel vials, entering the tunnel from the vial washer. This single row of vials is not pushed onto the tunnel's mesh conveyor until a measured amount of elapsed time has passed since the introduction of the previous row of vials. This design ensures that no horizontal pressure is applied to vials already moving on the conveyor. The minimum horizontal pressure required to feed each row of vials onto the conveyor effectively eliminates "crashing" of glass and prevents particulate formation, or vial breakage resulting from harsh glass-to-glass contact.

Aseptic Filling Machine/Rubber Stopping Machine and Isolator

Fill mass (volume) is controlled by means of eight mass flow meters, each of which supplies a single filling nozzle. All filling data are digitized and stored electronically. This enables the system to record the precise fill data including mass, vial number, and time, and to display this data on the control panel. A full summary of all filling data for each filled unit within each lot can be printed out on a daily basis. All product contact parts within the mass flow meters are composed of 316 L stainless steel. The mass flow meters are fully cleaned and sterilized in place obviating the need for manual aseptic connections within the wetted path. Handai-Biken engineers specified that in addition to the mass flow metering system, fill weights must also be taken gravimetrically. This system consists of eight load cells, which can perform the fill weight function in approximately 10 seconds. The gravimetric weight check system was originally used at 15-minute intervals throughout the full duration of each lot's filling operation. However, after sufficient experience with the mass flow system it was found that it was not necessary to check fill volumes gravimetrically throughout the filling process, because the flow metering system proved to be extremely accurate and reliable. Actual mass flow fill accuracies have been ±0.5%, which is well within the ±1% validation acceptance criterion established in the Handai-Biken user requirement specifications. At the present time, the mass flow filling control system is considered fully validated and fill volumes are checked by the load cells now only for reference purposes during setup.

The fill machine construction has a cantilevered balcony type design, so all maintenance can be performed from outside the isolator enclosure. Also, there is no equipment located under the filling needles allowing air to flow undisturbed to the air returns located at the floor of the machine. To further ensure minimal airflow disturbance, curved fill needles are used so that only these small cross-sectional area tubes are within the airflow above the vials. Thus, unlike most systems, flexible tubing and mechanical supports for the fill needles are located away from the vials and because the mass flow fill pumps are mounted externally the filling zone is remarkably uncluttered (Fig. 3).

Rubber Stopper Supply System

The rubber stopper supply system is one of the most important design features of this entire processing system. Handai-Biken and Shibuya Kogyo Co., Ltd. recognized that one of the most frequent routine interventions required in aseptic vial processing lines is to stage rubber stoppers and manually place them into the stopper feed hopper. In a filling system capable of line speeds of up to 400 vials/min, stopper supply can be labor intensive and batch processing of stoppers would require significant storage space after autoclaving. It was also determined that, at the stopper consumption rate required for this filling system, the use of a rapid transfer port or "Beta-Bag" system was not an ideal solution.

To address these issues, Shibuya engineered a stopper washing system that washes each stopper individually to ensure gentle handling and minimal particulate generation. The stopper washing system automatically feeds the stoppers into custom-designed stainless steel stopper cans, which are perforated for proper steam penetration during autoclaving. These cans are fed automatically into a dedicated autoclave in which all stoppers are sterilized using a validated moist heat process. After the cycle is complete, the autoclave is automatically unloaded using

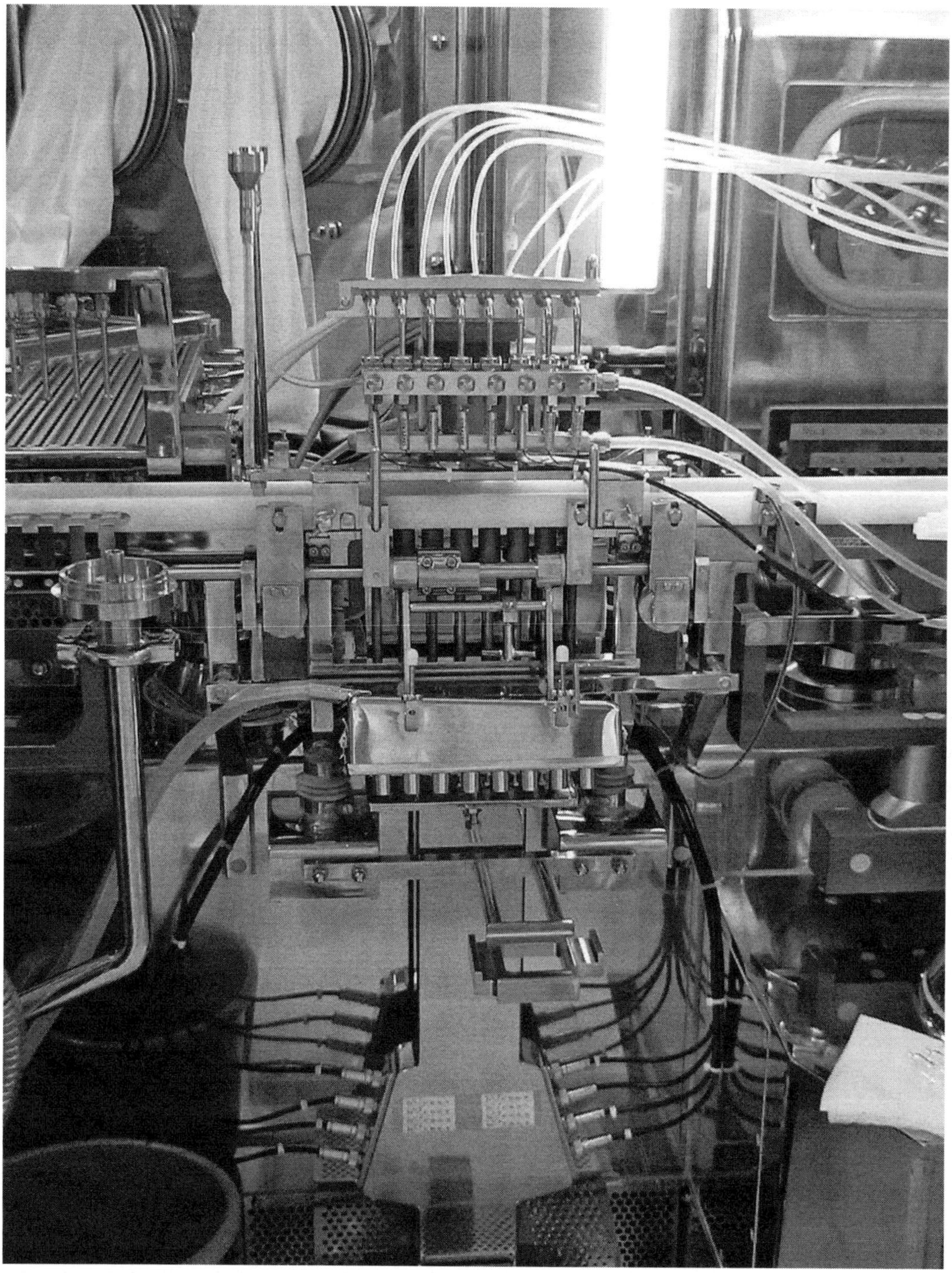

Figure 3 This photograph shows the 8 mass flow fill nozzles along with the S/CIP drain receptacle. The mass flow pumps are located outside the filling isolator on a separate skid. In the foreground of this photograph the built in VPHP decontaminated active air sampling head is visible.

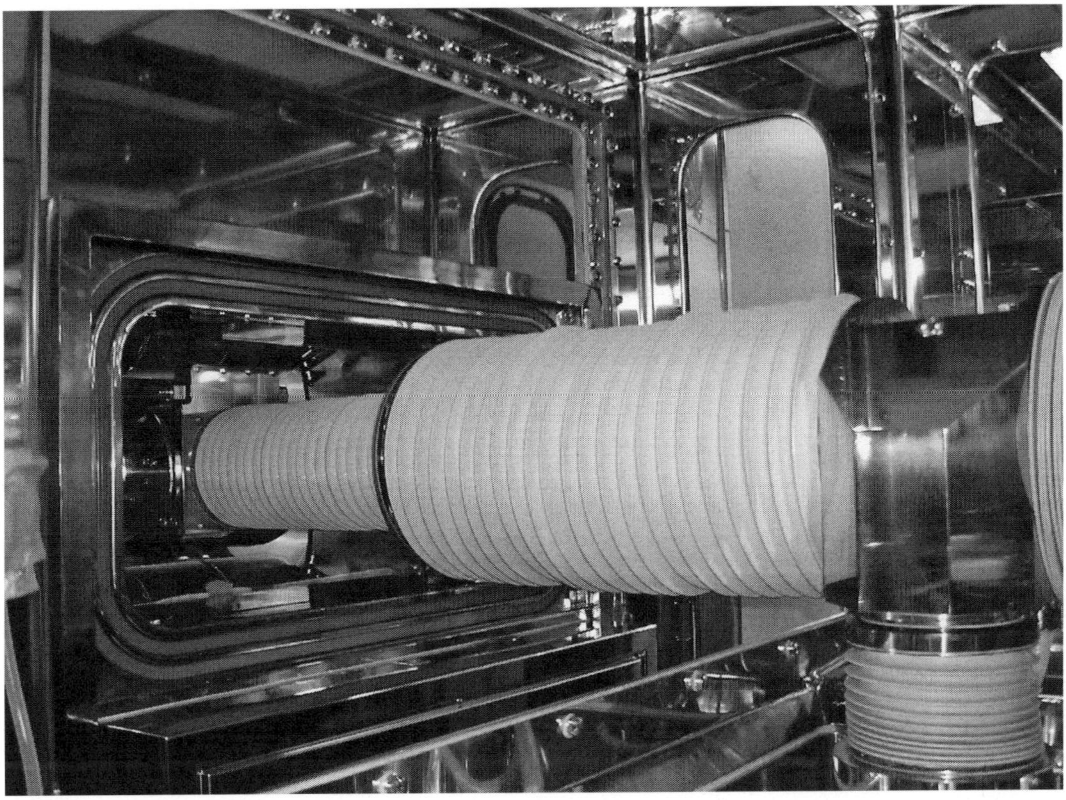

Figure 4 Robotic stopper supply system. This robot is designed and built to be fully VPHP resistant and to operate in ISO Class 5 environments. This is the first installation in which VPHP resistant robots were utilized.

robotics and the sterile stopper-filled cans are accumulated within a conveyor inside the stopper supply isolator. Robots automatically lift the cans and tip the stoppers into the hoppers when signaled to do so by sensors located on the stopper hopper (Fig. 4). Empty cans are returned to the autoclave, which serves as a pass box for transfer of these empty cans back to the loading side of the autoclave, where they are prepared for their next use.

To ensure smooth stopper feeding, eight separate parallel stopper tracks are used to feed the rubber plugs to the stoppering mechanism (Fig. 5). This means that at the high speed the line is capable of, no more than 50 stoppers/min are required to travel down any single stopper feed track. The stoppering mechanism itself has been designed to provide positive stopper seating with highly reproducible depth for lyophilization.

The authors believe that this automatic stopper preparation and feed system is a tremendous advantage over more conventional manual systems. This combination of automation and robotics eliminates potential ergonomic problems that have been known to exist in conventional isolators and also minimizes contamination risk by avoiding the use of gloved interventions. A further benefit to this approach is that it eliminates waste that would normally have to be removed from the isolator since there are no autoclave bags or wraps required for this stopper supply operation. This system has proven to be efficient and extremely reliable in day-to-day production operations.

The implementation of this stopper supply system also required the development of robots capable of withstanding vapor phase hydrogen peroxide decontamination. These robots do not contribute particulate contamination that would be considered significant in an ISO Class 5 environment. In fact, studies have determined that these robots would be suitable for use in an ISO Class 4 environment. This project represents the first use of vapor phase hydrogen peroxide-resistant isolators in the global pharmaceutical industry.

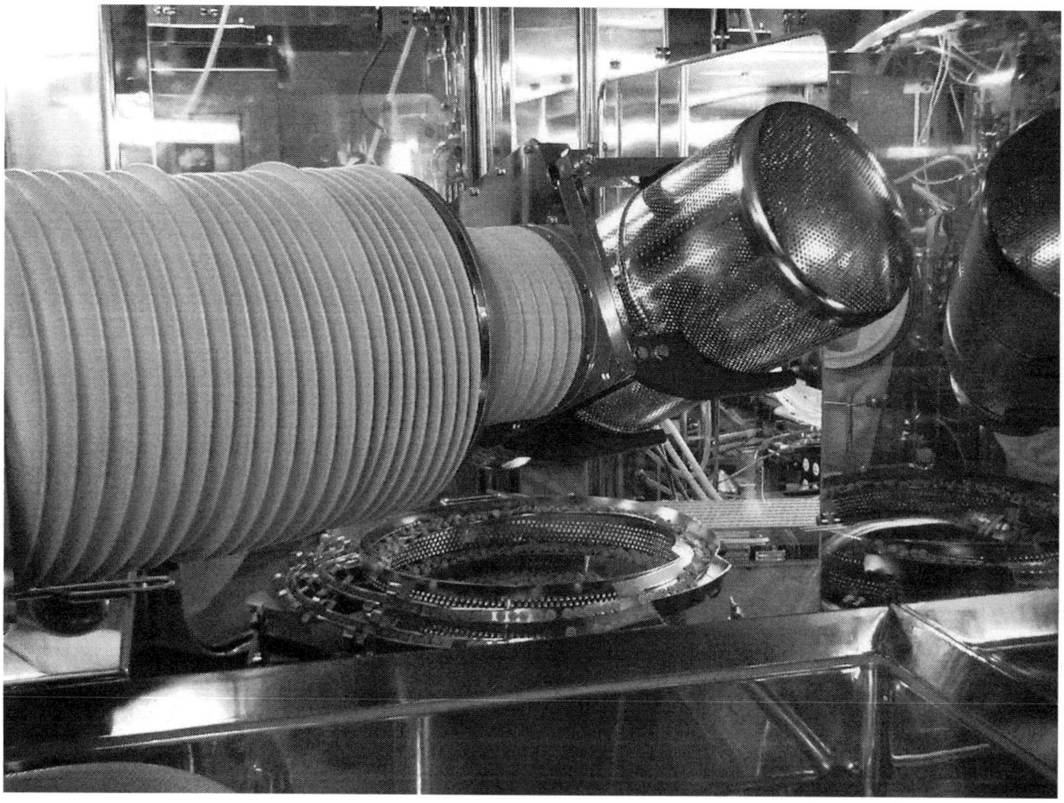

Figure 5 A view of the stopper supply robot as it doses sterilized stoppers into the feed hopper under validated and fully automated conditions.

Lyophilization/Aluminum Cap Sealing

Half-stoppered vials are conveyed from the stoppering unit in the filling isolator to the lyophilizer without exiting an isolator environment. All loading and unloading of the lyophilizer is fully automated and requires no operator interventions. At the end of the lyophilization process, the fully stoppered vials, once automatically unloaded from the lyophilizer, are conveyed to an aluminum cap applying and sealing station. This station is located within a unidirectional HEPA filtered clean booth, which meets ISO 5 conditions.

Environmental Monitoring Systems

Environmental microbiological air sampling systems are located within the isolator network and sites, which were carefully considered during the design process. The air sampling units are fully decontaminated with vapor phase hydrogen peroxide to minimize the possibility of false–positive results. HEPA filters mounted at the distal end of the supply system, external to the isolator, protect against contamination from the surrounding environment eliminating the possibility of adverse effects upon the isolator environment. Microbial sampling can be accomplished with good ease of use and with minimal risk of contamination in sample taking or handling. Additionally, the filling system is equipped with automatic electronic total particulate air monitoring at multiple locations.

Vital Production Statistics

The following are critical production statistics for the isolator-based vial filling system for vaccines:

1. Filling speeds: 400 vials/min for 2 mL vials and 200 vials/min for 7 mL vials. In the future, the system will be equipped to handle 10 mL vials.

2. Container types: Glass vials 2 and 7 mL (future 10 mL).
3. Stopper types: A total of five types of rubber stoppers was used: they include lyophilization stoppers for both 2 and 7 mL, and three different types of conventional stoppers for 2 mL vials.
4. Aluminum caps: Two types: one for 2 mL containers and another for 7 mL containers.
5. Product types filled: (*i*) Clear vaccine solution with a mean viscosity of 2 cP. (*ii*) Vaccine suspension, which will sediment without mixing.

SUMMARY

Japan has standards for aseptic processing and for validation of sterilization processes that are well harmonized with those in force in Europe and North America. Japan's aseptic processing guidance documents, which are available in English, comprehensively cover advanced aseptic processing systems such as isolators. The isolator-based aseptic filing line described in this article was conceived and built in Japan utilizing equipment sourced nearly exclusively from Japanese vendors. The authors believe that the filling system described in this article is fully state-of-the-art and will meet all global production quality and validation requirements for many years to come. Perhaps most significantly stopper feeding, the frequent routine intervention in most aseptic processes, and lyophilizer loading and unloading the most laborious intervention are fully automated and conducted within ISO 5 isolators.

According to the authors an important trend in aseptic manufacturing will be the elimination of human contamination and ease of operation in separative environments such as isolators.

The use of carefully designed automation and robotics reduces contamination risk by eliminating many interventions and also improve productivity and reliability. In the filling line described in this chapter, the automation and robotics have proven to be very reliable and have not caused increased maintenance downtime. We can envision a future in which the need for human operators for direct intervention in aseptic operations will be completely eliminated.

FURTHER READING

1. Japan PDA Task Force on Sterile Drug Products Produced by Aseptic Processing (with support from the Japanese Ministry of Health, Labor, and Welfare). Guidance for Industry—Sterile Drug Products Produced by Aseptic Processing, 2005.
2. Oshima Y, Yoshida S, Akers J. PasepT: A new concept in aseptic processing. In: Proceedings of the 36th R3 Nordic Symposium and 5th European Parenteral Conference; May 30–June 1, 2005; Linköping, Sweden.
3. Akers JE, Kokubo M, Oshima Y. The next generation of aseptic processing equipment. Pharm Technol 2006; 32–36.
4. U.S. Food and Drug Administration. Guidance for Industry. Sterile Drug Products Produced by Aseptic Processing—Current Good Manufacturing Practices. Rockville, MD: FDA, 2004.

35 Technological advancements in aseptic processing and the elimination of contamination risk

James E. Akers and Yoshi Izumi

There has been from the inception of aseptic processing an understanding among knowledgeable experts that a low level of contamination was to one degree or another inevitable. One needs only to consider relevant international regulatory standards and guidance to confirm this expectation of contamination. For example, neither EU Annex 1 nor the FDA's Guideline on Sterile Drugs Produced by Aseptic Processing (1,2) suggests that the recovery of viable contamination in monitoring should be an unexpected result. EU Annex 1 stated that in what is defined in that document as a Grade A environment, microbial content of air in environmental monitoring should average <1 CFU, this reflects that the expectation levels of residual contamination must be low, but it neither states nor implies that a zero recovery results are expected or required. Certainly regulations and guidance implies that the target for contamination recovery in process simulation tests and environmental monitoring is zero, but these documents make room for a rare low level contamination event because rationally, where conventional clean room aseptic processing is concerned, it is impractical to do otherwise. Similarly, the United States Pharmacopoeia (USP) chapter <1116>, which is undergoing revision (3), recommends a low, less than 1%, contamination incident rate for ISO 5 environments.

The reasons for this begrudging acceptance of the inevitability of contamination in the aseptic environment can be readily comprehended. During what can be termed the manned clean room era of aseptic processing, a period of time that roughly spans the last four decades, gowned human operators have been essential to the conduct of aseptic processing. In fact, the need for humans to be involved in aseptic processing necessitates a *human-scale* clean room. Simply put, a human-scale clean room is one that allows people to conduct the work of moving components and supplies to points-of-use, set up equipment, and make the necessary (and risk intensive) interventions that have always been essential in aseptic processing. Humans contribute contamination today just as they have throughout the entire period that manned operations have been required in aseptic processing (4).

Another unavoidable feature dictated by the presence of people working in close proximity to the process and hence product is that human-scale clean rooms need points of entry and exit for the personnel they require. These manned facilities also rely on manual disinfection of materials that may enter the aseptic operations area through airlocks of various designs. Although, in the modern human-scale clean room these entry points are typically fastidiously designed and carefully controlled they remain a secondary source of contamination. The risks associated with materials transfer are generally minor in comparison to human borne contamination. However, contamination entry at transfer points, such as gown rooms and airlocks, can still cause contamination problems that are difficult to reliably detect, very challenging to track, and that can put product at risk (5).

Certainly as evolutionary improvements in aseptic technology resulted in empirically better contamination control, regulatory expectations for the aseptic production of pharmaceutical products labeled sterile have continued to tighten. A perusal of either the current FDA guidance regarding aseptic processing or Annex 1 of the EU-GMP regulations clearly confirms that regulatory expectations are significantly more stringent than they were even a decade ago. The authors believe that this ongoing escalation in regulatory requirement for aseptic processing originates principally from the perceived need of regulatory authorities to encourage firms to make the closest approach possible to an absolute proof of sterility. Certainly, while it is clear from a scientific perspective that an absolute proof of sterility will always elude us, it nevertheless seems as though the conundrum in aseptic processing that arises from this immutable fact will persist. That conundrum can be stated quite simply, we label products *sterile* that are made in an environment acknowledged to be nonsterile. That nonsterile environment is occupied by necessity by operators who are often said to be "sterile gowned," but who are in reality mobile contamination generators who consistently slough microbial contamination while working (6).

That being said the wise course in strategic planning for aseptic processing operations must include consideration of not only current but also future regulatory requirements as well as product liability. Thus, logically it is prudent to consider not only contamination risk to the product, but also producer's risk in the event difficult to assess and resolve contamination issues should arise. It seems safe to suggest that a production system that has an exceedingly low likelihood of contamination risk in terms of media fill, sterility test or environmental monitoring would provide the greatest abatement of producer's risk in terms of both compliance and increasingly legal liability.

PRODUCTION EASE AND EFFICIENCY VERSUS CONTAMINATION RISK

In our experience, the strategic decision regarding the production environment for aseptic processing most commonly in 2009 hinges on a trade-off between state-of-the-art contamination control and perceived production ease and efficiency. Since at least the early 1990s, it has been recognized that isolator technology afforded contamination control advantages over conventional human-scale clean rooms. Put another way, it has been widely understood if not clearly stated that isolator technology was a powerful contamination risk abatement tool. However, although there have been numerous examples of successful implementation of isolator technology, the perception among firms conservative in adopting this technology is that it was difficult to design, hard to validate, and could result in severe compromises in terms of operating efficiency. Among the most prevalent concerns relating to efficiency have been difficulty in making adjustments intended to correct operational faults, ergonomic difficulties, problems in supply, and component movement into and out of the isolator.

There is an obvious irony in the supposed manufacturing inefficiency associated with the conduct of interventions in isolators or other separative technologies such as RABS. To whit, the easy access that conventional human-scale clean rooms afford to critical aseptic processing areas is in fact the principle source of risk in aseptic processing. So, the decision to maintain ease of access without the need to work through isolator or RABS separative technology increases risk (4,7).

Additionally, there have been fears regarding cumbersome (and lengthy) change over from one container size or configuration to another. These issues ultimately led to some isolator systems actually being decommissioned, and restricted access barrier systems (RABS) being considered as means of achieving most of the contamination control and risk abatement that isolators offer, while at the same time retaining some, or perhaps even most, of the human–machine interface advantages of a clean room. Again, ironically, the very intensive interventions required during changeover and set up are exceedingly risky, making the ease of access possible in a clean room very much a mixed blessing.

Turning back to RABS, this separative technology, unless it is the closed variety (which is operationally very much the same as an isolator) does not diminish contamination or producer's risk as effectively as isolators. So-called "open door" RABS certainly was the subject of considerable enthusiasm within industry a few short years ago; however, at present it is possible (perhaps likely) that this approach is best suited to the improvement of existing aseptic processes (8). So, while nearly all new installed aseptic pharmaceutical production systems embody some form of what can be called separative technologies such as isolator technology, RABS or even some combination thereof; the selection of environmental technology continues to be a major, perhaps even the major, point of discussion and debate during the conceptual design phase of aseptic production projects.

RISK AND ASEPTIC PRODUCTION EXPERIENCE

An important tool in studying risk as it relates to aseptic processing is to actively compare systems using different environmental management strategies as Katayama et al. have done (7). Their work indicates that facilities, which better minimize contamination risk arising from human operators, do, as expected, reduce the likelihood of microbiological contamination.

A widely held view within the pharmaceutical industry is that the technologies employed in the production of human and veterinary medicines labeled sterile must sit at the pinnacle of technological attainment in aseptic processing. The authors do not suggest that pharmaceutical/biopharmaceutical industry aseptic processing operations are in any way deficient in terms of user safety. However, we have found that the aseptic beverage industry has in many ways surpassed the pharmaceutical industry in aseptic technology. In the beverage industry, there is no debate at the present time regarding aseptic manufacturing environments. All such environments are separative enclosures or what known in pharmaceutical aseptic processing as isolators.

There are critical differences between the regulations for aseptic food/beverage production and those for pharmaceutical/biopharmaceutical aseptic processing. A good example of such a difference is the use of turbulent airflow systems instead of unidirectional (often erroneously referred to as "laminar") airflow. However, air entering the enclosure is always filtered through HEPA or in some cases ULPA filters. It is not surprising from a scientific and engineering viewpoint that turbulent airflow in the absence of personnel provides freedom from airborne contamination that is indistinguishable from that of unidirectional air supply. Certainly, the emphasis on unidirectional airflow in the pharmaceutical industry seems logical because it arises out of a perceived need to manage the movement of air and hence contamination streams within the aseptic production environment. However, if such contamination is very low or even completely absent, it is obvious that airstream management becomes a minor factor in the risk management puzzle, that is, "sterility assurance."

DECONTAMINATION OF THE ENCLOSURE OR ISOLATOR

Decontamination of the isolator in aseptic beverage filling is similar in all respects to the sporicidal treatments used in conjunction with pharmaceutical isolators. The most common agents used are hydrogen peroxide (H_2O_2) or a combination of H_2O_2 and peracetic acid. The equipment built, installed, and validated by Shibuya Kogyo Co. Ltd, with which the authors are very familiar, relies on H_2O_2 either in liquid form or vapor phase. As is the case with pharmaceutical isolators, decontamination efficacy is confirmed by biological indicator challenges conducted using bacterial spores, and the expectation is complete kill of the challenge spores. Typically, with food production the challenge organism is *Bacillus atropheus* rather than *Geobacillus stearothermophilus*, but the resistance profiles of these two spore-bearing organisms are not dissimilar. So, while the decontamination approaches are different the outcome is effectively the same. In the case of both beverage and pharmaceutical aseptic processing isolators, decontamination results in the complete absence of microbial contamination, as measured by any known environmental monitoring method.

WHY PRODUCE BEVERAGES ASEPTICALLY?

The reader may be wondering why a beverage would be aseptically produced? First, it must be realized that a great many beverages are at substantial risk from microbial contamination. Beverage formulations that are low acid or contain milk are, because of their nutrient content, quite susceptible to microbial contamination. In fact, in a very real sense these natural beverages, which can be nutrient rich, are much like filling a form of microbiological media each production run.

Also, aseptic processing as opposed to heat treatment to mitigate contamination risk can improve flavor, reduce the need for continuous cold storage in distribution/retail, and increase the shelf life of these contamination susceptible products. Aseptically filled beverages, since they do not contain anything in their formulation that is bacteriostatic or bacteriocidal, are spoilage evident. An interesting side effect of this contamination susceptibility is that it is often possible to get a very realistic picture regarding the likelihood of contamination appearing in the field. In the United States, the Food and Drug Administration regulates aseptic beverage production, both in terms of approval of manufacturing processes and ongoing plant inspection.

PROCESS DESCRIPTION AND BACKGROUND

In the 1990s, Shibuya Kogyo Co. Ltd developed a new range of equipment for the aseptic production of beverages in light, clear PET plastic bottles. There have been more than 30 such

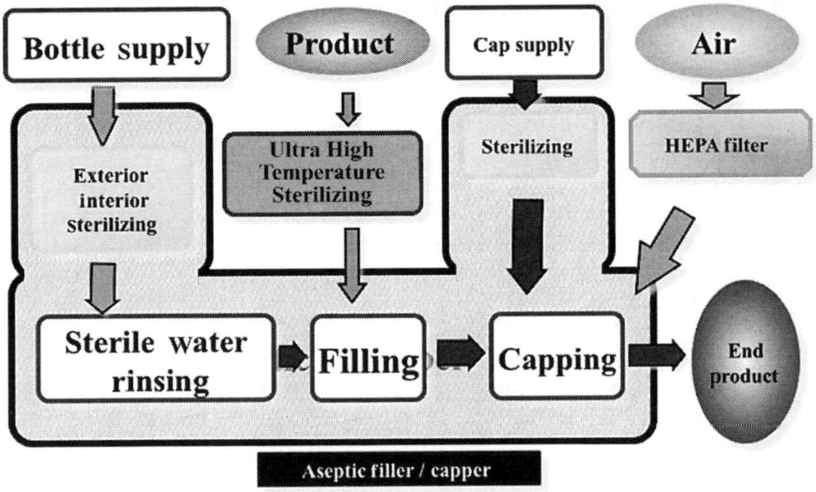

Figure 1 Process flow diagram for a typical aseptic PET bottle advanced aseptic processing system.

processing lines based on this concept installed and validated in both Asia and North America, and FDA approval has been achieved. In general, all of these installations hew to central technical principles; however, differences in size of container processed, line throughout speed, and container sterilization method do exist. A generalized process flow for aseptically filled beverages may be seen in Figure 1.

One of the key considerations from the outset was that these aseptic beverage processes would have to be capable of high output and long production run times. Unlike pharmaceuticals, the profit per unit associated with beverages is extremely low. Thus, aseptic processing lines must not only be very low risk in terms of microbial contamination, but they must also possess an extremely high level of mechanical and electronic reliability. The throughput speeds desired by customers have typically ranged from around 600 bottles/min to speeds as high as 1200 bottles/min. Given that the typical fill volume range for these products is approximately 300 mL to 2 L or more, the very high production output rates demand large multihead filling systems of rotary design. A gravimetric net weight filling system is included to ensure optimum fill accuracy control, a very important economic consideration. The size of these systems and the speed made it necessary that these systems be sufficiently stable in operation so that routine interventions are not required at all. In fact, given the rotary speed and mass, interventions could only be safely done if the equipment was fully stopped. Therefore, a key principle in equipment design must be stable and consistent operation without jams. The high level of automation and intervention free operation has the added benefit of reducing labor costs.

Also, prospective users desired extremely high rates of "uptime." Since 24/7 operations were expected, further emphasis on mechanical reliability and essentially perfect process and contamination control were critical requirements. As a result, the following requirement specifications were established:

1. The lightweight PET bottles would be neck handled to ensure stability at high speed through positive bottle control. Therefore, simple, reliable, and precise high quality grippers were designed to handle the speed and postfill weight of the bottles. These grippers can be easily changed out for service during infrequent process stoppages. The neck handling approach also makes it easy to convey bottles within the system without jams or misfeeds and to "hand off" bottles from one rotary station to another. As an added benefit, neck handling makes it possible to run several container sizes and shapes with no change parts required provided the neck and flange design on all bottles is the same.
2. The grippers that grasp the bottle at the neck within the filling section are attached to lever arms that act on load cells so that each bottle could be filled to a precise weight. Filling nozzles

and rates can be customized to minimize foaming. Fill data is output to a programmable logic controller (PLC)/computer as a permanent record.
3. Bottles and caps are sterilized in-line and enter the fill enclosure ready for use; thus only sterile materials enter the isolator and no human interventions are required to periodically introduce parts into the filling system. All component feeding is fully automatic. Bottles may be sterilized with H_2O_2, although more recently electron beam sterilization of bottles has been employed with superb results. Some systems have incorporated blow molding of the bottles, with sterilization occurring postmolding. Caps are also sterilized by H_2O_2. Bottle and cap sterilization is accomplished at a fast enough rate to keep up with filling speed.
4. Capping of filled bottles is done using a servo-capping system that tightens the caps to a predetermined torque value.
5. Any product that falls outside the established acceptance criteria for weight, cap torque or appearance is automatically rejected with no human intervention required.
6. The isolators can be considered during product use to be "gloveless," and gloves when installed cannot be used for intervention during production operations.
7. The entire fluid or wetted path through which the product passes on its way to the fill nozzles is both cleaned and sterilized in place (C/SIP). These C/SIP steps are fully automatic and thermocouples provide control and process monitoring during moist heat sterilization.
8. The isolator enclosure can also be "CIP'ed" using a cleaning process optimized for the product(s) being aseptically produced. The isolator enclosures are designed for optimal CIP efficacy. Spray ball location is carefully considered, as is effective drainage of cleaning solutions. The processing equipment is designed so that sensors and sensitive electronics are well protected from the CIP and decontamination processes for maximum reliability and longevity.

Figure 2 below provides a view through an isolator enclosure window into the filling section. Several bottles can be seen in various stages of gravimetric weight controlled filling. The rotary filler uses C/SIP capable positive displacement piston fillers, and may have as many as 128 filling heads.

A key operational objective in designing this advanced aseptic processing system is that it would require so little direct human interface in operation that it could operate essentially "lights out." As such, the human interface with the equipment is primarily at a PLC/computer video screen. Thus, a plant equipped with multiple fill lines of this design might require only

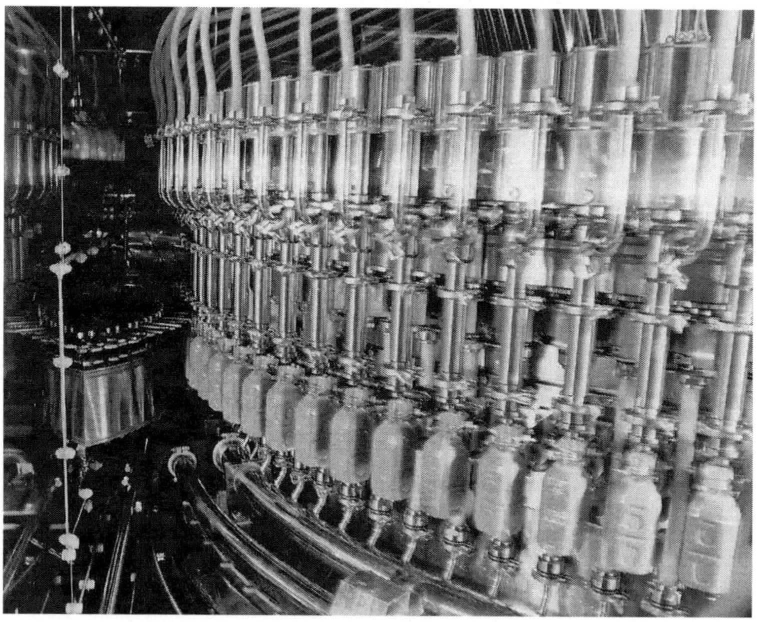

Figure 2 Internal view of PET high speed rotary aseptic filling isolator.

a small number of technicians and operators to control and monitor these advanced aseptic processing lines.

DIRECT APPLICABILITY TO ASEPTIC PHARMACEUTICAL MANUFACTURING

We believe that nearly all of the technology embodied in this highly automated, very high-speed aseptic beverage system can be directly applied to pharmaceutical manufacturing (Figs. 3 and 4). Neck handling, for example, is directly applicable to vial and plastic bottle manufacturing. Fully automated rubber stopper sterilization and feeding have been accomplished using a combination of automated sterilization and H_2O_2-resistant robotics systems. Vapor phase hydrogen peroxide parts feeders have also been developed and can be interfaced with decontamination pass boxes to allow fully automatic, contamination risk-free introduction of components such as caps, dropper tips, and bottles that are radiation sterilized in bags. In the near future, sterilization of plastic components in-line seems within reach.

CONCLUSION

The proof of any production process is in the quality of the end product. Variations on the basic aseptic beverage filling process described in this article have produced well over 4 billion containers without a single report of contamination. As previously mentioned, the products filled are not preserved and most are quite supportive of microbial growth. We believe this result, along with the very high yields obtained, clearly demonstrates the capability of highly automated and very advanced aseptic manufacturing systems to achieve very high levels of contamination risk abatement without compromising operational efficiency and reliability. These systems have the potential to not only revolutionize the manner in which aseptic processing

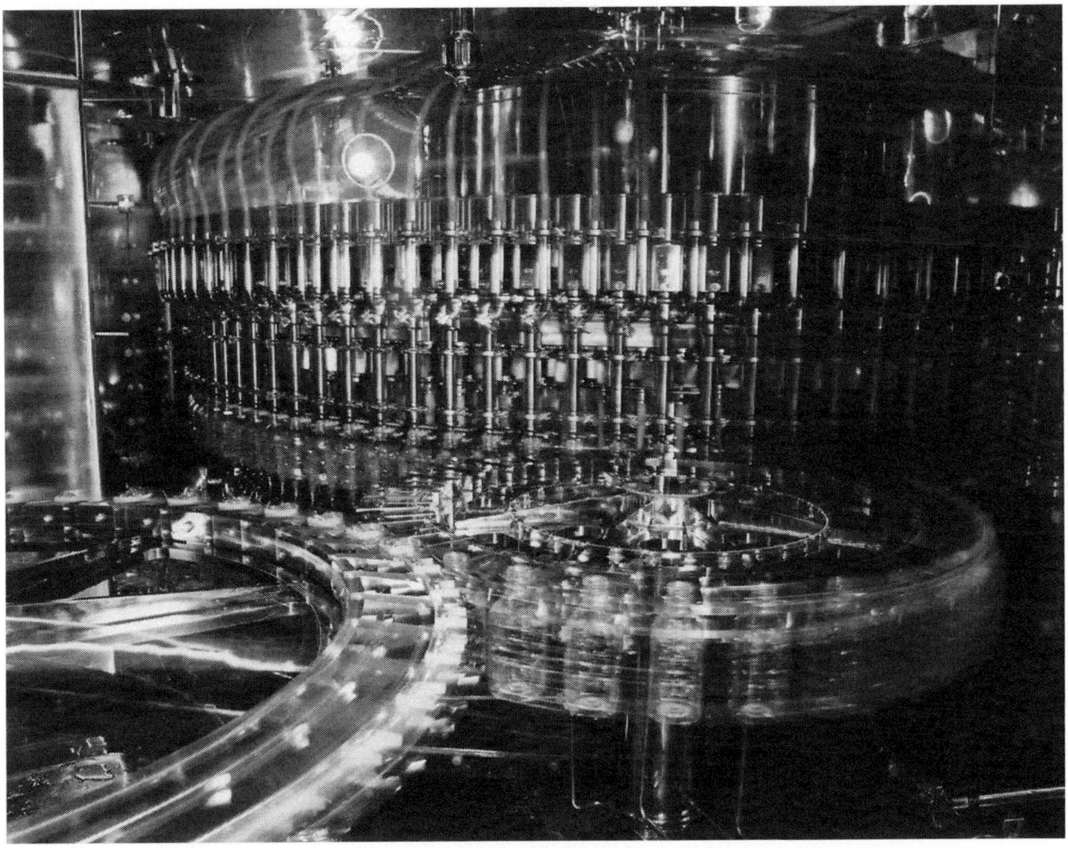

Figure 3 The filling section of a gloveless isolator-based high speed aseptic filling system capable of throughputs greater than 1,000 bottles/minute. The filling system is S/CIP and uses load cells for full automatic fill volume control on each container filled. These systems represent the pinnacle of current high speed advanced aseptic processing technologies.

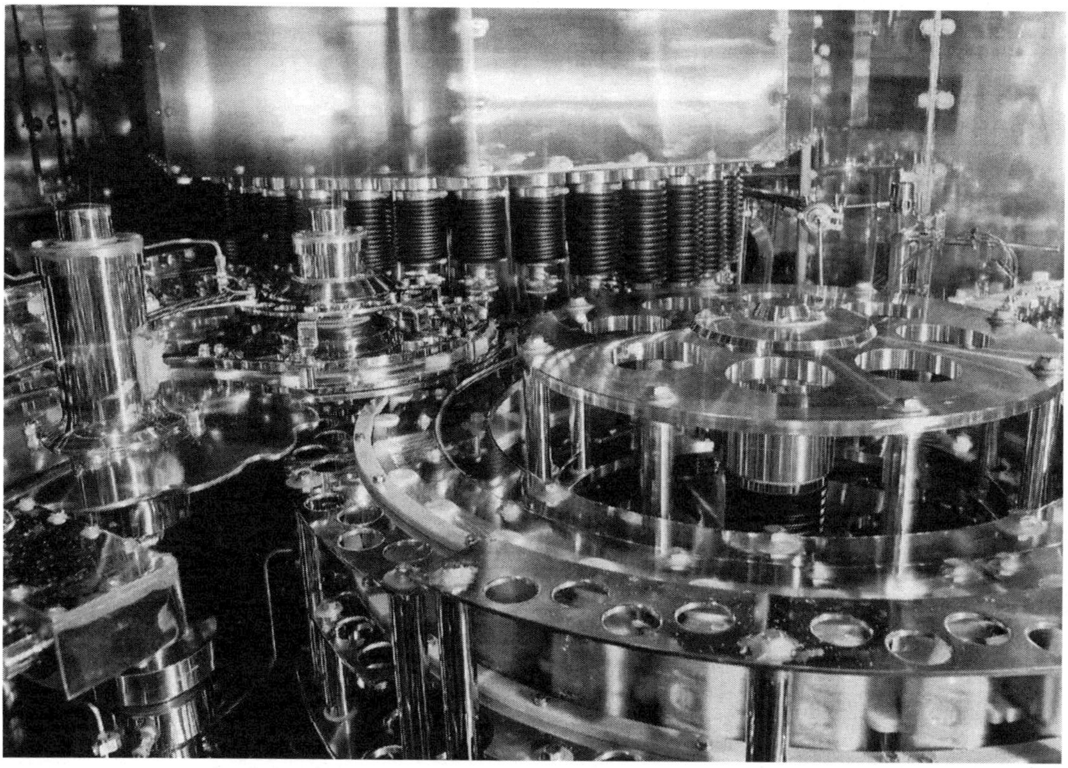

Figure 4 Servo controlled capping section of the PET aseptic bottling system. All caps are applied to a predetermined torque by PLC controlled servo motor capping stations and speeds of up to 1300 bottles/minute. Bottles that do not fall within cap torque specifications are automatically rejected without operator intervention.

is done, but also to completely change industry and regulatory thinking regarding process control, process validation, and environmental monitoring. In fact, environmental monitoring, where required, can also be fully automated using vapor phase hydrogen peroxide-resistant robotics. Fully advanced and optimized aseptic processing that comes very close to the theoretical limit regarding elimination of contamination risk is not only available in 2010, but it is very efficiently at work everyday supplying the optimum in microbiologically pure beverages and pharmaceutical products.

REFERENCES

1. Japan-PDA Task Force on Sterile Drug Products Produced by Aseptic Processing (with support from the Japanese Ministry of Health, Labor, and Welfare). Guidance for Industry—Sterile Drug Products Produced by Aseptic Processing, 2005.
2. Oshima Y, Yoshida S, Akers J. PasepT: A new concept in aseptic processing. In: Proceedings of the 36th R3 Nordic Symposium and 5th European Parenteral Conference; May 2005; Linköping, Sweden.
3. Akers JE, Kokubo M, Oshima Y. The next generation of aseptic processing equipment. Pharm Technol Aseptic Processing Supplement 2006; 30:32–36.
4. US Food and Drug Administration. Guidance for Industry. Sterile Drug Products Produced by Aseptic Processing—Current Good Manufacturing Practices. 2004.
5. Akers JE. An overview of advanced aseptic processing—And a few thoughts on implementation. In: Proceedings of the PDA Conference on Risk Management and Aseptic Processing; May 2008; Bethesda, MD.
6. Akers J, Tanimoto K, Kawata M. Aseptic processing the Japanese way. Pharmaceutical Manufacturing, June 2006; 4:23–27.
7. Katayama H, Toda A, Tokunaga Y, et al. Proposal for a new categorization of aseptic processing facilities based on risk assessment scores. PDA J Pharm Sci Technol 2008; 62(4):235–243.
8. Agalloco JP. Thinking inside the box—application of isolation technology for aseptic processing. Pharm Technol Aseptic Process Suppl 2006; 30(5):S8–S11.

36 Radiopharmaceutical filling line

Frank Mastromonica and Simon Steingart

When manufacturing radiopharmaceuticals there is always a need to think outside the box. The use of potent compounds for drug manufacturing does not lend itself easily to certain industry standards for manufacturing sterile products such as open vial filling and large clean room environments. When using radioactive isotopes in the manufacturing process, the issues of shielding, contamination, and airborne volatility must be taken into account. This does not mean that current Good Manufacturing Practices (cGMPs) are not carried out or followed when dealing with the manufacture of a radiopharmaceutical, but the industry must always try to be innovative and cutting edge in order to meet cGMPs considering the specialized needs of radiopharmaceutical manufacturing.

When this project was initiated, the use of isolator systems for manufacturing was new to GE Healthcare. In the past, manufacturing operations had always been performed under standard clean room environments with the use of considerable shielding to protect the workers. Under these conditions, operators have always incorporated as much radiation technique and aseptic technique as possible to maintain the crucial balance between cGMP and Health Physics regulations. The manufacturing of an aseptically filled Sr-82 Generator lends itself well to the use of isolation technology.

PROJECT REQUIREMENTS

The project required the transfer of technology for an older product, manufactured in a "Hot Cell" environment. It was evident from reviewing present manufacturing procedures that there would be a substantial need for upgrades to the systems in order to meet current regulatory expectations. From experience, we had the following assumptions:

- The methods for product transfer would need a technology upgrade.
- It would be difficult to manufacture a truly aseptic product in a "Hot Cell" due to cleaning issues.
- Large amounts of radioactive shielding would be needed.
- We had no existing clean room on site.

We felt that a novel use of isolation technology would be the best route for maintaining control of sterility while including the proper shielding needed to successfully produce this product. Before the project could go any further, we needed to ask a few questions.

- How much shielding would be needed?
- What type of air flow would be incorporated? Laminar? Turbulent? Negative pressure?
- Ergonomics: What issues would we encounter?
- Since the room the isolator would reside in was not classified, how would we control the environment where the isolator resides?

SHIELDING

With these questions in mind, we began with a rudimentary conceptual design. The manufacturing line began with a simple diagram of what we felt the manufacturing line should look like (Fig. 1). The concept for the manufacturing line would incorporate the use of three isolators. One isolator (*Cold Prep*) would be used for the preparation of materials prior to introduction of any radioactive materials. The second isolator would be used for filling and formulation (*Gray/Fill*), and a third isolator would be used for a staging area (*Airlock*) before packaging. All the isolators would incorporate turbulent flow. Since the isotope was not volatile and the filling would be performed transeptally, this seemed the most cost-effective way of creating ISO 5 environment manufacturing areas. The filling/formulation isolator would incorporate a dual isolator design. One part of the isolator would be used for the storage of the bulk solution, filling pumps and would be considered a "*Gray*" area incorporating high efficiency particulate air (HEPA) filtered

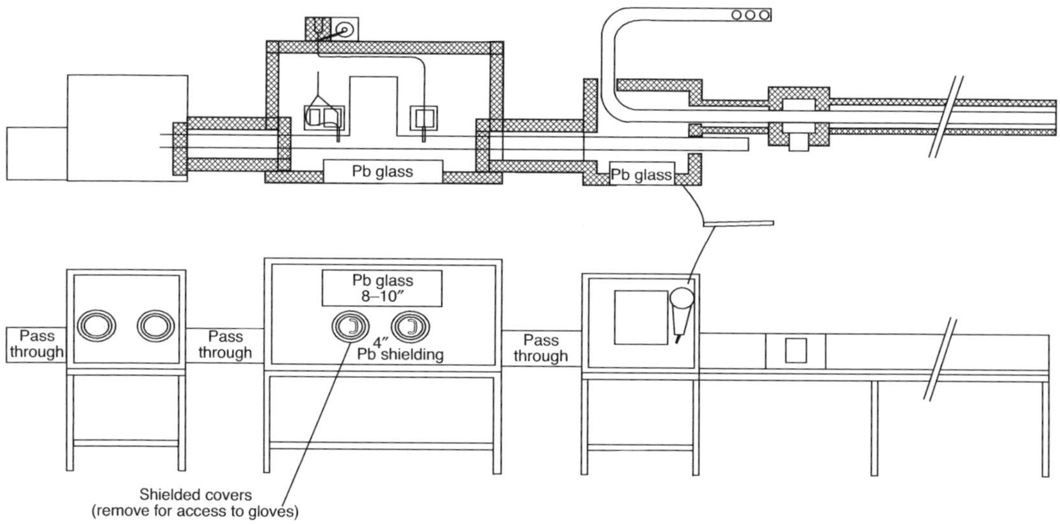

Figure 1 Initial concept for manufacturing line.

air under negative pressure. The aseptic "*Fill*" side would be positive turbulent flow (Class 100). The shielding concerns were handled by shielding the Fill/Gray and Airlock isolators with 4 in. of sheet lead. The lead was clad with an interior skin of 316 L SS and an outer skin of 304 SS. The Cold Prep isolator would be unshielded since no work with the radioactive isotope would be performed in it (therefore the name "*Cold*" Prep).

ERGONOMICS

The use of a mock up model was critical for confirming the ergonomics for the system. With the mock up in our facility, it gave us great insight into how the ergonomics would affect the manufacturing process. Dealing with the large shielding issues, the "mock up" gave us a means to identify the needs for automation, where to locate the RTPs (rapid transfer ports), where additional shelves would be needed, where to enlarge areas, and to try out the system with operators of different sizes. One issue was quite evident. Ergonomics in the *Fill/Gray* isolator (Fig. 2) would have to be sacrificed to protect that operator for the radiation hazards. In this isolator, we automated as much of the operations as possible. We also designed specialized tools for removing objects from the "Beta" canisters and placing the fill heads into the filling system. The *Cold Prep* isolator (Fig. 3) was enlarged to allow more than one operator to work at

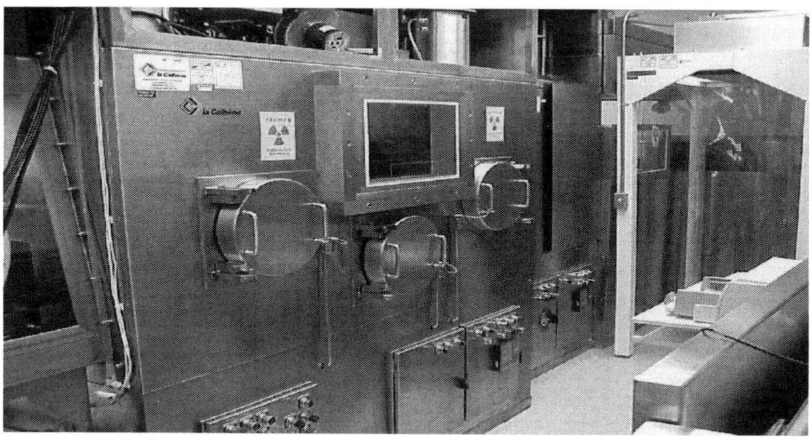

Figure 2 Sterile fill side of Fill/Gray isolator.

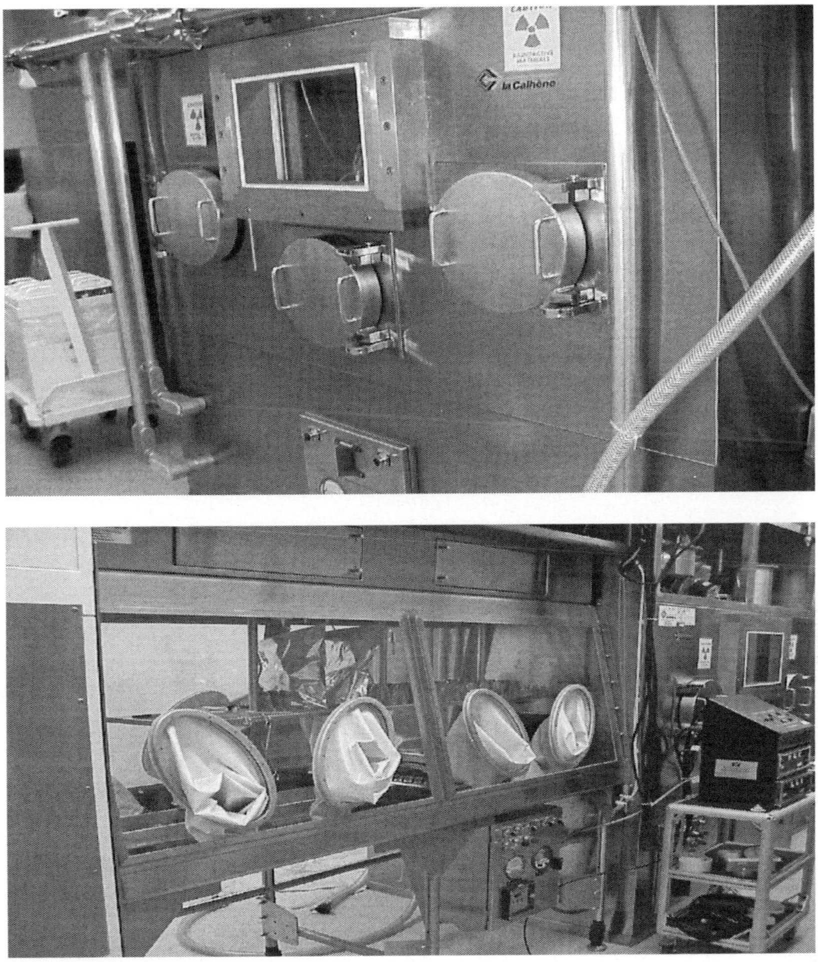

Figure 3 Cold Prep isolator.

the same time. The use of elliptical glove ports was incorporated. This allowed greater range of motion for operators of different heights. After a thorough evaluation, a final design was agreed upon. The changes made allowed us to meet cGMP requirements as well as maintaining Health Physics requirements for the protection of the operators from the radiation hazard.

FINAL DESIGN

In the final design (Fig. 4), the manufacturing line incorporated the original concept of three isolators in a linear format. The line was set for surface sterilization using vaporized hydrogen peroxide (VHP) to a sterility assurance level (SAL) to 10^{-6} with the isolators set up to be sterilized as either a single unit or as separate units. Additionally to protect the entry and exit of the manufacturing line, ISO 5 down flow hoods were attached to ISO 7 portable clean rooms (PCR) over the *Cold Prep* and *Airlock* isolators. Adding the ISO 7 allowed for the maintenance of a clean environment for aseptic preparations, clean entry, and exit from the isolators since the manufacturing line would be placed in a clean unclassified room. Each of the isolators would have its own control panel that allowed for the monitoring/operation of internal pressure, differential pressure between isolators, temperature, relative humidity, and door controls.

DECONTAMINATION METHOD/CYCLE/FREQUENCY

The method chosen for the decontamination of the radiopharmaceutical filling suite was VHP. The filling suite utilizes positive pressure supplied to each part of the isolator through the use

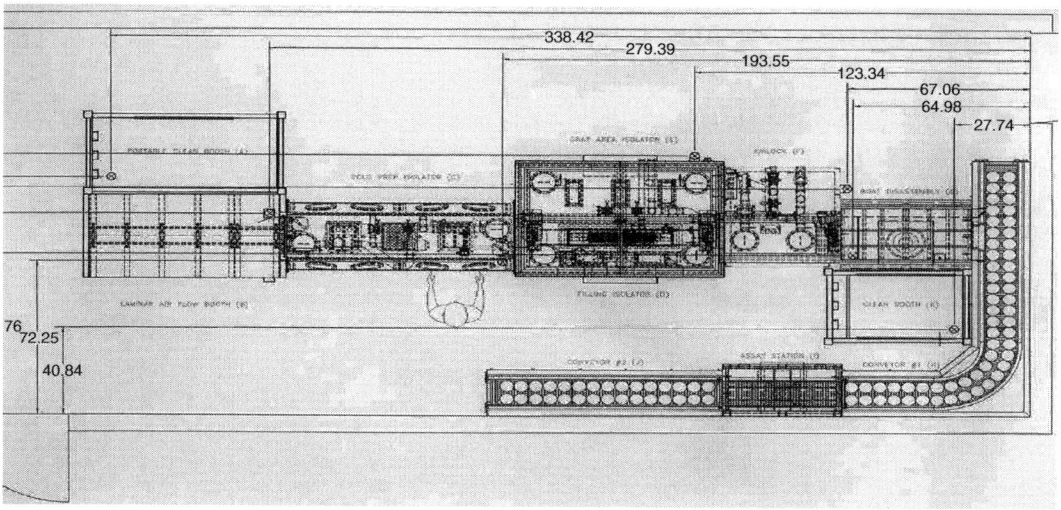

Figure 4 Final design incorporating PCR units at entry and exit.

of positive pressure blowers. The VHP-1000 Generator uses a closed loop method of decontamination for closed systems, eliminating the need for excess peroxide disposal and the risk of breaching containment through the introduction of human or chemical influences to the decontaminated environment. The decontamination cycles were loosely based on the STERIS guide and calculated using the total volume of the isolator and temperature as a starting point.

The VHP decontamination process utilizes five major phases: dehumidification, conditioning, decontamination, aeration, and regeneration. The dehumidification phase dries the isolator air through circulation of the air through a desiccant bed to remove any excess water vapor. This allows for a higher concentration of the VHP sterilant vapor. The conditioning phase introduces a higher injection rate of VHP sterilant to rapidly increase the concentration, which decreases the total cycle time by reaching the steady state concentration in the shortest overall time possible. The decontamination phase provides a consistent VHP concentration and water vapor concentration to the isolator based on a preprogramed calculated cycle. The aeration phase is performed at decontamination completion and helps degrade the VHP sterilant into oxygen and water by recirculating the isolators air through the desiccant bed of the VHP-1000 Generator. The Cold Prep isolator was fitted with a Guided Wave hydrogen peroxide concentration monitor. The concentration monitor was used in validation studies to document the levels of peroxide at a single point in the isolator. Since monitoring of the peroxide concentration is conducted at a single point, it was decided to use the equipment as a reference-only tool during manufacturing cycles.

The isolator must be aerated until a threshold limit value (TLV) of 1 PPM is achieved. The regeneration phase is conducted when the drying capacity of the generator desiccant falls to 10 hours (full drying capacity is 20 hours). This cycle is best performed over a weekend because it takes a total time of 18 hours for completion of this phase.

The filling suite is a custom-designed rigid-walled isolator system made up of three different isolators. Two of these isolators are lined with 4 in. of lead for worker protection.

The isolator system was installed in a room that has the ability to have its temperature controlled. Initial validation of the isolator cycles was conducted at three different air recirculation rates (18, 16, and 14 SCFM). These rates were chosen to take into account worst-case conditions. The 18 SCFM cycle was conducted because it represented the lowest concentration, the 16 SCFM the nominal concentration, and the 14 SCFM cycle the highest possible concentration. The 14 SCFM cycle would also be the cycle most likely to exhibit condensation.

During the cycle development validation studies, some isolator design flaws surfaced. For example, there was a lack of GMP ports to easily map out each isolator system with thermocouples to determine the isolator temperature and the placement of the VHP dispersion fans built into the isolator system. These fans are key to providing turbulent flow inside of the isolator to evenly disperse the VHP gas concentration within the system. There were several problems encountered with the calculated cycles for this system. Calculating the starting point for the cycle proved more difficult when compared with calculating the cycle of a standard flexible-walled transfer isolator. The STERIS guide does not account for a rigid-walled system and for any off-gassing of VHP from the isolator load during the aeration phase. The original cycle calculated called for a total of 137.8 g of hydrogen peroxide. Because of poor placement of the VHP dispersion fans and unsealed positive pressure blowers improper air/gas mixing resulted. In addition, due to poor blower design, the units would leak and required that the blowers remained on during VHP decontamination. These issues caused the final amount of hydrogen peroxide used at a 16 SCFM cycle to be 956.8 g, which almost met the maximum amount the generator's hydrogen peroxide reservoir would hold. Because of the high peroxide concentration, the aeration time was significantly increased, which significantly decreased the drying capacity of the generator desiccant. To solve this problem, aeration with the generator was kept at 60 minutes and aeration was continued through the facility's house exhaust system overnight.

In the spirit of continuous improvement, the cycle was improved upon in the following fashion: through Change Control, new sealed motor positive pressure blowers were sourced and installed along with added VHP dispersion fans. The cycle was then reworked and validated using a 12 SCFM recirculation rate as a worst-case test cycle and a 10 SCFM recirculation rate as a routine decontamination cycle. This was based on keeping the environment suitable for microcondensation of the VHP gas and not a dry process as previously thought. These changes resulted in a routine cycle that used 295 g of peroxide and a fast optimized cycle.

CONCLUSION

When this project was originally initiated, it introduced a large amount of innovation in ideas that brought the project team closer to cutting edge technology for manufacturing and delivering an aseptic process. Currently at GE Healthcare, there are numerous products and processes that use or incorporate Isolator Technology as its main source of control. The lessons learned from the design of this radiopharmaceutical filling suite have allowed us to be more innovative, improve on ergonomics, and protect the product and personnel better. Based on our experience this shows to be an effective method for manufacturing aseptically produced product.

37 Powder handling installation for high potent bulk pharmaceutical ingredients

Bert Brabants

APPLICATION

In 2003, a new powder handling installation was installed at the chemical production site in Geel, Belgium. This installation was used to obtain the correct particle size distribution for the most potent drugs manufactured at the site. It had a handling capacity of several dozen tonnes of product annually. Initially, approximately 30 different products were processed with the new installation.

REASONS FOR ISOLATION

The main reasons for using isolators are to protect the product (quality) and the operator.

Protection of the Product

The installation complies with EU Grade C,[1] which allows the handling of intermediate products for parenteral use. The installation needs to be completely sanitizable through an automated cleaning in place (CIP) after each campaign. Sterility is not required.

Protection of the Operator

The construction of this new installation heralded a new chapter in the field of safety. For the first time ever, instead of using personal protective equipment (PPE) to protect the operators from exposure to high potent active pharmaceutical ingredients (APIs), the installation itself will be shielded. As a consequence, the use of PPE to protect personnel will no longer be necessary.

The installation has a design exposure limit (DEL) of 50 ng/m^3. The eight-hour average ambient concentration of the product may not exceed this value.

The requirements with respect to operator protection are much more stringent than those required to protect the product (product quality). Hence, the main focus of this article will be on operator protection, and in doing so most product protection requirements are covered automatically. In case of conflicting requirements, operator safety was always put first due to the acute toxicity of most of our products. Of course, all product quality requirements are also needed to be met.

PROCESS DESCRIPTION

The new installation for handling high potent APIs consists of a process line containing, in succession, the following main components:

1. A delumper (hammer mill), which crushes the bulk solids that are too large to be milled.
2. An air classifier mill, which reduces the particle size down to 2 μm average size (Fig. 1).
3. A cyclone with a dust separator (or a second delumper), which separates the transporting gas and the powder.
4. A sieve to ensure that oversized particles are removed.
5. A tumbler, which eliminates the effect of separating particles of a different size during milling and sieving by homogenizing the product.
6. A packaging unit for 10-L drums with a double inner liner.

Schematically, the process looks as follows:

As shown in Figure 2, the installation consists of two vertical towers. Product can be fed into the installation at two points, that is, at the top of both towers. The rectangles in the diagram

[1] ISO 14644-1 class 7 (particles > 0.5 μm) + microbial requirements.

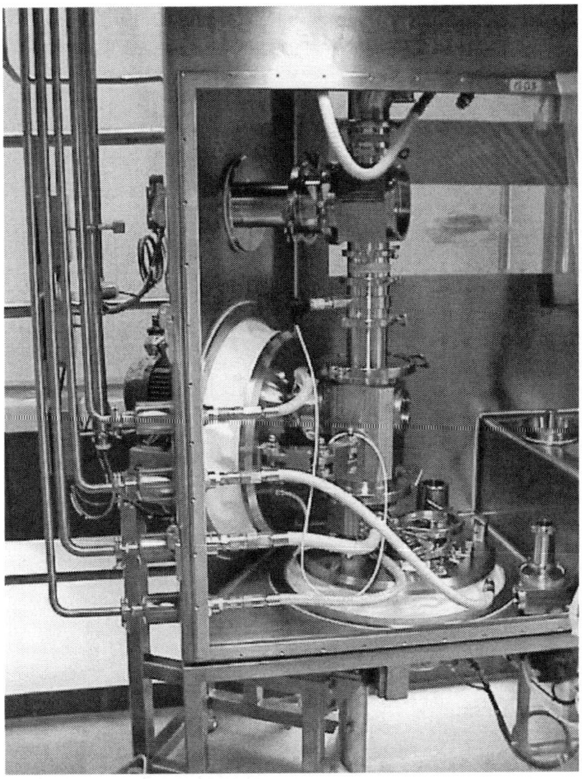

Figure 1 Air classifier mill with nitrogen connections.

represent the isolators. A total of seven isolators were required in order to encapsulate the entire process. At the time of design of the installation the use of isolators was judged indispensable. The alternative, a milling installation that could be cleaned entirely through CIP, was deemed unfeasible.

Since then, the technology of internally rinsed split butterfly valves has evolved significantly and could now be considered as an alternative for the feed isolators.

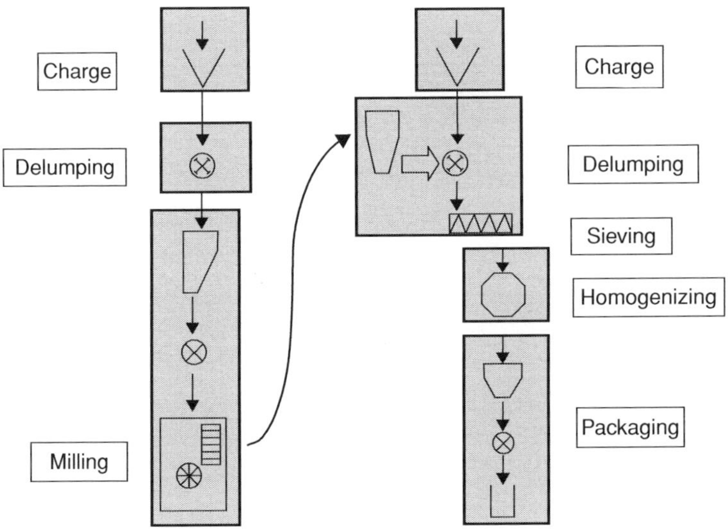

Figure 2 Schematic process flow diagram.

CLEANING

As the basic principle underlying the cleaning process, it was assumed that all parts of the installation must be CIP capable in order to eliminate the risk of contamination with API elsewhere on the site. Sanitization is done to obtain a maximum level of 100 CFU (colony forming unit)/m^3 in the gas phase and 25 CFU/m^3 on the surfaces of the isolators. The requirements for EU Grade C compliance impose standards in this regard.

Cleaning involves the use of two solvents: dimethylacetamide (DMA) and an ethanol–water (70/30%) solution. DMA was selected since all the APIs produced at the site are soluble in DMA. The ethanol solution serves as a disinfectant to achieve aseptic conditions. Specifying these two solvents as the only ones to come into contact with the installation has the added advantage since a larger range of plastics can be used in the installation. Inexpensive flexible silicones can be used to replace the polytetrafluoroethylene (PTFE) (stiff) and perfluoroelastomers (expensive) currently in use at the site.

Cleaning occurs via fixed spray balls and handspray guns. Sinks are also provided, which allow for some parts to be soaked in the solvent. The possibility of spraying nitrogen under high pressure with handspray guns allows for the glove boxes to be dried faster (by dispersing droplets).

The contaminated solvent is removed through gravity, collected in a tank and taken away for incineration.

MATERIAL TRANSFERS

The product is fed into the installation via rapid transfer ports (RTPs).

In order to empty the packaging isolator, the product is not filled in RTP canisters but in plastic bags made from a thermally welded continuous polyethylene liner; a cartridge had to be developed to serve as the carrier for the liner (Fig. 3). The connection between the liner and the cartridge needed to be completely leakproof. To this end, an RTP connection (ß port) was fixed to a large diameter tube to which the continuous liner is attached with several leakproof O-ring

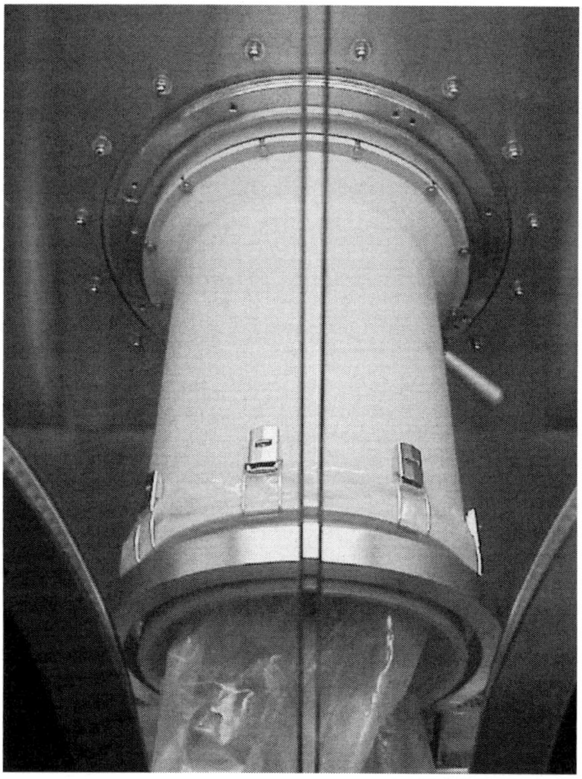

Figure 3 Cartridge with a finished liner photographed through the split in the door.

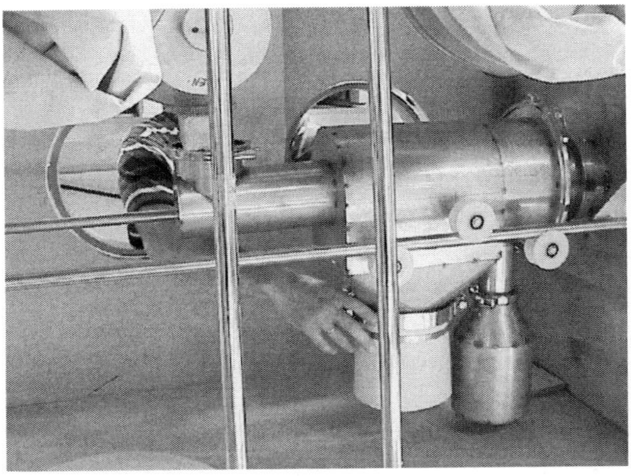

Figure 4 Mock-up of sieving isolator and sieving equipment on slides.

seals and clamps. This cartridge can be handled as a regular RTP canister both with regard to assembly and cleaning. If the end of the liner is reached during the packaging process, a new cartridge/liner assembly can be fitted within a sealed environment.

To prevent exposure to APIs in the event of a malfunction during the heat-sealing operation of the continuous liner, this part of the installation was placed in a cabinet with doors and an integral glove box. A fan ensures a constant negative pressure and an entry flow (through a crack between the doors) of approximately 140 Nm^3/hr, so that even in the event of an accidental release of powder into this enclosed space, exposure of staff will not occur.

CHALLENGES OWING TO CONTAINMENT REQUIREMENTS

This paragraph provides a more detailed description of the specific technical aspects related to handling of toxic APIs. Achieving a DEL of 50 ng/m^3 for a process of this magnitude and complexity requires an approach involving a battery of techniques, which together ensure that no powder is released into the work area or environment. Some of these techniques, such as the use of glove boxes and RTPs, have already proved their practical value (although not always achieving the required containment level). Other techniques were specifically designed for this installation out of pure need and have their origin in the exceptional combination of isolator technology with a relatively large milling installation that could not be housed in a single isolator because of its size.

In addition to the DEL of 50 ng/m^3, the principal containment requirements set for the installation are as follows:

- Maximum permissible leak rate of 10 nL/sec[2] for the isolators.
- Use of a *negative*[3] pressure of approximately −150 Pa on the isolators to prevent product migration in the event of leakage.
- In the event of glove fracture (Ø 35 cm), an entry velocity of 0.4 m/sec is expected to prevent contamination of the environment.
- Isolators fitted with safety glass.
- Outside the isolators, only permanent (welded) connections are to be used.

The next paragraphs will cover specific key areas related to the integration of a "traditional" milling and sieving process in isolators.

Ergonomic Aspects

When using relatively large devices in combination with isolators, it becomes important to consider the ergonomic aspects. For each isolator, at least one mock-up (Fig. 4) was constructed

[2] When conducting a helium leakage test at 500 Pa overpressure.

[3] Not allowed by European legislation in isolators used for sterile production.

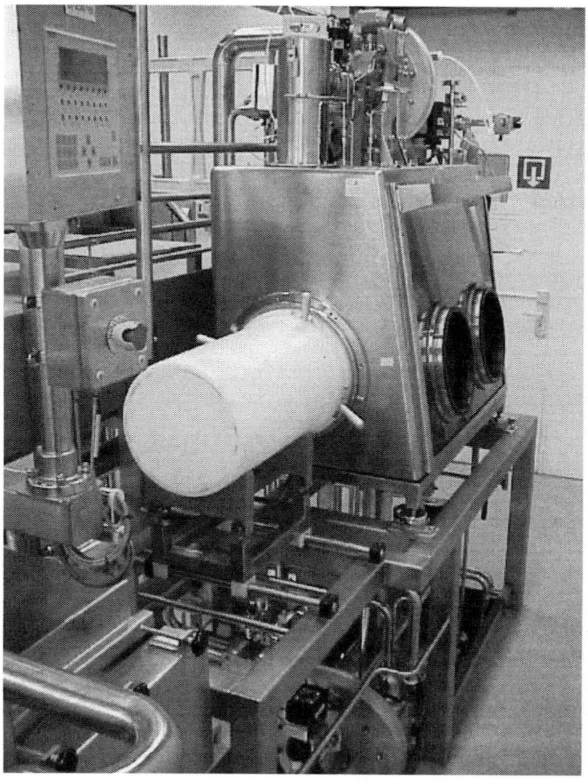

Figure 5 RTP canister on slide ready to be docked.

in wood and steel based on the design drawings. Structural models of the equipment were also made. This enabled operators, who will be using the installation, to check whether the required operations are justified from an ergonomic viewpoint.

Based on the outcomes of this test, many devices were mounted either on *hinges* or *slides* (Figs. 4 and 5), so they can be dismantled for cleaning without having to be lifted.

This was prompted by the consideration that lifting heavy objects while using glove boxes is not possible due to the operators' restricted freedom of movement. For ergonomic reasons, the RTP canister can likewise be brought to the isolator RTP port via a slide.

The construction and testing of the mock-up isolators and equipment were essential to the success of the project in view of the many operations that need to be performed with the equipment (assembly/dismantling for cleaning). A single, unworkable operation would render the entire installation unusable! Theoretical, ergonomic simulation models [NIOSH (National Institute for Occupational Safety and Health) and OWAS (Ovako Working Posture Analyzing System)] were found to be ineffective, as these models do not take the restricted freedom of movement, that working with glove boxes involves, into account. Moreover, the simulation methods cover only a few of the ergonomic aspects (carrying loads, repetitive movements) and give no conclusive data on such things as the reachability of parts and the practicability of operations with just one hand. The latter restriction, that is, the availability of only one hand for certain tasks owing to the use of glove boxes, resulted in a host of technical modifications.

Apart from the need to use stainless steel for the main structure, it was also deemed necessary to incorporate flexible connections in the powder transport piping. These flexible (silicone) connections can compensate minor deviations in the position of the individually supported isolators. Without these connections, the assembly of the installation would not have been possible.

The pipes and devices were specifically designed, again for ergonomic reasons, to be as light as possible. As a consequence, in contrast to the powder handling installations elsewhere on the site, the pipes do not have an explosion pressure shock–resistant design. To eliminate any explosion hazard, inertization of the system with nitrogen is therefore employed.

Isolator Transit Points and Pipe Conduits

The isolators contain shaft-driven devices. The motors are located outside the isolator (because of their poor cleanability and the limited space inside the isolators) so that a dust-tight, nitrogen purged shaft seal is required. A seal is also required on the pipe conduits between the isolators.

To prevent vibrations from the fast running motors being transmitted to the isolators, with potentially detrimental consequences such as leaks, noise nuisance, and loose vibrating connections, these motors were installed in a completely isolated position. The conduit through the isolator wall was also specially designed to prevent the transmission of vibrations. This was achieved by fitting a flexible ring (ethylene vinyl acetate copolymer) of approximately 15 cm wide, between the shaft seal of the motor and the isolator (see white rings on Figure 1).

Ventilation

Ventilation of the Isolator

As mentioned earlier, it was decided to inert the isolators in order to prevent dust explosions. This is done by constantly purging them with nitrogen gas. A needle valve on the feed line controls the nitrogen flow rate to between 3 and 4 air changes per hour. A fan on the isolator outlet regulates the (negative) pressure in the system. Each isolator has its own oxygen sensor, which will shut down the installation if the oxygen concentration rises above 5%. As the spent gas may be contaminated with powder, it is passed through two HEPA (high efficiency particulate arrestance) filters (EN 799, H13) connected in series before being exhausted to the atmosphere. Filter replacement is done according to the push–push principle[4] toward the isolator.

The fans on the isolators are greatly overdimensioned so that in case of a glove fracture they are able to achieve an entry velocity of 0.4 m/sec in order to prevent contamination of the environment.

The use of nitrogen for inertization of the process does have one disadvantage, however, as nitrogen leaks can cause suffocation by displacement of oxygen in the air. For that reason, oxygen meters have been installed at strategic points in the work environment; in the event of a reduced oxygen concentration the process is automatically shut down.

Ventilation of the Process

During the milling process, the mill consumes nitrogen at a rate of approximately 130 Nm^3/hr. Integration of a milling process and isolator technology causes the following problem. The nitrogen flow enters the classifier mill at a pressure of 4.2 bar(g).[5] However, isolators are built to withstand a pressure of barely 0.01 bar(g), which is 420 times[6] lower than the entry pressure in the classifier mill. Higher pressure levels, which could occur due to incorrect pressure readings, incorrect assembly of the installation, defective valves, etc., must therefore be avoided at all cost. The following precautions ensuing from a far-reaching hazard and operability analysis (HAZOP) are among the measures taken to this end:

- The start-up sequence tests for correct assembly explores the boundaries of the process parameters so that failures are detected before the API enters the installation.
- Use of redundant sensors (pressure readings) and actuators (valves) interfaced with a safety PLC.[7]

[4] These cylindrical filters are located in a straight tube mounted between the fan and the isolator. When the filter is saturated, this is detected by the high pressure drop across the filter. A third, clean filter is then pushed into the tube from the outside, causing the old, saturated filter to fall into the isolator.

[5] Relative pressure versus atmospheric pressure.

[6] Lowering this factor by reducing the supply pressure to the mill is technically unfeasible in this case due to the large dimensions of the supply pipes.

[7] A safety-PLC (or Safety Programmable Logic Controller) is a PLC with enhanced reliability according to standards IEC 61508, IEC 62061 or ISO 13849-1.

- Use of ultrafast valves to shut off the nitrogen supply in case of overpressure.
- The pressure in the milling and sieving installation usually spans several hundred millibars, but in this installation it is regulated precisely to the isolator pressure by a process fan. Consequently, any leaks in the equipment will have less impact on the pressure in the isolators.
- Wherever possible (e.g., during cleaning) the isolators are interconnected in order to maximize the volume (and hence minimize the pressure increase in the event of leakage).

PROJECT MANAGEMENT

The overall cost of the project was 5.9 million Euros.

The project timeline can be found in the table below.

May 2000	• Concept/mock-ups
October 2000	• Basic engineering
January 2001	• Detailed design
September 2001	• Start installation
April 2002	• Mechanical completion
August 2002	• Process start-up, validation
August 2003	• Hand over to client

FURTHER READING

1. Wood J. Containment in the Pharmaceutical Industry. New York: Marcel Dekker, 2000.
2. Gurney-Read P, Koch M. Guidelines for assessing the particulate containment performance of pharmaceutical equipment. Pharm Eng 2002; 22:55–59.

38 Isolator technology for aseptic filling of anti-cancer drugs

Paul Martin

INTRODUCTION

The Pierre Fabre Group is the third largest French pharmaceutical manufacturer and produces a number of essential medications. Pierre Fabre Medicament Production (Aquitaine Pharm International) is a pharmaceutical laboratory of the Pierre Fabre Group. A portion of the Pierre Fabre facility in Idron, South West of France, specializes in the production of sterile anti-cancer drugs. This facility offers contract manufacturing services to worldwide pharmaceutical business and has used isolation technology from the early 1990s. Pierre Fabre required a facility for the manufacture of its new anti-cancer injectable drug "Navelbine" and the 'new' technology of isolators was selected. This product (and other oncology drugs) presents unique challenges to manufacture because of its high toxicity, which requires that specific measures be undertaken to protect the production operators. The principle reasons for selection of isolators were to improve both aseptic processing and the protection of personnel and environment. The first stage of operation and the product it manufactured were FDA approved in 1993.

By the end of the century, a second production suite was built with somewhat different characteristics and improvements based on the first 10 years know-how on isolator usage for aseptic processing. The main objectives of the second suite were to fill six different products with a larger batch size for cost reduction.

The second generation suite was also dedicated to contract manufacturing servicing of liquid anti-cancer injectable formulation. This suite and the associated products were FDA approved in 2002.

In 2007, Pierre Fabre began to construct a new facility with two new production suites dedicated to anti-cancer freeze-dried injectable products. The third generation suites are utilized for products containing a high level of alcohol and are also dedicated to contract manufacturing. The primary objectives of the third set of suites are safety, quality, and operational flexibility. This latest suite and products were FDA approved in 2009. This chapter will summarize Pierre Fabre's experience collected over 18 years of aseptic manufacturing high potent drugs through the three different generations of production suites and isolation technology.

FIRST GENERATION CYTOTOXIC FACILITY (ATM-1 WORKSHOP) 1991–2000

For the first commercial scale production line, the project employed was essentially a conventional high speed filling line positioned within isolators. Pierre Fabre's concept was to have:

- Containment isolator at compounding in negative pressure
- Containment isolator at autoclave/filling/stoppering/capping in positive pressure
- Containment isolator in negative pressure for external decontamination of each vial
- Containment isolator with a combination of plastic rigid wall and soft wall isolators.

Figure 1 provides an overview of filling isolator with half-suit on filling machine.

Production Experience

During the first eight years of operation in suite # ATM-1, we manufactured five different products in three different vial sizes. Manufacturing was organized in campaigns of one to three weeks. One batch per day was filled or one batch over a week period depending on the filling volume. The total quantity of cytotoxic liquid injectables manufactured was approximately 11 million vials.

During filling, microbial air sampling on the filler was performed using three air samplers and two settle plate locations. The microbial specification was 0 CFU/m^3. We had a total of six out of specification results. Particle measurement with 3 Probes using continuous automatic

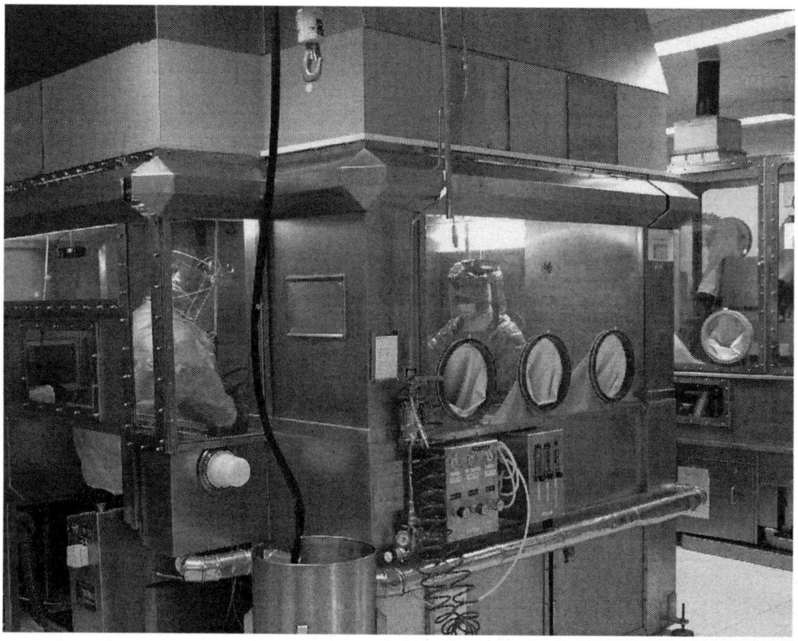

Figure 1 First generation filling isolator.

system during in activity was also performed, with limit of 75% of all samples indicating less than 100 particles of 0.5 μm/cubic foot. Occasional counts of 100 to 500 particles were recorded at the stopper feeder and discounted as being the result of the components themselves.

Media fills were performed using fills ranging from 3000 to 5000 vials under both anaerobic and aerobic conditions. During the operational period, more than 210,000 media fill vials were filled, and the results were "0" positive.

Format Change

During format changes, we performed

- Manual cleaning incorporating a neutralization agent for the drug
- Cleaning evaluation using swab and TOC
- Format change of the equipment/components as needed
- Manual bio decontamination using quaternary ammonium products
- Sanitization with liquid hydrogen peroxide at 15%
- Start of aseptic filling.

The average downtime per format change was three days.

Maintenance

During this period, significant replacement of line components was made including:

- 1 Rigid plastic wall isolator
- 3 Soft wall isolators
- 2 Rapid transfer port (RTP)
- 21 Half-suits.

Improvements Through 2000 in ATM-1 Workshop

To accommodate the manufacture of two new products, some improvements, mainly at filling and stoppering isolator level, were necessary on:

- Air patterns
- Leak tightness
- Decontamination by vaporized hydrogen peroxide (VHP)

- Introduction of glove leak testers
- Sterilization of cooling part of tunnel
- Modifications to the filling pump system.

Production

The suite manufactured two different products in two vial sizes. Manufacturing was conducted in campaign of three weeks duration. The total quantity of cytotoxic liquid injectables manufactured after the listed improvements in the system was approximately 6 million vials.

Results

The "Out of Specification" results obtained over a five-year period after the upgrades were as follows:

- Microbial results at filling—1 positive on glove
- Particle results—No further excursions over 100, 0.5 μm particles/ft^3.
- Media fills—6000 vials × 3 times per year at both anaerobic and aerobic conditions with simulation of worst-case scenario. A total of 90,000 media vials were filled with "0" positive.

SECOND GENERATION OF CYTOTOXIC FACILITY (ATM-2 WORKSHOP) 2000–2008

The new workshop was built, based on the same concepts as the first one. The main objective for the new line was a cost reduction of product price by

- No more half-suits on filling line only glove boxes (Fig. 2)
- Maintain half-suits only at compounding (Fig. 3)
- Use of a high speed filling line
- Batch size increase
- More flexibility in operation
- Reductions in format change/sterilization cycle times.

A period of two years was necessary for the construction and qualification of this second generation workshop (Fig. 2).

Production Experience

The second generation line manufactured four different products in a total of seven unique vial sizes. Manufacturing campaigns were maintained at three weeks duration. The total quantity of units manufactured over the first five years for this new line approximated 6 million vials.

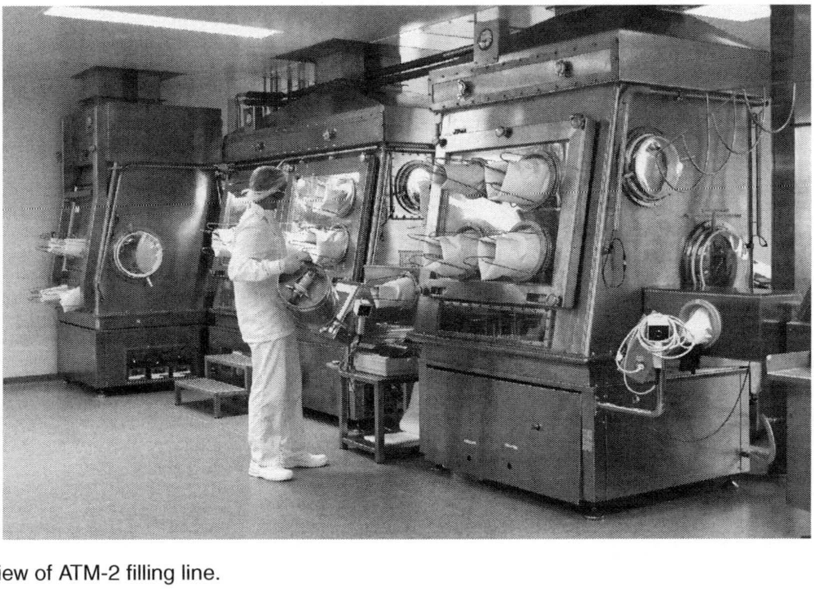

Figure 2 View of ATM-2 filling line.

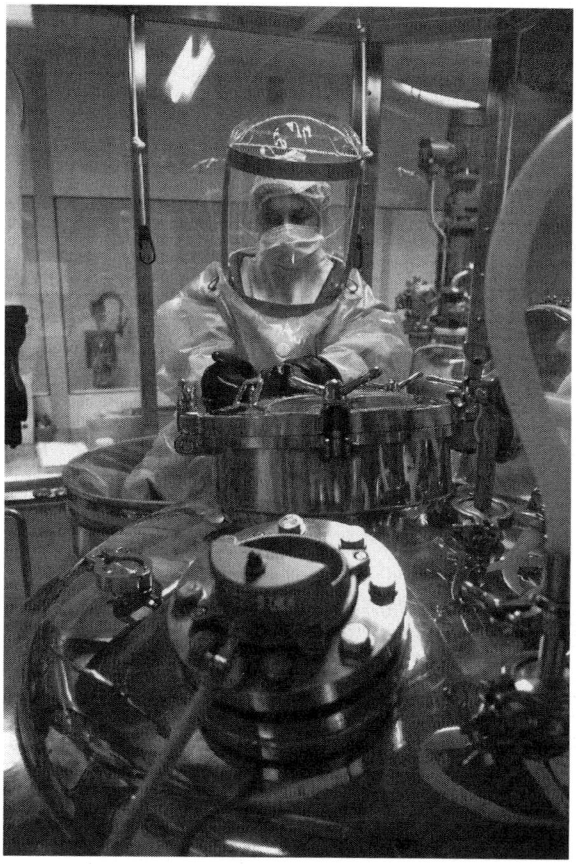

Figure 3 View of ATM-2 compounding.

The bacteriological monitoring results for that period were

- 2 positives on gloves
- 1 positive on settle plate (which led to a single batch rejection)
- All particle monitoring results are conformed to specifications.

The media fill sizes ranged from 25,000 vials for the 1-mL format to 15,000 vials for the 10-mL format. The studies were again performed using both anaerobic and aerobic conditions with simulation of worst-case scenario. A total of 250,000 media fill containers were examined, with "0" positive.

THIRD GENERATION OF CYTOTOXIC FACILITY (ATM-3 AND ATM-4 WORKSHOPS) 2007–2014

Our newest generation of cytotoxic suite has been built to manufacture new products with the following specific characteristics:

- Non soluble in water
- Highly potent and aggressive
- Specific freeze-dried conditions
- Temperature/oxygen and humidity sensitive
- Specific cleaning requirements.

The project goal was to have

- High speed filling line
- High speed sanitization
- Quick surface cleaning

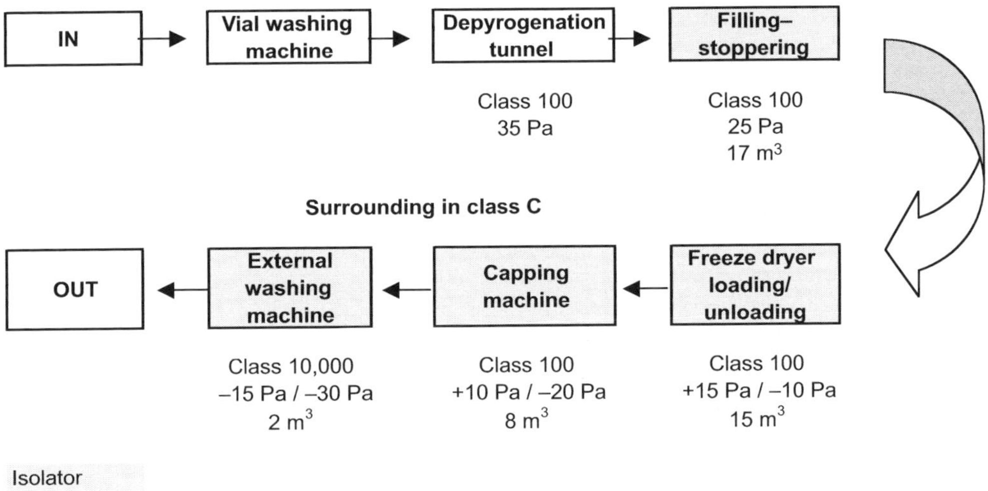

Figure 4 Third generation fill suite design concept.

- High speed format change
- Explosion proof equipment
- Temperature/oxygen/relative humidity regulation.

For this project, Pierre Fabre decided on the following:

- Conduct a risk analysis of the current isolator suites (ATM-1 and ATM-2 workshops)
- Integration of the operating experience from the older fill lines
- Keep the overall system as simple as possible
- Study degradation working modes for all process steps.

The third generation production suite concept is shown in Figure 4.

During filling operations, all of the isolators are maintained under positive pressure to keep sterility as a first priority. During unloading of the freeze-dryer, capping, and external washing of vials, the relevant isolators are under negative pressure to minimize hazard risks to the operator.

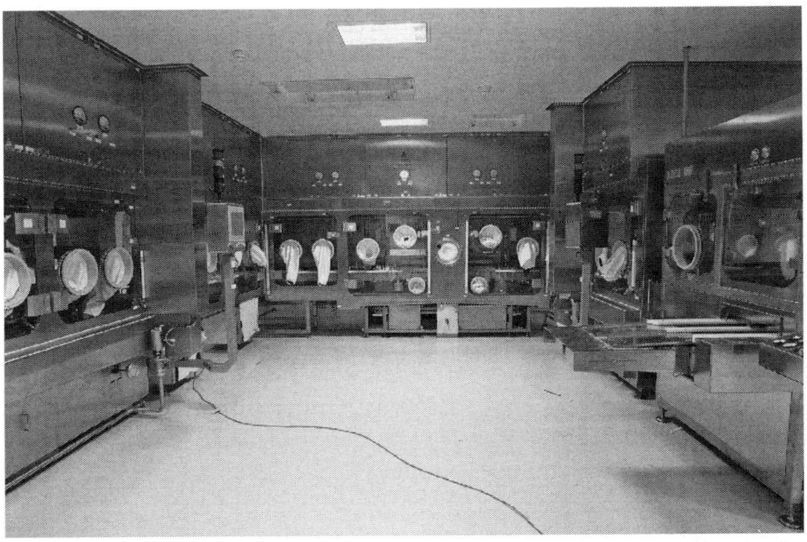

Figure 5 View of new ATM-3 filling line.

Technical Characteristics of the Third Generation Isolators

Humidity/Temperature

The specification for humidity is <10%, at temperatures of 20 to 35°C ± 1°C. This is necessary to avoid evaporation of the product solvent and to maintain the product at a low water concentration. This created some difficulties with static electricity that needed to be solved.

Explosion Proof Production Suite

As the solvent system uses 100% of Tertiary Butyl Alcohol as an excipient, there was a requirement to avoid any spark potential and vapor concentration zone. The considerations in the design for explosion proof operation were

- To prioritize sterility assurance first
- To use an AMDEC "Analyse des Modes de Défaillance et de leur Criticité" (HAZOP—hazard and operability analysis) risk analysis
- To leverage in depth Pièrre Fabre's knowledge of isolator-based sterile manufacturing
- To minimize the isolator volume
- To use vacuum and/or nitrogen in place of air in the critical zone of processing
- To have automated control of the production process and the safety management.

Isolator Cleaning and Decontamination

It was realized that for this system successful cleaning would be very difficult to achieve and several specific requirements were established.

- Guarantee of protection of operating staff
- Prevention of cross-contamination
- A "No Retention" design
- A "No Touch" system for waste recovery.

The means to address these objectives was to develop a washing in place (WIP) system inside each isolator (Fig. 6). Isolator WIP is performed with Water for Injection at 40°C, through static nozzles. It is an automatic WIP and draining system that is fully sanitized after each usage. The main characteristics of WIP system are as follows:

- Isolator internal walls and air ducts (from diffuser membrane to filter bag in–bag out)
- Use of spray nozzle (a total of >300 locations)
- Use of Water for Injection and detergent (final rinsing with Water for Injection)
- Automatic cycle of 30 minutes per isolator
- Manual operation with spray gun also in 30 minutes
- 4 isolators/volume 20 m^3
- Water for Injection consumption—8000 L
- Acceptance criteria—presence of active in rinsing water at <5 PPM.

The main characteristics of post WIP drying are: WIP piping dried by air flush, isolators dried by air recirculation for a duration of three hours with target RH level of 40%.

Pre-VHP Sanitization

The biodecontamination is manually performed over a three-hour period using a sanitizing agent (changed each month).

Isolator Decontamination by VHP

After WIP, isolator decontamination is completed by VHP, using built-in systems, performed with slow motion of the equipment with VHP consumption and monitoring on concentration based on SKAN isolator supplier system. The main characteristics of the VHP decontamination are as follows:

- Constant temperature/initial relative humidity at 30% concentration
- Set up during one hour, followed by the leak testing of the isolators (one hour) Class 3 ISO 10648-2, by constant pressure

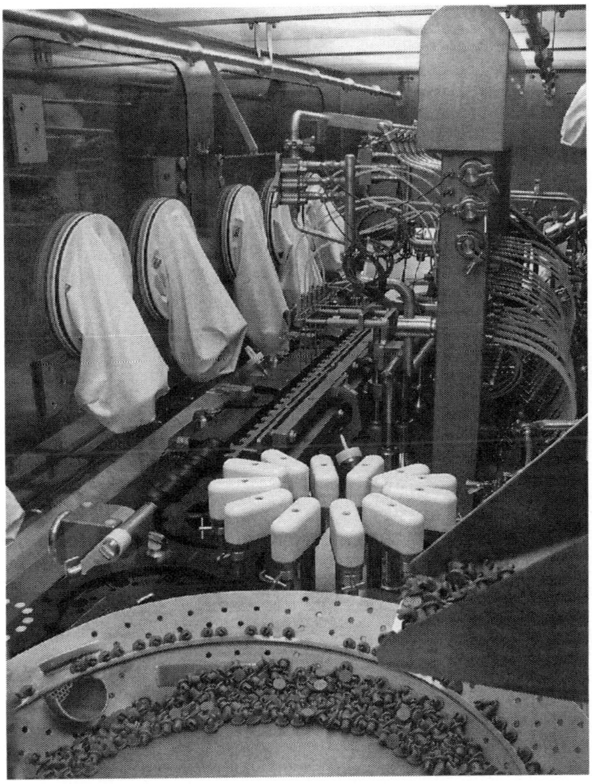

Figure 6 View of WIP inside filling isolator.

- VHP injection for two hours
- Aeration for three hours
- Criteria: in air sampling, H_2O_2 residual <1 PPM.

Glove leak test is performed on 30 gloves (a five-hour process) (4 gloves and sleeves at a time).

Freeze-Drying: Loading and Unloading

The freeze-drying loading/unloading system is a new generation of loader, very compact, fully adjustable by row or pack loads, and easy to clean (Fig. 7). The isolator width is very small (80 cm). The loading system provides

- A regulated product temperature
- An adjustable HR and pressure ($\pm$) of isolator
- A low temperature loading.

Freeze-Drying

The potent compounds are controlled during every step of the process. The nitrogen cover is permanent with pressure equilibrium between isolator and the lyophilizer chamber. CIP of the lyophilizer is performed by Water for Injection at 85°C with the possibility of specific detergent usage. Defrosting of the condenser is performed under vacuum.

Impact on Other Equipments

The suite utilizes a specific drying in the steam autoclave for rubber stopper treatment to ensure lower moisture content to avoid transfer of moisture from stopper to product. Specially designed equipments for stopper handling with custom RTP transfer have been developed. Capping is done in sterile environment isolator with flip off cape sterilized by autoclave. External washing of one hundred percent of vials after capping is done with Purified Water to guarantee no PPM

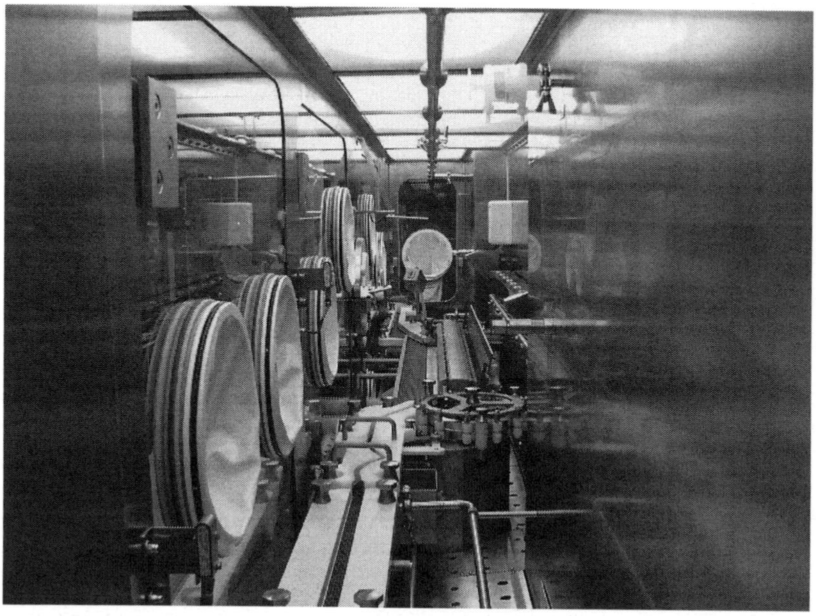

Figure 7 View of isolator at automatic load/unload system of freeze-drier.

of active on outside of vial, for safety during handling of vial at visual inspection and at usage in hospital.

Liquid Waste Control

In order to ensure worker safety it was essential to take care of liquid waste recovery and treatment. The system affords the following:

- "No touch" by vacuum transfer
- A No valves or connectors design
- Dedicated network for liquid wastes
- Specific draining valves for safe transfer
- Specific storage tanks 2 × 10 m^3
- Treatment on special resin material for alkaloid waste, and incineration for all the other types of waste.

Process Sequence

After each batch of product or change of product, the following steps are undertaken for all the isolators:

- WIP
- Drying
- Glove leak test
- Biodecontamination
- Leak test
- VHP decontamination.

This is all accomplished by an automatic system with an average duration of 24 hours.

Specific Developments

The improvements in the third generation of isolator in comparison with the two earlier other suites are as follows:

- Humidity and temperature control and regulation
- Explosion proof compliance

- Easy cleaning and sterilization design
- Easy change format
- Specific freezing conditions
- Built-in VHP
- Safety and redundant equipment and instrumentation
- Automatic waste recovery.

CONCLUSION

Isolation technology has really fundamental advantages over other approaches for aseptic filling:

1. Relative to conventional aseptic filling

   It is the BEST for aseptic processing and very well adapted to high value products.

2. To RABS technology

   It is a MUST for high potent drugs.

It guarantees a higher level of sterility confidence as well as safety for both operators and for the environment. Pierre Fabre has some of the broadest experience worldwide with over 18 years of using isolator technology for aseptic filling of high potent drugs. Our strategy is to propose to partners for contract manufacturing a service with a high level of performance using such technology. Our main objective is always turned to the future, what technology innovation to do for future product in a future environmental and safety conditions.

39 RABS case study

Jörg Zimmermann

INTRODUCTION

The development of isolators and RABS (restricted access barrier systems) was started at the end of the 1980s and beginning of the 1990s, almost in parallel.

While isolators were developed for critical operations based on the experience gained in the nuclear power industry, RABS development took conventional clean room technologies one step further. Early on, the main obstacles to the introduction of isolators were the challenges in validating the "sterilization" or, rather, decontamination cycles for the units. When this issue was solved, the development focused more on rapid decontamination for better utilization of the lines by achieving quick turnaround. For RABS, the challenge lay in the missing definition of RABS with widely different ways of operating the various RABS designs.

In 2005, triggered by a request from the FDA, a group of industrial professionals within ISPE (International Society of Pharmaceutical Engineering) worked out a concise definition of RABS (1): The main building blocks of this definition are as follows:

- Rigid wall enclosure
- ISO 5 Unidirectional Airflow environment
- Gloves for setup and interventions
- Automation of the process wherever possible
- Sterilization of all equipment
- High-level disinfection (i.e., sporicidal disinfection)
- Rare open-door interventions.

When this definition was published, the debate continued on the inclusion of "rare open-door interventions under protocol." This was seen as a way out of proper aseptic technology, allowing for inclusion of bad practice.

DESIGN APPROACH TO RABS

When the decision for a new production line for fill-finish operations is taken at a pharmaceutical company, the following points should be considered on a very high level before proceeding further:

- What kind of products are to be filled? Recombinant protein, cytotoxic, vaccine, chemical entity, etc.
- What kind of container system is to be filled? Vial, prefilled syringe, bag, blow-fill-seal container, etc.
- Can the product be terminally sterilized?
- What kind of volume will production have at full capacity?
- Is focus on high volume/high throughput, but limited variability?
- Is focus on flexibility for different products, container sizes, and types?
- What approach does the companies' quality unit adopt to aseptic processing?
- Is there a company policy in place for questions of this nature?

These questions need to be discussed very thoroughly at the outset, since the decisions taken at this stage will determine the direction the entire project will then pursue. Universal decision trees do not exist; however, some facts automatically lead to certain decisions. For example, if a cytotoxic product is to be filled where operator protection becomes equally important as protection of the product from contamination, a well-designed isolator facility should be taken into due consideration. The same may be said for radiopharmaceuticals or early stage development with compounds where the toxicological profile is not yet known.

If it is not clear, however, as to which products and container sizes the facility will be filling in a few years time, a more flexible, yet safe approach should be adopted. Here, a RABS might well be the best choice.

In the next step, the footprint available and the potential machine designs, coupled with the process design, will be evaluated. What level of automation is desired or possible? How will material be transferred to the classified areas?

In an iterative process, machine and room layout will be optimized. Usually, a team of engineers, operators as well as quality functions work together at this stage.

An important and very helpful step in this development will be mock-up studies—once the general machine design has been agreed upon. Quite often, plywood is used to simulate the barrier of either the RABS or isolator. Going through the paces of regular operation of the line and interventions, the design is refined with the positioning of the gloves in the machine cover, as well as the position of individual functions on the filling machine (i.e., sampling points such as particle probes, active air sampling, and removal of rejected material, and jammed stoppers). Other requirements are as follows:

- Cleanability of the machine
- Accessibility for interventions
- Accessibility for maintenance
- Visibility from outside for supervision
- Avoidance of turbulent airflows caused by machine design
- Absorption of cleansing/disinfection agents to surfaces to be avoided
- No contact of processing aids with the product (grease, etc.)
- Sterile filtration of air from pneumatic actuators
- Format parts should be steam sterilizable wherever possible
- Easy set up of format parts (snap-fit-secure)
- Reduce risk of cuts to gloves by avoiding sharp edges, etc.

It can be readily seen that a great deal of the design requirements do not differ very much between an isolator and a RABS.

QUALIFICATION OF RABS

In a RABS system, the room is usually built as a conventional clean room with extensive unidirectional airflow coverage. The machine with its cover is placed under this flow. For the qualification of the room, all the parameters have to be considered for a conventional clean room. These include air exchange rates, high efficiency particulate absorbing (HEPA)-filter retention rates, room recovery, airflow velocity, pressure differential, airflow visualization under dynamic conditions, and so on. Airflow visualization is of extreme importance, as the pressure differential between inside and outside the machine cover can be of the great significance. The machine cover is not an airtight enclosure as in an isolator and has to be qualified accordingly. This is also one of the fundamental challenges when the machine cover is subsequently modified or adapted.

As is the case with all aseptic fill-finish operations, the pinnacle of qualification is the media fill challenge before the line is handed over to production. With RABS and its high level of automation, a relatively high number of units will be filled.

OPERATION OF RABS

Gloves play a very important role in RABS operation. The material for the gloves can vary. Hypalon, bromobutyl, and ethylene propylene diene monomer rubber (EPDM) are used. The method of sterilization or decontamination may also vary. While some users will apply only an alcoholic wipe to the already installed sterile gloves, others will use steam-sterilized or gamma-irradiated gloves. Finally, integrity testing the gloves can also be done in various ways—from just visual inspection of the already installed gloves to pressure decay testing of installed gloves, or off-line testing.

In best practice RABS, all setup activities and interventions during operation are performed with the barrier closed and the gloves in place. An exception may be the installation of oversized equipment such as vibrator bowls. One way of doing it is to use double-bagged, steam-sterilized gloves that are fitted to the barrier for each batch. During installation, a visual

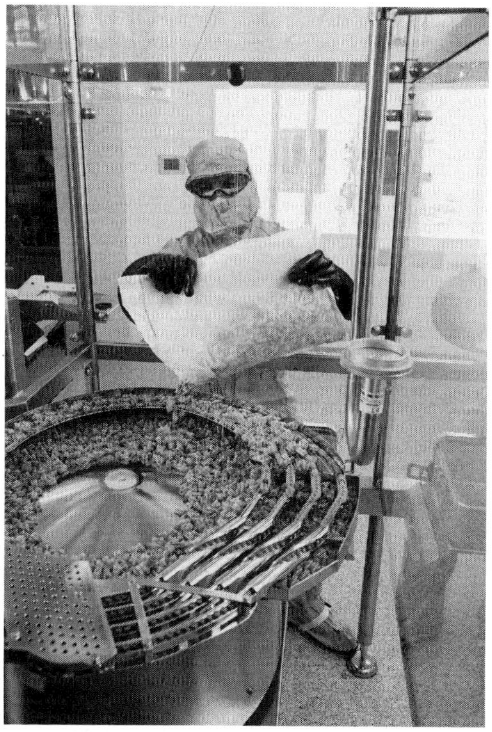

Figure 1 All work on the machines is performed with sterile gloves using glove ports. Persons, machines, and surroundings are clearly separated from each other. *Source*: Courtesy of Vetter Pharma-Fertigung GmbH & Co. KG.

check for integrity is done by the operator. Since the RABS is positioned in a class A/B area with the operator in B, and based on the proper qualification of air overflowing from A to B through the glove ports, removal of an individual glove may be justified, should this visual inspection fail. It is advisable to take microbiological fingerprint samples beforehand. This sampling should also be standard procedure at the end of a batch before removal of the gloves, and cleaning and disinfection of the line.

A simple way of testing the gloves for integrity after use is the pressure decay test. The gloves are fitted to an off-line glove port with a manometer. The glove is then inflated, for example, to 350 Pa, and the pressure observed for 10 minutes. Based on the qualification work, an acceptable pressure decay could be NMT 50 Pa.

Following this test, the gloves are cleaned, wrapped in sterilizable bags, and autoclaved for the next use. It is advisable to track the number and types of uses (which batch, which glove port) for every glove. This, of course, will necessitate that the gloves are individually numbered (Fig. 1).

With proper design of the barrier and proper positioning of the gloves, it should be possible to operate the RABS in the closed mode. In best practice RABS; an open-door intervention will lead into full line cleaning, cleaning and disinfection before continuation of the batch. The prerequisite is therefore a well-running, well-maintained machine to avoid such occurrences.

CASE STUDY: VETTER FACILITY LANGENARGEN

Vetter Pharma Fertigung GmbH & Co. KG is a pure contract manufacturing organization, specialized in the field of fill-finish operations of aseptically prefilled systems. These include vials, syringes, cartridges, and special systems like dual-chamber syringes Vetter LyoJect® (Fig. 2).

As an early adaptor and developer of RABS, Vetter has now more than 15 years experience in operating RABS-based clean rooms. The combination of maximum automation with extreme flexibility makes RABS a very attractive proposition for contract manufacturing organizations. The site in Langenargen on Lake Constance in southernmost Germany was developed by Vetter in the early 1990s. There are currently five production lines installed with space for more expansion.

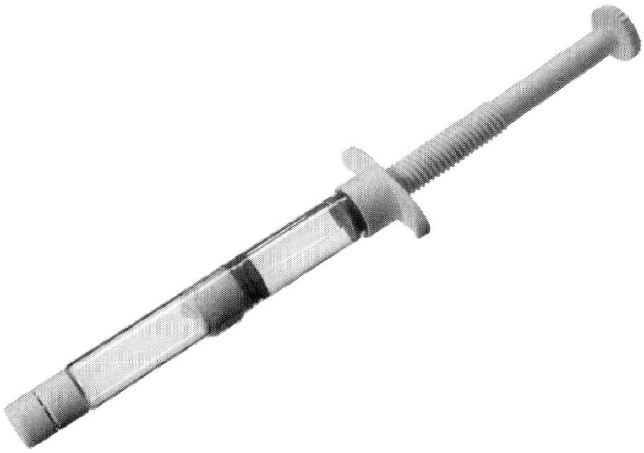

Figure 2 Recombinant proteins or monoclonal antibodies require more sophisticated packaging, such as the dual-chamber syringe Vetter Lyo-Ject®. *Source*: Courtesy of Vetter Pharma-Fertigung GmbH & Co. KG.

The first line was built in 1993 to 1996 and was designed to fill dual-chamber cartridges and syringes Vetter LyoJect®. In the Vetter LyoJect® syringe, a unique system of combining a lyophilized product and diluent in one syringe has been developed. Just before administration, the product is reconstituted via a bypass. With no risk of mixing-up the diluents and minimized hold-up volume, this is particularly suitable for high-value drugs in small doses. The filling process on this production line VLA1/2 was designed with focus on automation. This includes robot transfers of trays holding syringes, and automated loading and unloading of lyophilizers. To make best use of lyophilizer capacity, filling of active solution and filling of diluent are split into two discreet operations on either side of the double-door, pass-through lyophilizers. The line has been running FDA approved products in various presentations since 1998, and has been inspected and reinspected by international authorities almost on a yearly basis (Fig. 3).

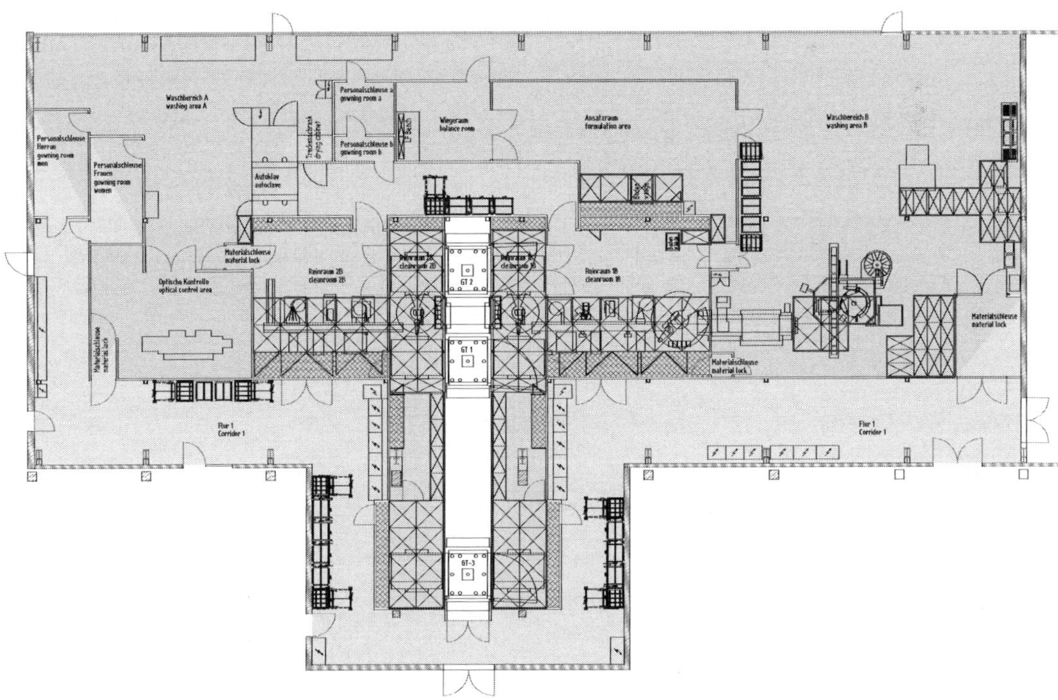

Figure 3 Layout of fill-finish lines VLA1/2 for syringes Vetter Lyo-Ject®. *Source*: Courtesy of Vetter Pharma-Fertigung GmbH & Co. KG.

In the next development stage, two lines for liquid prefilled syringes were installed in the building from 1999 to 2001. Both lines use the bulk process, where the components are purchased untreated from the vendor, and are washed, siliconized, and sterilized on-site. This is accomplished for all components, be they glass syringes, plastic components, or rubber stoppers. Line VLA3 is equipped with a dry heat sterilization tunnel for luer-lock or tip-cap syringes. Line VLA4 is equipped with an autoclave for the sterilization of stake-needle syringes.

Both lines are also fully automated to avoid manual transportation steps altogether. The syringes are transported fully automatically all the way from syringe washing machine infeed to the outfeed of the fully stoppered and filled syringes from the clean room.

Finally, line 5 is a small vial line for both liquid and lyophilized vials, which was put into operation in 2006. In total, the five filling lines represent a capacity of approximately 100 million units annually.

Media Fills

From 1996 to 2008, a grand total of 2,500,000 units were filled in media fill process simulations. Only three individual units were ever found contaminated in three separate runs. With the associated investigations, clear and plausible root causes for these contaminations were found and corrective action duly taken. One example for corrective action was introducing steam-sterilized goggles for the operators. Prior to the first contaminated unit, operators would not use goggles during the fill operation as the barrier was deemed good enough a protection.

Sterility Testing

In the operation of the site, there has never been a positive sterility test result.

Environmental Monitoring

During routine operation, approximately 30,000 microbiological samples are taken in the core Grade A area of the machine per year. These consist of settle plates, active-air monitoring using gelatin membrane filtration method, glove fingerprints, and machine contact plates. On an average, only a maximum of five of these samplings have resulted in a deviation per year. Particulate monitoring is carried out as continuous monitoring at both the 0.5 and 5 μm sizes with up to five sampling points per fill line. These sampling points have been carefully selected based on risk analysis, so that the locations are representative of the process. With the sampling being once/minute for 24 hr/day, approximately 40 million data points are generated per year. Out of these, again a maximum of 5 excursions lead to a deviation. These data go to show how well the environment can be controlled in a RABS installation.

For the "no open-doors" policy to be applied, the processes must run as smoothly as possible. As a daily key performance indicator, the technical availability is measured as the percentage of interruptions/downtimes due to technical errors in relation to the total available fill time. If the value falls below 95% of technical availability (or more than 5% of technical downtime), a failure mode and effect analysis (FMEA) of the process is performed with production, engineering, and quality unit being included.

The aseptic processes are evaluated as a continuous effort. Optimization in cleaning and sanitization, in handling of components, and monitoring is carried out on a regular basis.

RETROFITTING EXISTING CLEAN ROOMS TO RABS

Existing conventional clean rooms can be retrofitted to a RABS to a certain extent. As always, retrofits require some compromises, but our experience shows that it is worthwhile. For the case study presented here, one of the clean rooms at Vetter's Ravensburg facility was upgraded. Upgrade focus was on two areas: the machine cover and glove positioning, as well as extension of the HEPA-filter ceiling. The project was carried out in two steps:

First, the HEPA-filter ceiling surface was increased to enable safer handing around the machine. Since this required the clean room to be opened and modified, the process was requalified at the end of a six-week downtime. A media fill was carried out before production, carried on with the existing machine and machine cover. The time to rebuild the room was used to conduct mock-up studies with plywood machine covers. The operators and engineers of the line united to optimize the machine covers, and reposition the gloves. The final covers were then built in the workshop, and fitted to the line four months later. Again, the line was fully requalified, with airflow pattern visualization being a major part.

Finally, a new media fill validation was carried out with three consecutive runs. When the project had been approved by senior management, the regulatory implications were evaluated parallel to the engineering work. For a contract manufacturer, communication with the authorities and customers was of utmost importance and a great deal of attention was paid to details in this.

Although some compromises had to be made, the overall benefit of upgrading an existing room to RABS is that this is a modification to an existing facility, and can be readily handled as an annual product review item with the authorities. As always, it does, however, help to discuss these changes well in advance, so as not to take the regulators by surprise.

For our case study, the total running time of the project was less than 12 months, with two three to four weeks downtimes of the line. Investments were in the range of €500,000.

PROS AND CONS OF RABS

With relatively large areas of highly classified areas, that is, Grade A and B, the operating costs of a RABS might be higher than for an isolator. This also includes higher costs for gowning and monitoring the area. This has to be balanced with the higher usability of the line plus very quick changeovers from format to format and product to product. Cleaning and disinfecting is manual in most cases with RABS, while isolators have fully automated decontamination. Some people believe that these manual processes are difficult to validate, however, in the performance of the RABS lines as outlined in section "Retrofitting Existing Clean Rooms to RABS", there is daily verification of the clean status of the rooms. A best practice RABS provides a very safe process while being very flexible at the same time.

CONCLUSION

Many attempts have been made to compare and contrast RABS and isolators—to show the superiority of the one over the other. In the end, there is no one right answer. Invariably, there are a host of aspects to be taken into consideration, and the decision to use either RABS or isolator has to be made on a case-to-case basis. In the final analysis, the product, the process, and the company requirements have to neatly dovetail.

In this chapter, Vetter's experience using RABS is outlined. The data given here represent the status of knowledge within the company that, of course, might well not be applicable in all detail to other companies and projects. For Vetter Pharma, however, the question of "RABS or isolator?" has been answered by RABS having been adopted for the 9 fill-finish lines that have been introduced in the course of the last 10 years.

REFERENCE

1. Lysfjord, J. Restricted access barrier system (RABS) for aseptic processing. Pharmaceutical Engineering. November/December 2005:25(6):116–117, 120.

40 Innovation in aseptic processing: case study through the development of a new technology

Benoît Verjans

INTRODUCTION

As many drugs can be administered only through systemic way, due either to patient condition or due to bioavailability of the drug itself, the continued availability of existing drugs and development of new parenteral formulations remain a must in the pharmaceutical industry. Among parenterals, aseptically filled drugs are more and more common, especially since many of the new biological drugs cannot resist terminal sterilization.

Four major issues can be pointed out, being related to injectable drugs in general or to aseptically filled drugs in particular.

The first issue is patient safety. In contrast to terminal sterilization, aseptic processing does not guarantee a complete absence of bacterial presence and, thus its potential, proliferation inside a liquid solution. In case of such contamination, patient life is at risk as it can face septic shock and death. The presence of operators in the vast majority of aseptic processes means that the greatest source of potential microbial is ever present.

The second issue raised more specifically for vaccines is that the presence of preservatives, such as thimerosal in vaccines, has been challenged by various governmental organizations such as the Food and Drug Administration (FDA), the Center for Disease Control (CDC), and the National Institute for Health (NIH) in the early 2000s (1). As a result, vaccines manufacturers took the decision to withdraw preservatives from vaccines, eliminating the last safety barrier in case of presence of single bacteria.

The third issue is counterfeiting, a new threat, which has started to rise and in particular to target injectable products. The main driver to sell counterfeited injectable is that huge benefits can be achieved on selling high price vials. Several counterfeit batches of expensive biologics have already been identified and withdrawn by the FDA. Counterfeiting is a major issue on various points of view:

- Economic point of view: It is estimated that about 10% of worldwide drugs are counterfeited, generating a revenue loss of more than 32 billion USD. Counterfeiting is so severe that it can reach up to 50% of drugs sold in some countries such as Nigeria (2).
- Patient quality point of view: The quality of counterfeited drugs is seriously impaired. In some cases, the active ingredient is not present or not at the right dosage, leading to the lack of treatment and worsening of condition. For example, 2500 people died in Nigeria from meningitis among 25,000 people being vaccinated with a counterfeited vaccine without antigen inside. This patient risk is not specific to the third world countries and happens in developed countries such as the United States. The most well-known case is the contamination of Tim Fagan, a recent transplanted teenager who has been contaminated by a poor quality copy of the Amgen's drug Epogen. As a result, a law, named Tim Fagan's law, has been approved and has reinforced the legal actions against counterfeiting companies and people.

In parallel to counterfeiting, bioterrorism became a real issue since September 11, 2001 when people realized that terrorist can develop multiple ways to attack Western countries.[1]

The fourth driver was based on experience with glass vial filling in an isolator. The equipment used has reached such a level of complexity that each produced batch requires not only high resources in qualified human resources for operation and maintenance but also in quality assurance/quality control support. The complexity is driven by the washing, siliconization

[1] Glass vials, being very easy to copy, are good candidates to carry viruses and other biological weapons.

and sterilization of vials and stoppers, the high-speed filling/stoppering, and the high-speed aluminum capping. As a result, both operating expenses and investment for equipment, large utility production units, and building space have exploded. For example, a filling line under isolator with a nominal capacity of 42,000 vials/hr needs approximately 300 m^2 of class C (or class ISO 8) clean room, and overall equipment price would exceed 10 MM EUR.

These four issues triggered GSK Biologicals to investigate a new technology for aseptic filling of injectable drugs and created Aseptic Technologies to address this objective. After analysis of these issues, Aseptic Technologies determined that it was possible to create a new technology that would be able to address all these issues. This means that the technology should

- Provide a top-class sterility assurance level during operation
- Provide a reinforced security against counterfeiting and bioterrorism
- Simplify aseptic filling processes and operations.

THE CLOSED VIAL CONCEPT

The solution identified to address the three points described above is the Crystal® or Closed Vial technology (3,4). The concept is based on a closed container that can be filled through a heat resealable stopper (initial technology licensed from Medinstill Inc.) and, to simplify the process, a presterilized container is provided stoppered and ready-to-fill.

The vial is made of cyclo olefin copolymer (COC) whereas the stopper is made of thermoplastic elastomer. The latter is mandatory to allow heat resealing. For example, classic rubber stopper would burn under heat source but not reseal.

The vial manufacturing consists in three major steps:

- The two main elements of the vial are molded in class 100/ISO 5 to ensure the cleanness of the inside of the vial. They are molded at the same time and robots perform assembly of the two elements. Thanks to the specific shape of the stopper adapted to the vial body, the assembly strength is sufficient to hold them together. Thanks to rapid closing, the air entrapped inside the vial is from class 100/ISO 5 environment.
- The second step consists in the addition of top and bottom rings to secure closure integrity. This is completed on a rotary table with tight visual control of presence and positioning of each element to ensure rejection of any vials with missing or misplaced part. The vials are then packed in polypropylene akylux boxes and double wrapped in polyethylene bags. This packaging is the packaging used for loading the vials on the filling line (see below).
- The third step is the sterilization of the closed vial. As there is no glass, gamma-irradiation at minimum 25 kGray is entirely appropriate to ensure that the vial is sterile without altering its color. At the end of those three steps, the vial is clean and sterile and therefore ready-to-fill once delivered to the pharmaceutical manufacturing site.

The vial filling process consists in five major steps:

- The loading is performed on tables equipped with long arms to perform box opening and vial loading on accumulation table. By keeping the operator away from the vial, risk of contamination of the outside of the vial is minimized.
- Nevertheless, as it is not possible to exclude an operator mistake resulting in a contamination on the stopper, the vial can be processed through an e-beam to resterilize the stopper surface. Effectively, this surface is the most critical one because it will be penetrated by the needle during the piercing process (see next step). The e-beam delivers a dose of 25 kGray of beta irradiation on the stopper. This dose is sufficient to resterilize the surface, but penetrate not in depth in the material (irradiation dose is maintained to a depth of 30 μm and then starts to decrease rapidly).
- The vial is then filled with a pencil point needle that has been designed to
  - Minimize particle generation during piercing
  - Avoid coring of the stopper leading to large particles and absence of material necessary for optimal laser resealing
  - Dispense smoothly the liquid with a 30° angle, thanks to lateral holes
  - Eliminate overpressure due to liquid filling in a closed container, thanks to ventilation slots located on the needle sides at the height of the stopper.

- After filling, the vial is immediately resealed by a focused laser beam. The laser system has multiple functionalities to ensure optimal resealing of the piercing trace:
  - A flat-top curve lens that provides an equal distribution of the energy on the entire area hit by the laser to avoid both burn spots and low energy spots.
  - A feedback system that detects the presence and the intensity of the laser shot. This system is a Process Analytical Technology (PAT) to perform 100% check of the quality of the resealing.
- The final step is the capping of the vial. Thanks to plastic molding, the capping is made by snap fitting of polyethylene caps. A simple pressure is sufficient to ensure capping. The cap has the unique ability to ensure additional closure integrity at the level of the stopper surface. This closure integrity is achieved, thanks to a rib located on the inner face of the cap and that is pressing on the stopper. Therefore, the stopper surface is kept in the same class environment as the one around the capping station; and maintained until used by the medical practitioner.

An additional step can be added to address counterfeiting as a specific marking with either radio frequency identification (RFID) chip or laser marking. The RFID can be placed simply during capping. It can be easily located on the inner face of the cap and therefore be entrapped between the cap and the vial during capping. A simple coding station can be located before exiting the filling line. As a result, a secured RFID is coded before any operator could touch the vial.

The laser marking process has been designed on the same concept of having a coded vial coming out of the line. The marking can be made on the top ring lateral side that offers a surface big enough to perform either alpha-numeric coding or 2D matrix coding, again, before the vial exits the filling line.

Obviously, the Closed Vial technology introduces both new filling technologies and a new container. Therefore, to ensure that the technology is suitable for injectable drugs, it has been fully studied and validated to ensure that it meets all requirements from authorities regarding approval of container and filling process. Both the European and US Pharmacopeia provide mandatory detailed tests for polymeric materials such as material characterization, acceptable level of endotoxins and particle, and closure integrity tests. All of these tests have been performed successfully and, in addition, detailed extractable and leachable studies have been conducted to assess in depth the materials in contact with the injectable drug.

The final proof of robustness was the performance of a media fill inside a nonclassified environment. To that end, two prototype lines located in a workshop have been used to fill over 25,000 closed vials with media and none has been contaminated. Overall, over 100,000 vials have been filled without contamination.

ENVIRONMENT REQUIRED DURING THE VARIOUS MANUFACTURING STEPS

On one hand, to ensure that the Closed Vial technology meets the latest requirements from authorities regarding aseptic drug production, a high-quality environment must be continuously provided during all steps of production. On the other hand, the Closed Vial technology ensures by itself a better safety for the patient (e.g., the container is permanently closed during all filling operation). Therefore, through the use of quality by design this technology allows for the simplification of many processes, including the environment during both vial manufacturing process and vial filling process.

Environment During Vial Manufacturing

The cleanliness of the inside of the vial is a major concern, as it is closed before use and there is no opportunity to withdraw particles and endotoxins after container closing. Sterility is not an immediate concern at that time as the gamma sterilization will penetrate thoroughly all parts of the vial, but bioburden should be also minimized to avoid endotoxin generation. To ensure that cleanliness, the vials are molded in class 100/Grade A/ISO 5 environment. Operator presence during operation is strictly forbidden and environmental monitoring is permanent. Inside the room, the only equipment present are the molds, the robots to pick and assemble both vial parts,

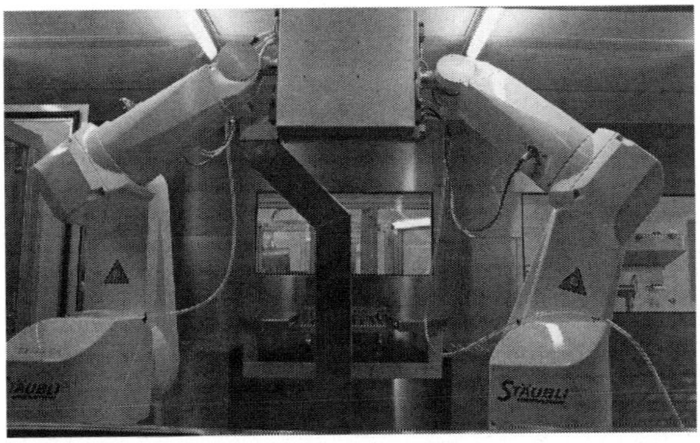

Figure 1 Illustration of the clean room class 100/Grade A/ISO 5 used for vial body and stopper molding, followed by robot assembly.

and a vibrating rail that deliver vials outside this room once closed (Fig. 1). Special care has been put on the design of the room.

- The concept of molding machine is designed with a mold and mold plates in an overhang "cantilever" position. Only the mold, the supporting platens, and the tie bars are located inside the clean room whereas the rest of the machine is outside. As the mold is opening, clean air can flush through the open space, with no underlying machine frame or component disturbing the flow. Special care is devoted to details, like cooling water hoses and electrical connections located under the mold.
- The molds are operating without addition of any additive to facilitate exit of parts. These additives are considered as a source of contaminants such as leachables and particles.
- The robot hands have been designed to touch only the noncritical surfaces of the vial parts. All robot surfaces are easily cleaned and grippers (difficult to clean) have been avoided. The component holding is done by cavities in the flat hand front surface, with vacuum in the center of this cavity.
- The selected robots are suitable for operation in high classification clean rooms, as usual in the semiconductor industry (class 10/ISO 4).

After molding and assembly of the two parts, they are transferred to a class 10,000/ISO 7 environment suitable for further automatic assembly and packaging. It is critical that the inside of the vial is not exposed to this room. Therefore, the assembled vial body–stopper is inspected with camera to ensure that the stopper is properly in place. Any unit with a missing stopper or partially lifted stopper is discarded. The vial handling systems have been designed to avoid risk of marks and scratches on the highly transparent body surfaces, allowing a free view for inspection for particles after filling. High tech CMM (Coordinate Measurement Machine) are also used to periodically evaluate all critical dimensions.

The result of the above practices is a vial where visible particles are totally absent; the level of subvisible particles is extremely low and difficult to measure. Also bioburden has been found to be zero on all tested samples.

Environment During Vial Filling

At this step, the vial remains permanently closed and therefore the risk of contamination due to the presence of bacteria in the environment is very low. As shown in Figure 2, when the needle is piercing the vial, the stopper remains tight on the needle surface. This effect has a wiping effect keeping potential contaminant out of the vial. The biggest risk is located at the level of the holes dispensing the liquid. This concept of the vial staying closed at all times means that the vial can be considered as "an isolator at item level."

The environment around the filling area is provided with an isolation system: the CVFS (Closed Vial Filling System). In this chapter, the main characteristics of this system are described.

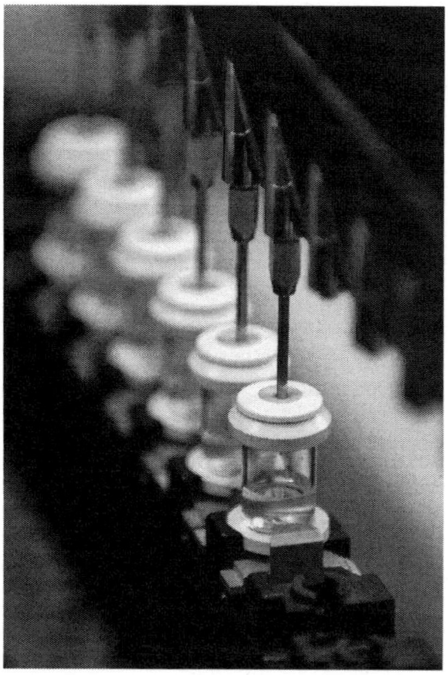

Figure 2 Piercing of the vial showing the tight contact between stopper and needle.

The CVFS is defined as: "An aseptic filling system providing an environment achieving uncompromised Class 100/Grade A/ISO 5 protection that surrounds containers which are delivered closed and sterile inside, are filled through their stoppers and then immediately re-sealed to preclude the possibility of microbial ingress."

The key characteristics of a CVFS have been defined using a "quality by design" process and can be summarized as:

- *Surrounding environment*: Surrounding room classification should be class 100,000/Grade C/ISO 8 minimum in operation.
- *Enclosure system*: Operators must be separated from aseptic processing operations by rigid walls to ensure complete physical separation. No door opening is allowed during operations and is allowed only after line clearance. To prevent unintentional opening, the doors are interlocked and linked to alarm systems. In case of door opening, all materials still present inside the CVFS (empty vials, filled vials, bulk in fluid path, caps, etc.) are discarded. The rigid wall is equipped with glove ports and rapid transfer ports (RTP) to allow manual intervention and component transfer such as needle, solution, or caps. The ceiling is equipped with HEPA filters to supply continuously unidirectional airflow from the ceiling of the enclosure. The environmental control system operates primarily on the principle of aerodynamic separation (air overspill) as defined in ISO 14644-7. An open bottom with air exit inside the surrounding environment is appropriate for classical products. For highly potent and/or toxic products, a closed bottom is recommended to maintain operator protection.
- *Entry of closed and sterile containers*: The vials can be entered either through closed systems such as beta-bags connected to RTP or polyethylene bags treated in a vapor hydrogen peroxide (VHP) airlock. These systems are adapted for small quantities of vials due to productivity limitations. For high-speed lines, a manual opening can be performed. As the line can be installed in a class 100,000/Grade C/ ISO 8 and the design cannot exclude unintentional contamination of the stopper surface; surface sterilization is mandatory before entering the CVFS. This can be achieved with an e-beam as described above.
- *Sanitization and environment quality in the enclosure system:* "High-level disinfection" of all nonproduct contact surfaces is achieved with an appropriate sporicidal agent before batch manufacture. All the product contact surfaces, such as fluid path, are sterilized in an autoclave and entered through RTP.

KEY ADVANTAGES OF THE CLOSED VIAL TECHNOLOGY OVER THE CLASSICAL GLASS VIAL TECHNOLOGY

As a reminder, Aseptic Technologies was interested to improve the aseptic filling on three major axes:

- Offer a better solution to the patient to reduce risk of contamination that demand being exacerbated by the withdrawal of preservatives
- Improve supply chain to reduce counterfeiting and bioterrorism risks
- Leverage a solution that is less complicated and less expensive compared with current glass vial technology.

The expectations placed on the Closed Vial technology can be summarized in two words: safer and easier. This chapter details how the technology can be proved to provide a better solution compared with glass vial.

Safer

The Closed Vial concept is the essence of reduction of patient risk due to contamination, as the inside of the sterile vial is never exposed to the environment. Thus, it is impossible for a contaminant to penetrate and proliferate inside the container in contact with the liquid product. With the glass vial technology, vials can be exposed for up to 20 to 30 minutes after depyrogenization, from exit of the hot air tunnel up to stoppering station. This exposure could lead to ingress of living organisms that can be present inside the manned environment. The situation with stoppers is even worse as stoppers are often loaded for a full batch, which means that stopper surface can be exposed several hours. These risks have been minimized by increased usage of systems such as isolators and restricted access barrier systems (RABS) but such systems do not guarantee a 100% protection of the product against contamination.

With respect to the fill needle, it is impossible to avoid exposure to the environment, but the Closed Vial technology offers an additional safety point which is the wiping of the needle by the very flexible material of the stopper. Moreover, the design of the equipment has taken into account the most critical current good manufacturing practices (cGMP) requirements. In particular, care has been taken to avoid as much as possible the presence of equipment above the needle to minimize airflow pattern turbulences.

Particle studies have shown that the entire process (including vial manufacturing, piercing, laser resealing, and 23-gauge needle piercing to collect the liquid) generates half the amount of particles with the closed vial compared with glass vial. This particle reduction is obtained thanks to a production process that is made in a class 100/ISO 5 environment and by using noncoring needle to pierce the vial. The use of molded plastic materials allows the introduction of new features to improve closure integrity (right angle snap fit assembly) or to facilitate particle inspection (elevated bottom), all contributing in attaining top-level quality for the product. In addition, the use of plastic cap provides additional closure integrity at the level of the stopper surface. The protection of the piercing trace is an important health issue, as cleaning of stopper is frequently inadequately performed by health care professionals. This can range from absence of cleaning or light wiping that is not sufficient to eliminate bacteria. Local infections have been often shown due to needle contamination when the product is collected from the vial.

Regarding supply chain, a safer solution is achieved through both secure coding and shock resistance (the plastic vials are less susceptible to breakage as compared with glass).

Easier

The Closed Vial technology substantially simplifies the aseptic filling process for the pharmaceutical manufacturers. In particular, the key simplifications are the elimination of the preparation steps mandatory for glass vials and rubber stopper. These steps include washing, siliconization, and sterilization. Other simplification are the elimination of the high-speed stoppering under aseptic conditions, the replacement of the aluminum cap crimping by snap fit of plastic cap, and the use of the CVFS in place of isolator.

As a result of the simplifications, the validation requirements are also reduced. In particular, validation efforts required for water for injection used for vial body and stopper washing can be eliminated. The new technologies introduced, that is, e-beam sterilization and laser resealing are relatively easy to validate and are performed for each batch. All these simplification have been shown to reduce the total cost of operation, thanks to reduction in operating expenses (fewer operators are needed, less validation work should be performed, only limited electricity and no water for injection is needed, etc.), a better productivity (less residual volume, less vial breakage, etc.), and a reduction of investment (smaller clean room, less expensive equipment,~etc.).

The technology also proved to be easier for health care professionals. A market study conducted with 246 professionals in hospitals (doctors, nurses, and hospital pharmacists, both in Europe and United States) has shown that 87% of them expressed a preference for the closed vial versus 7% for the glass vial. The main reasons pointed out are the ease to vial handling, vial opening, stopper piercing, and liquid collection. Other sources of preference were an unbreakable vial and a better asepsis for the patient (especially the protection of the piercing area).

In conclusion, the Closed Vial technology has not only proved itself as a suitable technology for the aseptic filling of injectable drugs but also provides a series of advantages to answer the most recent challenges faced by this industry.

REFERENCES

1. CDC. Joint Statement on Thimerosal. Centers for Disease Control and Prevention. MMWR 1999; 48(26):563–565.
2. World Health Organization (WHO). Factsheet 275. WHO, 2003.
3. Verjans B, Thilly J, Vandecasserie C. A new concept in aseptic filling: closed-vial technology. Pharm Technol 2005; 18:S24–S29.
4. Thilly J, Conrad D, Vandecasserie C. Aseptic filling of closed, ready to fill containers. Pharm Eng 2006; 26:66–74.

41 Isolated robotics

Christopher Procyshyn

INTRODUCTION

Medicines are manufactured because they have a profound effect on the lives of humans. When administered appropriately, medicines can improve lives enormously and save countless lives. Administered inappropriately, these same products can effect devastating consequences for the individual. And, as the health care industry develops more effective and specific therapies, these properties are enhanced and intensified with the ultimate goal of creation of the most specific and potent molecules achievable. Unintentionally, due to their own biological nature, humans working to produce these medicines may either harm or be harmed by these same therapeutic products.

Thus, there are diametrically opposite forces acting between the interests of the medicine and those humans working to produce it. And nowhere are these forces more evident than in the production of injectable drug products.

Complicating matters are the significant and growing classes of aseptically handled drug products that must be produced with presterilized components, as they are incapable of withstanding sterilization conditions. These aseptic products represent the added hazard for the potential of contaminating organisms, either from the process or the manufacturing environment, to be directly injected into the recipient patient. And so, it is a logical conclusion that ultimately the product and manufacturing personnel require complete and absolute separation.

In practice, this separation of people from product has been the subject of a great deal of deliberation and varied degrees of success. With the advent of clean room technology and high efficiency air filtration systems, the focus of product quality centered on the management of these human activities in an otherwise clean environment. Humans, with their inherent microbial flora present on all exposed surfaces of their bodies, provide the largest source of contamination. So long as the human and the environment were controlled and monitored appropriately, sterility of the product could be satisfactorily assured to industry conventions. However, for both the sanitization and operation of the clean room, human behavior was the determining factor between success and failure. This leaves a level of risk that is increasingly unacceptable to regulators and the public, and indeed unnecessary.

Conventionally, manufacturing processes and machines have been historically derived from some form of previously manual practices. In almost all situations, some level of human intervention remained as necessary to keep the machines working smoothly and efficiency optimized. These design concepts were the basis for today's filling technologies for pharmaceutical products, and represent an appropriate solution for the period in which they were created. Unfortunately, this time has largely passed.

Today, the accepted pinnacle of process and personnel separation is isolation technology. Isolators represent a hermetically sealed environment, commonly decontaminated with oxidizing agents, that yields a sterile and integral processing space. The earliest usage of isolator technology was generally limited to manual processes utilizing integral gloves or half-suits as the interfacing surfaces. Although clearly superior to conventional clean room operations, this need for manual intervention left significant room for improvement, both in quality and speed.

Throughout the supply chain of human therapeutics, from chemical or biological synthesis through drug product manufacturing and the clinic, there is a move toward automation of previously open and/or manual processes. This presents the opportunity to re-evaluate methods and practices to achieve cost-effective high-quality solutions, and learn from other industries' experience in modernization and automation.

ROBOTICS

The first digitally programmed and operated robot was the Unimate (1), built for hazardous environment use by General Motors in 1961 at their parts plant in Trenton, NJ. It was designed for the movement of hot metal die castings, a dangerous task for human operators due to the heat, exhaust gases from casting, and risk of lost limbs in the stacking process. It was highly successful, and within a short period other companies purchased similar systems and expanded the use of robotics into applications such as welding and other dangerous processes.

This represents a history of experience in robotics for the automotive industry of nearly 40 years. Robots are indeed ubiquitous in the automotive industry, having spawned a wide array of designs and applications. In turn, this demand has created markets for high-quality components and software, pushing capabilities of robotic systems well beyond the limits of human dexterity and reproducibility, to near perfection. As car models and parts evolve continuously from model year to the next, robotics has demonstrated its relative strength in adaptability to new processes and parts. This adaptability has enabled the creation of multiproduct assembly plants, able to change between vehicle models with brief changeover periods.

Such success has owed much to the development of microprocessor technology. The leaps in data processing and transmission in the semiconductor industry have enabled a rapid increase in the sophistication and speed of robotic systems. This synergy in computing power and the demands of the electronics industry has also served to bring about significant cost reductions for robots. Today, inexpensive and readily available computing power largely exceeds the demands of robot designers. This has created a wealth of possibilities to developers, with a suitable cost of goods for most markets. As a result, robotics is undergoing a revolution in its development, pushing into new applications and environments.

> . . . the emergence of the robotics industry, which is developing in much the same way that the computer business did 30 years ago. Think of the manufacturing robots currently used on automobile assembly lines as the equivalent of yesterday's mainframes. Bill Gates (2)

However, due to multitude of contributing factors, robotics has seen relatively limited installations in aseptic applications in the pharmaceutical industry. Historically, with relatively few manufacturing cost pressures, relatively high barriers to regulatory acceptance, and a high cost of implementation, pharmaceutical companies traditionally have opted for more basic and generally manual processes. However, increasing pressures on profitability for drug companies, combined with the increasing regulatory scrutiny on injectable products, have resulted in significant interest in the field of robotics of late.

ISOLATED ROBOTICS

Most notable has been the application of robotics within the confines of isolator technology. This combination of technologies promises the complete containment of product and process, with a level of precision and speed unattainable with manual labor. Robots have been used in isolator systems in a variety of applications such as environmental monitoring (3), fluid dispensing, and

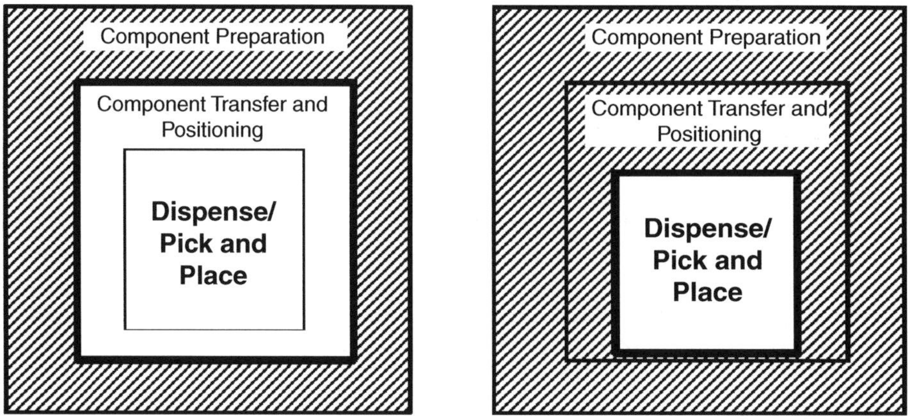

Figure 1 Zone diagram for material processing. Sterilization is defined as the solid black line in the figure. *Source:* Courtesy of Vanrx Pharmasystems.

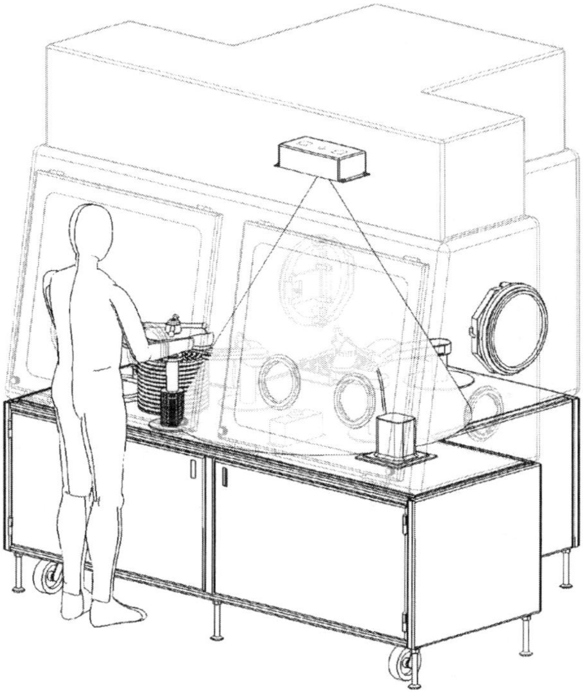

Figure 2 Design sketch of vision-guided robotic filling system. *Source:* Courtesy of Vanrx Pharmasystems.

material transfer. These systems have eliminated the need for intervention by human operators through the use of integral gloves attached to the isolator.

However, due to unique aspects of isolator technology not present in most other operating environments, technical hurdles have been encountered in the application of isolated robotics. Commonly, hydrogen peroxide vapor is used to oxidize and destroy microbial contamination within the isolated space. This presents a challenge for the corrosion of electronic components by the peroxide vapor, as well as the overall hermetic sealing of the system. Very few classes of robots have been designed to operate in a hermetic environment, and do so in a clean, particle-free manner.

Clean room robots have been employed since the late 1970s in the semiconductor industry for the handling and processing of silicon wafers. Inherent in any mechanical process is some degree of particle generation due to friction. The clean room robot designs have routinely employed internal vacuum systems to remove particles, thus drawing air from the operating environment through the robot and then exhausted to the external environment. Although this strategy has been successful in the wafer processing industry, it presents challenges in the application of isolated robotics. Venting of peroxide vapor during processing is undesirable, and the maintenance of filtered internal air pressure during operations often difficult and complex to control. Manufacturers have employed various strategies to mitigate these issues, ranging from catalytic degradation of peroxide exhaust from the robot to various seal mechanisms within the robot arm itself.

DEVELOPMENT OF AN ISOLATED ROBOTIC ASEPTIC FILLING SYSTEM

Technology in and of itself often lacks true impact without a detailed and thoughtful analysis of the user experience with it. The tools and components exist to build an almost limitless variety of technological solutions, but only those that truly speak to the user needs and leave the individual with a satisfactory experience have made a lasting impression. This pursuit of form and function is at the heart of modern industrial design.

It's not just what it looks like and feels like. Design is how it works. Steve Jobs

Getting the Design Right and the Right Design. Bill Buxton (4)

Industrial design is an applied art in which the usability and manufacturability are the central considerations of a product and its creation. It comprises a process in which concepts are screened and refined to best achieve the goals of the product, ideally as a preface to the engineering of the product, but with the involvement of a variety of disciplines and perspectives. These perspectives range from the technical and numerical requirements to the overall aesthetics of the product. Prime examples of industrial design include such manufacturing icons as the Volkswagen Beetle and Apple Ipod. These are the products that employed available technologies, but with deep consideration for the user experience and cost-efficiency in manufacture.

Design has been a continuing challenge with isolator systems. One common expression within the field is that "no two isolators are the same," reflecting the historically custom nature of isolator implementations. Compounding this is the absolute criticality in design consideration for issues such as material ingress and egress, airflow, ergonomics, instrumentation, and monitoring. Not surprisingly, the history of implementation has been one of varied degrees of success. Complete systems have been scrapped for failing to meet user requirements or chosen validation criteria, while others have long histories of flawless aseptic operations.

One must understand a process well to perform it successfully, but one must understand a process completely to automate it. It is also true that with any automation project, design flaws are lasting and repetitive.

As a demonstration of the potential of isolated robotics in an industrially designed application, a project was initiated to design, construct, and validate a fully robotic isolated filling system. The overarching purpose of the project was to develop a system that provided the adaptability of conventional manual filling, with the quality and precision of the best isolated filling systems. After careful debate and consideration, the goals of the project were defined as follows:

- All motion must be digitally controlled and operated, wherever possible
- Design a system to fill any conventional vial or syringe
  - 1 mLto 1000 mL contained volume
- Stopper vials or syringes in line with filling
- Aseptically and/or contained processing
  - 20 units per minute
- No change parts required, other than fill tubing and needle
- No aseptic interventions necessary.

As an additional exercise in the design, a risk assessment of processes steps was performed using industry standardized metrics. From this analysis, key risk factors were identified that were to be minimized or eliminated from the operations of the system. These include the jamming or tipping of vials and stoppers, the need for gloved interventions during aseptic operations, and the elimination of all but essential movement within the isolator.

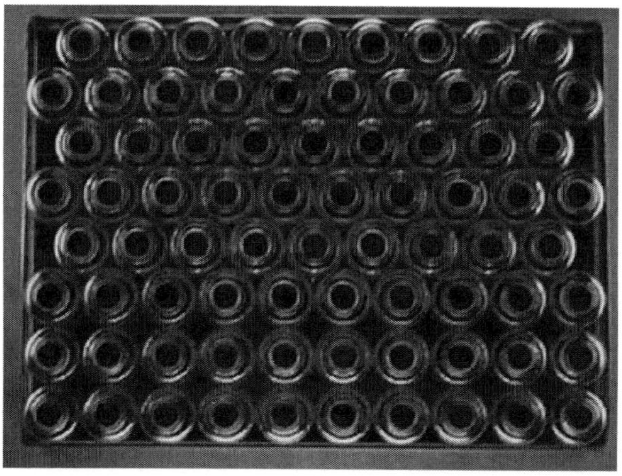

Figure 3 Overhead digital image of vial tray. *Source:* Courtesy of Vanrx Pharmasystems.

Most prominent of the technical challenges in the project is the necessity for adaptation to different vial and syringe formats without the use mechanical change parts or fixtures. This requirement necessitates the need for a variable position filling and stoppering system. As these motions are inherently planar, it is an ideal application for a 3-axis robotics.

Within the automotive industry, the predominant method of placement of devices is from predetermined positions or fixtures, in which parts are either placed in specific known locations repeatedly or are located in a defined area through the use of sensors. This fixturing reduces the robotic motion to that of simple pick and place. It also eliminates extraneous movement, as the consistent picking of components relies on fixed location. Vial and stopper components, which are trayed in fixed positions, may then be reliably located without concern of machinability or lubrication for fluid motion.

With the mindset of shrinking the size and scope of the aseptic field, it is advantageous to perform as many unit operations prior to sterilization as possible. Thus, the steps between sterilization and ultimate sealing of the filled dosage are kept to an absolute minimum. Trays or cassettes filled with vials or stoppers must be assembled and sterilized, and transported from the sterilizer to an interface isolator. From this interface isolator, trays are then robotically loaded into the filling system for processing. This is very similar to conventional handling of nested syringes, which are processed and transferred in a comparable fashion.

This concept reduces the movement of the vials from continuous motion to a single placement in the tray. The center of gravity and frictional coefficient of the vials, normally the largest source of problems for vial movement, are eliminated as significant factors in machinability. For a batch of 3000 units of 5 mL vials containing 100 units each, this strategy obviously reduces the motion steps from 3000 to a total of 30.

As there are a multitude of vial and syringe sizes and shapes, it was decided to incorporate a pervasive companion to robotic technology in the modern manufacturing environment, machine vision. Vision technology involves the digital imaging of objects to generate patterns and shapes from which to generate locational data and analyze this data for patterns. This can be used to make decisions on acceptability of parts, in terms of dimensional aspects, color, defects, and composition. With modern computing power, this analysis can be performed in well under 100 msec, thus suitable for most applications. This affords the ability for the robot to receive data about the position, condition, and acceptability of an object. With proper logic, this data can be used to direct operations of the robot and therefore increase the intelligence and adaptability of the process.

To enable such decision making, a set of key characteristics of the product to be analyzed must be developed. In the filling application, it was noted that while vial size and shape varied considerably, internal neck diameters were relatively conserved within the various sizes of

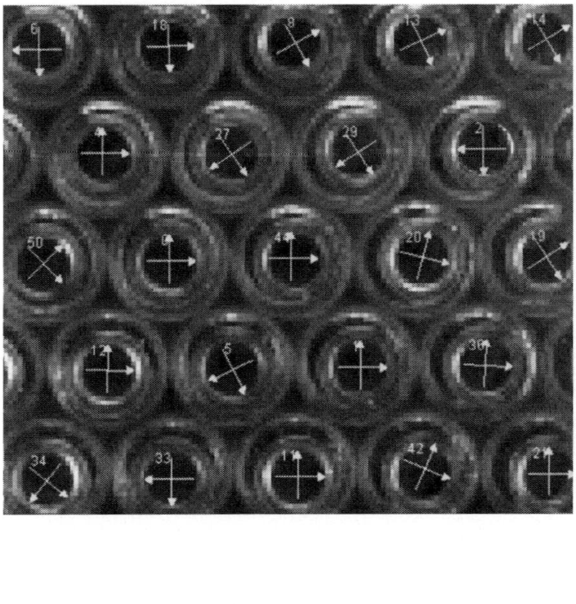

Figure 4 Pattern recognition image analysis with centerpoint determinations. *Source:* Courtesy of Vanrx Pharmasystems.

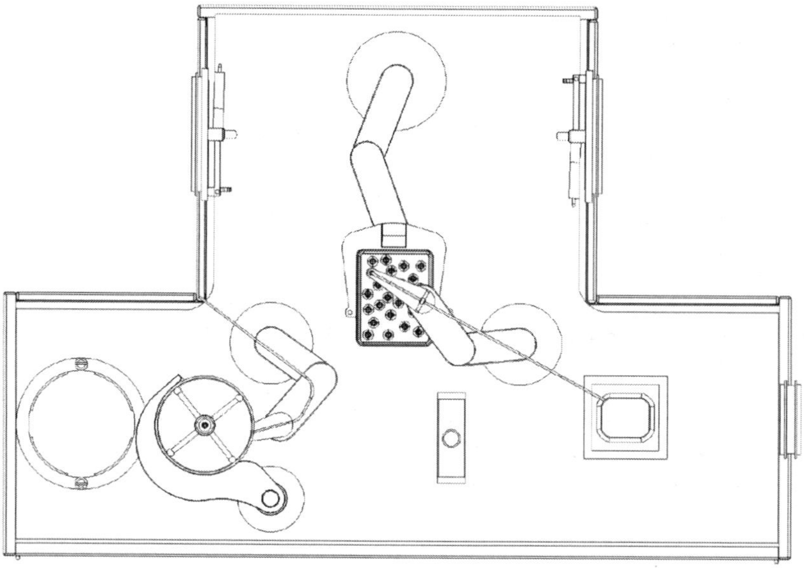

Figure 5 Overhead schematic of vision-guided robotic filling system. *Source:* Courtesy of Vanrx Pharmasystems.

commercially available stoppers. Further, as vials and syringes are generally cylindrical and symmetrical, a determination of the coordinates of the center of the inner diameter of the container would yield sufficient data to enable robotic interaction. Thus, vision data from an overhead camera system combined with pattern recognition technology yield a map of the available containers within the defined space.

Thus, trayed vials may be imaged from overhead and the individual vials x and y coordinates determined. This yields an adaptive system for quick changeover, and uses a technology that may remotely sense and provide no source of particles or contamination within the isolator.

With the positional map generated for each tray of containers and stoppers, the robotic arms may perform the common tasks of pick and placement as well as fluid dispensing without the need for complex movements or other movement of containers. This eliminates a major cause for system jams and the need for human interventions.

Stopper placement is achieved in a similar manner, with fixturing of individual components and pick and place to the resultant vial position map. As stoppers retain a circular shape, and are generally limited to a much smaller variety of sizes, fixturing in specially designed trays was chosen.

By creating a fully configurable filling head–container interface, which is the interfacing of two robot arms, the range of fill volumes possible is limited only by the overall size of the chosen tray and z-axis range of the robotics. Through proper dimensional planning, it is a relatively easy task to accommodate the desired range of 1 mL to 1000 mL. For an adaptable small volume filler, this is a significant advantage over prior systems. These systems often required multiple filling units to achieve this range, as the fixed nature of the filling and stoppering heads often limited the overall height of a machinable container.

Beyond the central motions of filling and stoppering, ancillary steps in production often create difficulties in automation. A common issue encountered in filling isolator applications is the need to calibrate the dispensing volumes from the filling pump. As the filling head is normally stationary, this is typically achieved by removing filled units as samples. These samples are gravimetrically measured and the fill data used to recalibrate the pump system. However, the simple removal of samples from the filling line is a complex motion that often requires multiple axes of motion and an egress from the isolated space. This creates problems for the maintenance of an integral system, as well as for proper placement and storage of sample units.

Manufacturers have addressed this issue through a variety of means, from online mass flow sensors contained with the product fluid path to hard automation that removes vials and places them onto a balance adjacent to the filling area. Although technically sufficient, these methods are often complex and expensive to implement, and result in additional maintenance and operational issues.

Through the use of a robotically positioned filling head, it becomes possible to incorporate a pump calibration step, which measures the output of the pump directly from the filling needle, rather than through sampling of filled units. This removes the need to store or remove sample units from the isolator, and reduces the mechanical complexity of the ancillary systems. Through the use of an appropriate electronic balance, the fill weight can be measured from the needle in replicates and the data processed. The recalibration data are then transmitted back to the filling pump in a manner of seconds, and filling operations continued. This eliminates the need to remove vials from the trays and creates opportunities for spills and tipped vials.

A further benefit of the robotic architecture of the filling system is its physical simplicity within the isolated space. Simply put, there are only a minimum of parts and structure within the isolator. Often the systems required to move containers and perform processing steps are complex, with many corners and moving parts that represent difficult locations to clean and adequately expose to decontaminating agents. By maintaining a simple and streamlined layout inside the isolator, there is less area to contain and more thorough ability to ensure cleanliness and effective decontamination.

This exercise in design focuses on the breakdown of movement and function to their most basic elements. By exploiting the computing power and speed of modern microprocessors, the precision and throughput necessary to obsolete manual filling is achieved. However, it is also a demonstration of how proper design requires a mix of disciplines. The design priorities and tools applied include aspects of basic microbiological techniques, mechatronics, as well as conventional process engineering principles. This holistic approach to design better reflects the collective knowledge necessary to make form meet function, and indeed make the design work.

FUTURE CONCEPTS

As can be seen from the above example, process technologies exist in a variety of industries with applicability to aseptic pharmaceutical production. Technologies in development today will enable the solutions of tomorrow, and given the dramatic improvement in mechatronics technology, it is foreseeable that the future facility will be unmanned.

Current technologies that show promise for aseptic applications include the concept of bin-picking vision systems (5). This technology involves three-dimensional imaging of parts randomly placed in a hopper or bin. Vision systems then correlate multiple images to identify the orientation and identity of the part and calculate the path for the robot to properly pick and place the part. This involves sophisticated algorithms, but removes the necessity of fixturing parts prior to processing. Objects such as stoppers or other components may be simply loaded

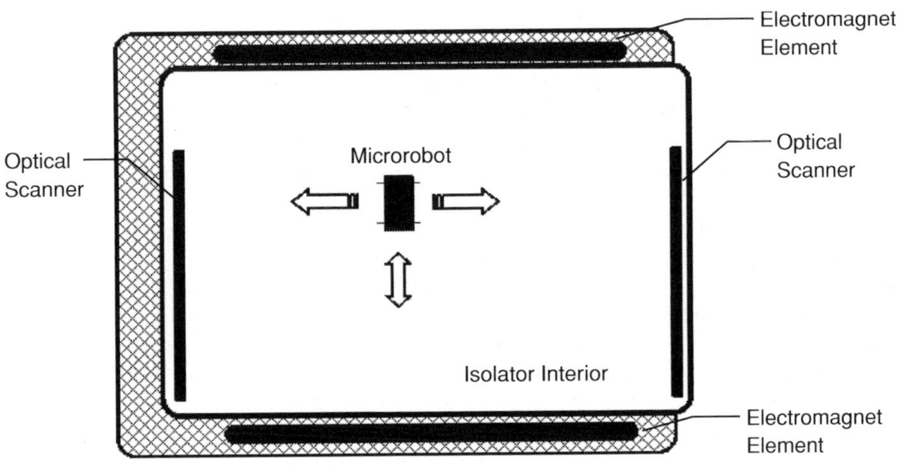

Figure 6 Isolator-based magnetic levitation robotic schematic. *Source:* Courtesy of Vanrx Pharmasystems.

through a port in an isolator to a bin, and simply picked up by a robot as any human might, however, with significantly more speed, accuracy, and cleanliness.

Another such promising area of research lies in the field of magnetic levitation robotics (6). Like a virtual magic trick, complex electromagnetic fields are modulated from both above and below a small robot, or microrobot, which is then guided through the use of positional sensors. These sensors determine the coordinates of the microrobot, and transmit in a feedback loop to the electromagnetic array to drive the microrobot directionally, as programmed. Such a device enables noncontact control, as they are able to penetrate stainless steel sheet metal, thus simplifying the mechanics inside the isolator.

These microrobots have incorporated pincer-type end effects for pick and place, with submicron precision. Thus, complex and delicate manipulations can be performed in a fully sealed and remote manner. This technology is ideally suited to clean or hazardous environments, as it has no moving parts beyond the actual microrobot itself.

SUMMARY

Given the criticality in what products and processes aseptic pharmaceutical manufacturing involves, demands are such that systems operate in near perfection. With the advances in microprocessor and robotic technologies, many new applications are possible to remove the human element from aseptic production. However, given this criticality along with the complexity of such sophisticated systems, the conventional methods of custom fabrication of individual pharmaceutical isolator systems seemed destined to become history. In order to meet the requirements of the future with the technologies of the future, heavy emphasis must be placed on design and functionality. As well, it will become a financial necessity to not reinvent the wheel for each installation. Thus, product-focused technology developers have an opportunity to lead the efforts to build the safe and efficient aseptic manufacturing systems for tomorrow's medicines.

REFERENCES

1. Nof SY. Handbook of Industrial Robotics. 2nd ed. New York, NY: John Wiley & Sons, 1999:3–5.
2. Gates B. A robot in every home. Sci Am 2007(Jan):58–65.
3. Deguchi M, Akers J, Yoshida S, et al. Development of an advanced high speed aseptic filling system. PDA J Pharm Sci Technol 2003; 57(1):43–48.
4. Tohidi M, Buxton W, Baecker R, et al. Getting the right design and the design right. Paper presented at: Conference on Human Factors in Computing Systems, CHI 2006; April 2006; 22–27; Montréal, Québec, Canada.
5. Ranky PG. Advanced machine vision systems and application examples. Sensor Rev. 2003; 23(3):242–245(4).
6. Shameli SE, Khamesee MB, Huissoon JP. Real-time control of a magnetic levitation device based on instantaneous modeling of magnetic field. J Mechatronics 2008; 18(10):536–544.

42 The future of aseptic processing

James Agalloco and James Akers

The opening chapter of this book reviewed the history of aseptic processing technology starting with its origins in the works of Lister and culminating with an overview of the more advanced technologies for aseptic processing presently available. The chapters that followed addressed some of the innovative technical solutions currently available for aseptic processing. Most of the technologies included in this book embody the full spirit of our suggested definition of advanced aseptic processing:

> An advanced aseptic process is one in which direct intervention with open product containers or exposed product contact surfaces by operators wearing conventional cleanroom garments is not required and never permitted (1).

However, we would commit an egregious error if we were to suggest that further improvements in aseptic processing beyond those included in this text are not possible. Despite the substantial performance enhancements witnessed by the new technologies now coming into expanded use across our industry we are confident that further development is not only possible but also highly likely.

To understand our perspective, one must accept that aseptic processing technology has not yet reached its apogee. The declassification of the high efficiency particulate air (HEPA) filter in the 1950s resulted in the manned aseptic processing area that is still the predominant approach for aseptic processing. Its capability had improved substantially over the years, and it was not until the introduction of isolation technology in the early 1990s that a demonstrably superior environment for aseptic processing became available. The performance differences between manned clean rooms and isolation technology are substantial; nevertheless it took some time for the industry to acknowledge the superior capability of isolators. Our initial enthusiasm for isolation systems was perhaps beyond the understanding of others, but in the last 20 years isolators have increasingly become the technology of choice for aseptic processing (2). Restricted access barrier systems (RABS) in their most evolved form offer many of the same performance improvements of isolators along with similar validation and operational requirements. It seems near certain to us that future aseptic processing systems will be developed with isolation concepts throughout. We expect the appearance of future systems to be somewhat different from isolators, which to many in this industry resemble miniature clean rooms. This resemblance is only superficial, clean rooms have people and isolators do not, a difference of truly meaningful significance.

The distinction between today's advanced system and those we envision for the future lies at the very core of what isolation technology provides for aseptic processing (and in the area of potent compound containment as well for that matter). Isolators outperform manned processing systems primarily through the removal of personnel from the critical environment where the aseptic process is performed. That single design feature provides the greatest performance improvement: the elimination of human borne viable and nonviable contamination.

The gradual improvements in manned aseptic processing in the past were the result of a series of modest changes: improved equipment, better air systems, more robust and comfortable gowning materials, and simple barriers that served to reduce the need for and impact of operators within the critical zone. The industry has long acknowledged the primacy of personnel as contamination sources and the refinements made to manned aseptic processing largely focused on minimizing the human impact (3,4). Isolation technology addressed this through placement of the operators in an environment physically separate from the sterile field with a defined pressure differential providing an extra measure of protection (5). RABS designs approach this same concept (at least where open door interventions are prohibited) with the separation of personnel improved by designed air overspill from critical zone to the surrounding manned environment (6,7). As a consequence of the change in operator location, these advanced systems are being increasingly chosen for both new installations and facility renovations.

The technology changes in aseptic processing that led to the advanced aseptic processing designs described in this text gradually moved the operator farther from the critical zone. Isolators and closed RABS take this somewhat further by placing the operator in an environment separate from that of the critical zone; however, with few exceptions these systems require a substantial amount of human involvement to execute the core processes performed within. Unfortunately, the vast majority of the currently available aseptic processing systems, even those that meet the definition of advanced aseptic processing, still rely heavily on operators. Some of the activities commonly performed by operators in even the most advanced of present day systems include:

- Initial adjustment of the internal equipment to accommodate specific containers and or closures
- Connection of the product delivery line to the liquid filling systems (powder fillers require intervention throughout the process for product replenishment)
- Replenishment of containers (in some instances) and closures during the process
- Periodic collection of environmental monitoring samples during the process
- Corrective interventions addressing missfeeds, container breakage, leaks, etc.

In the most evolved designs, most if not all of, the interventional activities can be eliminated and the system operates devoid of human involvement. These more capable systems operating without personnel represent the future of aseptic processing.

Personnel execute a variety of tasks supporting the operation of equipment and systems utilized for aseptic processing. The operation of aseptic processing equipment requires operators to perform interventional activities of two prevalent kinds:

- Inherent—An intervention that is an integral part of the aseptic process required for either setup, routine operation and/or monitoring, for example, aseptic assembly, container replenishment, and environmental sampling. Inherent interventions are required by batch record, procedure, or work instruction for the proper conduct of the aseptic process.
- Corrective—An intervention that is performed to correct or adjust an aseptic process during its execution. These may not occur with the same frequency (or at all) in the aseptic process. Examples include such activities as: clearing component missfeed, stopping leaks, adjusting sensors, and replacing equipment components.

Beyond the critical zone, the operators perform additional supportive activities including transfer of materials within the background aseptic environment and cleaning and decontamination of the aseptic processing area. To realize our vision of aseptic processing without the need for an operator, whether in an aseptic gown, RABS or isolator glove or half-suit, future systems will have to accommodate or eliminate all of these operator tasks. The operational means to attain this future are at hand and include: automation/robotics and isolation working in concert to completely eliminate personnel during the aseptic process. Perhaps more critical to realizing the future, we envision the redefinition of our regulatory and compendial expectations with respect to aseptic processing. It is essential that the key elements to our vision be properly coordinated; improvements in one area without concurrent progress in another will detract from the outcome. There must be synergy among them to attain the next level of performance.

AUTOMATION/ROBOTICS

Central to the removal of personnel from the aseptic process must be the complete elimination of the manual tasks they perform within and around the process equipment. There have been significant strides in this area over the last 50+ years. The introduction of the HEPA filter allowed for machines to be used for the core aseptic filling/sealing activity and there has been steady progress with filling machine design that has gradually reduced the need for manual interventions. The steady improvements in aseptic processing performance over this period are in part a consequence of advances in equipment design, reliability, and sophistication.

While these refinements have dramatically reduced the need for operator intervention it has not resulted in eliminating the need for it.

To bring aseptic processing equipment to the next level of performance a greater degree of system integration/automation is needed. We envision that the next generation of equipment will operate without direct personnel involvement through features such as:

- Elimination of all interventions (routine and corrective) through proper automation, robotic manipulation, and application of PAT
- Integrated clean-in-place and sterilize-in-place capabilities for all product contact surfaces (nonproduct contact cleaning would be avoided by the elimination of product spillage), or the implementation of single-use technology in a manner that obviates the need for human intervention
- In-line weight verification of all filled containers and automated adjustment at fill speed as needed
- Continuous verification of container integrity and confirmation on all containers at fill speed
- Continuous monitoring and adjustment of critical process parameters and variables (PAT)
- Automated component infeed and filled/sealed container discharge without contamination ingress
- Automated environmental monitoring of isolator internal air and surfaces[1]
- Automated setup and transition from clean-in-place or sterilize-in-place to aseptic filling to accommodate product and/or component changeover
- Self-clearing filling and component handling systems for continuous jam-free operation
- No container, no fill to eliminate spillage
- Integrated inspection for particles, fill volume, product appearance, etc.

This level of automation, robotics, and overall system integration may seem overwhelming, but is becoming commonplace in other industries such as automotive and electronics. Comparable applications in the food industry for aseptic filling of beverages are already operational. These systems and those envisioned for the pharmaceutical industry would be capable of essentially continuous operation over lengthy periods or campaigns. The speed of these systems need not be overwhelming (although some fully automated aseptic beverage systems operate at >1000 U/min) because equipment downtime would be minimal, and 24/7 operations would provide ample capacity.

It must be recognized that the level of automation described above does not imply that these future systems operate at high speed. The production of clinical supplies, small lots, and low volume products can be successfully accomplished with equipment addressing the absence of personnel involvement without the requirements for high throughput.

ISOLATION TECHNOLOGY

In order to execute an aseptic process, the background environment must be decontaminated to ensure microbial levels are sufficiently low. The use of automated systems as described earlier eliminates the need for personnel in proximity to the critical zone greatly reducing the contamination potential. The use of isolation technology providing aseptic conditions surrounding the automated system should provide ample means to ensure control over the environment. The isolators envisioned would be effectively decontaminated by automated means to ensure effective control over the environment. The environmental control capability of present day isolators is such that suitable aseptic environments can be maintained over lengthy periods without intermediate decontamination. The elimination of personnel and carefully controlled automated introduction of materials and components ensure that the likelihood of contamination entering the enclosure is consistently extremely low. In operation they would incorporate automated sterilization and/or decontamination systems to accommodate material and component infeed. Discharge of components would be similarly protected by fail-safe systems designed to

[1] The elimination of environmental monitoring could be considered; however, this would entail a major shift in compliance and regulatory thinking. The first systems of this type would include provision for monitoring, with its eventual elimination a strong possibility.

preclude microbial ingress. These elements are already available on many present day isolator systems so their application to the next generation of technology is easily accommodated.

We expect that in the next generation designs it will be difficult to identify the isolator. Many of the present-day aseptic isolators are originally designed to essentially surround the existing filling equipment that had been located in manned clean rooms. In more recent system, there has been greater integration between the filler and the isolator, but the basic concept is still that the isolator is first and foremost an environment surrounding a piece of equipment. We anticipate that in future systems the critical zone where the aseptic process is performed will be located in the midst of the automated equipment described earlier. Any suggestion that it is a mini clean room will no longer be apparent. With that change the last vestiges of the clean room will disappear. The new machines will not have gloves; no access to the critical zone will be necessary for setup, operation, cleaning, and decontamination and thus gloves will no longer be required. The absence of personnel activity anywhere proximate to the aseptic process allows for some further differences. Unidirectional air flow and high rates of air exchange will no longer be necessary for the operation of the system, as their intent in clean rooms was to eliminate human-derived contamination. With the complete absence of personnel within these systems, the complexity and cost associated with these features is unnecessary as there will no longer be any human contamination to eliminate.

There is an element of the current controls for aseptic processing that will likely linger for some period of time in these future systems. Environmental monitoring is considered one of the essential controls for aseptic processing. The requirements for monitoring of viable and total particulate established when manned clean rooms were the prevalent and perhaps only means for production of aseptically manufactured products. In those environments, the potential microbial insult to the aseptic process was substantial and monitoring was necessary to help establish that the aseptic process was suitably controlled. With the passage of time, the environmental conditions surrounding the critical zone gradually improved, and then took a quantum leap forward with the introduction of isolation technology. Present day isolators because of their decontamination methods and constant pressure differential to their surroundings provide environmental controls such that the detection of microbial contamination has become a rare event. In the automated and isolated aseptic processing systems of the future, the scientific value of microbiological environmental monitoring is low enough to call the entire practice into question. While the initial systems may include some capability to monitor microbial and particle contamination, there is really little value to that monitoring especially for microorganisms. Long-term monitoring of these systems is likely to be predominantly parametric: drawing information from the equipment itself during its operation.

REGULATORY/COMPENDIAL EXPECTATIONS

The global health care industry is highly regulated, and nowhere are those regulations more demanding than where aseptically manufactured products are produced. The controls and precepts in place today were largely developed based on the realities of manned clean rooms. Regulatory guidance focused on isolators and RABS are largely nonexistent. If the potential of the next generation of aseptic filling is to be fully realized, regulatory and compendial constraints must be minimized. Controls and expectations developed for yesterday's technologies embody requirements that are of little or no value in the process control of present day advanced aseptic processing and will be completely inappropriate for those described in this chapter. Some form of regulation will of course be required, but the profound differences in system capability for these future systems are such that controls required should be markedly different from those currently in use. New essential controls to operate these systems in the future have yet to be defined as the systems themselves are largely conceptual at this time, nevertheless they are likely to be quite different from those currently in place. Without a willingness to adjust their expectations, regulators will only serve as a brake on the promised technological advances that are available for aseptic processing.

CONCLUSION

Simply put, the next generation of aseptic processing system will eliminate the need for any personnel involvement during the cleaning, sterilization, setup, operation and monitoring of the process. The means to conduct all of these activities will be performed by automated means eliminating the operator's presence anywhere in the process. The aseptic processing capabilities of these systems will likely approach those of terminal sterilization, however, since they would operate in an exclusionary rather than lethal manner and any such comparison is likely to draw the ire of regulators. These systems already exist in the food industry with multiple billions of units of aseptically filled foods, primarily beverages, having already been produced using the same concepts. Their application for aseptic processing in the health care industry only awaits a firm willing to apply the technology.

FURTHER READING

1. Akers J, Agalloco J, Madsen R. What is advanced aseptic processing. Pharmaceutical Manufacturing 2006; 4(2):25–27.
2. Lysfjord JP, Porter M. Barrier isolator history and trends–2008 final data. Pharmaceutical Engineering 2009:50–55.
3. Agalloco J, Gordon B. Current practices in the use of media fills in the validation of aseptic processing. J Parenter Sci Technol 1987; 41(4):128–141.
4. Avallone H. Current regulatory issues regarding parenteral inspections. J Parenter Sci Technol 1989; 43(1):3–7.
5. PDA, TR #34 Design and validation of isolator systems for the manufacturing and testing of health care products. PDA J Pharma Sci Technol 2001; 55(5 suppl).
6. ISO 14644-7. Separative Enclosures. 2004.
7. ISPE. Definition of a RABS. August 2005.

Appendix I—extracts of IQ, OQ, and PQ protocols for filling isolator

INSTALLATION QUALIFICATION PROTOCOL EXTRACT

1 Purpose

1.1 Installation qualification—Verify that the filling isolator and its corresponding utilities have been installed in accordance with design specifications and manufacturers' recommendations.

1.2 This protocol will define the inspection procedures, documentation, references, specifications, and acceptance criteria used to establish that the filling isolator is installed properly.

2 General Requirements

2.1 All documentation requirements defined in each section of the protocol must be completed.

2.2 Test instruments must be calibrated per XXX's Calibration Program and be documented.

2.3 If any of the acceptance criteria in this protocol are not met due to equipment malfunction or operator error the cause of failure will be documented. Testing for data collection affected by the failure may be repeated. Modification of the equipment may be required for successful validation. Changes or additions will be documented in an addendum to this protocol.

3 System Description

The liquid filling system consists of eight volumetric pumps that deliver the appropriate amount of product solution to filling stations in the machine. A small holding tank located outside the filling isolator assures consistent head pressure to the pumps. A transport mechanism moves the containers through the liquid filler. The design of the isolator system allows access to the filling line via glove ports and rapid transfer ports (RTP). The filler has a dedicated air handling unit and interconnecting ductwork.

4 Acceptance Criteria

4.1 Equipment installation qualification acceptance criteria are defined in the Test Functions section of this protocol.

4.2 In the event that a test function does not meet its acceptance criteria, a Deviation Notice Form must be completed. This form will describe the nature of the deviation, the impact, and corrective action taken, if needed.

5 References

This protocol conforms to the applicable guidelines of the publications listed below. Each publication shall be the latest revision and addendum in effect on the date the respective protocol is approved for execution unless noted otherwise.

5.1 Specifications and drawings

5.2 United States Code of Federal Regulations (CFR)

5.3 Food and Drug Administration (FDA) guidelines and standards

5.4 Other industry standards.

6 Protocol Execution

The installation of the filling isolator will be verified by reviewing the equipment installed and documenting the conditions found on copies of the Test Functions Data Sheets and attachments of this protocol or other equivalent means that shall be referenced in the data sheets. The findings will be utilized to document that the system, as installed, conforms to design requirements.

7 Protocol Final Report

7.1 Deviations

Any discrepancies from the design, drawings, manufacturer's specification, listed operational criteria, or other documents defining the quality attributes of the filling isolator must be fully described on the Deviation Notice form. The completed form, describing the conditions and recommended corrective action, will be reviewed by a quality unit and engineering. A decision to requalify, take corrective action, or accept the deviation will be made.

7.2 Final Report

Upon completion of the field execution of the subject protocol, prepare a protocol final report. This final report is intended to be a narrative of the filling isolator conformance to acceptance criteria. Test data will be presented, discussed, and conclusions drawn. Ensure that the required protocol data sheets and attachments have been completed. Verify that any discrepancies are documented and logged deviations are completed with approved corrective measures.

8 IQ Test Functions

8.1 Identification of executor(s)

All executors involved with this protocol are to record name, signature, and initials/date.

8.2 Documentation

Documentation listed below is verified to be present and adequate.

Document description	**Document name/number/ location**	**Initial/date**
Purchase orders		
Equipment manuals		
Spare parts list for mechanical equipment and instruments including manufacturer name, model number, description, cost, and quantities. Ensure the following are available upon the start-up for the filling isolator:		
Component manufacturers catalog information and manuals		
HVAC filter list		
Lubricants list		
Documentation of materials of construction		
A list of applicable drawings such as piping and instrument drawings (P&IDs), assembly drawings, component drawings, control system layout, electrical schematics, pneumatic system drawings, and PLC I/O wiring diagrams		
A list of all instruments and control devices including tag numbers, manufacturer name and model, serial number, calibration dates		
Softcopy and annotated hard copy from all programmable devices where applicable. List each programmable device and date of current program version		
Name and version of software package used during the development, documentation, and testing of programmable devices		
Factory test procedures and reports		

8.3 Drawings Verification—Drawings/P&IDs below are intended to reflect the equipment "as-built." Verify the accuracy of these drawings.

Drawing Name	Drawing Number	Verified (yes/no)	Initial/Date
Drawing A			
Drawing B			
. . .			
Drawing N			

8.4 Procedures

Copies of draft standard operating procedures for the execution of the following tasks shall be included in the IQ report. These procedures shall be approved after the completion of the appropriate operational qualification (OQ) and performance qualification (PQ) studies, with the exception of calibration procedures that must be approved prior to the completion of the IQ.

Calibration	SOP title/number	Approval date	Revision no.
Procedures to indicate traceability to National Institute of Standards and Technology (NIST) where possible			
Cleaning	SOP title/number	Revision no.	Revision no.
Procedures to include specifics of system cleaning, interior, exterior, materials, supplies, frequency, etc.			
Maintenance	SOP title/number	Approval date	Revision no.
Procedures to include all required functions: daily, weekly, quarterly, each batch, each use, etc.			
Setup and decontamination	SOP title/number	Approval date	Revision no.
Procedures to include all items to be placed into the unit and their preparation and position within the isolator during the process. Wrappings, orientation, etc. to be defined in the procedures. To include detailed procedure for decontamination			
Environmental monitoring	SOP title/number	Approval date	Revision no.
Procedures to include sampling methods, locations, frequency, and proposed initial limits. Any relevant reference standard operating procedures (SOPs) should also be listed for environmental monitoring			
Operation and use	SOP title/number	Approval date	Revision no.
Procedures to include the isolator and all functions of the equipment installed within			

8.5 Calibration verification

Calibrations listed below are verified to have been performed and documented.

Pressure monitor	**As found**	**Acceptable Yes/No**	**Initial/date**
Instrument name			
Instrument number			
Model number			
Use range			
Accuracy			
Calibration method			
Calibrated by			
Calibration date			

Make-up air velocity sensor	**As found**	**Acceptable Yes/No**	**Initial/date**
Air velocity sensor			
Recirculation air velocity sensor			
Humidity sensor			
Oxygen sensor			
Temperature sensor			

8.6 Machine Utilities

Dehumidified air	**As found**	**Acceptable Yes/No**	**Initial/date**
System identification			
Static pressure			
System dew point			
Block valve location			
Block valve identification			
Duct size			
Duct material of construction			
Prefilter manufacturer			
Prefilter type/model			
Prefilter rating			
Prefilter surface area			
Prefilter material			
Filter manufacturer			
Filter type/model			
Filter rating			
Filter surface area			
Filter material			
Maximum flow rate			
Supply temperature			
Qualification report reference			
Drawing reference			

Similar detailed information is required on process compressed air, nitrogen, instrument air, hot water, chilled water, drains, and electrical service. Details of these were intentionally omitted in this appendix.

8.7 System Components

Make-up blower	**As found**	**Acceptable Yes/No**	**Initial/date**
On/off switch			
Voltage			
Amperage			
Motor size (HP)			
Rotation			
Manufacturer			
Model number			
Circuit breaker			
Breaker location			
Breaker identification			
Variable speed controller			
Controller range			
Exhaust air blower			
Recirculation blower			

8.8 HVAC System Components and Performance

Prefilter	**As found**	**Acceptable Yes/No**	**Initial/date**
Description			
Manufacturer			
Materials of construction			
Filter size			
Rated efficiency			
Gasket material			

Comparable information should be provided on all filters installed on the isolator.

8.9 Design Specifications

Seq. #	**Design specifications**	**As found (if deviation is found note here and reference deviation notice form #)**	**Acceptable Yes or No**	**Initial/date**
1	Germ-free environment exists for the component transfer/aseptic filling			
2	All machine components and isolator are easy to clean			
3	All machine components and isolator are vaporized hydrogen peroxide (VHP) compatible			

(Continued)

4	Isolator is maintained under positive pressure			
5	Access to the module is through glove ports and an RTP			

9 Deviation Notice Form

Deviation number___________

OPERATIONAL QUALIFICATION PROTOCOL EXTRACT

1 Purpose

1.1 Operational qualification—Verify that the filling isolator and its corresponding subcomponents consistently and reliably operate in accordance with design specifications and manufacturers' recommendations.

1.2 This protocol will define the testing/inspection procedures, documentation, references, specifications, and acceptance criteria used to establish that the filling isolator operates properly.

2 General Requirements

2.1 All documentation requirements defined in each section of the protocol must be completed.

2.2 Test instruments must be calibrated per XXX's Calibration Program and be documented.

2.3 If any of the acceptance criteria in this protocol are not met due to equipment malfunction or operator error the cause of failure will be documented. Testing for data collection affected by the failure may be repeated. Modification of the equipment may be required for successful validation. Changes or additions will be documented in an addendum to this protocol.

3 System Description

3.1 The liquid filling system consists of eight volumetric pumps that deliver the appropriate amount of product solution to filling stations in the machine. A small holding tank located outside the filling isolator assures consistent head pressure to the pumps. A transport mechanism moves the containers through the liquid filler. The design of the isolator system allows access to the filling line via glove ports and RTP. The filler has a dedicated air handling unit and interconnecting ductwork. *This document outlines the OQ requirements for the filling isolator and associated items only*. Separate qualification documents have been prepared that cover the other modules and the VHP 1000 generators. Similarly, the qualification for the overall control system has been placed in a separate document. Some of the required studies may be performed simultaneously in multiple systems.

4 Acceptance Criteria

4.1 Equipment OQ acceptance criteria are defined in the Test Functions section of this protocol.

4.2 In the event that a test function does not meet its acceptance criteria, a Deviation Notice Form must be completed. This form will describe the nature of the deviation, the impact, and corrective action taken, if needed.

5 References

5.1 This protocol conforms to the applicable guidelines of the publications listed below. Each publication shall be the latest revision and addendum in effect on the date the respective protocol is approved for execution unless noted otherwise.

5.1.1 Specifications and drawing

5.1.2 United States Code of Federal Regulations (CFR)

5.1.3 Food and Drug Administration (FDA) guidelines and standards

5.1.4 Other industry standards.

6 Protocol Execution

6.1 The operational of the filling isolator will be verified by testing the equipment installed, and documenting the conditions found on copies of the Test Functions Data Sheets and attachments of this protocol or other equivalent means that shall be referenced in the data sheets. The findings will be utilized to document that the system operation conforms to design requirements.

7 Protocol Final Report

7.1 Deviations—Any discrepancies from the design, drawings, manufacturer's specification, listed operational criteria, or other documents defining the quality attributes of the filling isolator must be fully described on the Deviation Notice form. The completed form, describing the conditions and recommended corrective action, will be reviewed by a quality unit and Engineering. A decision to requalify, take corrective action, or accept the deviation will be made.

7.2 Final report—Upon completion of the field execution or the subject protocol, prepare a protocol final report. This final report is intended to be a narrative of the Powder Loading Module of the filling line/isolator system conformance to acceptance criteria. Test data will be presented, discussed, and conclusions drawn. Ensure that the required protocol data sheets and attachments have been completed. Verify that any discrepancies are documented and logged deviations are completed with approved corrective measures.

8 OQ Test Functions

8.1 Identification of executor(s)—All executors involved with this protocol are to record name, signature, and initials/date.

8.2 Validation test instruments

Instrument name/number	Manufacturer name, model, and serial number	Calibration date	Calibration due date	Initial/date
Dioctyl phthalate (DOP) generator or equivalent				

8.3 Validation test materials

When test materials are used to operate, the system/equipment includes available information such as description, manufacturer, lot number, part number, manufacture date, and release date.

Description	Manufacturer name, lot number, part number, manufacture date (as available)	Release date	Initial/date
DOP			

9 OQ Testing

9.1 HEPA Filter Integrity

Test the HEPA filter integrity. If using the DOP method, aerate 100 mg/L of DOP on the upstream of each HEPA filter. Scan the downstream side of each filter. An acceptable filter will retain 99.99% of the DOP supplied to the upstream side. Filters not passing the DOP test can be repaired provided the size of the repair does not exceed Institute of Environmental Sciences and Technology (IEST) requirements for HEPA filters. Diagram the location of the repaired leak on a grid and file with this protocol.

Filter	Report number	Date of test	Test result	Approval
Inlet HEPA #1				

9.2 Isolator Particle Counts

Determine the particle count within the isolator at eight locations using a particle counter. Counts shall be taken for particles in the range of 0.5 to 50 microns in triplicate at each location. The unit is acceptable if samples at each location confirm the unit's ability to maintain Class 100 conditions with all the machinery at rest. Filters not passing the particulate test can be repaired provided the size of the repair does not exceed IEST requirements for HEPA filters.

Location	Report number	Date of test	Test result	Approval
Location #1				

9.3 Air Velocity

Determine the velocity of the air discharged from the internal HEPAs. Test the air velocity 6″ from the filter face and at work heights using an anemometer, or equivalent device, while the isolator is closed. Test all HEPA modules and report the minimum, maximum, and average velocity for each module. The air velocity shall be approximately 0.45 ± 0.09 m/sec at the work height (wh).

Location	Date of test	Minimum	Maximum	Average	Approval

9.4 Air Changes

Calculate the number of air changes in the filling isolator while closed. Utilize readings 6 in. from the filter face in these calculations.

Air changes per hour based on average outlet airflow:____________________

9.5 Unidirectional Flow Patterning

Determine the direction of the airflow inside the isolator as it is installed with the liquid filling equipment. Using smoke sticks or equivalent, observe the airflow pattern within the isolator and around the equipment. Photographs or videotape may be used to document the results of this study. The airflow should be unidirectional within the isolator and over the equipment.

Location	Date of test	Performed by	Flow pattern	Approval
Fill zone				

9.6 Static Pressure

Determine the static pressure in the isolator relative to the surrounding room under normal operating conditions. Measure the static pressure over a one minute period.

Location	Date of test	Expected value	Actual value	Approval

9.7 Ammonia Leak Test

Determine the leak tightness of the isolator. Place a small container (less than 1 L) of ammonium hydroxide in the interior of the isolator along with a glass or plastic beaker. Close all of the openings to the isolator. Raise the internal pressure in the isolator to its intended normal operating pressure. Maintain circulation of the air inside the isolator throughout the conduct of this test. Using gloves open the ammonium hydroxide bottle and pour approximately 100 mL into the beaker. Allow the unit to operate for five minutes. Obtain a LaCalhene ammonia detection cloth (bright yellow). Before the test, verify the sensitivity of the cloth by opening a small aperture in the isolator (i.e., DOP injection port) and hold the cloth over the opening for 30 seconds. The cloth should change color. If no color change is observed, carefully smell the air leaving the isolator for the presence of ammonia. Once ammonia has been detected, recheck the aperture with the detection cloth. If the cloth still does not change color, replace the cloth and repeat the cloth sensitivity test. Using the passing detection cloth, hold the cloth along the seams, gaskets, glove ports, and other joints on the system for approximately 30 seconds. If a leak is present, a slight blue color will appear on the cloth. When leaks are detected their location should be noted for later correction. The absence of color changes confirms the integrity of the isolator.

Note: The cloth should be protected from exposure to light and air that decreases its usable life. Store the cloths in their original packages.

Location	Date of test	Color change Yes/No	Approval
RTP end			

9.8 Pressure Drop Test

Note: Reference American Glovebox Society, Guideline for Gloveboxes, AGS-G001-1994, p. 118.

Determine the pressure drop within the pressurized isolator over a period of time. Pressurize the system to its intended normal operating pressure (40 Pa). Seal off all inlets and outlets to the isolator. Record the initial pressure and start time. Wait one hour and record the final pressure and time. During the conduct of the test, the isolator must be maintained at constant temperature. A temperature change of more than 0.5°C during the course of the test will invalidate the test. Isolator internal temperatures shall be recorded at multiple locations within the isolator and the associated ductwork. It is acceptable to place thermocouples on the exterior of the isolator; however, the thermocouples must measure surface temperature and be well insulated from the surrounding environment. The total internal volume of the isolator must be known in order to perform this test.

Data	Results	Date of test	Approval
Internal volume of the isolator	V (ft^2)		
Initial pressure (absolute)	P_s (in H_2O)		
Starting time	t_s		
Average temperature at start	T_s (K)		
Final pressure (absolute)	P_f (in H_2O)		
Finish time	t_f		
Average temperature at finish	T_f (K)		

Q = leak rate (ft^3/hr) $= 60/(t_f - t_s) \times [(P_f \times V \times T_s)/(P_s \times T_f) - V]$

If Q is less than 0.5% of the total volume of the isolator, the system is acceptable.

$Q/V =$ ________________ (maximum of 0.005)

Results: Pass Fail

9.9 Safety Systems

Determine the noise level, the emergency stops, and interlocks on the system.

(a) Noise level—Measure the noise levels at a distance of 1 m from the equipment while it is in full operation. The noise level shall be not more than 80 dBA at a 1 m distance from the equipment.

Location	Results	Date of test	Approval
	dBA		

(b) Emergency stops—Confirm the functionality of the emergency stops.

Location	Results	Date of test	Approval

(c) Interlocks—Confirm the operation of the glove interlocks that will stop the equipment operation with a defined period of time when a glove is entered. Also confirm other system interlocks.

Location	Date of test	Interlocked	Time to activate	Approval
Fill isolator glove #3				

9.10 System Operation

Confirm the operation of the isolator system blowers, pressure monitor, and oxygen sensor as well as the operation of the powder loading equipment.

(a) Blowers–Test with pressure controller set at 40 Pa and 100 Pa and the isolator set for normal operation.

Blower	RPM 40 Pa in operation	RPM 100 Pa in operation	FPM 40 Pa blower inlet (range)	FPM 100 Pa blower inlet (range)	Approval
Recirculation blower					

(b) Pressure monitor

Location	High pressure alarm set point	High pressure alarm confirmed	Low pressure alarm set point	Low pressure alarm confirmed	Approval

9.11 Purge System

Determine the oxygen concentration within the isolator over a period of time. Purge the system of oxygen with nitrogen and confirm that a final oxygen concentration of less than 0.5% can be achieved in the system. Maintain the system inert for a period of one hour and observe oxygen concentration over that period.

Data	Record values below	Approval
Date of test		
Initial oxygen concentration (%)		
Start time		
Final oxygen concentration (%)		

9.12 Room Temperature Distribution (Operation)

Note: This study may be performed with the Isolator Temperature Distribution (Operational) study, section 9.13.

Determine the cold spot location in the isolator room over the course of a normal workday. Isolator external temperatures shall be recorded at multiple locations outside the isolator and the associated ductwork. The thermocouples must measure surface temperature of the isolator and be insulated from the surrounding environment. The study shall be performed in a single trial over a 24-hour period. The minimum and maximum temperatures in the room shall be recorded. This study is for informational purposes only but the desired temperature range is 20°C ± 3°C.

Data	Results (°C)	Location
Room temperature minimum		
Next lowest temperature		
Next lowest temperature		
Next lowest temperature		
Next lowest temperature		
Room temperature maximum		

9.13 Isolator Temperature Distribution (Operational)
Note: This study may be performed with the Room Temperature Distribution (Operational) study, section 9.12.

Determine the temperature uniformity within the isolator unit under normal operating conditions. Isolator internal temperatures shall be recorded at multiple locations within the isolator and the associated ductwork. All internally installed equipment in the isolator shall be operational during this test. Thermocouples in the isolator are positioned to measure air temperature at work level locations. The study shall be performed over a 24-hour period. The minimum and maximum temperatures in the room shall be recorded concurrently with the performance of this test. The internal pressure in the isolator shall be measured over the same time period as the temperature distribution study. This study is for informational purposes only but the desired temperature range is 22°C ± 3°C and the pressure differential relative to the surrounding room is +40 Pa.

Data	Results (°C or Pa)	Location
Isolator temperature minimum		
Isolator temperature maximum		
Room temperature minimum		
Room temperature maximum		
Maximum differential pressure		
Minimum differential pressure		

9.14 Isolator Temperature Distribution (Decontamination)
Determine the cold spot location within the isolator unit at the completion of the conditioning phase of the hydrogen peroxide sterilization process. Isolator internal temperatures shall be recorded at multiple locations within the isolator and the associated ductwork. All internally installed equipment in the isolator shall be operational during this test. It is acceptable to place thermocouples on the exterior of the isolator in the conduct of this test; however, the thermocouples must measure surface temperature of the isolator and be insulated from the surrounding environment. The study shall be performed in triplicate. The minimum and maximum temperatures in the room shall be recorded concurrently with the performance of this test. This study is for informational purposes only.

Data	Run #1	Run #2	Run #3
Isolator temperature minimum (°C)			
Location			
Room temperature minimum (°C)			
Location			
Room temperature maximum (°C)			
Location			

9.15 Operation of Connectors

Confirm the satisfactory operation of all connectors between the fill isolator and all transfer isolators.

Filling isolator to transfer isolator #1____________________

Filling isolator to transfer isolator #2____________________

Result: Pass or Fail

PERFORMANCE QUALIFICATION PROTOCOL EXTRACT

1 Purpose

1.1 Performance qualification—(a) Verify that the filling isolator can be decontaminated with VHP and that the germ-free environment in the isolators can be maintained over a defined period of time, confirmed via (b) environmental monitoring. Also, to (c) verify that the filling equipment operates according to design specifications on a consistent basis.

1.2 This protocol will define the testing/inspection procedures, documentation, references, specifications, and acceptance criteria used to establish that the filling isolator operates properly.

2 General Requirements

2.1 All documentation requirements defined in each section of the protocol must be completed.

2.2 Test instruments must be calibrated per XXX's Calibration Program and be documented.

2.3 If any of the acceptance criteria in this protocol are not met due to equipment malfunction or operator error, the cause of failure will be documented. Testing for data collection affected by the failure may be repeated. Modification of the equipment may be required for successful validation. Changes or additions will be documented in an addendum to this protocol.

3 System Description

The liquid filling system consists of eight volumetric pumps that deliver the appropriate amount of product solution to filling stations in the machine. A small holding tank located outside the filling isolator assures consistent head pressure to the pumps. A transport mechanism moves the containers through the liquid filler. The design of the isolator system allows access to the filling line via glove ports and RTP. The filler has a dedicated air handling unit and interconnecting ductwork. The isolator is decontaminated using hydrogen peroxide provided by the AMSCO/STERIS VHP 1000 generators and is located in a Class 100,000 environment.

This document outlines the PQ requirements for the filling line/isolator system.

4 Acceptance Criteria

4.1 Equipment PQ acceptance criteria are defined in the Test Functions section of this protocol.

4.2 In the event that a test function does not meet its acceptance criteria, a Deviation Notice Form must be completed. This form will describe the nature of the deviation, the impact, and corrective action taken, if needed.

5 References

This protocol conforms to the applicable guidelines of the publications listed below. Each publication shall be the latest revision and addendum in effect on the date the respective protocol is approved for execution unless noted otherwise.

5.1 Specifications and drawings
5.2 United States Code of Federal Regulations (CFR)
5.3 Food and Drug Administration (FDA) guidelines and standards
5.4 Other industry standards.

6 Protocol Execution

The performance of the filling isolator will be verified by performing various tests and documenting the conditions found on copies of the Test Functions Data Sheets and attachments of this protocol or other equivalent means that shall be referenced in the data sheets. The findings will be utilized to document that the system performance conforms to design requirements and can be used to perform sterility tests.

7 Protocol Final Report

7.1 Deviations

Any discrepancies from the design, drawings, manufacturer's specification, listed performance criteria, or other documents defining the quality attributes of the filling isolator must be fully described on the Deviation Notice form. The completed form, describing the conditions and recommended corrective action, will be reviewed by a quality unit and engineering. A decision to requalify, take corrective action, or accept the deviation will be made.

7.2 Final Report

Upon completion of the field execution or the subject protocol, prepare a protocol final report. This final report is intended to be a narrative of the filling isolator conformance to acceptance criteria. Test data will be presented, discussed, and conclusions drawn. Ensure that the required protocol data sheets and attachments have been completed, signed, and approved. Verify that any discrepancies are documented and logged deviations are completed with approved corrective measures.

8 PQ Test Functions

8.1 Identification of executor(s)—All executors involved with this protocol are to record name, signature, and initials/date.

8.2 Test instruments

If test instruments are used to support this protocol, record equipment information below.

Instrument name/number	Manufacturer name, model, and serial number	Calibration date	Calibration due date	Initial/date

8.3 Test Materials

When test materials are used to operate the system/equipment, it includes available information such as description, manufacturer, lot number, part number, manufacture date, and release date.

Description	Manufacturer name, lot number, part number, manufacture date (as available)	Expiration date	Initial/date

8.4 PQ Testing

8.4.1 Isolator Particle Counts (at rest)

Determine the particle count within the filling isolator in an at-rest condition as per Federal Standard 209E for Class 100 areas with unidirectional airflow. The minimum number of sampling locations per module will be determined and counts shall be taken for particles in the range of 0.5 to 5.0 microns in triplicate at each location. The isolator is acceptable if it maintains Class 100 conditions per Federal Standard 209E with the machinery at rest. Attach the particle count report with sampling location diagrams to the final report.

Location	Acceptance criteria	Actual response	Pass/Fail	Initial/date
Fill zone	Meets Class 100 conditions		P F	

8.4.2 Setup and Decontamination Validation of the Isolator

Perform three consecutive biological indicator challenge studies in the Filling Isolator. Record the results on *Attachment #1*.

Overview: The cycle design for this validation study requires complete inactivation of VHP-resistant biological indicators (BIs). *Geobacillus stearothermophilus* spores have been determined to be the most resistant to VHP by various investigators. Therefore, *G. stearothermophilus* BIs at an initial population of at least 10^4 spores per strip will be used. The use of this BI organism provides a significant margin of safety since it is more resistant than typical environmental bioburden. Test indicators must show no growth after incubation for a minimum of seven days at 55°C to 60°C, and the positive control must show growth within seven days at 55°C to 60°C.

8.4.3 Environmental Monitoring

Ensure that the filling isolator will maintain a "germ-free" environment after VHP decontamination. Record the results on *Attachment #2*.

Overview: The fill isolator shall be monitored during process simulations using the routine environmental monitoring sampling procedures. In addition, at the conclusion of the process simulation studies, swab and RODAC© samples shall be taken at locations proximate to intervention locations. Consider intervention location from the setup, operation, and environmental monitoring of the isolator in the selection of sampling sites.

8.4.4 Validation of Cleaning

Perform the cleaning of the isolator interior and associated equipment. Record results.

Overview: The fill isolator shall be monitored following the preparation of the initial batches produced. At the conclusion of the first production campaign, swab samples shall be taken at locations proximate to intervention locations. Consider intervention location from the setup, operation, and environmental monitoring of the isolator in selection of the sampling sites.

8.4.5 Overall System Operational Check

Perform a series of three system operational checks after the system has been VHP decontaminated. Set up the liquid filling machines according to SOPs Use filter sterilized water for injection (WFI) and operate the system according to SOP. Fill the largest and smallest container intended for the filling isolator. A minimum of 5000 units shall be filled. Stoppages, interruptions, and other issues shall be comparable to performance on manned filling rooms at the XXX facility for similar containers.

8.4.6 Media Fill Tests

A minimum of three media fill process simulation tests will be conducted to demonstrate the ability of the filling isolator to manufacture sterile product under anticipated production conditions. The container will be filled with the volume specified in XXX's process simulation plan for container using sterile Soybean Casein Digest Medium (SCDM). Equipment sterilization and setup will be done as per production SOPs.

Sufficient containers will be filled so that a minimum of 5000 media filled units are incubated. Incubation will be conducted for 14 days at 25°C to 30°C. Ten units taken randomly at the end of the incubation period will be tested for growth promotion against each of the growth promotion organisms required by USP Chapter <71> for SCDM. Each of the test units must satisfy the USP requirements for growth promotion.

Media fill test	Date of test	Acceptance criteria	Growth promotion Pass/Fail	MFT result Pass/Fail	Initial/date
SCDM No. 1		0/5000	P F	P F	
SCMD No. 2		0/5000	P F	P F	
SCDM No. 3		0/5000	P F	P F	

Note: The above tests may be run on consecutive days, but in each case all equipment must be sterilized and set up prior to conducting the media fill test.

9 Deviation Notice Form
Deviation number__________

Index